STEWART'S OPERATIVE UROLOGY

Volume One

THE KIDNEYS, ADRENAL GLANDS, and RETROPERITONEUM

Second Edition

STEWART'S OPERATIVE UROLOGY

Volume One

THE KIDNEYS, ADRENAL GLANDS, and RETROPERITONEUM

Second Edition

Senior Editor

ANDREW C. NOVICK, M.D.
Chairman, Department of Urology
The Cleveland Clinic Foundation
Cleveland, Ohio

Associate Editors

STEVAN B. STREEM, M.D.
Department of Urology
The Cleveland Clinic Foundation
Cleveland, Ohio

J. EDSON PONTES, M.D.
Department of Urology
The Cleveland Clinic Foundation
Cleveland, Ohio

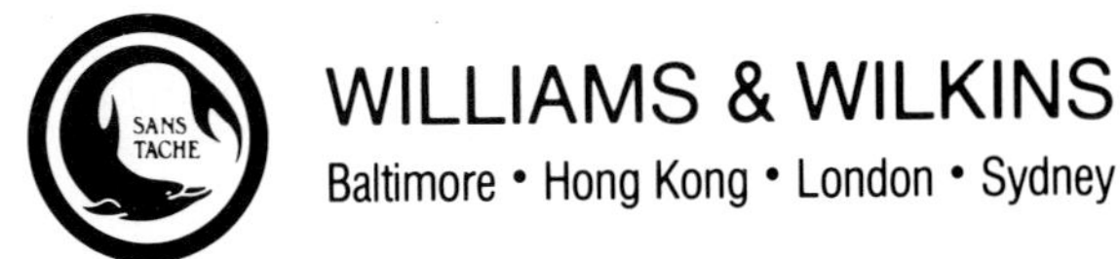

WILLIAMS & WILKINS
Baltimore • Hong Kong • London • Sydney

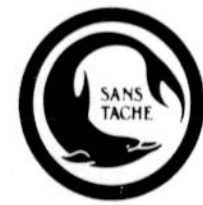

Editor: Kimberly M. Kist
Associate Editor: Victoria M. Vaughn
Copy Editor: Klementyna L. Bryte and Shelley Potler
Design: Bob Och
Production: Theda Harris

428 East Preston Street
Baltimore, Maryland 21202, USA

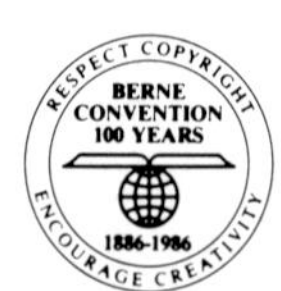

Accurate indications, adverse reactions, and dosage schedules for drugs are provided in this book, but it is possible that they may change. The reader is urged to review the package information data of the manufacturers of the medications mentioned.

Printed in the United States of America

First Edition 1975

Library of Congress Cataloging-in-Publication Data

Stewart's Operative urology / senior editor, Andrew C. Novick,
associate editors, Stevan B. Streem, J. Edson Pontes. — 2nd ed.
p. cm.
Vol. 1 is a rev. ed. of: Operative urology : the kidneys, adrenal glands, and retroperitoneum / edited by Bruce H. Stewart. c1975.
Vol. 2 is a rev. ed. of: Operative urology : lower urinary tract, pelvic structures, and male reproductive system / edited by Bruce H. Stewart. c1982.
Includes bibliographies and indexes.
Contents: v. 1. The kidneys, adrenal glands, and retroperitoneum — v. 2. Lower urinary tract, pelvic structures, and male reproductive system.
ISBN 0-683-06589-0
1. Genito-urinary organs—Surgery. 2. Generative organs, Male—Surgery. I. Novick, Andrew C. II. Streem, Stevan B. III. Pontes, J. Edson IV. Stewart, Bruce H. V. Operative urology.
RD571.S74 1989
617'.46—dc19 88-17124
CIP

Preface to the Second Edition

The first edition of *Operative Urology*, published in 1975 and 1982 as two separate volumes, was extremely well received by urology residents, practitioners, and academicians. The strength of this work was in providing detailed, well-illustrated, step-by-step instruction in the performance of all major operations within our specialty. In the preface to the first edition, Dr. Stewart wrote: ''With the passage of time, many of the procedures described herein will undoubtedly become obsolete. Our greatest satisfaction will come when future advances in surgery make necessary a major revision of this text.'' There is little doubt that the surgical approach to many urologic problems has changed significantly during the past several years. It is our hope that this expanded second edition of *Stewart's Operative Urology* will provide a complete compendium of modern urologic operations in the same effective style and format as the outstanding first edition.

This work is also intended to honor the memory of a dear friend and colleague, Bruce H. Stewart, M.D. With his untimely passing, the urologic community lost one of its most talented clinicians and educators. Those of us who hadd the privilege of working with Dr. Stewart considered him to be a role model and, to this day, we are guided by his teachings and practices. The publication of the first edition of *Operative Urology* was one of Dr. Stewart's most gratifying accomplishments. At the time of his death, he was planning a new edition and had begun to revise the chapters on adrenal surgery. The second edition of Stewart's Operative Urology includes contributions from many former residents and colleagues of Dr. Stewart whose efforts blend together in a fitting tribute to him.

Andrew D. Novick, M.D.
for the Editors

Preface to the First Edition

Over a century has passed since the basic contributions of John Hunter, Crawford Long, and Lord Lister transformed surgery into a sound science as well as a delicate art. A number of great surgeons in later decades established general principles of management which are still valid today. As more knowledge was gained, surgical subspecialties evolved and grew, and textbooks were published covering these specialized areas of endeavour. This was particularly true in urology, which has expanded tremendously in depth and sophistication during recent years.

It is not the purpose of this book to review all of the available procedures for dealing surgically with various diseases of the kidneys, adrenals and supravesical retroperitoneum. Nor is it our intention to describe in detail the nature and management of major diseases involving these structures. Rather, we have attempted to assemble and portray those procedures that experience has led us to believe are most suitable in dealing with abnormalities of this somewhat limited and often controversial area.

Selection of what we judge to be procedures of choice comes not only from evaluation of the work of surgeons world-wide, but also from a rich heritage gained from our predecessors at The Cleveland Clinic Foundation. The early work of Crile and Lower, followed by that of Higgins, Engel, Poutasse and Turnbull, has provided an inspiring background for the present authors.

The procedures described herein reflect the surgical training all urology residents now receive at The Cleveland Clinic Foundation. It is our feeling that modern urologists should be thoroughly familiar with the great vessels and their branches, and be able to use vascular techniques whenever indicated. Likewise, the general principles of intestinal surgery should be understood and incorporated into various urinary tract reconstructive procedures whenever necessary. Close cooperation with intestinal and vascular surgeons, when necessary in difficult cases, may well provide the margin between success and failure.

This book will present a philosophy of operative urology which should be of particular value to the resident in training. Hopefully, it will also provide the experienced urologist with ideas on technique that he can incorporate into an already established surgical armamentarium. With the passage of time many of the procedures described herein will undoubtedly become obsolete. Our greatest satisfaction will come when future advances in surgery make necessary a major revision of this text.

Bruce H. Stewart, M.D.

Cleveland, Ohio

Acknowledgments

The editors acknowledge with deep appreciation the efforts and expertise of all contributing authors to this text. We are grateful for the continued support of the Cleveland Clinic Foundation and, in particular, for the outstanding work of our Medical Illustrations Department. We are indebted to Ms. Cynthia Rogers and Ms. Sally Kickel for their untiring secretarial assistance. Finally, our special thanks go to Victoria Vaughn, Kim Kist, and the staff of Williams & Wilkins for their patience and guidance along the road to publication.

Contributors

Contributors From Cleveland Clinic Foundation

Peter N. Bretan, Jr., M.D.
Department of Urology

Michael A. Geisinger, M.D.
Section of Vascular and Interventional Radiology
Department of Diagnostic Radiology

Ernest E. Hodge, M.D.
Department of Urology

Robert Kay, M.D.
Head, Section of Pediatric Urology
Department of Urology

Ian C. Lavery, M.D.
Department of Colon and Rectal Surgery

Drogo K. Montague, M.D.
Head, Section of Urodynamics and Prosthetic Surgery
Department of Urology

James E. Montie, M.D.
Department of Urology
Cleveland Clinic Foundation—Florida

Andrew C. Novick, M.D.
Chairman, Department of Urology

J. Edson Pontes
Head, Section of Urologic Oncology
Department of Urology

Barbara Risius, M.D.
Section of Vascular and Interventional Radiology
Department of Diagnostic Radiology

Steven W. Siegel, M.D.
Department of Urology

Bruce H. Stewart, M.D. (deceased)
Former Chairman, Division of Surgery
Department of Urology

Ralph A. Straffon, M.D.
Vice Chairman, Board of Governors
Chief of Staff
Department of Urology

Stevan B. Streem, M.D.
Head, Section of Stone Disease and Endourology
Department of Urology

Anthony J. Thomas, Jr., M.D.
Head, Section of Male Infertility
Department of Urology

Margaret G. Zelch, M.D.
Head, Section of Vascular and Interventional Radiology
Department of Diagnostic Radiology

Contributors From Other Institutions

Lynn H. W. Banowsky, M.D.
Chief, Renal Transplantation
Humana Hospital
San Antonio, Texas

John M. Barry, M.D.
Professor of Surgery
Chairman, Division of Urology
Director, Section of Surgical Transplantation
Oregon Health Sciences University
Portland, Oregon

Charles J. Devine, Jr., M.D.
Professor of Urology
Eastern Virginia Medical School
Norfolk, Virginia

Patrick C. Devine, M.D.
Professor of Urology
Eastern Virginia Medical School
Norfolk, Virginia

John P. Donohue, M.D.
Professor and Chairman
Department of Urology
Indiana University Medical Center
Indianapolis, Indiana

Thomas R. Hatch, M.D.
Assistant Professor
Division of Urology
Oregon Health Sciences University
Portland, Oregon

Thomas R. Hefty, M.D.
Assistant Professor
Division of Urology
Oregon Health Sciences Center
Portland, Oregon

Charles E. Horton, M.D.
Professor of Plastic Surgery
Eastern Virginia Medical School
Norfolk, Virginia

Eric A. Klein, M.D.
Fellow, Urology Service
Memorial Sloan-Kettering Cancer Center
New York, New York

James S. Krieger, M.D.
Emeritus, Cleveland Clinic Foundation
Sanibel, Florida

Richard M. Lewis, M.D.
Assistant Professor
Division of Urology and Division of Immunology and Organ Transplantation
University of Texas Health Science Center
Houston, Texas

John A. Libertino, M.D.
Chairman, Division of Surgery
Department of Urology
Lahey Clinic
Boston, Massachusetts

Michael J. Malone
Chief Resident
Department of Urology
Lahey Clinic
Boston, Massachusetts

Michael Marberger, M.D.
Professor, Department of Urology
Rudolfstiftung Hospital
Vienna, Austria

Jack W. McAninch, M.D.
Professor of Urology
University of California
Chief of Urology
San Francisco General Hospital
San Francisco, California

Mark J. Noble, M.D.
Associate Professor, Section of Urology
Department of Surgery
University of Kansas Medical Center
Attending Staff Urologist
Kansas City Veterans Administration Hospital
Kansas City, Kansas

Donald E. Novicki, M.D.
Associate Professor of Surgery (Urology)
University of Texas Health Science Center
San Antonio, Texas

Joseph Ortenberg, M.D.
Assistant Professor
Departments of Urology and Pediatrics
Louisiana School of Medicine
New Orleans, Louisiana

Lester Persky, M.D.
Clinical Professor
University of South Florida
Tampa, Florida

James M. Pierce, Jr., M.D.
Professor and Chairman
Department of Urology
Wayne State University
Detroit, Michigan

Martin I. Resnick, M.D.
Professor and Chairman
Division of Urology
Case Western Reserve University
School of Medicine
Cleveland, Ohio

J. Patrick Spirnak, M.D.
Assistant Professor
Division of Urologic Surgery
Case Western Reserve University
Director, Urology
Metropolitan General Hospital
Cleveland, Ohio

Contents

VOLUME ONE

Section 4. Surgery for Renal Calculous Disease

Section 5. Surgery for Other Benign Renal Disorders

Section 6. Renal Vascular Surgery

Section 7. Renal Transplantation

Section 8. Operative Procedures in the Retroperitoneum

Section 9. Supravesical Urinary Diversion

VOLUME TWO

Section 10. General Information

Section 11. Operations Upon the Bladdder

Section 12. Operations Upon the Prostate Gland

Section 13. Operations Upon Paravesical Structures

Section 14. Operations Upon the Urethra

Section 15. Operations Upon the Genitalia

SECTION 1

General Information

CHAPTER 1

Surgical Anatomy

LYNN H. W. BANOWSKY

RETROPERITONEAL SPACE AND ITS CONTENTS

The retroperitoneal space lies between the peritoneum anteriorly and the posterior parietal wall of the abdominal cavity; it is conveniently divided into lumbar and iliac regions. Extending from the 12th thoracic vertebra and 12th rib to the base of the sacrum and iliac crest is the lumbar portion of the retroperitoneum. The lateral border is the lateral margin of the quadratus lumborum muscle and the floor is composed of the remainder of the quadratus lumborum and the psoas major muscles. Principal contents of the lumbar portion of the retroperitoneal space are the abdominal aorta, inferior vena cava, adrenal glands, second portion of the duodenum, kidneys, ureters, gonadal vessels, and the paraaortic lymphatic network.

The iliac portion of the retroperitoneal space is covered anteriorly by peritoneum and the anterior and lateral walls of the abdomen. Superiorly, the boundary of the iliac portion of the retroperitoneum is the lumbar region of the retroperitoneum, while the inferior boundary is provided by the pelvis. The significant structures coursing through the iliac area of the retroperitoneum are the iliac vessels, ureters, gonadal vessels, iliac lymphatics, and the genitofemoral nerve.

Abdominal Aorta

The abdominal aorta is the continuation of the thoracic aorta and enters the retroperitoneal space by passing through the aortic hiatus of the diaphragm in front of the lower border of the 12th thoracic vertebra. The aorta then descends through the retroperitoneal space slightly to the left of the midline and terminates over the body of the 4th lumbar vertebra by dividing into the right and left common iliac arteries. During this descent, it transcribes a slightly forward convex curve.

At its origin, the abdominal aorta may have a diameter in excess of 2 cm. This diameter is markedly reduced after the first major branches leave the proximal one-third of the aorta. Distal to the renal arteries, the lumen maintains a relatively constant diameter to its termination. The abdominal aorta gives off the following paired and unpaired branches: inferior phrenic arteries, celiac axis, middle adrenal arteries, superior mesenteric artery, renal arteries, gonadal arteries, lumbar arteries, inferior mesenteric artery, middle sacral artery, and common iliac arteries.

Inferior Vena Cava

The inferior vena cava is formed by the junction of the right and left common iliac veins. The bifurcation of the vena cava occurs at a lower level (L-5) than the aortic bifurcation. As the inferior vena cava passes upward, it is slightly to the right of the midline. When it reaches the liver, the inferior vena cava enters a groove in the liver's posterior surface and then leaves the retroperitoneal space by perforating the diaphragm between the median and right portions of the central tendon.

Retroperitoneal Lymphatics

The retroperitoneal lymphatics consist of the iliac and paraaortic lymph nodes. The iliac lymphatic channels follow the iliac vessels and ultimately drain into the paraaortic lymphatics. They receive the drainage of the lower extremities, pelvic contents, and parts of the external genitalia.

The paraaortic lymphatics represent the most abundant lymphatic network in the body. These lymph nodes lie in superficial and deep planes on all sides of the aorta and vena cava. They receive the lymph drainage from the testes, intestines, kidneys, adrenals, and iliac lymphatic system. As the lymphatic channels converge at the level of L-2, three lymphatic trunks are formed, the right and left lumbar lymphatic trunks, and the intestinal lymphatic trunk. A union of these three trunks forms a triangular-shaped structure, the cisterna chyli, which lies in front of the body of the 2nd lumbar vertebra and to the right side and behind the aorta. The cisterna chyli drains into the thoracic duct, which subsequently enters the subclavian vein.

The primary and preferential lymphatic drainage of the testicles is to the preaortic, precanal, and aortic canal nodes near the level of the renal hilum, the embryologic origin of the testicles. Lymphatic drainage from the right testes goes to both precanal, preaortic, and aortocanal nodes. The left testes drains primarily to the pre- and paraaortic lymph nodes. While

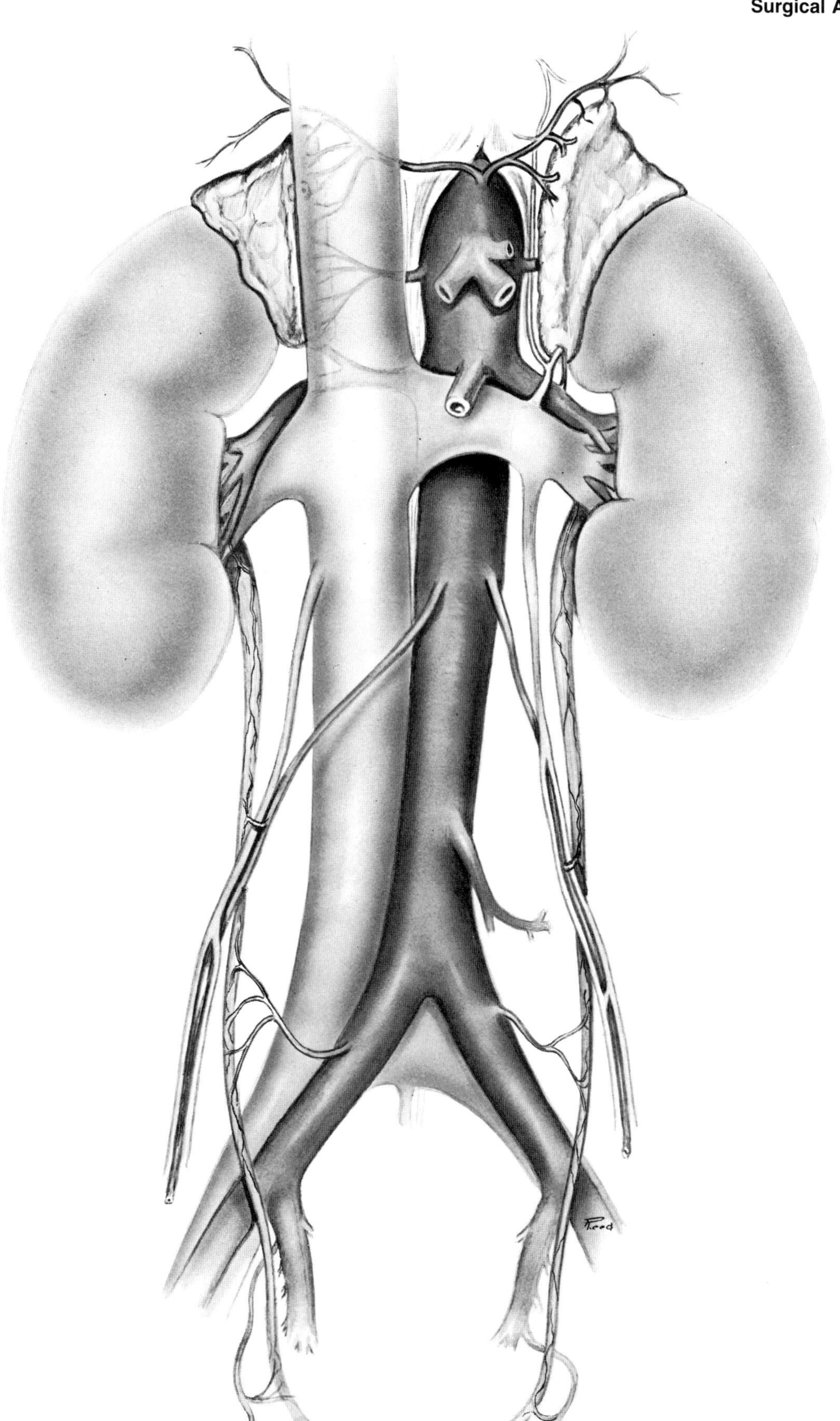

Figure 1.1. The abdominal aorta, inferior vena cava, and the major branches of these two great vessels.

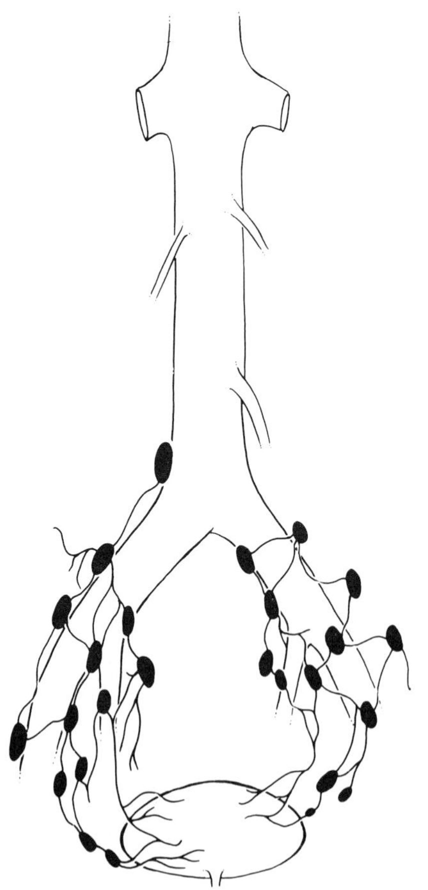

Figure 1.2. The lymphatic drainage of the bladder.

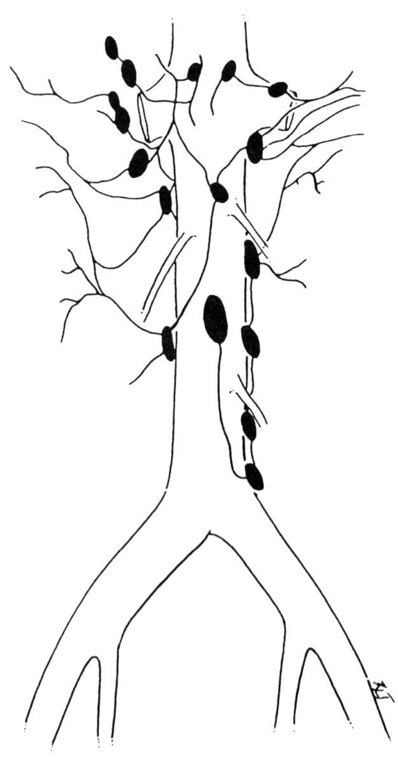

Figure 1.4. The lymphatic drainage of the kidney and ureters.

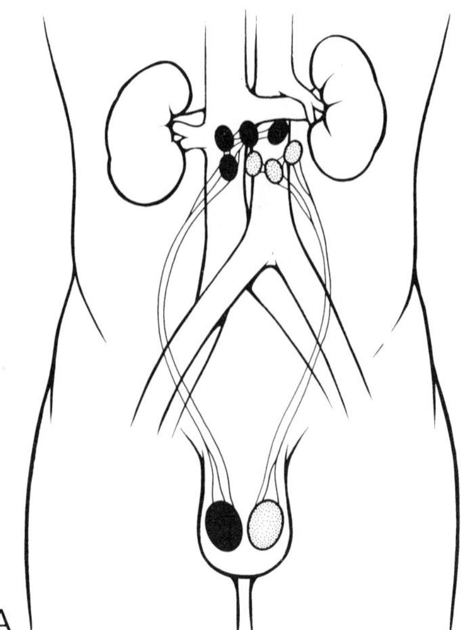

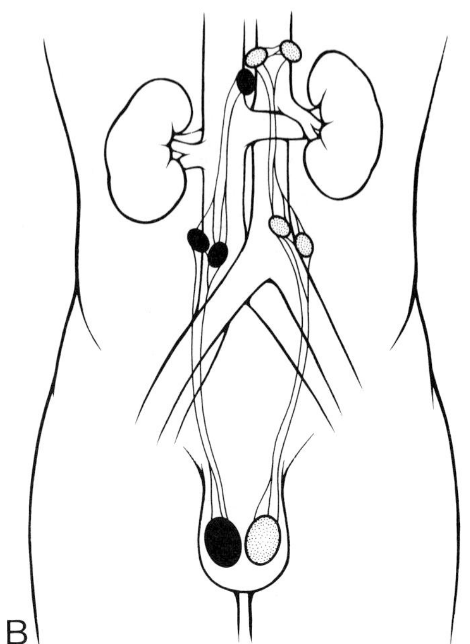

Figure 1.3. **A,** primary and preferred lymphatic drainage of right and left testicle. **B,** secondary or alternate lymphatic drainage of right and left testicle.

there is crossover drainage from both testicles, crossover is much more likely to go from right to left. There can also be bilateral retrograde filling of lower lumbar nodes and antegrade filling bilaterally to the thoracic duct and left supraclavicular area. In an elegant study, Donohue demonstrated suprahilar lymphatic drainage. This is not a preferred drainage route, however, and only assumes significance in testicular carcinomas of high stage.

A knowledge of this lymphatic network is necessary in the performance of extirpative surgery in the treatment of cancer of the bladder, kidney, testes, and ureter.

ADRENAL GLANDS

Gross Description

The adrenal glands are two small flattened structures residing in the retroperitoneal space superior and medial to the anterior upper surface of each kidney. Both adrenal glands have a distinctive bright yellow color and average 3.0–5.0 cm in length, 2.5–3.0 cm in width, and 4.0–6.0 mm in thickness. The average weight of a single gland is 3.0–5.0 gm. The right adrenal gland is slightly smaller than the left and is more triangular in shape, bearing resemblance to a cocked hat.

Embryologic Development

Each adrenal gland is composed of a cortex and medulla that are functionally and histologically distinct and are derived from separate embryologic origins. In fish, the adrenal cortex and medulla exist as two separate organs. As one progresses up the evolutionary chain, the two glands become more intimately involved culminating in mammals with the cortex enveloping the medulla and the two components being contained within a common sheath.

The adrenal cortex develops from mesoderm that arises from the same region that supplies the testicular interstitial cells or the ovarian thecal cells. This common origin accounts for the occasional occurrence of adrenal cortical rests within the gonads. The cortex is significantly larger than the medulla, accounting for 90% of the total weight of the gland. When the adrenal gland is seen surgically, it is the cortex that is responsible for its rich yellow color. Ectopic adrenal cortical tissue can be found adjacent to the adrenal gland, beneath the renal capsule, or in the liver.

The medulla is composed of chromaffin tissue derived from ectoderm of the neural crest. Adrenal medulla and paraganglion cells, thus, have a common embryologic origin; this common origin accounts for the possible occurrence of ectopic adrenal medullary tissue at any point along the sympathetic chain. Ectopic adrenal medullary tissue is responsible for the origin of at least 10% of pheochromocytomas and an even higher percentage of neuroblastomas. The medullary tissue is soft, pulpy, and a dark red or brown color. This part of the gland is extremely vascular and has numerous anastomosing venous sinusoids that directly bathe the medullary cells. This rich medullary vascular system accounts for the very high rate of blood flow through the gland, which averages 6–7 ml/gm of tissue/min.

Anatomic Relationships

Posteriorly, the right adrenal gland rests on the crus of the diaphragm and the anterior medial surface of the upper pole of the right kidney. Anteriorly, it is covered by the liver and inferiorly, it is bounded by the right renal artery and renal vein. The right adrenal gland has an important relationship with the inferior vena cava that not only supplies the medial relationship with the adrenal gland, but also covers the anterior portion of a significant part of the gland. Surgical exposure and removal of the right adrenal gland is more difficult than that of the left because of this close proximity to the inferior vena cava and because of the very short main right adrenal vein that empties directly into the vena cava.

The left adrenal gland is larger and more semilunar in shape than the right. Posteriorly, the left adrenal lies over the crus of the diaphragm and against the medial anterior surface of the upper pole of the left kidney. Anteriorly, it is crossed by the pancreas and the splenic artery and is separated from the stomach by the lesser sac. The spleen may be in contact with the superlateral portion of the left adrenal gland. Medially lies the aorta, although this is not an intimate relationship. Inferiorly, the boundary is established by the left renal artery and vein. For the above relationships, see Figure 1.5.

The fascial covering of both adrenal glands is provided by a superior extension of Gerota's fascia. As Gerota's fascia leaves the upper pole of each kidney, the anterior and posterior layers fuse into a single fascial sheet. This single sheet then splits again into anterior and posterior layers to encompass the adrenal gland. The sharing of this common but separate fascial covering by both the kidney and adrenal glands is surgically significant in two ways: the superior area of fusion between the kidney and adrenal helps prevent the inadvertent removal of the adrenal during nephrectomy and, when surgery on the adrenal is done, the common fascial covering allows the surgeon to pull the more superiorly placed adrenal down to a more accessible location by applying downward traction at the upper pole of the kidney.

Nerve Supply

The nerve supply to the adrenals is derived primarily from the splanchnics and is cholinergic in type. Stimulation causes discharge of medullary hormones and has little if any effect on the cortex.

Lymphatic Drainage

Lymphatic drainage of both the right and left adrenal glands is primarily into the lateral aortic lymph nodes.

Arterial Supply

The arterial supply is the same for the right and left adrenal gland and comes from three sources: the superior adrenal artery, which is a branch of the inferior phrenic artery; the middle adrenal artery, which is a branch directly from the aorta; and the inferior adrenal artery, which is a branch of the renal artery. All of these branches are quite small and form a complex intercommunicating arcade around the margins of the gland. From this arcade, numerous small branches, sometimes as many as 50–60 branches, penetrate the adrenal cor-

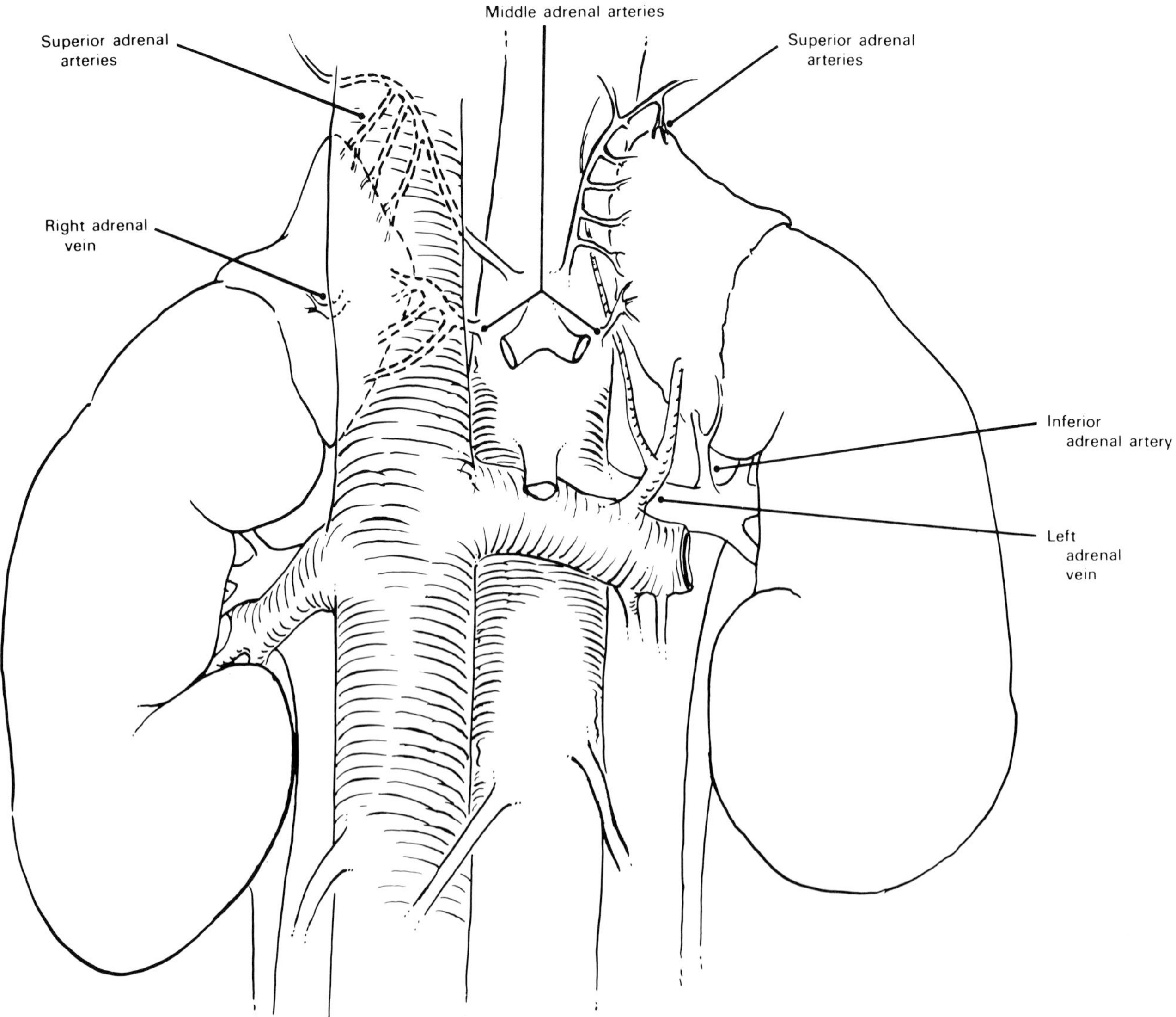

Figure 1.5. The arterial supply and venous drainage of the right and left adrenal glands. Note the relationship between the right adrenal gland and the inferior vena cava. The major arterial blood supply of the right adrenal gland is usually provided by the right inferior adrenal artery, which arises from the proximal one-third of the right renal artery. These vessels are overlain by the right renal vein and vena cava, not shown in this illustration.

tex to nourish the gland. In spite of the rather innocuous appearance of this periadrenal arterial arcade, all this tissue should be ligated or secured with clips during adrenal mobilization to avoid unnecessary hemorrhage. The least developed portion of the arcade is around the lateral aspect of the gland.

Venous Drainage

The venous drainage is different for the two adrenal glands and does not correspond on either side to the arterial supply. Both glands are drained by a central main adrenal vein that runs the entire length of the gland and exits at the adrenal hilum. The main vein is fed by tributaries that enter in such a manner that on adrenal phlebogram, the venous network appears similar to the veins in a leaf. The main right adrenal vein is extremely short and directly enters the posterolateral aspect of the inferior vena cava. The main left adrenal vein is significantly longer and enters the superior aspect of the left renal vein.

KIDNEYS

General Description

The kidneys are paired vital organs located on either side of the vertebral column in the lumbar fossa of the retroperitoneal space. Kidneys in mature adults will vary in length from 11.0–14.0 cm, in width from 5.0–7.5 cm, and in thickness from 2.5–3.0 cm. The weight of a single kidney in adult males is between 125.0 and 170.0 gm and, in adult females, from 115.0–155.0 gm. The average left kidney is usually 0.5 cm longer than the right and assumes a more cephalad position.

Each kidney is surrounded by a layer of fat that, in turn, is covered by a distinct fascial layer—the fascia of Gerota. Gerota's fascia is more developed posteriorly than anteriorly. This fascia is almost completely fused above and lateral to the kidney, while medially and to a greater extent inferiorly, the process of fusion is not complete. These areas of incomplete fusion of Gerota's fascia assume clinical importance in determining possible routes of spread of perinephric bleeding or infection. The kidney is also partially fixed by these points of fusion in Gerota's fascia; however, the main attachments of the kidney are the renal artery and vein.

Embryologic Development

The embryologic development of the kidney requires the multiple processes of development, degeneration, migration, union, and rotation. Three successive excretory systems (pronephros, mesonephros, and metanephros) are formed from the intermediate mesoderm. The pronephros and mesonephros undergo degeneration and are present at birth only as the Wolffian duct system.

The definitive kidney is formed by a union of the metanephric duct and mesoderm from the nephrogenic cord. The metanephric duct forms the ureter, renal pelvis, calyces, and collecting tubules. The vascular and excretory components of the kidney are formed by the mesoderm of the nephrogenic cord. The metanephric duct must migrate cephalad, before the union with the nephrogenic mesoderm occurs. After this union occurs, a process of development ensues that terminates approximately 1 month before birth, with functioning nephrons and a patent drainage system.

During the process of development, the embryonic kidney continues its cephalad migration, from the level of L-4 to its ultimate resting place at L-1. As the kidney moves from its pelvic position, it also undergoes a process of rotation in two different planes. The dorsal border rotates 90° to become the convex lateral border and the superior poles converge toward the midline, whereas the lower poles become more divergent, thus, giving the renal orientation that is present at birth.

Anatomic Relationships

A small segment of the anterior medial surface of the right kidney is in contact with the right adrenal gland. The major anterior relationships of the right kidney, however, are the liver that overlies the upper two-thirds of the anterior surface and the hepatic flexure of the colon that overlies the lower one-third. The second portion of the duodenum lies over the right renal hilum. The anterior surface of the kidney beneath the liver is the only area covered by peritoneum.

A small segment of the anterior medial surface of the left kidney is also covered by the left adrenal gland. The spleen, body of the pancreas, stomach, and splenic flexure of the colon also overlie the anterior surface of the left kidney. The area of the kidney beneath the small intestine, the spleen, and the stomach is covered by peritoneum.

Posteriorly, both kidneys lie on the psoas major and quadratus lumborum muscles. They are also in relationship with the medial and lateral lumbocostal arches and the tendon of the transversus abdominus. Posteriorly and superiorly, the upper pole of each kidney is in contact with the diaphragm.

Renal Arterial Supply

Both the right and left renal arteries arise from the lateral surface of the aorta at a point just distal to the superior mesenteric artery. The origin of the right renal artery is slightly more posterior than that of the left renal artery. The right renal artery is also longer than the left and reaches the right kidney by passing behind the inferior vena cava. There are two small but important branches arising from the main renal artery: the inferior adrenal artery and the artery that supplies the renal pelvis and upper ureter.

Each kidney can be divided into four constant vascular segments. The origin of the vessels supplying these segments may vary, although the anatomic position of the segments always remains constant. These four segments are the apical or superior, anterior, posterior, and basilar or inferior.

Five branches of the renal artery supply these four anatomic segments. Each segmental artery is an end-artery, with no collateral circulation. The apical artery is a very short branch and supplies both the anterior and posterior surfaces of the apical segment. The basilar artery is usually the first branch of the renal artery, but has the most variable origin. Like the apical artery, the basilar artery supplies both the anterior and posterior surfaces of its segment. The anterior segment is the largest segment and is supplied by two branches, one to the superior portion of the segment and one to the inferior portion. Although called the anterior segment, this segment extends beyond the midplane of the kidney onto the posterior surface. Once this is appreciated, one readily sees that Brödel's line is not in an avascular plane and that a surgical incision through this line would needlessly devascularize a significant portion of the kidney. The true avascular line is at the junction of the anterior and posterior segments and is on the posterior surface of the kidney. The posterior segment is supplied by a single artery. In order to perform renal surgery safely, a working knowledge of the intrarenal vascular supply is mandatory.

Renal Venous Drainage

The left and right renal veins both terminate in the lateral aspect of the inferior vena cava. The left renal vein is both longer (60–110 mm) and has a much thicker muscular layer than the right renal vein. Two important nonrenal branches empty into the left renal vein; inferiorly, the gonadal vein empties into the left renal vein and superiorly, the left adrenal vein terminates into the left renal vein. In a significant number of instances, one or even two large lumbar veins will empty into the posterior surface of the renal vein. Failure to be aware of the potential presence of these posterior lumbar veins can lead to dangerous hemorrhage during mobilization of the left renal vein. It is these three branches (adrenal, gonadal, and lumbar) that allow for temporary occlusion of the left renal vein at or near its entrance into the vena cava with minimal changes in renal function. This is very important an-

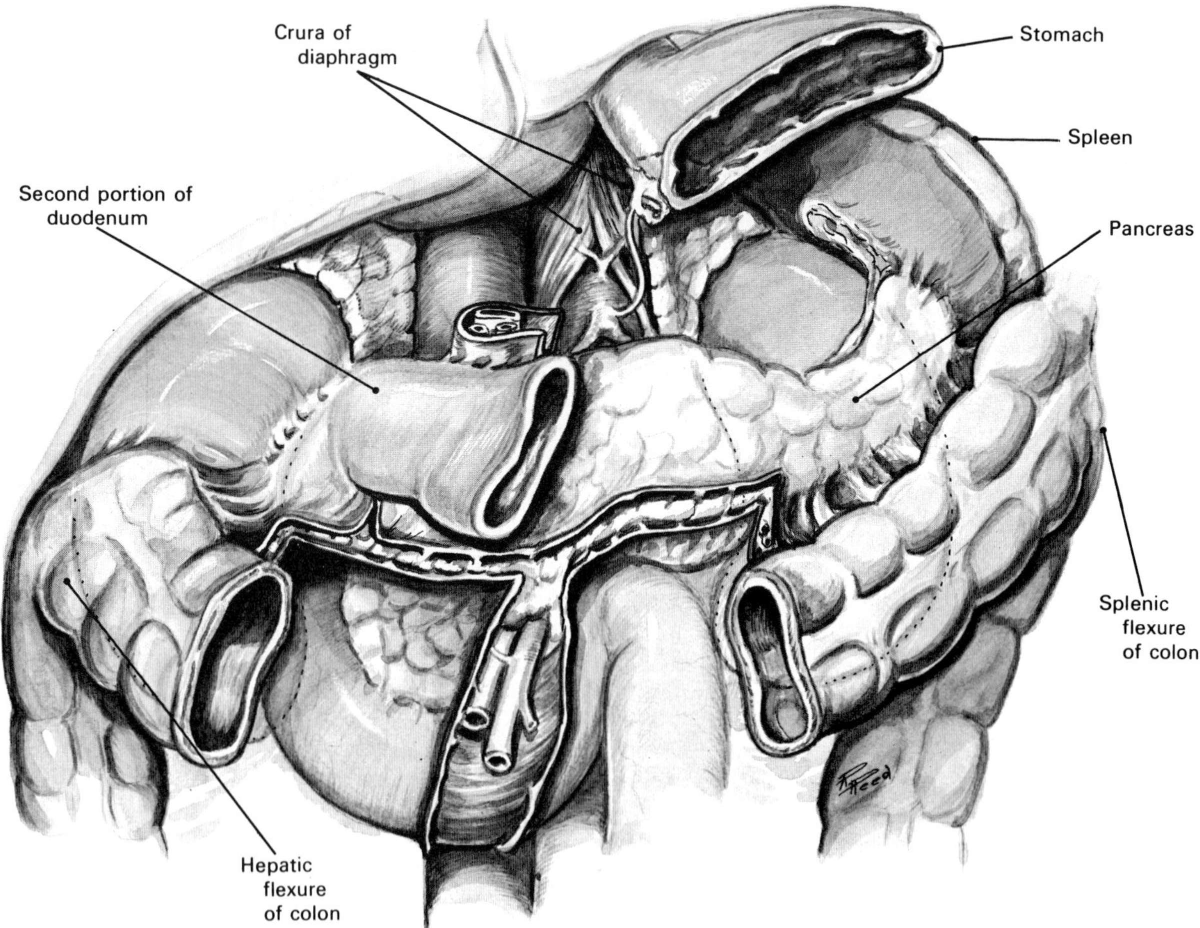

Figure 1.6. The anatomic relationship of the kidneys and adrenal glands to surrounding structures. The liver is retracted superiorly in this illustration.

atomic consideration; for example, when one must extract tumor thrombus from the inferior vena cava.

The right renal vein is shorter than the left and has a much less-developed muscular wall. There are no significant branches that consistently empty into the right renal vein. A valve and, consequently, a very thin area in the vein's wall is frequently present at the right renal vein's entrance into the inferior vena cava. This is of surgical importance when doing a right donor nephrectomy for renal transplantation. Unless a small cuff of vena cava is excised at the vein's entrance into the cava, the already short right renal vein will have to be further reduced in length as the thin area in the renal vein containing the valve must be excised because it does not hold sutures well and is prone to tear.

Multiple Renal Arteries and Veins

Unilateral multiple renal arteries occur in approximately 23% of the population. In 10% of the people, the multiple arteries will be bilateral. Multiple renal arteries are more common on the left side. Frequently, the smaller of the two vessels supplies the basilar segment of the kidney and gives off the important branch that supplies the renal pelvis and upper ureter. A significant distinction needs to be made between multiple renal arteries and accessory renal arteries. Multiple renal arteries always supply one of the vascular segments of the kidney and ligation of one of these vessels will result in the loss of one of the kidney's four vascular segments. Accessory renal arteries do *not* supply a vascular segment of the kidney but rather a very small portion of a segment. These accessory renal arteries can usually be ligated safely without devascularizing a significant portion of renal parenchyma. Accessory renal arteries are more common around the upper pole of the kidney and represent branches of the renal, phrenic, or adrenal arteries.

Multiple renal veins are less common than multiple renal arteries. Duplication of the left renal vein is quite rare. However, division of the single vein in its course to the inferior vena cava is not uncommon. The renal vein, when splitting, sends one branch anterior and one branch posterior to the aorta. Both branches then enter the inferior vena cava separately.

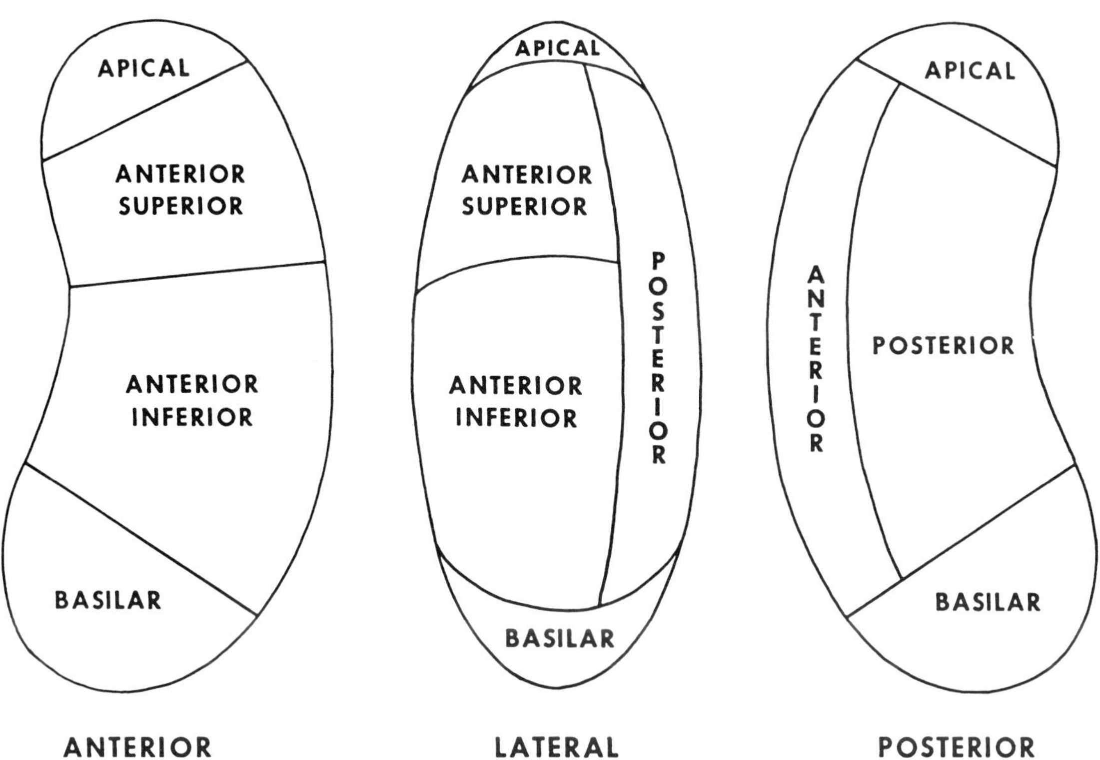

Figure 1.7. The vascular segments of the left kidney, as shown in the anterior, lateral, and posterior projections.

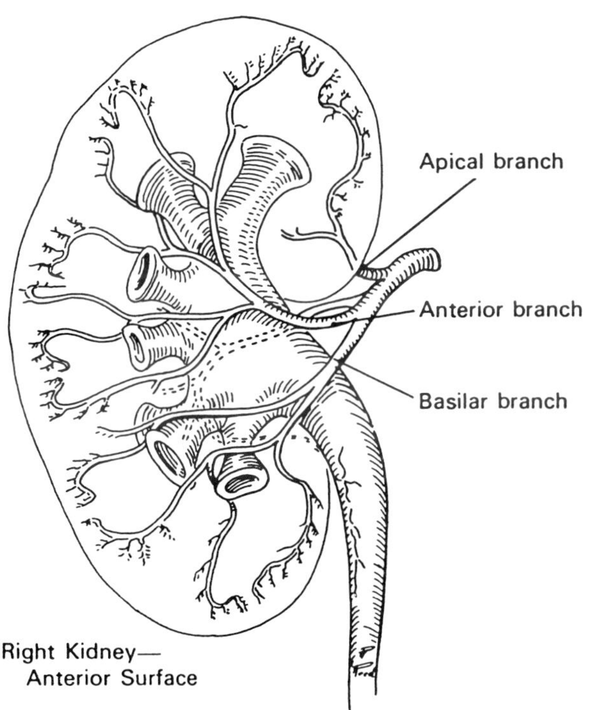

Figure 1.8. The intrarenal course and relationship to the anterior calyces of the apical, basilar, and anterior segmental arteries. Note the short length of the apical branch. The posterior branch is shown by a *broken line*.

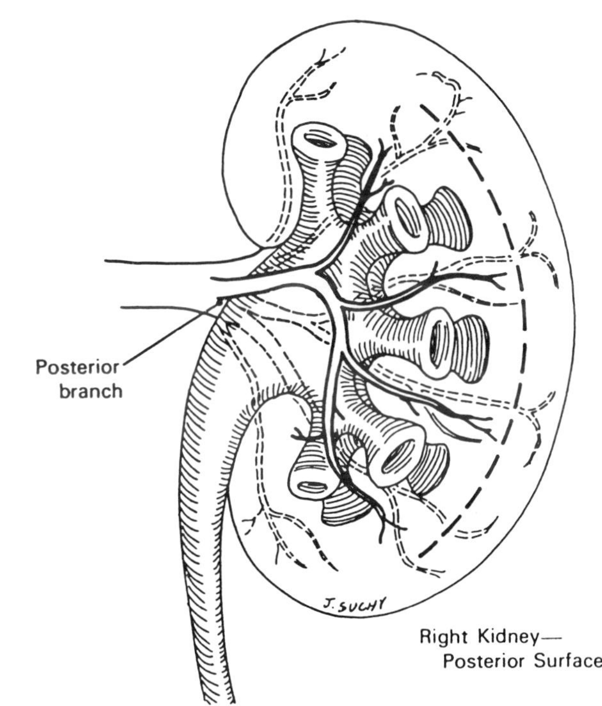

Figure 1.9. The branch of the renal artery supplying the posterior segment of the kidney passes along the posterior surface of the renal pelvis and then divides into smaller branches that course between the posterior calyces. The apical, basilar, and anterior branches are shown by *broken lines*.

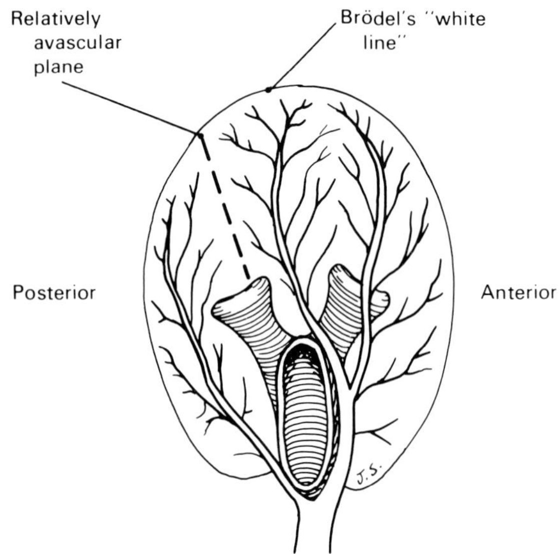

Figure 1.10. The true intersection of the anterior and posterior branches of the renal artery lies well within the posterior surface of the kidney and is shown by the *broken line*. This is posterior to the midlateral plane of the kidney and Brödel's "white line."

URETER

General Description and Structure

The ureter is a tube-like structure of unequal diameter that describes a gentle reverse S curve from its beginning at the ureteropelvic junction to its termination in the urinary bladder. This structure is composed of three separate layers: an outer fibrous layer, a middle muscular layer, and an inner mucosal layer of transitional epithelium. The muscular layer has a distinctive arrangement of its fibers—the outer and inner layers are longitudinally arranged fibers, and the middle are circular fibers.

The ureter varies in length from 28–34 cm, with the right ureter usually 1 cm shorter than the left. Three physiologic areas of constriction exist along the ureter: the ureteropelvic junction, with an average diameter of 2 mm; the point where the ureter crosses the iliac vessels, with an average diameter of 4 mm; and the ureterovesical junction, with a variable diameter of 1–5 mm. The abdominal portion of the ureter has an average diameter of 10 mm compared to the pelvic portion of the ureter which averages 5 mm.

Anatomic Relationships

The ureter courses medially as it leaves the ureteropelvic junction and lies on the medial aspect of the psoas major

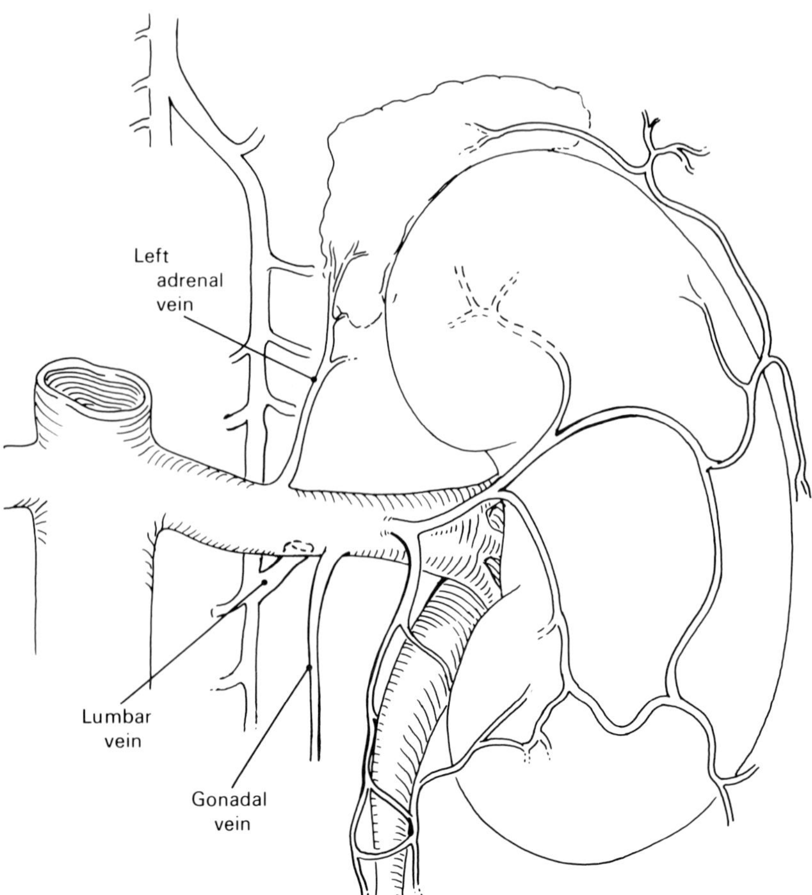

Figure 1.11. Branches of the left renal vein.

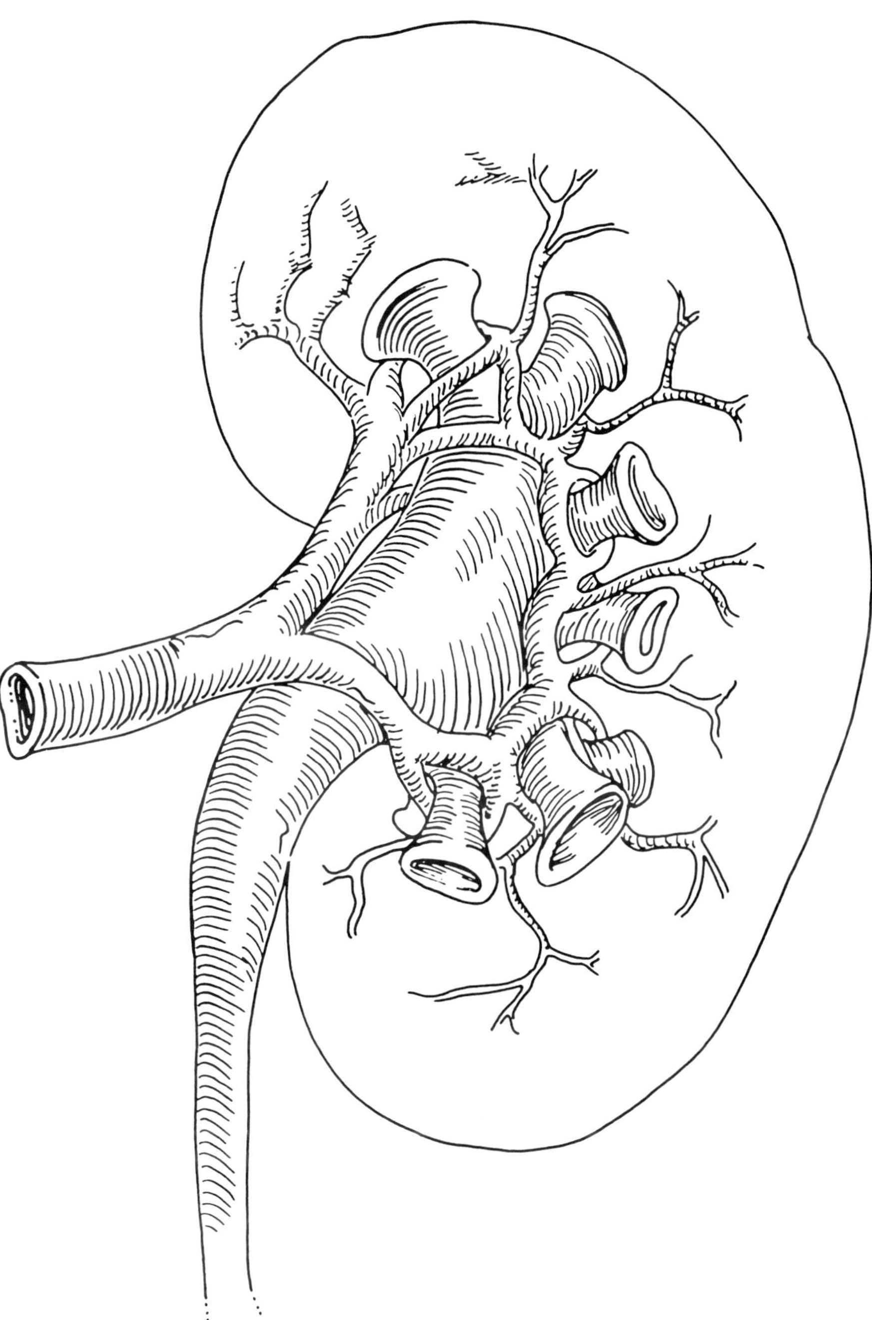

Figure 1.12. The intrarenal venous drainage, shown here for the left kidney, in general parallels the arterial blood supply and lies just outside the renal pelvis, infundibula, and calyces. The renal venous drainage system differs significantly from the arterial blood supply of the kidney in that the intrarenal branches intercommunicate freely between the various renal segments. Ligation of a major branch of the renal vein, therefore, will not result in segmental infarction of the kidney because collateral venous blood supply will provide adequate drainage.

muscle. It then descends in virtually a straight line adjacent to the transverse processes of the lumbar vertebrae. Just proximal to its midpoint, the ureter crosses under the gonadal vessels. The abdominal portion of the ureter ends and the pelvic portion begins where the ureter crosses over the iliac vessels, usually at the point of bifurcation of the common iliac artery.

Once the ureter begins its pelvic course, it follows the hypogastric artery and transcribes a gentle lateral curve along the wall of the bony pelvis. Opposite the lower part of the greater sciatic foramen, the ureter again turns medially and reaches the lateral angle of the bladder. At this point, it crosses under the vas deferens and is in close proximity to the upper end of the seminal vesicle. The ureter then enters the bladder obliquely and courses submucosally for 2–3 cm, ending in the ureteral orifice. During the ureters' pelvic course, they lie closest together over the sacroiliac joint, being only 4–5 cm apart, and are most divergent at the level of the ischial spines.

In its descent, the right ureter is behind the second portion of the duodenum, lateral to the inferior vena cava, and crossed by the right colic and ileocolic vessels. The left ureter is crossed by the left colic vessels, descends parallel to the aorta, and passed under the pelvic mesocolon.

The relationships of the pelvic ureter are somewhat different in the female. In the female pelvis, the ureter lies in the posterior border of the ovarian fossa, passes forward and beneath the lower part of the broad ligament, lateral to the cervix, and is closely associated with the upper vagina. At this point, the uterine artery passes in front of the ureter on its way to the cervix.

Ureteral Blood Supply

Urologists have long been aware of the tenuous nature of the blood supply of the ureter. Devascularization of the ureter could result in either the formation of a urinary fistula or the late complication of ureteral obstruction from stenosis secondary to the formation of scar tissue. A working knowledge of the ureteral arterial supply allows safe surgical mobilization and/or repair of the ureter under most clinical conditions. To avoid ischemic injury to the ureter, one must avoid damage to the main ureteral arterial supply, the ureteral branch arising from the renal artery, and stripping of the ureteral adventitia.

The ureter derives its arterial blood supply from adjacent arteries along its path to the bladder. The main tributary supplying the upper ureter is a ureteral branch arising from the main renal artery (see Fig. 1.13). As the ureter descends toward the bladder, it picks up additional branches from the gonadal artery, aorta, hypogastric artery, vasal artery, and vesical arteries.

There is a free anastomosis of all these vessels in the ureteral adventitia that allows all of the arterial networks, regardless of origin, to intercommunicate. This rich and interlocking system of anastomosis explains how the ureter may be surgically freed from its bed, or divided, and still remain viable as long as the adventitia is left intact.

Nerve Supply

Painful stimuli are transmitted by the autonomic nervous system to the levels of T-12 and L-2 and along with iliohypogastric, ilioinguinal, and external spermatic branch of the genitofemoral nerves. Thus, pain is referred from the flank to the inguinal region and scrotum. Ureteral peristalsis is stimulated by urine stretching the muscular coat of the ureter. At the present time, peristalsis is believed to be independent of the autonomic nervous system.

RETROPERITONEAL NERVES

Lumbar Plexus

The lumbar plexus is located anterior to the transverse process of the lumbar vertebrae deep within the psoas muscle and is formed by the ventral rami of the first three lumbar nerves and, at times, by part of the 4th lumbar nerve. Three significant branches of the lumbar plexus course through the lumbar portion of the retroperitoneal space: the iliohypogastric nerve, the ilioinguinal nerve, and the lateral femoral cutaneous nerve of the thigh. The genitofemoral nerve is also a branch of the lumbar plexus and crosses the iliac portion of the retroperitoneal space.

The iliohypogastric nerve has its origin from the 1st lumbar nerves, with a frequent contribution from the 12th thoracic nerve. It penetrates the superolateral aspect of the psoas major muscle, crosses the quadratus lumborum muscle, and penetrates the transversus abdominus muscle near the iliac crest. It is a motor nerve to the abdominal musculature.

The ilioinguinal nerve also emerges from the lateral aspect of the psoas major muscle and has a similar, though inferior, course to the iliohypogastric nerve. This nerve traverses the inguinal canal and, in men, supplies the cutaneous innervation of the medial aspect of the thigh and the anterior part of the scrotum. In women, it supplies the medial aspect of the thigh, as well as the mons pubis and labia majora.

The lateral femoral cutaneous nerve is derived from the posterior branches of the 2nd and 3rd lumbar nerves. It also emerges from the lateral margin of the psoas major muscle, but at a more inferior position than the ilioinguinal and iliohypogastric. It crosses the iliacus muscle on its way to the lateral margin of the inguinal ligament.

Sympathetic Nervous System

The sympathetic nervous system consists of two ganglionated nerve trunks, one on either side of the midline, that extend from the base of the skull to the coccyx. The lumbar portion of this chain resides within the retroperitoneal space. In addition, branches of the thoracic sympathetic chain enter the retroperitoneal space.

The lumbar portion of the sympathetic chain consists of four ganglia, connected by intervening portions of the sympathetic nerve trunk. This chain lies anterior to the vertebral column along the medial border of the psoas muscle. On the left side, the chain is overlain by the abdominal aorta and, on the right, by the inferior vena cava.

The celiac ganglion is comprised of two masses of ganglionic tissue approximately 2 cm in diameter, firm in consistency and whitish in color, lying in close approximation to the ventral and lateral surface of the abdominal aorta, at the level of the 1st lumbar vertebra. The ganglia are somewhat irregular in shape, partly dispersed into several small ganglionic masses, and connected with each other across the midline by a dense network of nerve bundles. The aorticorenal and superior mesenteric ganglia are smaller ganglionic masses slightly detached from the caudal portion of the celiac ganglion. The aorticorenal ganglion lies at the origin of the renal artery and the superior mesenteric ganglion lies at the origin of the superior mesenteric artery.

The roots of these ganglia are the splanchnic nerves. The greater splanchnic nerve is formed by branches of the 5th–9th or 10th thoracic ganglia, descends obliquely on the anterior surface of the thoracic vertebral bodies, and penetrates

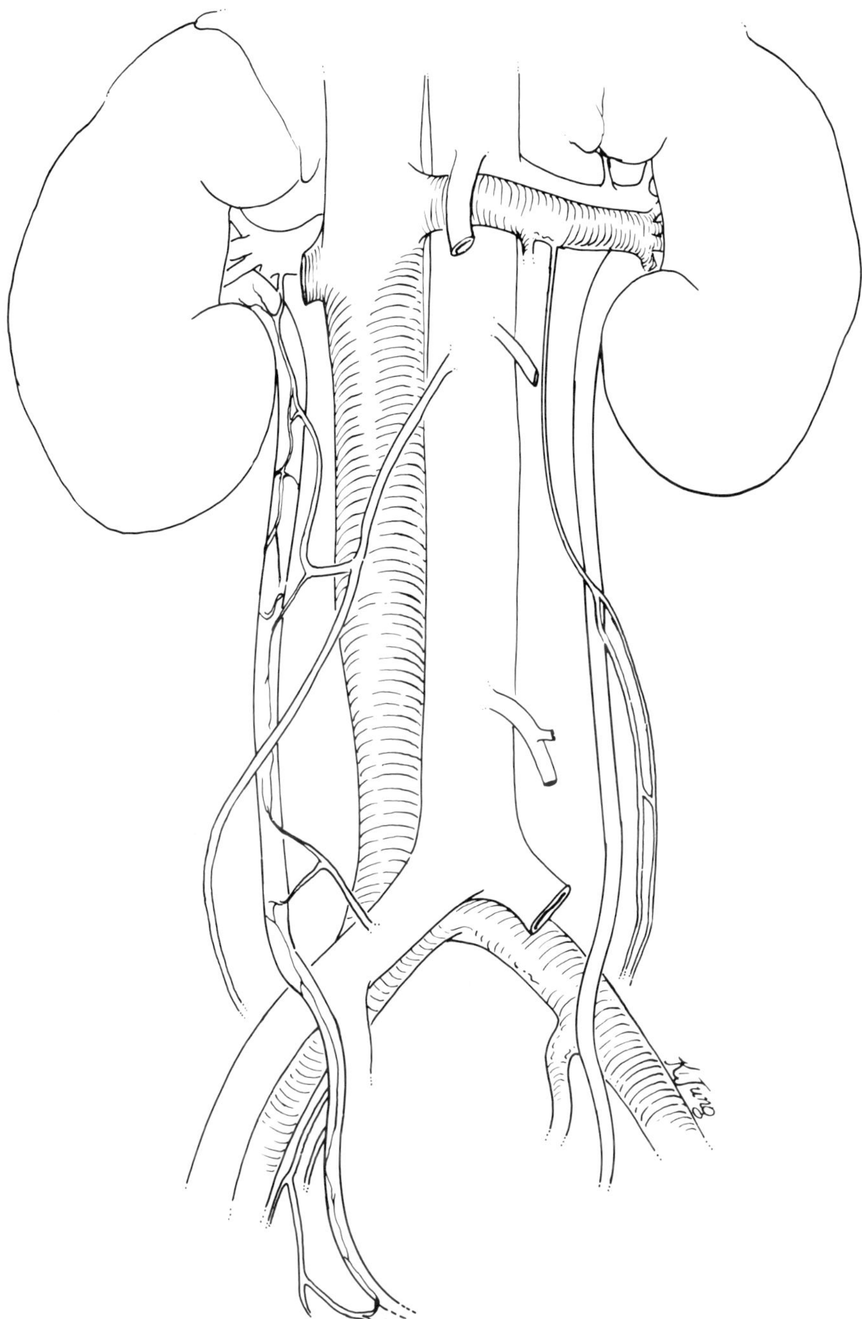

Figure 1.13. Major arterial supply of the ureter, here illustrated on right.

the crus of the diaphragm to enter the retroperitoneal space. It enters the dorsal and lateral margins of the main celiac ganglion but also sends branches to the aorticorenal and superior mesenteric ganglia.

The lesser spanchnic nerve is formed by filaments from the 9th and 10th thoracic ganglia. It pierces the diaphragm just below the greater splanchnic nerve and terminates in the aorticorenal ganglion.

The lowest (least) splanchnic nerve has been said to join the renal plexus. However, this nerve is difficult, if not impossible, to identify either at surgery or in the anatomy laboratory. From a practical standpoint, removal of all nerve fibers of the renal plexus that overlie the main renal artery and adjacent aorta is sufficient to obliterate the function of the least splanchnic nerve.

The splanchnic nerves contain preganglionic fibers from the

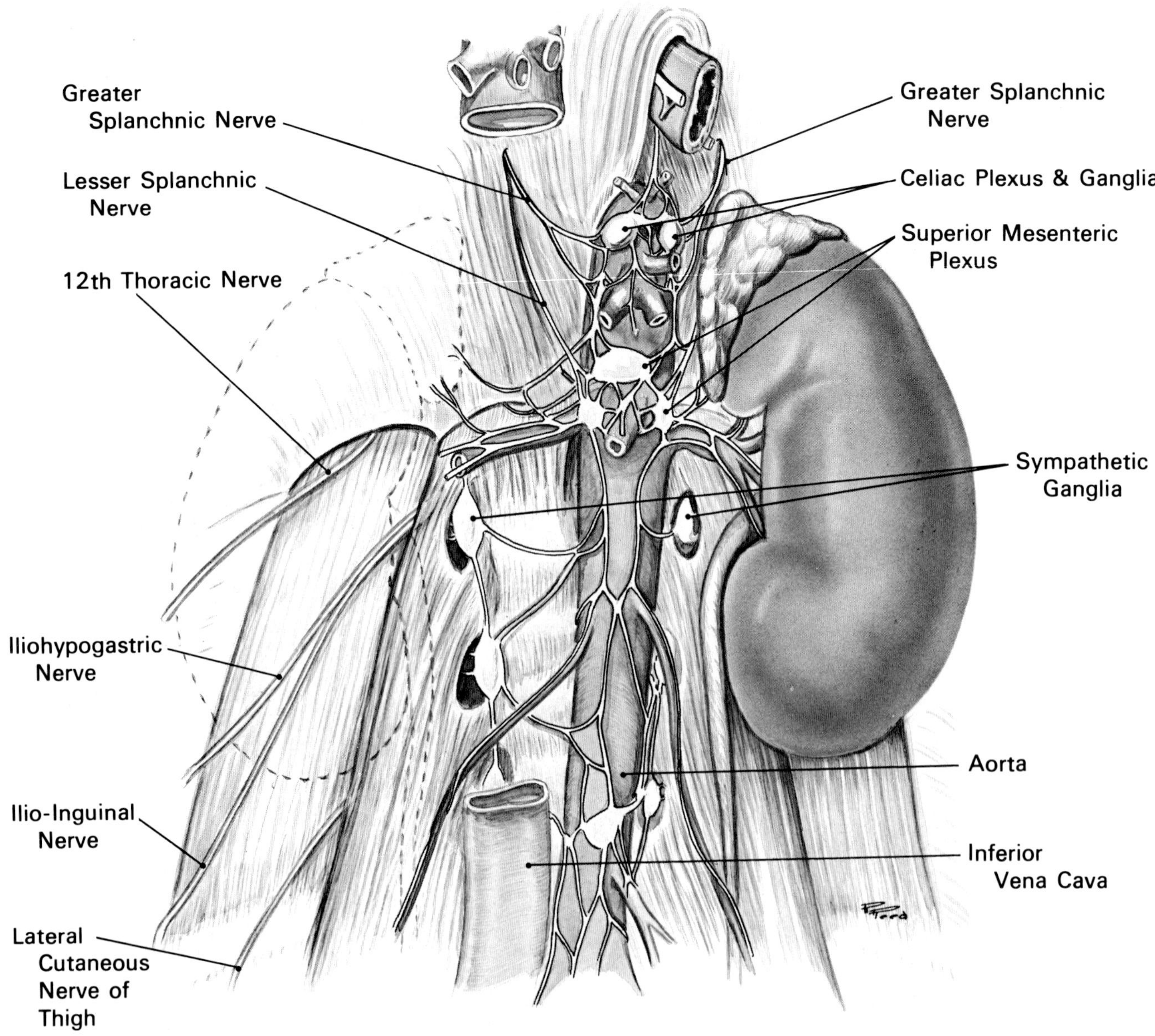

Figure 1.14. Nerves in the lumbar portion of the retroperitoneal space.

lower 6th or 7th thoracic spinal cord segments, which pass to the sympathetic trunk without synapses. The post-ganglionic fibers arising in the celiac ganglia form an extensive plexus of nerve bundles and fibers that branch off into subsidiary plexuses, following the major branches of the abdominal aorta.

Suggested Readings

Arey LB: *Developmental Anatomy,* 6th ed. Philadelphia, WB Saunders, 1954.

Atlas of Descriptive Human Anatomy, 7th English ed. New York, Harper Publishing, 1957.

Bassett DL: A Stereoscopic Atlas of Human Anatomy. Section 5, The Abdomen. View Master Reels, 143–152. Portland, OR, Sawyers Inc.

Callander's Surgical Anatomy, 4th ed. Philadelphia, WB Saunders, 1958.

Cunningham's Textbook of Anatomy, 9th ed., London, Oxford University Press, 1951.

Donohue JP, Zachary JM, Maynard R: Distribution of nodal metastases in nonseminomatous testis cancer. *J Urol* 128:315, 1982.

Glenn JF, Boyce WH (eds): *Urologic Surgery,* 1st ed. New York, Harper & Row, 1969.

Goss CM (ed): *Gray's Anatomy,* 28th ed. Philadelphia, Lea & Febiger, 1969.

Grant JC: *Atlas of Anatomy,* 6th ed. Baltimore, The Williams & Wilkins Co., 1972.

Gray's Anatomy, 35th British ed. Philadelphia, WB Saunders, 1973.

Pernkopf E: *Atlas of Topographical and Applied Human Anatomy,* Vol. II. Philadelphia, WB Saunders, 1963.

Woodbourne RT: *Essentials of Human Anatomy,* 5th ed. London, Oxford University Press, 1973.

CHAPTER 2

Surgical Incisions

DROGO K. MONTAGUE

GENERAL CONSIDERATIONS

The most important and obvious factor in the selection of an operative approach is the operation to be performed. Using the kidney as an example, simple nephrectomies, renal biopsies, unroofing of renal cysts, pyelolithotomies, and nephrolithotomies are usually best performed through a flank or other type of extraperitoneal incision. In contrast, we feel that radical nephrectomies and renal vascular operations are usually best performed through an anterior transperitoneal incision.

The actual pathology involved also needs to be considered. Most radical nephrectomies can be accomplished easily through a subcostal transperitoneal incision. However, if there is bilateral involvement, a bilateral subcostal incision may be required. Moreover, if there is a large upper pole lesion, an 11th rib transabdominal incision or even a thoracoabdominal incision may be the optimal approach.

Concurrent pathology or other operations to be performed may also determine the operative approach. For example, in the case of a renal cell carcinoma with a solitary pulmonary metastasis, a thoracoabdominal incision may result in the removal of the primary tumor and also the metastasis. Occasionally, the urologic surgeon is called upon, to do a procedure in a patient in whom some form of intraabdominal surgery also needs to be done. The urologic procedure may be carried out transabdominally, and if the patient is doing well, the other elective intraabdominal surgery may be performed by the general surgeon.

Body habitus is also an important consideration in the selection of an operative approach. A nephroureterectomy in a relatively thin person may be accomplished through a single modified flank incision with a downward extension. In the more obese patient, two separate incisions may be required for this operation.

Physical abnormalities in the patient, such as kyphoscoliosis or severe pulmonary disease, may dictate that certain approaches, such as the standard flank approach, not be used.

Finally, in certain operations that can be done through more than one incision, it is often advantageous to choose an alternative approach if the patient has had previous surgery through the more standard approach.

The flank incisions have as a principal advantage the fact that the peritoneal cavity is not entered. The period of ileus after surgery is somewhat less in most flank than in most intraperitoneal procedures. In addition, urinary drainage is confined to the retroperitoneum. The flank approaches are particularly useful in the obese patient, as most of the panniculus falls forward, making this incision relatively straightforward even in the very large person. The principal disadvantage of the flank incision is that exposure in the area of the renal pedicle is not as good as with anterior transperitoneal approaches. In addition, the flank incision may prove, as already mentioned, unsuitable for the patient with scoliosis or severe pulmonary problems.

The converse of what has been stated about the flank approach proves true for the anterior approach. The principal advantage of this procedure is that exposure in the area of the renal pedicle, with proper use of a Bookwalter ring retractor (Codman and Shurtleff, Inc., Randolph, MA), is excellent. We use this approach almost exclusively for radical nephrectomies, renal vascular procedures, and most adrenal procedures; it is particularly important in operations for pheochromocytoma, as these tumors may be multiple or in ectopic locations. The principal disadvantages of the anterior approach are the somewhat longer period of postoperative ileus and the possible long-term complication of intraabdominal adhesions leading to bowel obstruction.

The midline abdominal approach has ease of performance as its principal advantage. The peritoneal cavity is quickly entered and closure is likewise quickly effected. The principal disadvantage is the relatively high incidence of hernia formation. The paramedian incision gives essentially the same exposure and does not have the higher incidence of hernia formation but takes longer to perform and close.

The Gibson incision, with the modification that will subsequently be described, has the advantage of very good exposure of the bladder and lower ureteral area as well as the area of the iliac vessels. With the modification, it is easy to perform and involves a minimum of muscle division. If necessary, it can be extended upward to allow relatively good access to the ipsilateral renal area.

The posterior lumbar approaches have as a principal advantage the ease of execution and the relative comfort and return to early eating for the patient in the immediate postoperative period. The principal disadvantage is that exposure with these incisions is quite limited, particularly with respect to the blood supply of either the adrenal gland or the kidney. In addition, the posterior lumbar approaches, if undertaken for adrenal operations, require a simultaneous bilateral approach if both adrenal areas are to be examined.

FLANK APPROACHES

Subcostal Flank Incision

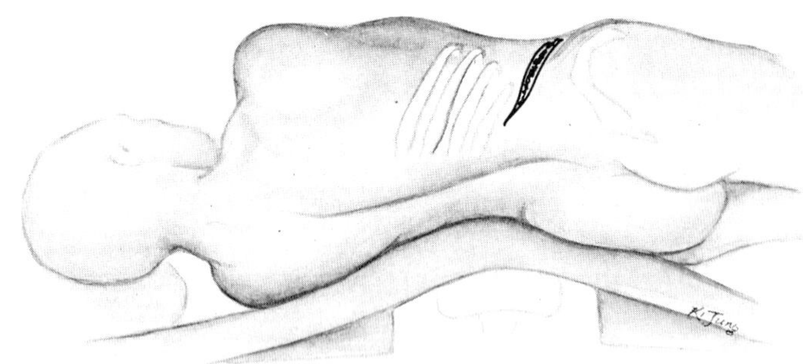

Figure 2.1. The patient is in the lateral position, with the table broken and the kidney rest up. Notice that the patient is positioned so that the center of the kidney rest is just below the tip of the 12th rib. The outlines of the 10th, 11th, and 12th ribs can be seen, as well as the outline of the iliac crest. The incision begins approximately 1 fingerbreadth below and parallel to the 12th rib and extends toward the umbilicus.

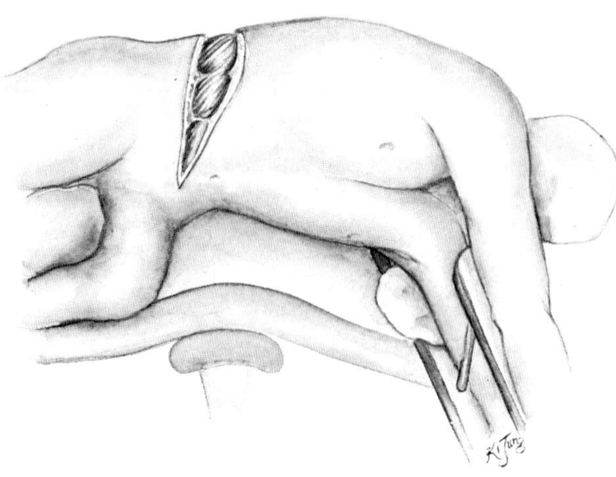

Figure 2.2. Note that for the lower extremities the lowermost limb is flexed at the hip and at the knee while the uppermost limb is extended. A pillow is placed between the thighs. Care is taken to make certain that no portion of either lower extremity is left unsupported or that any undue pressure is applied against any portion of the lower extremity. The patient's upper extremities are supported by a double-arm board, again making certain that adequate padding has been employed. A rolled towel is placed in the lowermost axilla to guard against a brachial palsy. Note the anterior extension of the incision. The length of this anterior extension is determined by the operation being performed. Where considerable exposure is needed, the incision can be extended to the midpoint of the opposite rectus muscle.

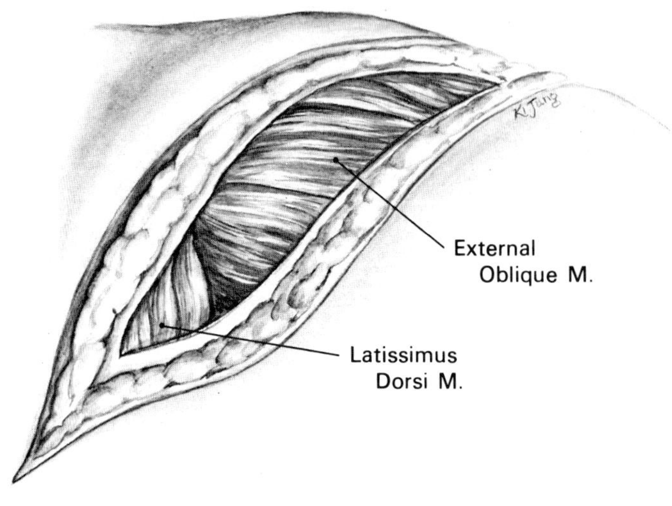

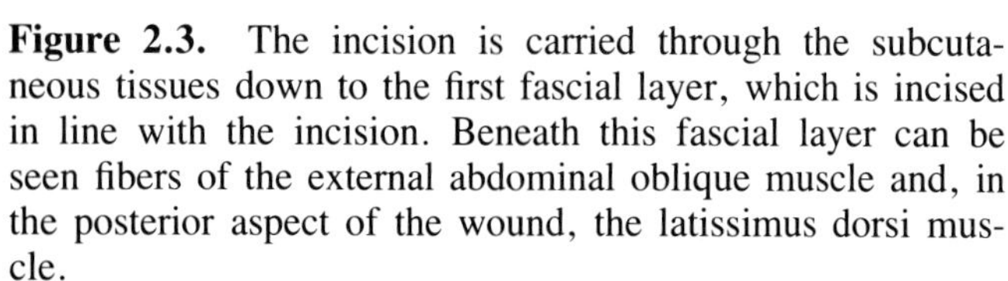

Figure 2.3. The incision is carried through the subcutaneous tissues down to the first fascial layer, which is incised in line with the incision. Beneath this fascial layer can be seen fibers of the external abdominal oblique muscle and, in the posterior aspect of the wound, the latissimus dorsi muscle.

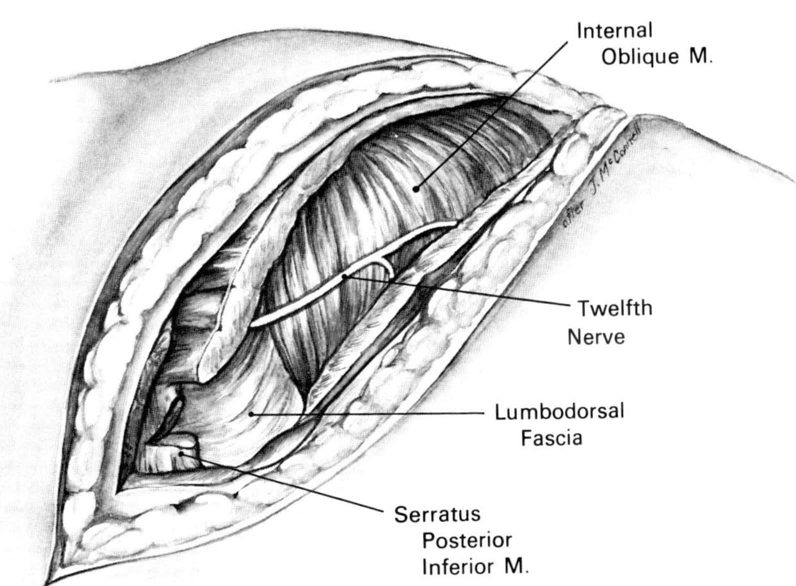

Figure 2.4. The external abdominal oblique muscle and a portion of the latissimus dorsi are divided in line with the incision. The 12th nerve is then identified, dissected free from surrounding structures, and retracted out of the way. Beneath the latissimus dorsi muscle, the serratus posterior inferior can sometimes be seen, and if necessary, a portion of this may be divided. The lumbodorsal fascia lies immediately beneath the divided latissimus dorsi muscle. Anterior to this is the internal abdominal oblique muscle, which is transected in line with the incision.

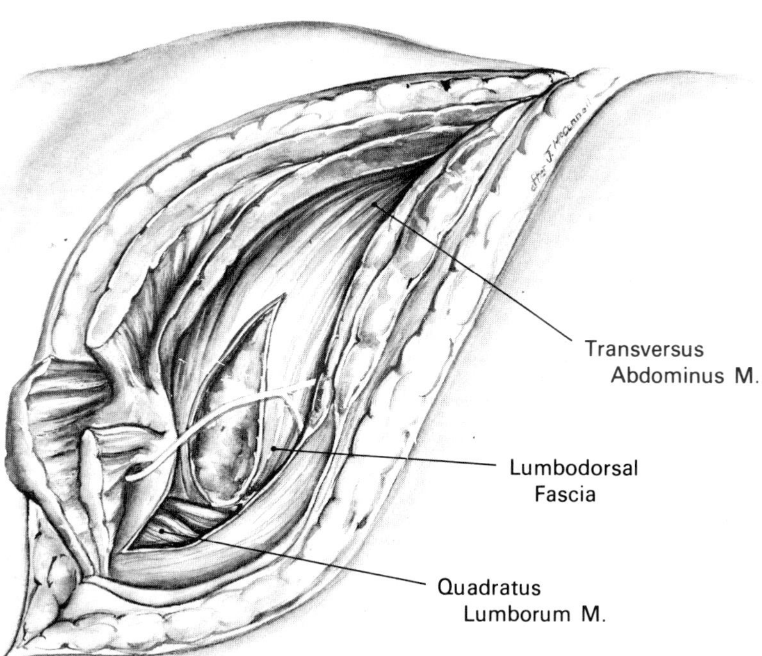

Figure 2.5. In the posterior aspect of the wound the lumbodorsal (thoracolumbar) fascia is sharply divided, allowing entrance to the retroperitoneal space. Either the transversus abdominis muscle can then be divided in line with the incision or its fibers may be separated. Care is taken to push the peritoneum off the undersurface of the transversus abdominis fascia, and the peritoneum and its contents are retracted medially, avoiding entry into the peritoneal cavity.

Eleventh Rib Flank Incision

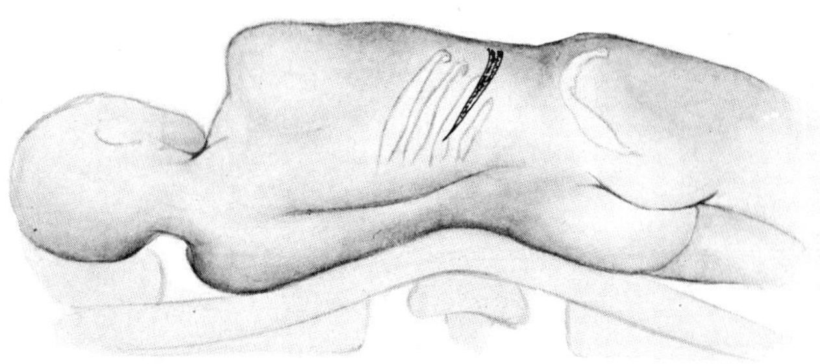

Figure 2.6. The patient is positioned as for a subcostal flank incision. The incision begins back at the angle of the 11th rib and is carried off the tip of the 11th rib toward a point just above the umbilicus.

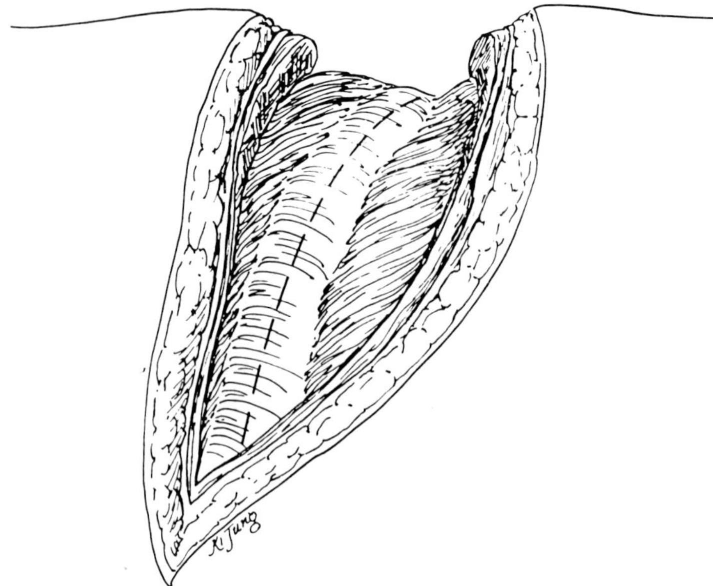

Figure 2.7. The incision is carried down to the fascia, which is incised in line with the incision. The latissimus dorsi muscles are partially divided into the posterior aspect of the incision. The incision is then carried down to the surface of the rib where the periosteum is incised with a scalpel for the full length of the exposed rib.

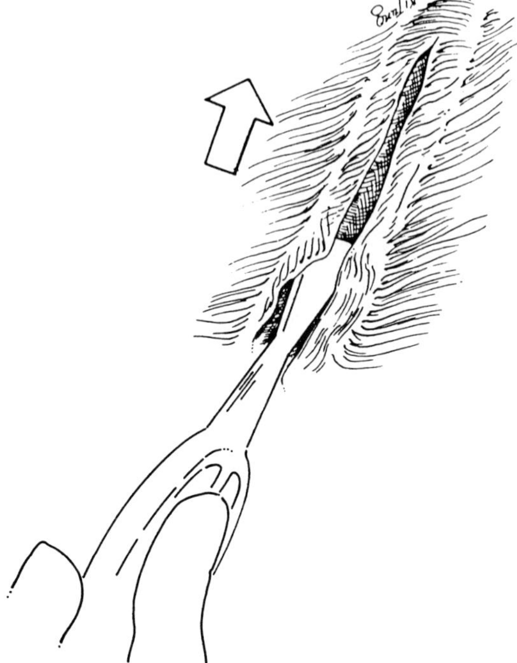

Figure 2.8. A periosteal elevator is used to strip back the periosteum and, thus, remove the attachments of the external abdominal oblique muscle from the rib. This also frees the attachments of the intercostal muscles.

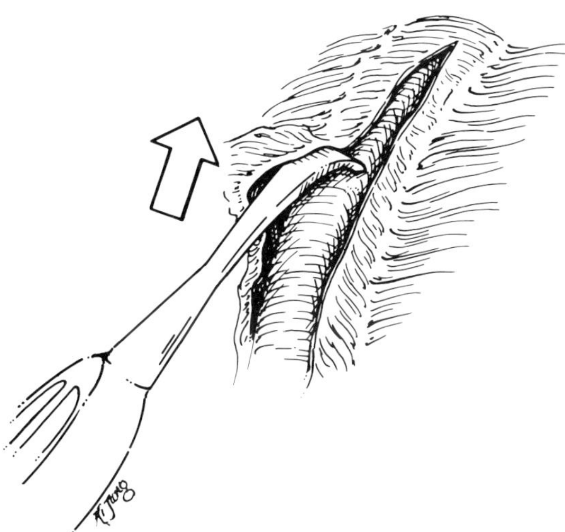

Figure 2.9. Generally, these muscles can best be detached by employing the periosteal elevator on the upper surface of the rib in a direction toward the midline of the abdomen.

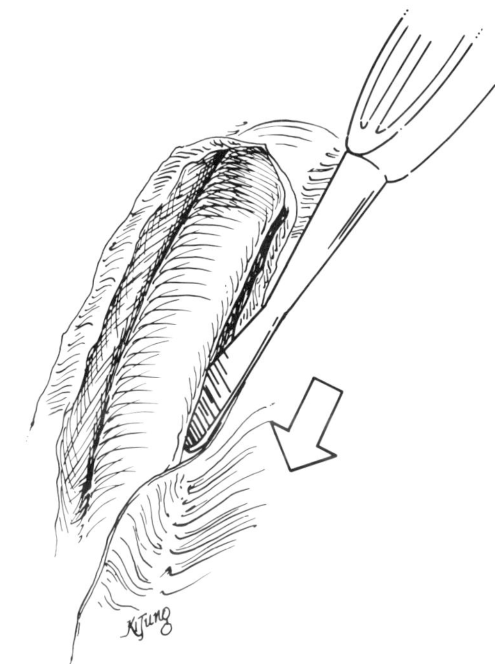

Figure 2.10. On the lower surface of the rib, the elevator is directed toward the posterior aspect of the incision. Care is taken to avoid damage to the neurovascular bundle along the inferior margin of the rib. By following the old adage ''up on the down side, and down on the up side,'' the periosteal elevator is used to strip away the fibers of the intercostal muscles and fascia without damaging adjacent neurovascular structures.

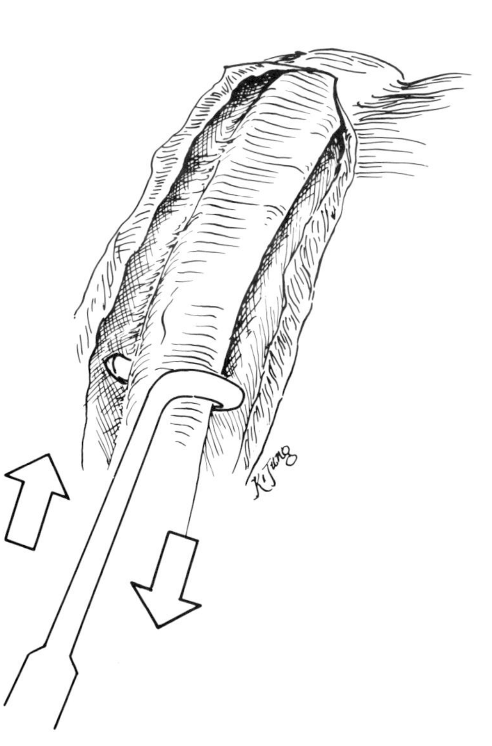

Figure 2.11. A Doyen rib elevator is slipped beneath the rib to free it from its underlying attachments.

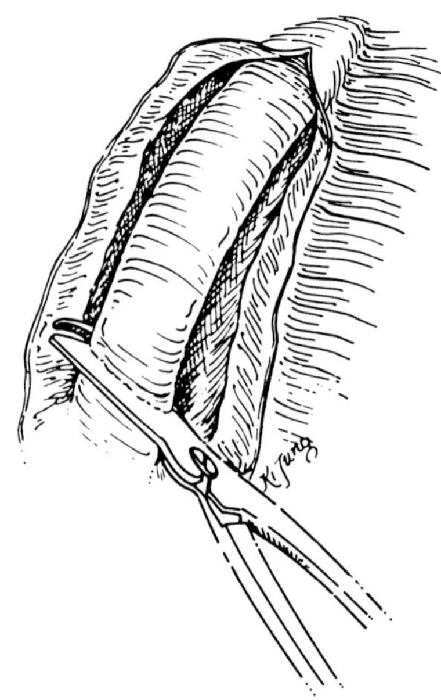

Figure 2.12. A rib cutter is used to divide the rib as far back as the exposure will permit.

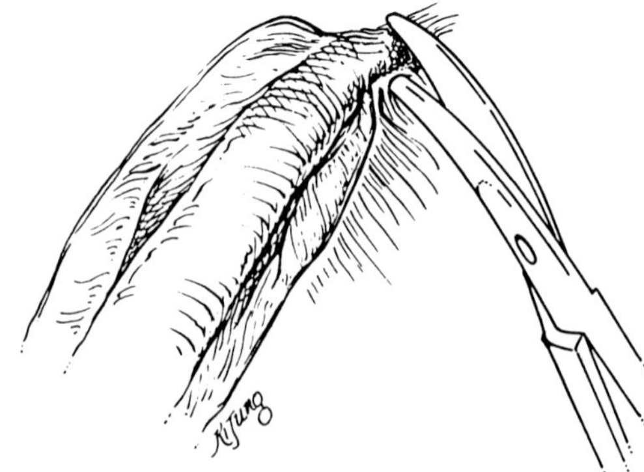

Figure 2.13. The rib remains attached only by fibrous attachments at its tip; these are cut with heavy scissors. The cut surface of the rib is inspected for bony spicules, which are removed with a rongeur. In all aspects of the 11th rib resection, care is taken to avoid entry into the pleura, which lies immediately beneath the posterior aspect of the resected rib.

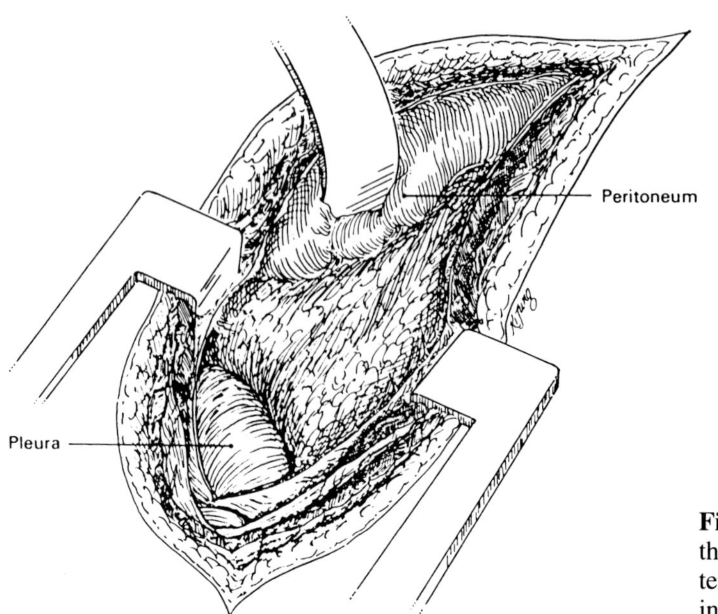

Figure 2.14. The retroperitoneal space is entered through the bed of the 11th rib, and the remaining muscle layers anteriorly are divided, as was described in the subcostal flank incision.

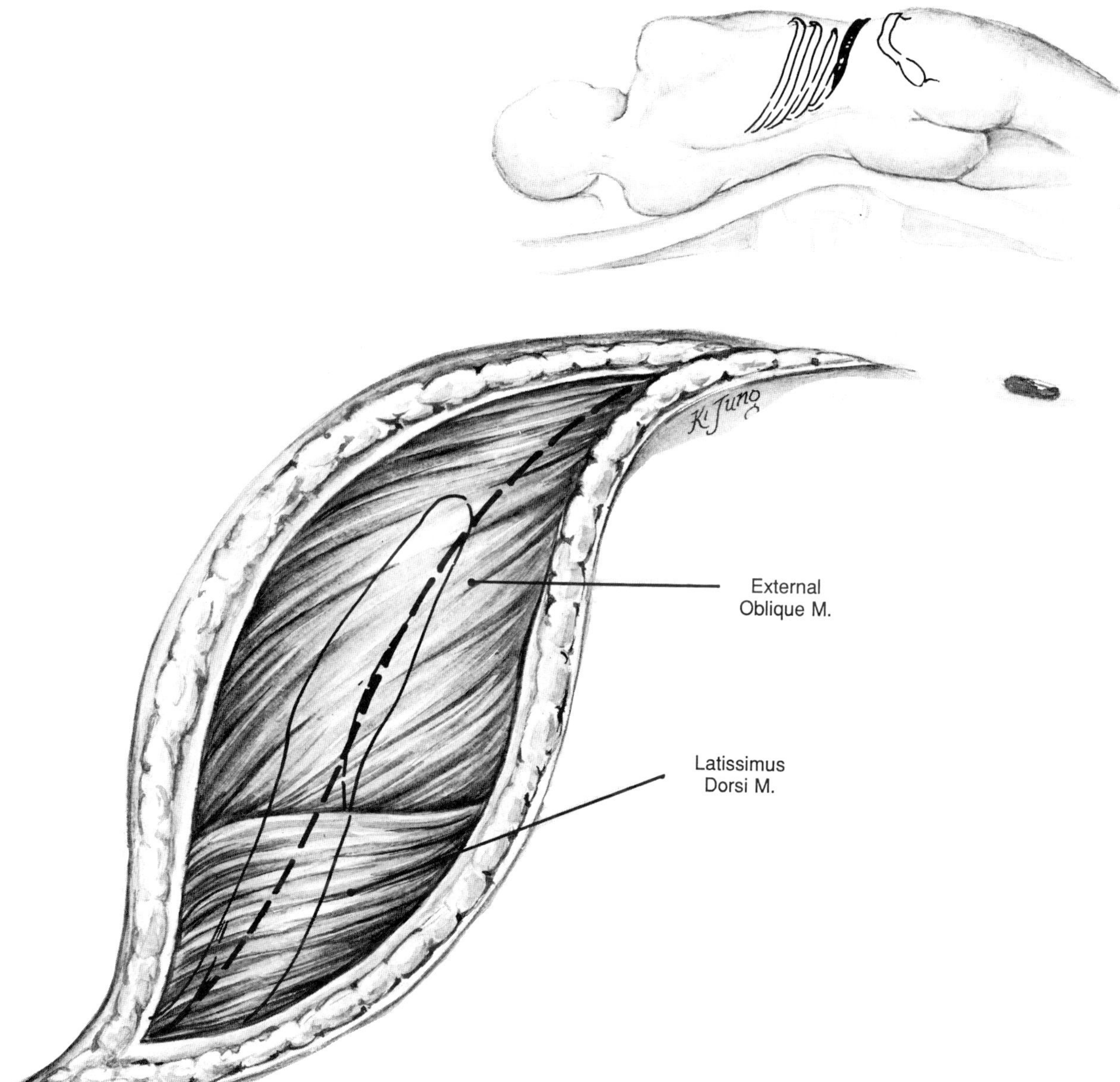

Figure 2.15. The positioning is the same as for the other flank incisions. The incision is begun back near the angle of the 12th rib and is carried off the tip of the 12th rib anteriorly to a point above the umbilicus. The rib is resected as in the 11th rib flank incision, except that a smaller portion of rib is removed and there is less danger of injuring pleura. The remainder of the incision is the same as for the other flank approaches.

Modified Flank Incision with Downward Extension

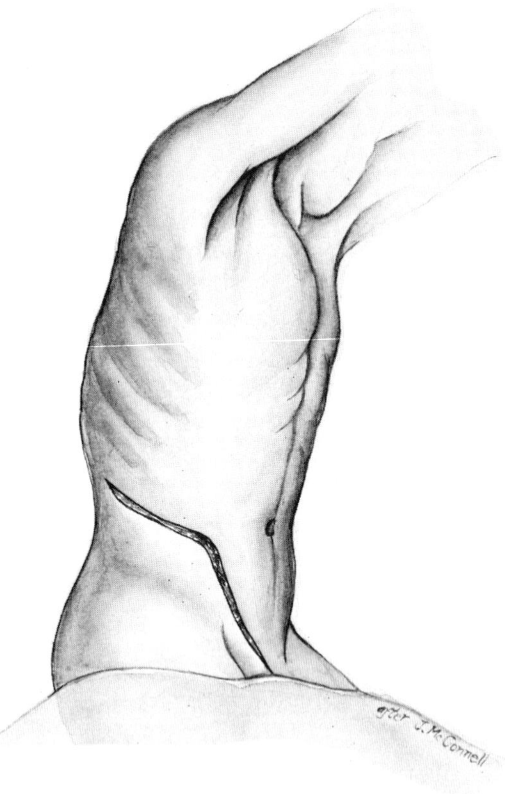

Figure 2.16. This incision is employed primarily for nephroureterectomies in persons who are relatively thin. The patient is placed in a semioblique position with a rolled sheet placed lengthwise beneath the flank. The incision shown is a subcostal incision, but either a 12th or an 11th rib incision can also be employed. The incision begins approximately 1 fingerbreadth below the 12th rib, is carried parallel to the rib toward the umbilicus, and then with a gradual turn, the incision is extended downward along the lateral border of the rectus muscle to the lower quadrant of the abdomen. The incision can be extended to the pubis, as shown, or carried across the midline 2 fingerbreadths above the pubis.

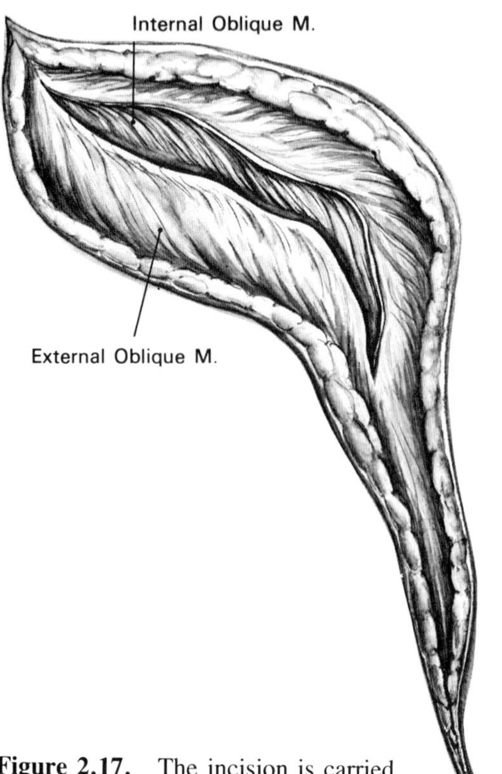

Figure 2.17. The incision is carried down to the fascia, which is incised to the lateral border of the rectus muscle.

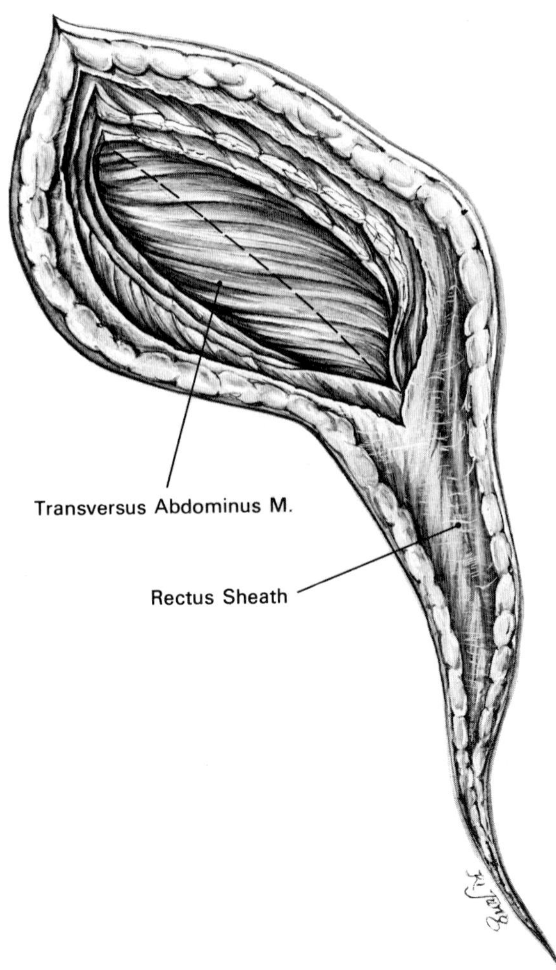

Figure 2.18. The retroperitoneal space is entered, as was described for the previous flank incisions, and the external abdominal oblique and internal abdominal oblique muscles are divided. The transversus abdominis muscle is shown about to be transected. In this incision the rectus muscle is not divided.

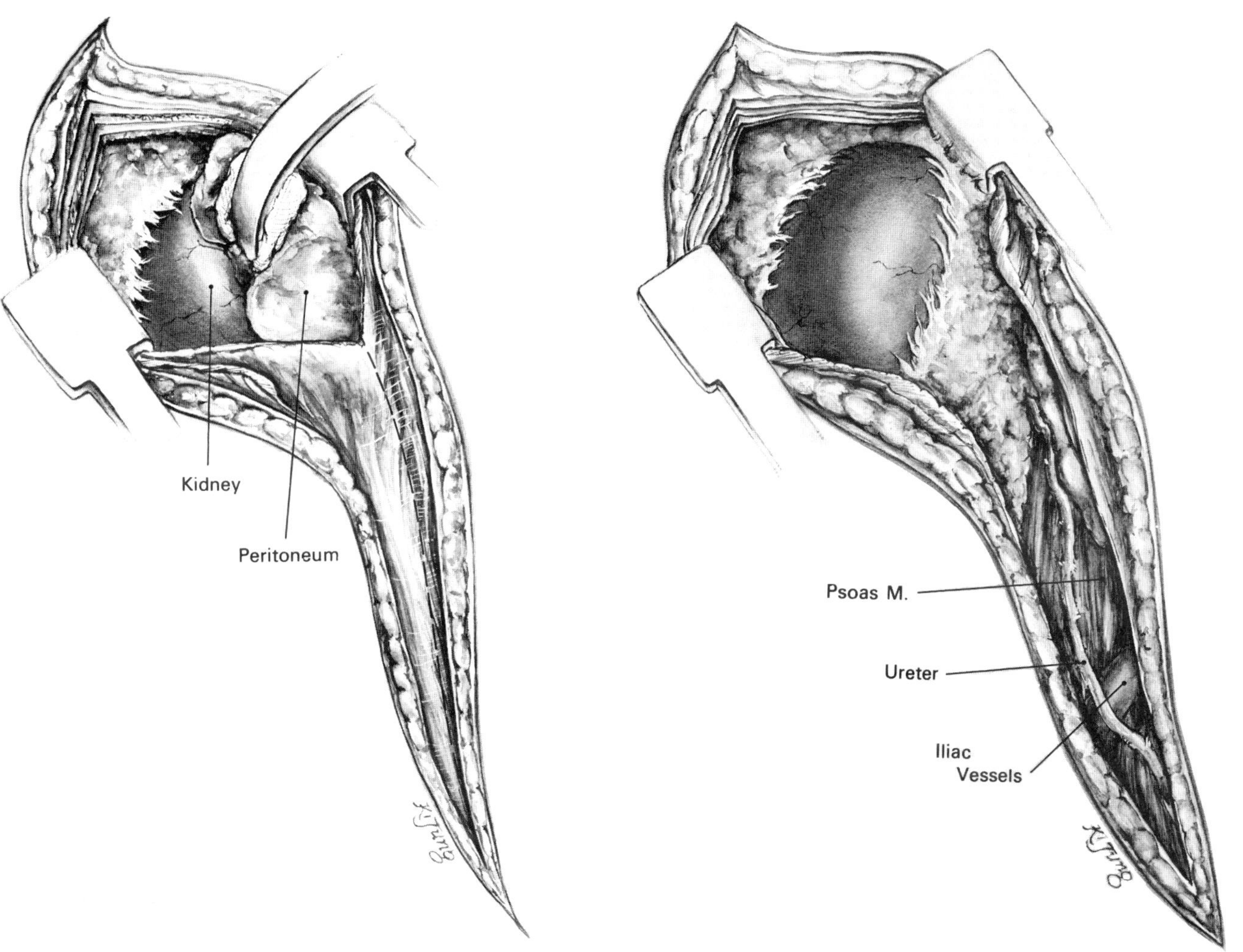

Figure 2.19. At the lateral border of the rectus muscle, the incision turns downward. The fusion of fascia along the lateral border of the rectus muscle is incised after pushing the peritoneum downward. This is a relatively avascular plane. The peritoneum is then retracted medially.

Figure 2.20. The completed incision shows good exposure of the kidney and the entire length of the ureter.

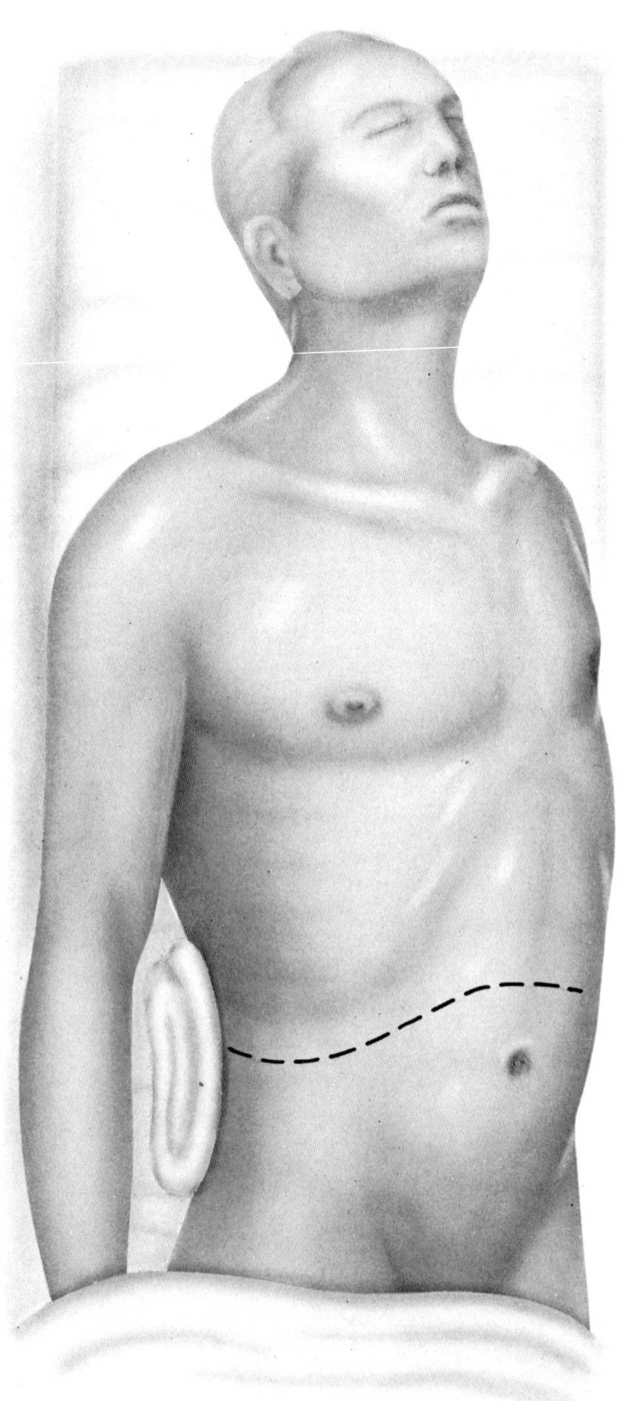

ANTERIOR APPROACHES
Unilateral Subcostal Incision

Figure 2.21. The patient is in the supine position with a rolled sheet beneath the upper lumbar spine. The incision begins approximately 1–2 fingerbreadths below the costal margin in the anterior axillary line and then extends with a gentle curve across the midline, ending at the midpoint of the opposite rectus muscle. The incision is carried through the subcutaneous tissues to the anterior fascia, which is divided in the direction of the incision.

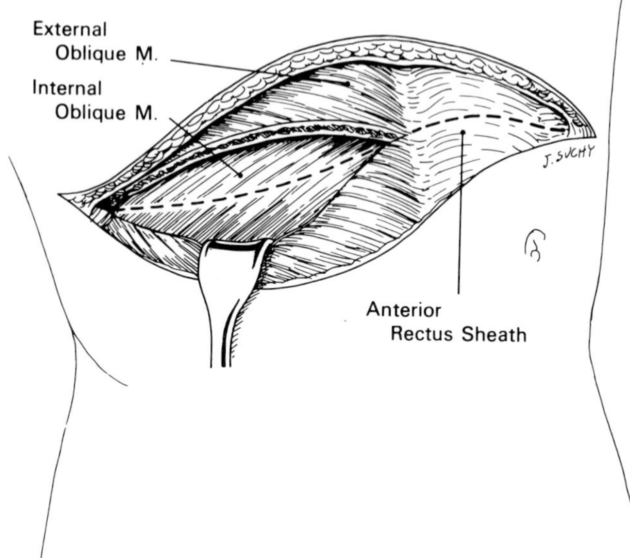

Figure 2.22. In the lateral aspect of the incision, a portion of the latissimus dorsi muscle has been divided. The external abdominal oblique muscle is likewise divided, exposing the fibers of the internal abdominal oblique muscle. The rectus muscle are in the medial portion of the incision.

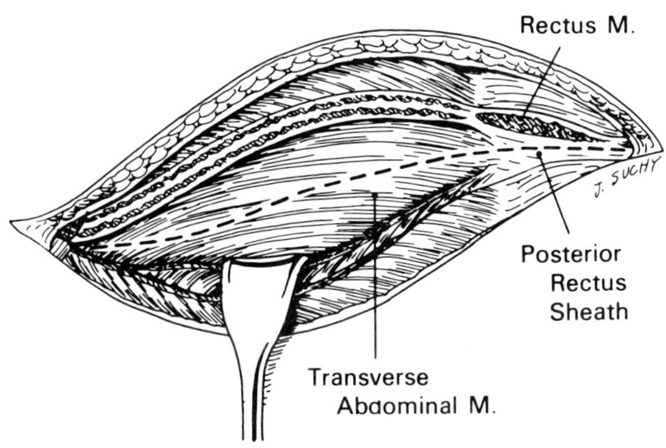

Figure 2.23. The rectus muscle is divided, exposing the posterior rectus sheath. The internal abdominal oblique muscle is divided, exposing the transversus abdominis muscle.

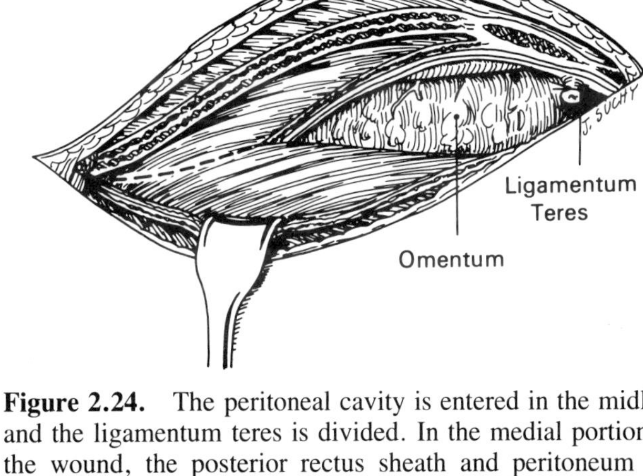

Figure 2.24. The peritoneal cavity is entered in the midline and the ligamentum teres is divided. In the medial portion of the wound, the posterior rectus sheath and peritoneum are incised, and in the lateral portion of the wound, the transversus abdominis muscle, fascia, and peritoneum are incised.

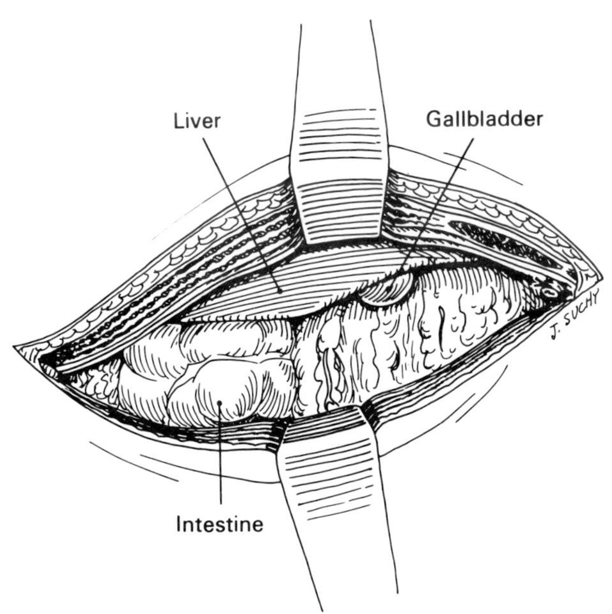

Figure 2.25. The completed exposure shows the liver, gallbladder, and transverse colon.

Bilateral Subcostal Incision

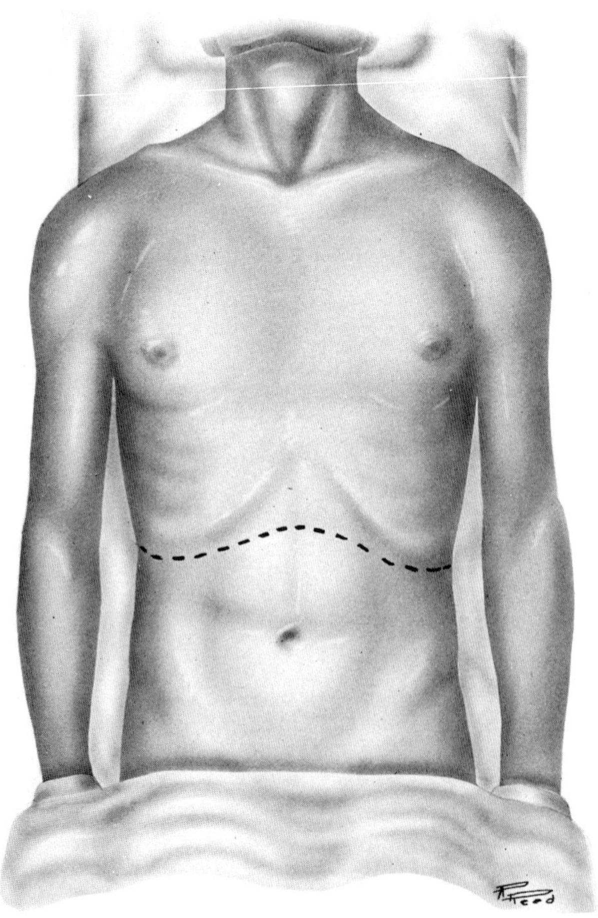

Figure 2.26. The incision is outlined as for the unilateral subcostal incision, except that it extends from one anterior axillary line to the opposite anterior axillary line, with a gentle curve upward as it crosses the midline.

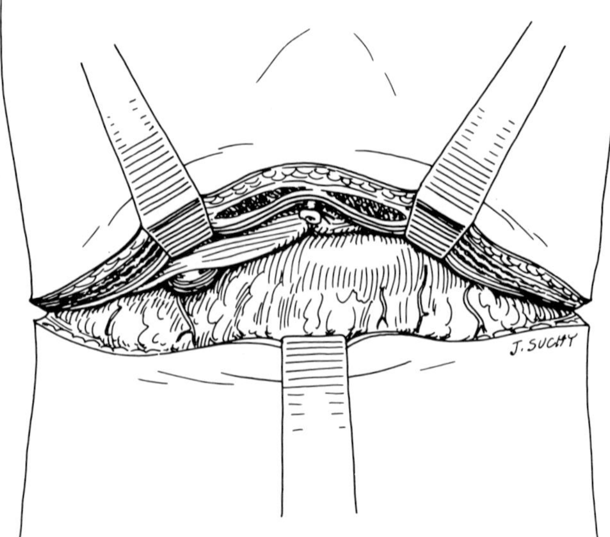

Figure 2.27. The incision is made as described for the unilateral subcostal incision, except that both sides are involved. The completed incision is shown. Along the upper extent of the incision, the divided rectus muscles, and lateral to the rectus muscles, the divided external abdominal oblique, internal abdominal oblique, and transversus abdominis muscle layers can be seen. Note that in the midline the only layers present are skin, subcutaneous tissue, and the fascia and peritoneum, which are fused together.

Anterior Extraperitoneal Incision

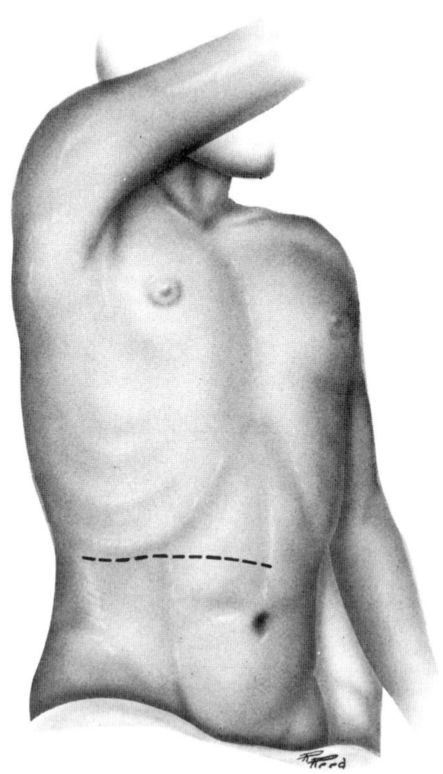

Figure 2.28. The patient is shown in a semioblique position with a rolled sheet beneath the side in which the incision is to be made. The incision is outlined.

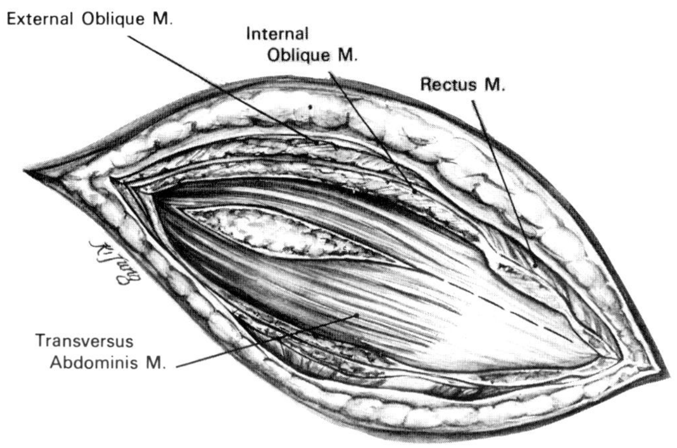

Figure 2.29. The muscle layers are divided as they are for a unilateral subcostal incision, except that the peritoneal cavity is not entered. This figure shows the rectus muscles divided with the posterior rectus sheath beneath them. The external abdominal oblique, internal abdominal oblique, and transversus abdominis muscles are likewise divided. The peritoneum lies beneath them.

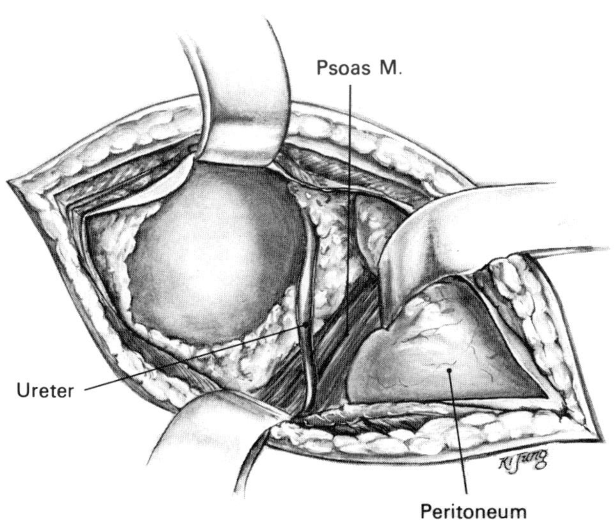

Figure 2.30. After the peritoneum has been separated from the undersurface of the rectus sheath, the rectus sheath is divided and the peritoneal contents are retracted medially, giving access to the retroperitoneal space.

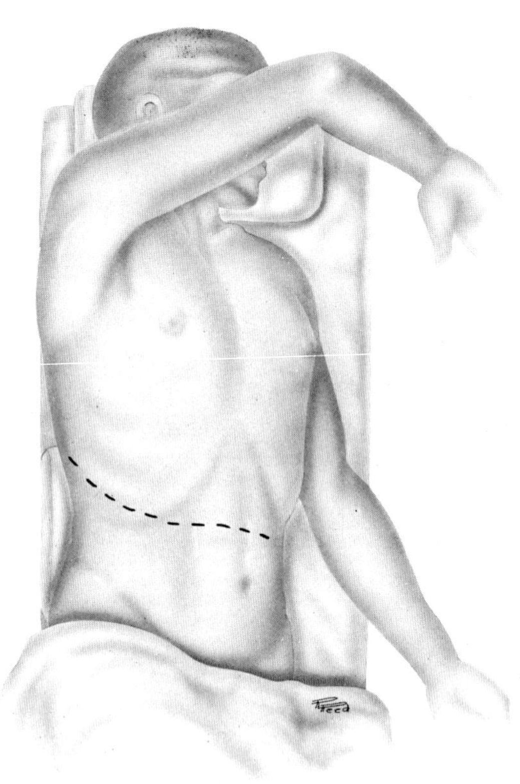

Eleventh Rib Transperitoneal Incision

Figure 2.31. The patient is positioned as for the anterior extraperitoneal incision previously described. The incision begins as far back on the 11th rib as the positioning will permit and extends along the 11th rib, off its tip, and across the midline to the midpoint of the opposite rectus muscle. The incision crosses the midline at a point approximately midway between the xiphoid and the umbilicus.

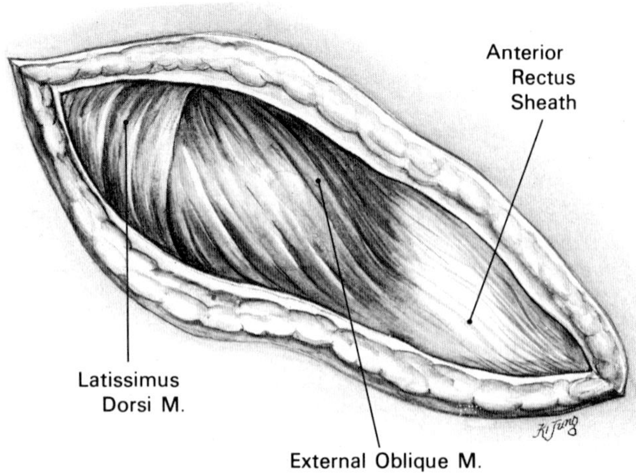

Figure 2.32. This figure shows the first fascial layer divided in line with the incision. In the posterior aspect of the wound are the fibers of the latissimus dorsi muscle running perpendicularly to the ribs. Just anterior to this are the fibers of the external abdominal oblique muscle originating from the ribs and coursing obliquely down to the crest of the ilium. At the medial aspect of the incision are the rectus muscles.

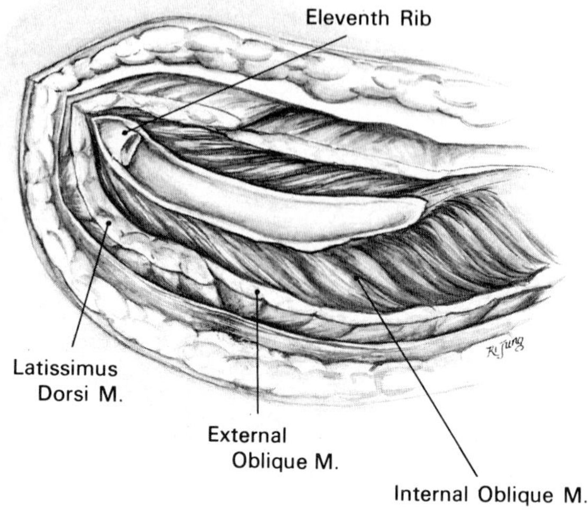

Figure 2.33. The latissimus dorsi muscle is divided and the 11th rib is resected, as previously described in the 11th rib flank incision. Care is taken to avoid damage to the neurovascular bundle along the inferior margin of the rib.

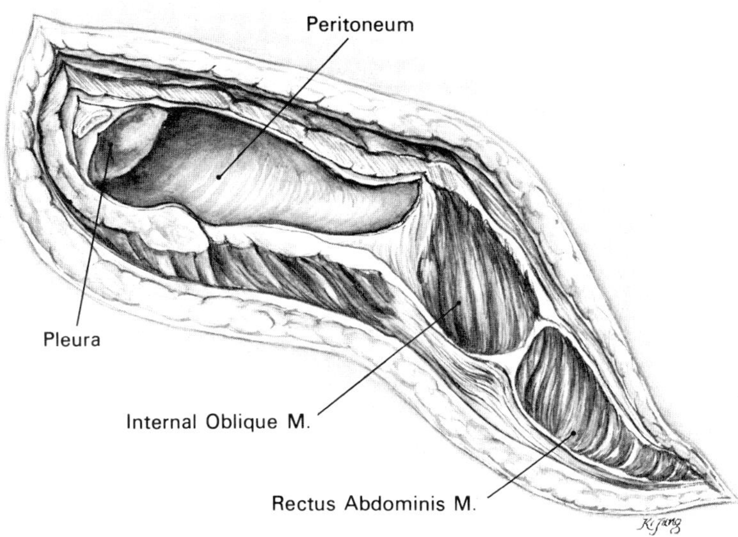

Figure 2.34. The retroperitoneal space is then entered through the bed of the rib, with care being taken to avoid damage to the pleura posteriorly. After identification the pleura may be pushed posteriorly. Anteriorly, the rectus muscles are divided and the external abdominal oblique, internal abdominal oblique, and transversus abdominis are divided in line with the incision.

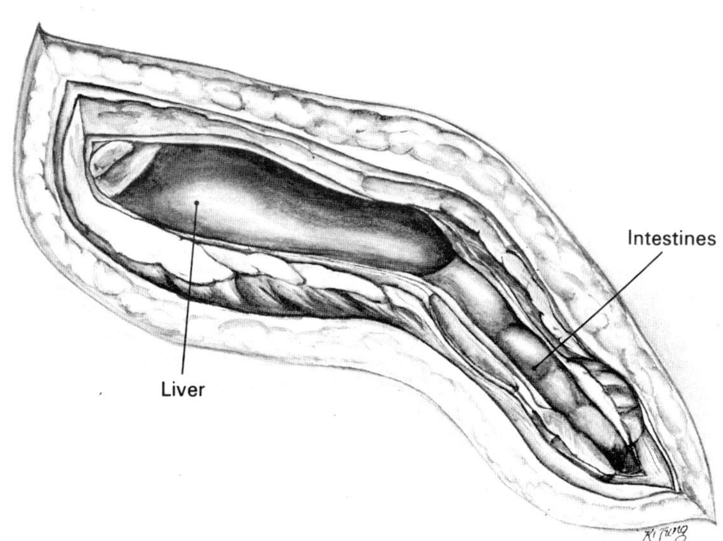

Figure 2.35. This figure shows the completed division of the muscle layers. The peritoneal cavity is entered for the entire length of the incision.

Midline Upper Abdominal Incision

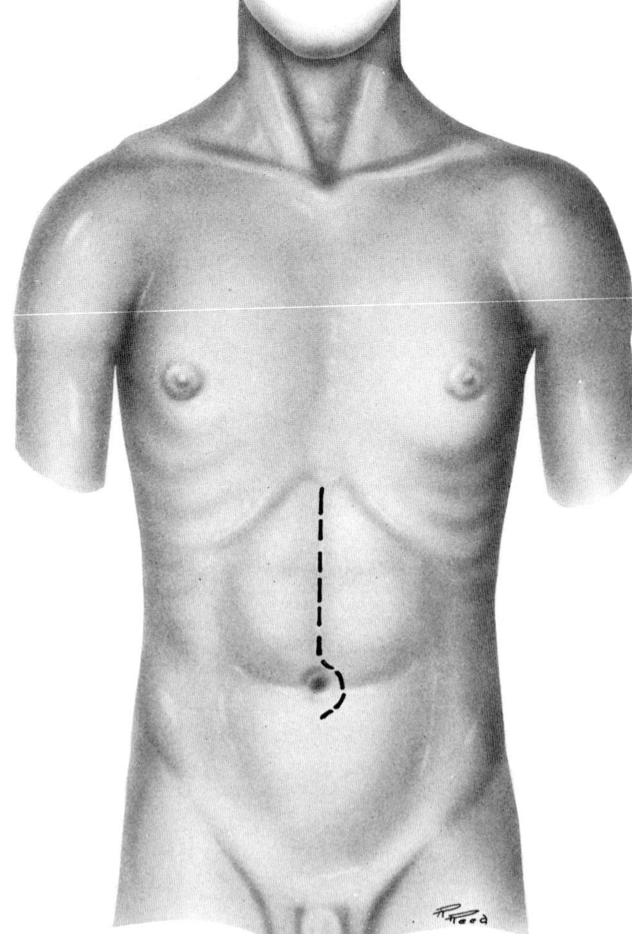

Figure 2.36. The patient is shown in the supine position with the incision extending from the xiphoid to the umbilicus. The incision can be extended around the umbilicus to either side if necessary.

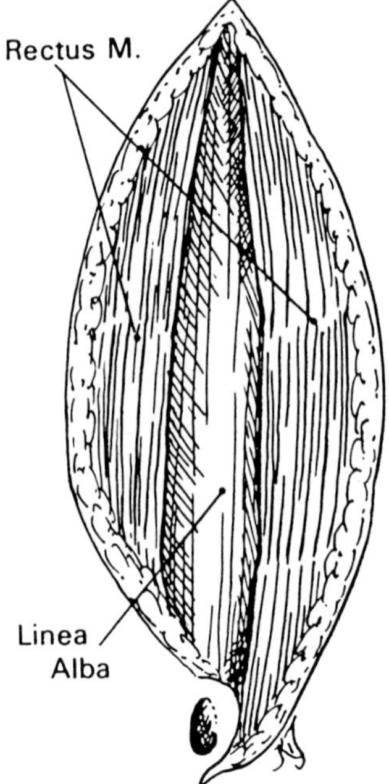

Figure 2.37. The incision is carried down through the subcutaneous tissues to the fascia. The rectus muscles can be seen on either side of the midline fusion of fascia (linea alba).

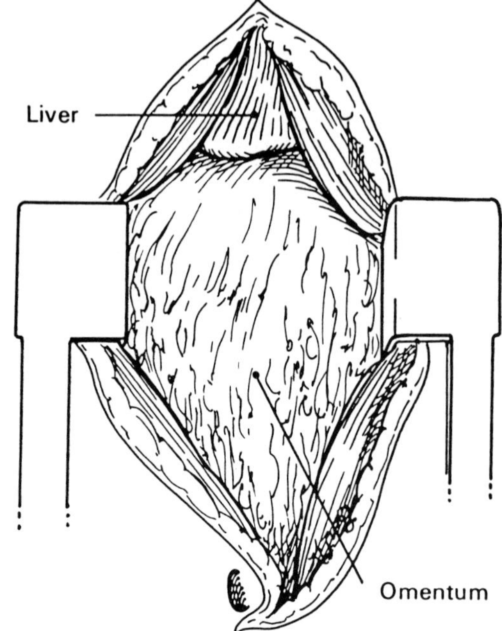

Figure 2.38. The midline fusion of the fascia and peritoneum is divided to enter the peritoneal cavity.

Midline Lower Abdominal Incision

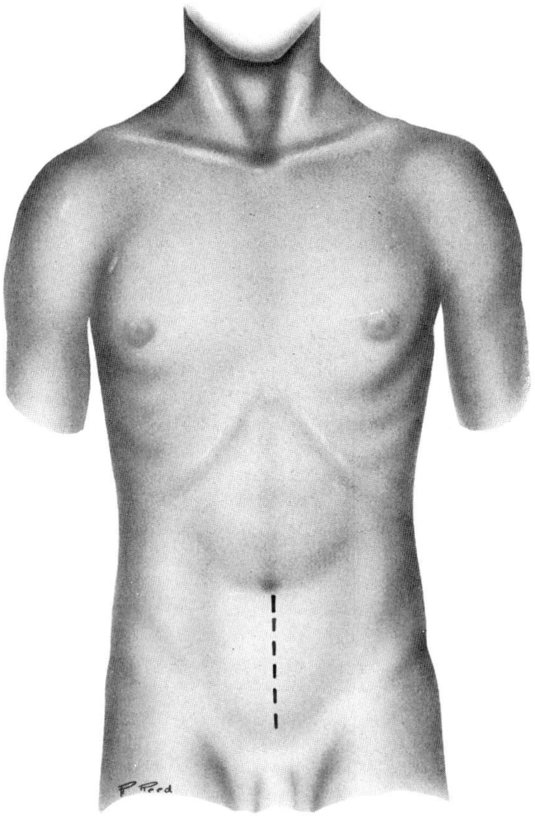

Figure 2.39. The patient is in the supine position. The incision is outlined from the umbilicus down to the symphysis pubis.

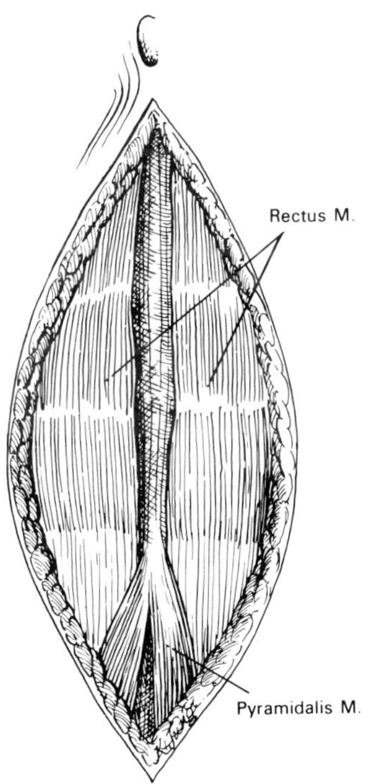

Figure 2.40. The subcutaneous tissues are divided, exposing the fascia. In the lower margin of the incision the pyramidalis muscles, and inconstant finding, are seen.

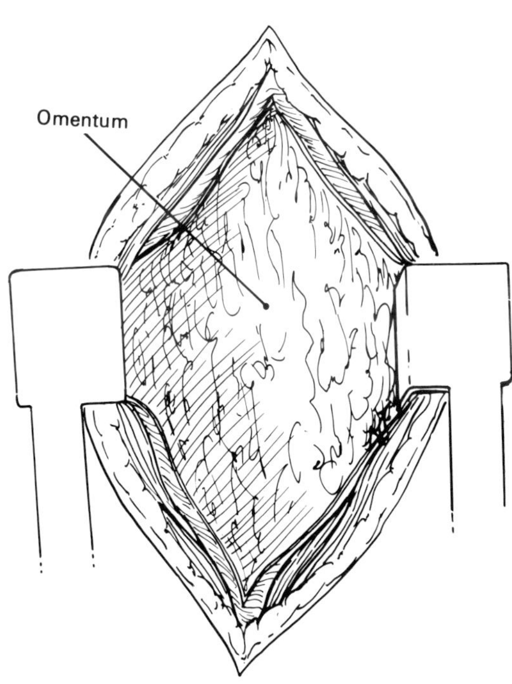

Figure 2.41. The fascia and peritoneum are divided along the midline linea alba to gain access to the peritoneal cavity.

Xiphoid to Pubis Midline Abdominal Incision

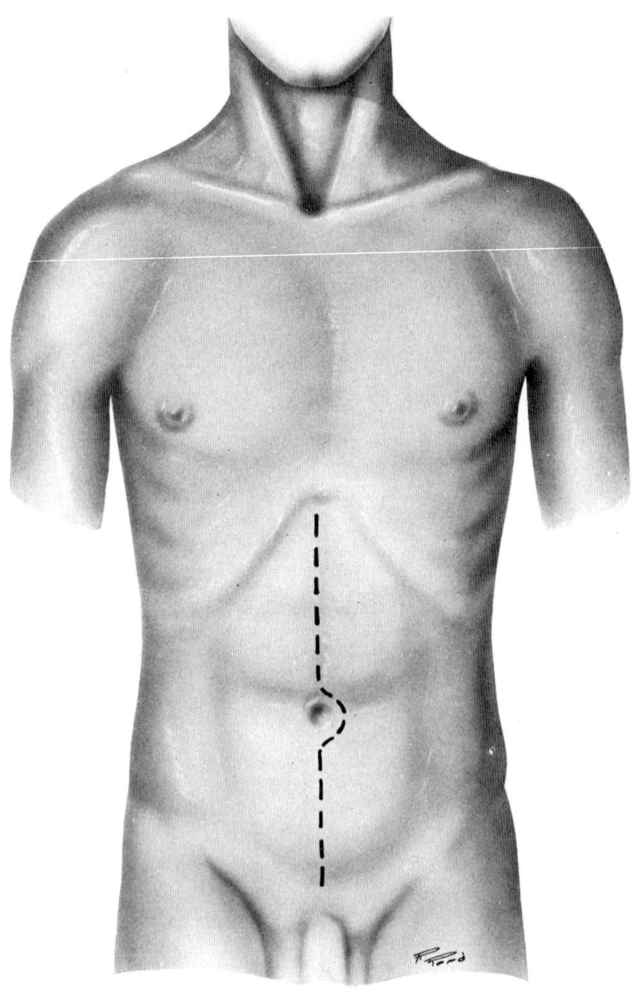

Figure 2.42. This is a combination of the upper abdominal midline incision and the lower abdominal midline incision. The figure shows the patient in the supine position with the incision being outlined. The incision can be carried around either side of the umbilicus. The remainder of the incision is made as described for the upper and lower abdominal midline incisions.

Paramedian Incision

The incision described is a lower abdominal paramedian incision. It is used in operations where a stoma is created so that the subsequent scar will not lie beneath the faceplate of the urinary appliance (see chapters 22 and 23).

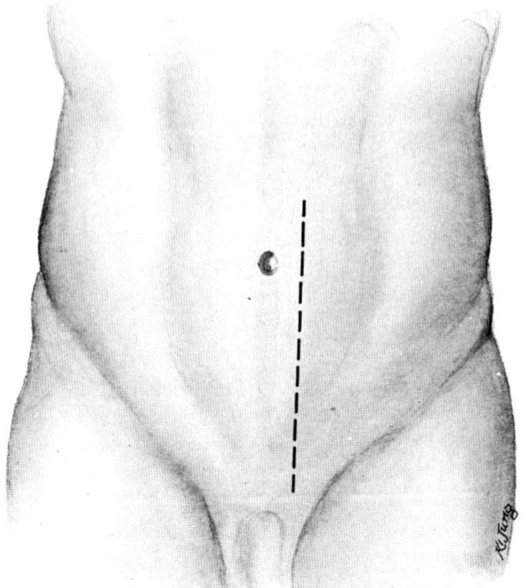

Figure 2.43. The patient is in the supine position. The incision is outlined over the belly of one of the rectus muscles approximately 2–3 fingerbreadths from the midline. It can be extended above the umbilicus. Inferiorly, it is carried down to the pubis.

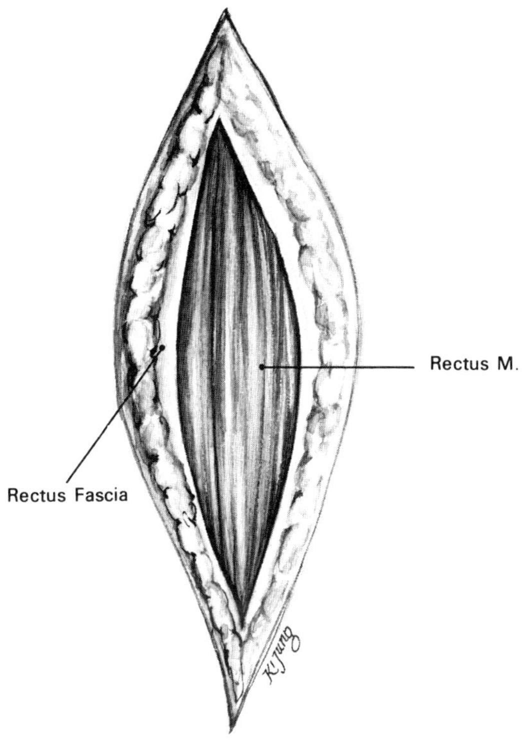

Figure 2.44. The subcutaneous tissues and the anterior rectus fascia are divided, revealing the underlying rectus muscle.

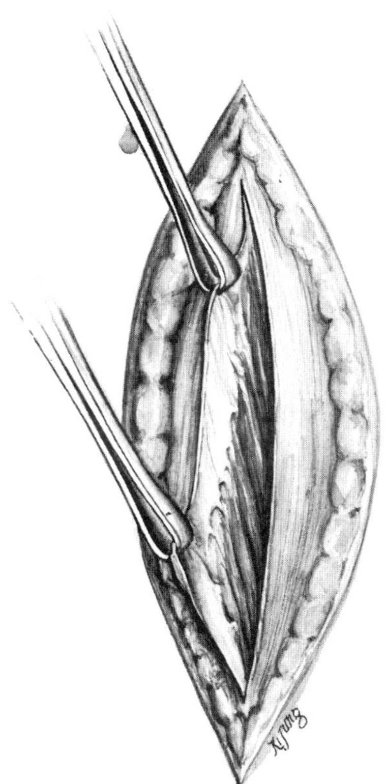

Figure 2.45. Allis clamps are placed on the medial edge of the transected rectus fascia and upward traction is applied. The fascia is dissected off the rectus muscle toward the midline of the abdomen.

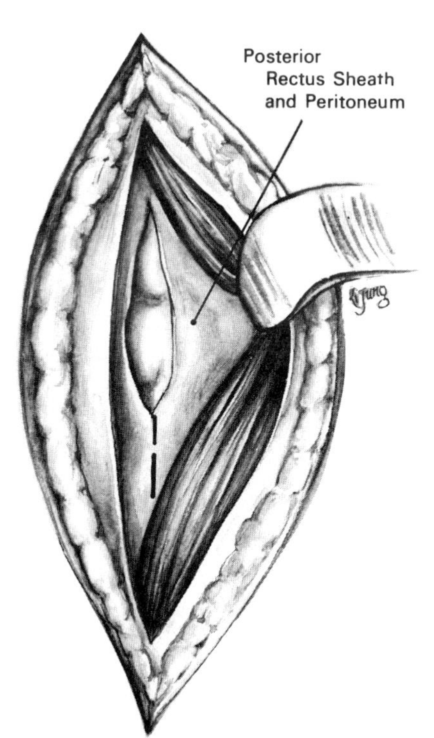

Figure 2.46. When the midline of the abdomen is reached, the rectus muscle is retracted laterally, and the posterior rectus sheath and peritoneum are transected to gain entrance to the peritoneal cavity.

Modified Gibson Incision

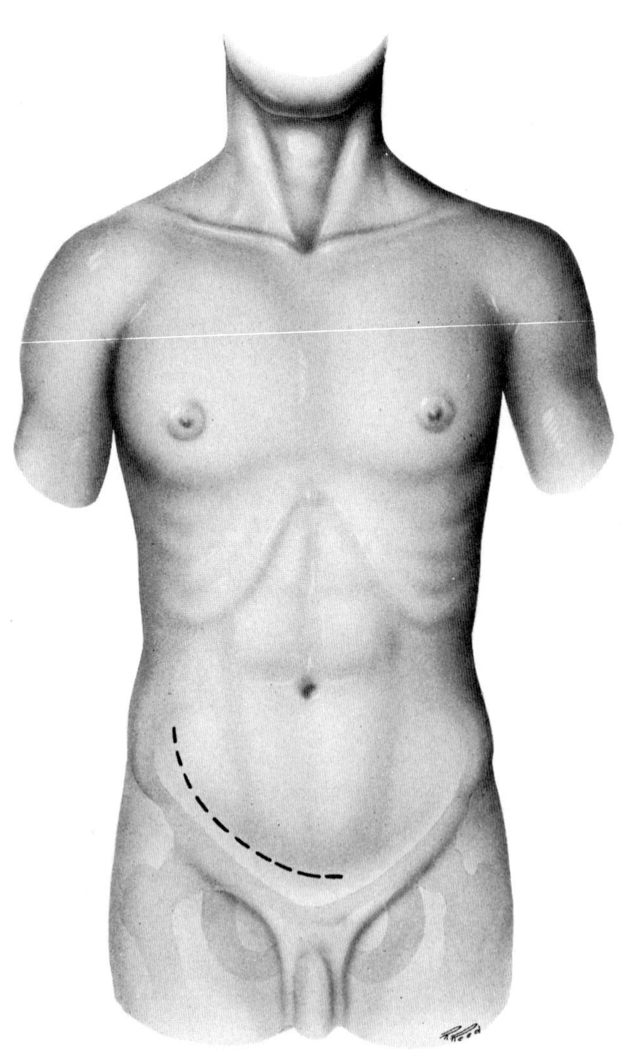

Figure 2.47. The patient is in the supine position. A curvilinear incision is made in the lower quadrant of the abdomen. It is 2 fingerbreadths medial to the anterosuperior iliac spine and 2 fingerbreadths above the symphysis pubis. It extends across the midline and, at its opposite end, may have an upward extension parallel to the midline of the abdomen.

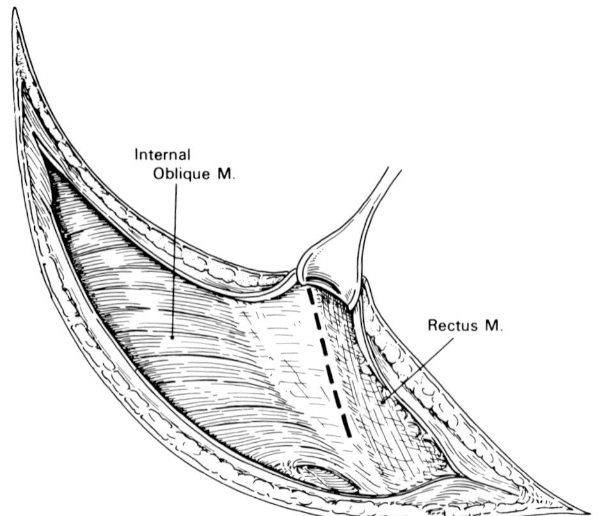

Figure 2.48. The incision is made down to the aponeurosis of the external abdominal oblique muscle. This aponeurosis is then incised in the direction of the incision. The cut aponeurosis is retracted upward, and the fusion of fascia at the lateral border of the rectus muscle is incised upward as far as the retraction will permit. This is a relatively avascular plane. Care must be taken to push down the underlying peritoneum so that the peritoneal cavity is not inadvertently entered.

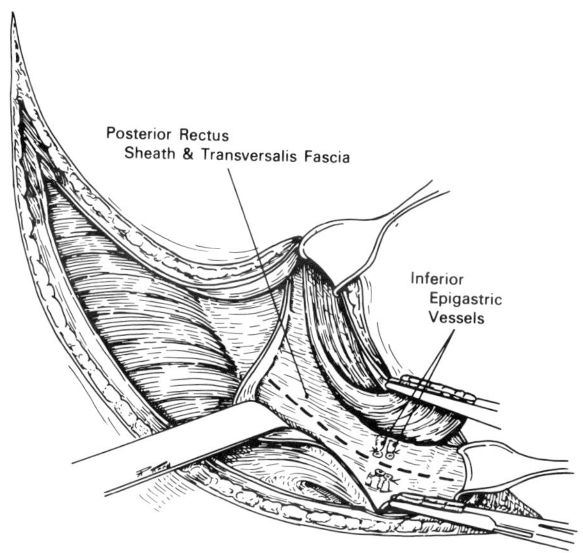

Figure 2.49. The rectus muscle itself can be treated in one of three ways. It may be retracted medially. If more medial exposure is needed, the lateral portion of its tendonous attachment to the pubis may be transected. If still further medical exposure is required, the entire tendonous attachment to the pubis may be transected as shown. The inferior epigastric vessels are indentified beneath the rectus muscle at its inferolateral portion and are divided. The transversalis fascia is then incised in the direction of the incision, and the retroperitoneal space is entered with the peritoneum being swept medially to gain access to this space.

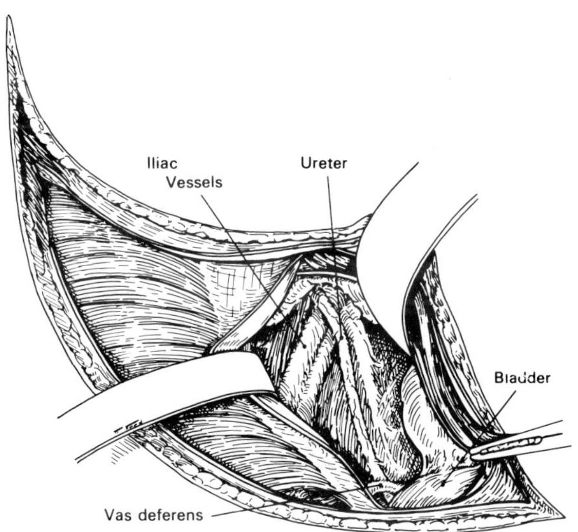

Figure 2.50. The peritoneal envelope is retracted in an upward and medial direction, exposing the iliac vessels and the patient's ureter. The bladder and the vas deferens can be seen in the lower aspect of the wound. To gain maximum exposure, it may be necessary to extend the incision laterally and upward into the internal oblique muscle. In addition, the vas deferens and associated round ligament structures may be transected and ligated to gain better exposure of the bladder and distal iliac vessels.

THORACOABDOMINAL APPROACH

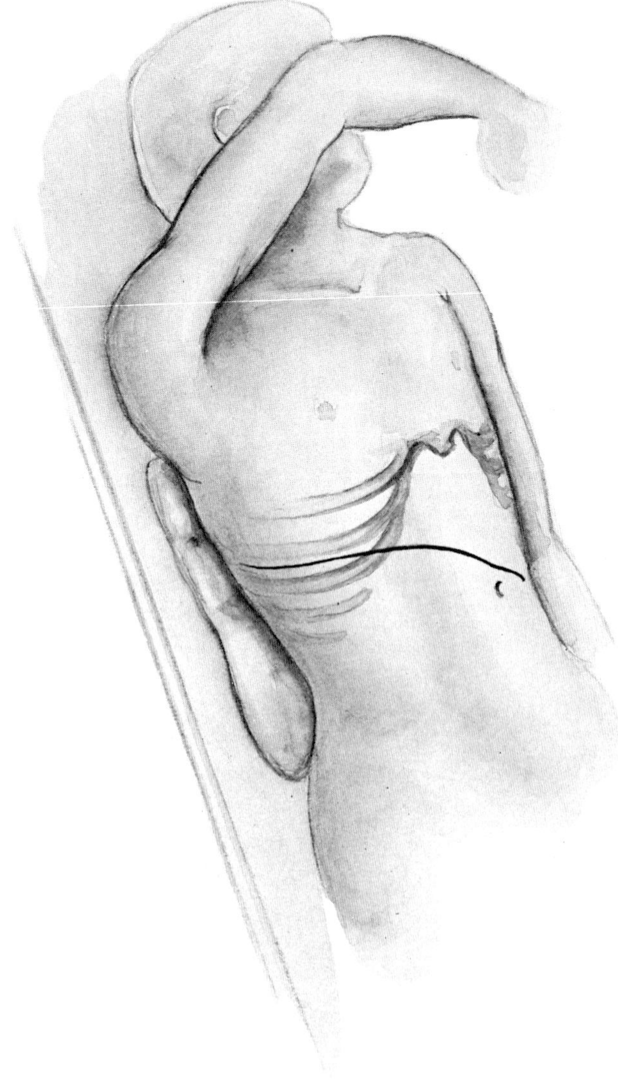

Figure 2.51. The patient is placed in a semioblique position with a rolled sheet placed longitudinally beneath the flank. The incision is begun in the 9th intercostal space near the angle of the rib and is carried across the costal margin to the midpoint of the opposite rectus muscle just above the umbilicus. As an alternative, this incision may be made through the bed of the 9th or the 10th rib.

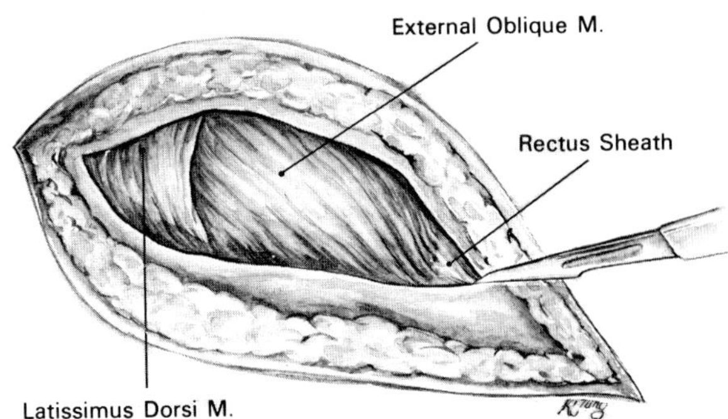

Figure 2.52. The incision is carried down to the fascia, which is divided in the direction of the incision.

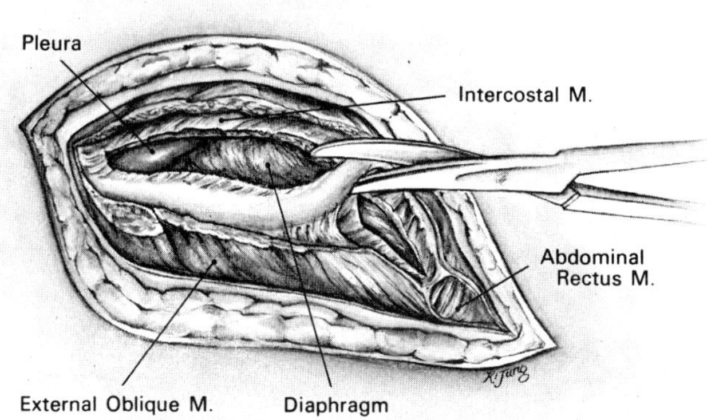

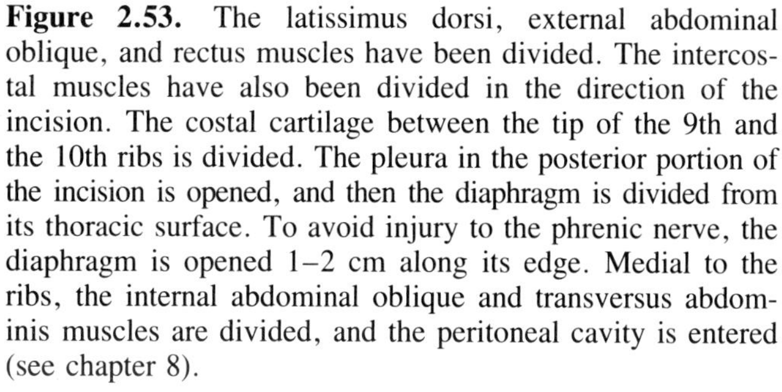

Figure 2.53. The latissimus dorsi, external abdominal oblique, and rectus muscles have been divided. The intercostal muscles have also been divided in the direction of the incision. The costal cartilage between the tip of the 9th and the 10th ribs is divided. The pleura in the posterior portion of the incision is opened, and then the diaphragm is divided from its thoracic surface. To avoid injury to the phrenic nerve, the diaphragm is opened 1–2 cm along its edge. Medial to the ribs, the internal abdominal oblique and transversus abdominis muscles are divided, and the peritoneal cavity is entered (see chapter 8).

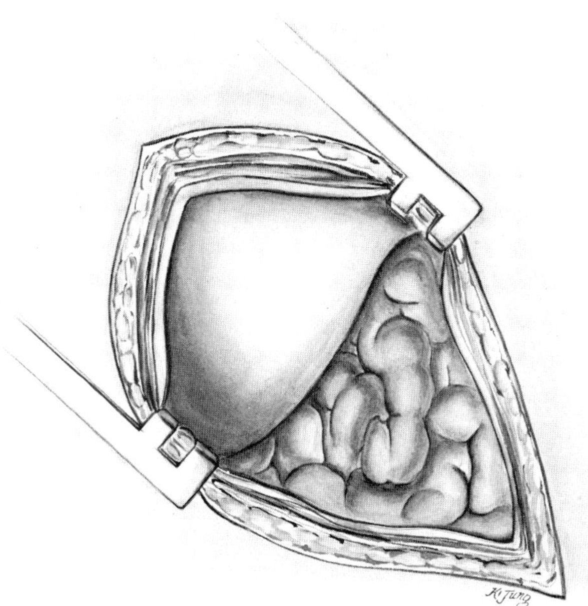

Figure 2.54. Exposure can then be maintained with the rib-spreading Finochietto retractor.

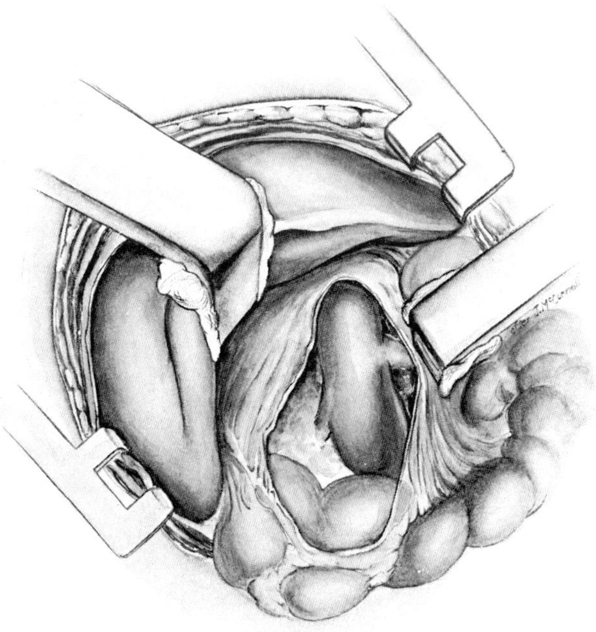

Figure 2.55. The liver is retracted upward and the colon downward, allowing access to the retroperitoneal space.

POSTERIOR APPROACHES

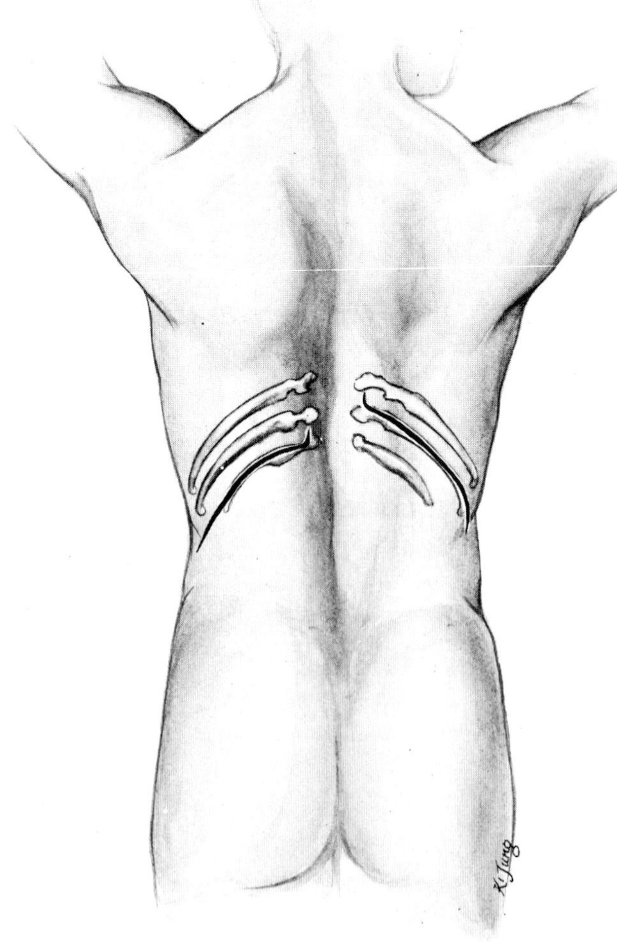

Figure 2.56. The patient is placed in the prone position with the operating table flexed beneath the lower rib cage. If necessary, the kidney rest can be elevated to give further flexion. The incision can be made over either the 12th rib as shown on the patient's left, or the 11th rib, as shown on the patient's right.

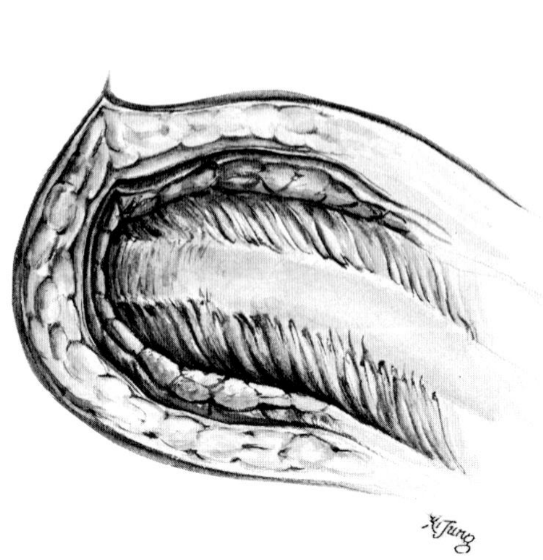

Figure 2.57. The incision is carried down to the periosteum of the rib.

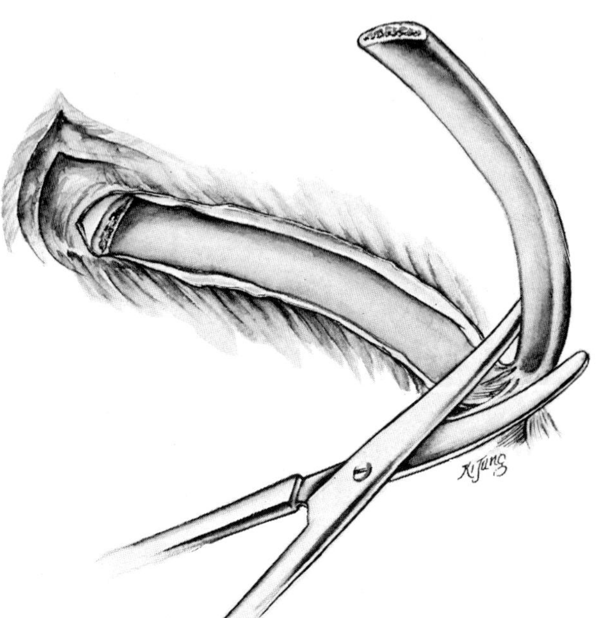

Figure 2.58. The rib is resected subperiosteally, as described for the 11th rib flank incision.

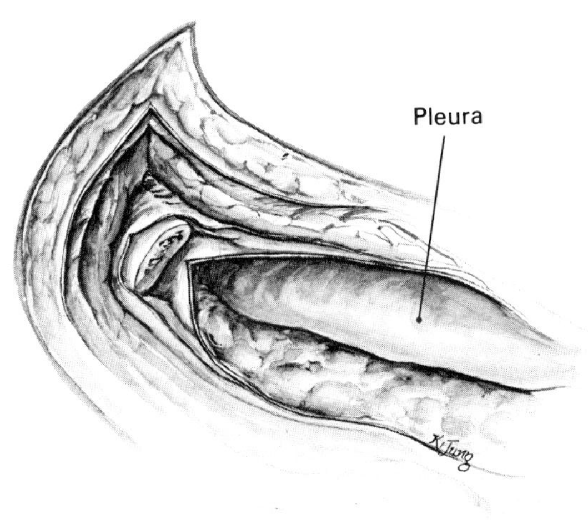

Figure 2.59. After removal of the rib, the periosteum in the bed of the rib is incised, exposing the pleura above and diaphragm beneath the pleura.

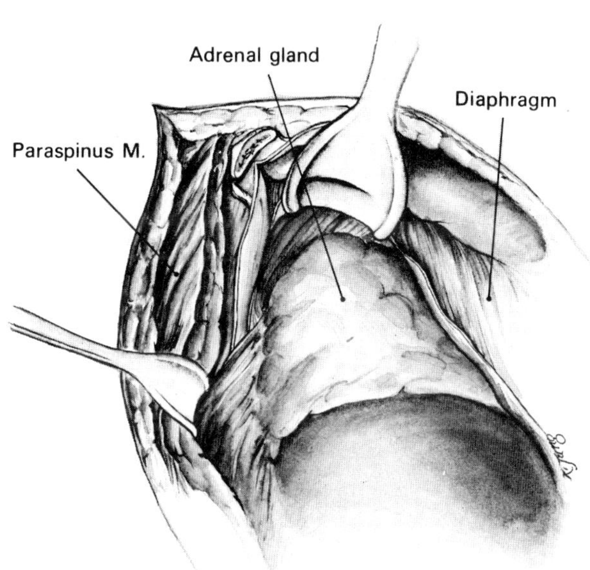

Figure 2.60. The diaphragm and the pleura are then retracted superiorly and the paraspinous muscles are retracted medially, exposing the adrenal gland and the upper pole of the kidney. In some cases, the diaphragm and pleura are directly incised to expose the adrenal gland (see chapter 6).

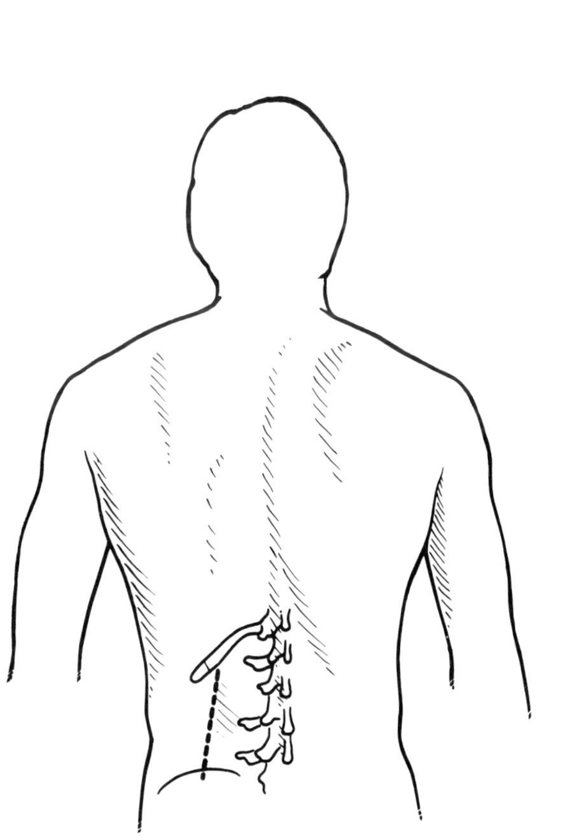

Figure 2.61. A dorsal lumbotomy incision provides adequate exposure of the lower portion of the kidney and upper ureter. The incision is made at the lateral border of the paraspinous muscles and extends from the 12th rib to the iliac crest.

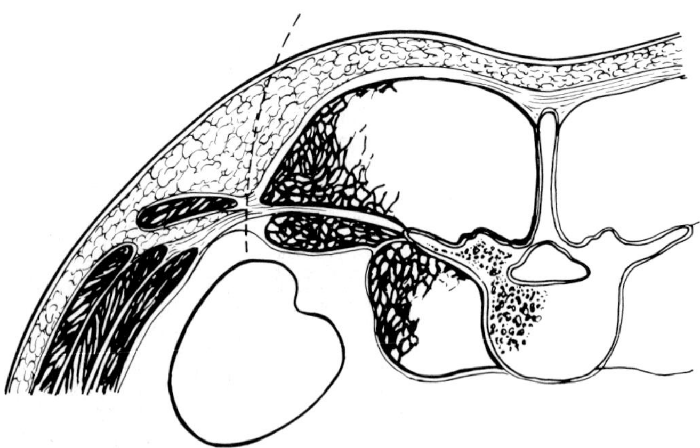

Figure 2.62. The dashed line indicates the pathway for the incision, which begins at the lateral margin of the sacrospinalis muscle and proceeds between the latissimus dorsi muscle laterally and the quadratus lumborum muscle medially. The thoracolumbar fascia is incised, the retroperitoneum is entered, and the kidney, surrounded by Gerota's fascia, is encountered.

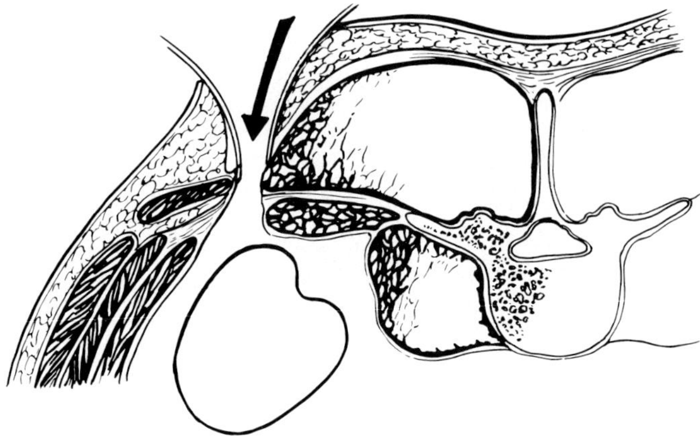

Figure 2.63. Adequate exposure can be obtained by hand-held retractors.

Suggested Readings

Bodner H, Briskin HJ: Subdiaphragmatic renal exposure by resection of the eleventh rib. *Urol Cutan Rev* 54:272, 1950.

Chute R, Baron JA, Jr, Olsson CA: The transverse upper abdominal "chevron" incision in urological surgery. *J Urol* 99:528, 1968.

Chute R, Soutter L, Kerr WS, Jr: Value of thoraco-abdominal incision in removal of kidney tumors. *N Engl J Med* 241:951, 1949.

Culp OS: Anterior nepthro-ureterectomy, advantages and limitations of a single incision. *J Urol* 85:193, 1961.

Glenn JF: Surgery of the adrenal glands. In Glenn JF, Boyce WH (eds): *Urologic Surgery*. New York, Harper & Row, 1969, pp. 16–30.

Grayhack JT, Graham JB: Surgery of the kidney. In Glenn JF, Boyce WH (eds): *Urologic Surgery*. New York, Harper & Row, 1969, pp. 42–62.

Hess E: Resection of the rib in renal operations. *J Urol* 42:943, 1939.

Lyon R: An anterior extraperitoneal incision for kidney surgery. *J Urol* 79:383, 1958.

Mayo WJ: The incision for the lumbar exposure of the kidney. *Ann Surg* 55:63, 1912.

Nagamatsu G: Dorso-lumbar approach to the kidney and adrenal with osteoplastic flap. *J Urol* 63:569, 1950.

Poutasse EF: Anterior approach to the upper urinary tracts. *J Urol* 85:199, 1961.

Presman D: Eleventh intercostal space incision for renal surgery. *J Urol* 74:578, 1955.

Robson CJ: Radical nephrectomy for renal cell carcinoma. *J Urol* 89:37, 1963.

Smith DP: An anchored mechanical retractor. *Am J Surg* 83:717, 1952.

Stewart BH, Hewitt CB, Kiser WS, Straffon RA: Anterior transperitoneal operative approach to the kidney. *Cleve Clin Q* 36:123, 1969.

Young HH, Davis DM: Operations on the kidney. *Young's Practice of Urology*, Vol. II. Philadelphia, WB Saunders, 1926, pp. 276–279.

CHAPTER 3

Basic Techniques of Vascular Surgery

LYNN H. W. BANOWSKY

Vascular surgery has evolved as a surgical discipline over a relatively short period of time (50–60 years). This rapid development was made possible not only by the creativity and courage of many surgical pioneers, but also by numerous advances in the surgical sciences that have included improved anesthesia, type-specific blood transfusions, anticoagulants, antibiotics, angiography, and synthetic vascular grafts. All of these, once available, permitted the surgical correction of ischemia in organs and extremities.

Lessons learned during the evolution of vascular surgery have enabled it to become a respected surgical specialty and promoted the growth and development of virtually every other surgical discipline. Urologic surgery, as it is known today, would be more modest in scope if the capability did not exist safely to dissect, control, ligate, repair, and temporarily occlude important blood vessels. These skills are necessary for a large number of frequently performed urologic operations, e.g., radical nephrectomy, partial nephrectomy, repair of renal injuries, and retroperitoneal lymphadenectomy. Performing vascular anastomoses successfully has allowed renal revascularization, renal allotransplantation, renal autotransplantation, and creation of vascular access for hemodialysis to become clinical realities.

Proficiency in performing urologic operations such as those just mentioned is contingent on a thorough understanding and working knowledge of the basic principles of vascular surgery. Such proficiency is mandatory if surgical capabilities and opportunities as a specialty are to grow. Acquiring proficiency in vascular surgery requires the learning of technical skills *and* a proper mental attitude. When performing a vascular anastomosis, the first operation is the best and, frequently, the only legitimate opportunity for establishing normal flow through the involved vessel. Mental discipline is necessary to insist on precision, avoid the temptation of short cuts, and preserve the tenacity required for tedious, complex operations. The purpose of this chapter is to provide the foundation for beginning to learn vascular surgery as it relates to the specialty of urology.

VASCULAR INSTRUMENTS

As experience with various types of surgery is gained, instruments that are uniquely suited for specific tasks are developed. Rather than being an affectation, the use of vascular instruments is a necessity in performing surgery on blood vessels. The common denominator for these instruments is their ability to grasp or occlude blood vessels without crushing or injuring them. A basic set of vascular instruments should include forceps, needle holders, scissors, and occlusive clamps. Although it is not a specialized instrument, the right-angle clamp is unusually helpful in dissecting and mobilizing the posterior wall of a vessel.

Surgical Loupes

Surgical loupes of 2.5 × are a great aid in vascular surgery. The slight magnification of the operative field afforded by these wide-angled loupes allows for safer dissection and more accurate suture placement.

Needle Holders

Vascular needle holders should have fine tips and diamond jaws for grasping small delicate needles without bending or slipping (Fig. 3.1). Needle holders with large jaws can either damage the needle or obscure the surgeon's vision, making precise suture placement more difficult. For suturing very small vessels, a Jacobson needle holder is preferred. This instrument is held like a pen or pencil and allows very fine movements that are controlled by the fingers rather than the wrist.

Forceps

Two types of vascular forceps are commonly used. A forceps used for dissecting and mobilizing vessels will be slightly heavier than the forceps used for vascular anastomosis (Fig. 3.2A and B). All vascular forceps allow the surgeon to grasp the vessel firmly without simultaneously crushing the wall. This is accomplished by fine interdigitating teeth or serrations in the forceps jaws.

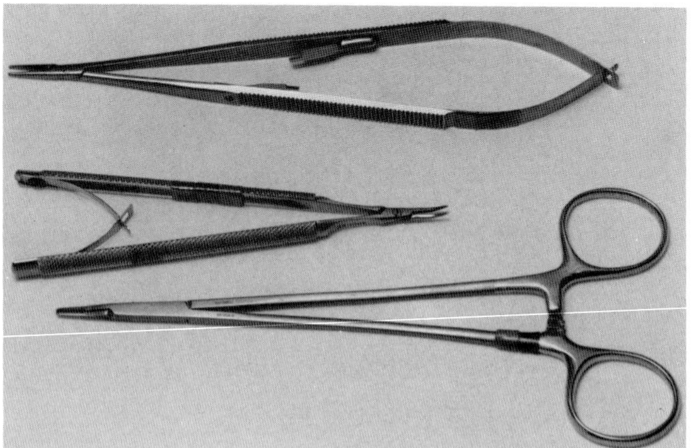

Figure 3.1. Three types of vascular needle holders. *Top* to *bottom*—Jacobsen, microvascular, and standard diamond jaw needle holder.

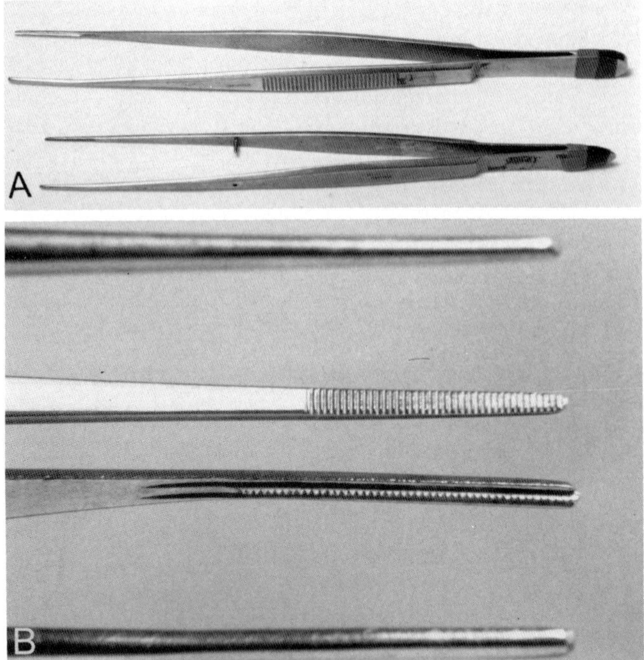

Figure 3.2. **A,** two types of vascular forceps. The smaller pair is used during the vascular anastomosis. **B,** a close-up view of the jaws, showing the interdigitating teeth and serrations.

Vascular Clamps

Vascular clamps are used to occlude a vessel temporarily without crushing or damaging the wall. The clamp must be atraumatic and, at the same time, capable of securely grasping the vessel so that no slippage occurs. As with the vascular forceps, this is accomplished by fine interdigitating teeth or serrations on the jaws of the clamp. Vascular clamps that are capable of either partially or totally occluding the lumen of a vessel are also available.

Totally occlusive clamps are used when it is necessary to stop flow entirely through a vessel. These clamps can be obtained in a variety of shapes and angles (Fig. 3.3). For securing small vessels, branches of a vessel, or a vessel where exposure is limited, bulldog clamps are invaluable. These clamps have no handles, and tension is maintained by a spring. The most desirable bulldog clamps have a mechanism for adjusting the tension so it will be appropriate for the size of the vessel to be clamped. These clamps can be acquired in a variety of sizes and shapes (Fig. 3.4).

In some circumstances, it is desirable to occlude only part of the vessel lumen so that flow is not completely interrupted. In this setting, a partial-occlusion clamp should be used. These clamps are best suited for reasonably large vessels and their greatest applicability is in partially occluding the aorta or vena cava. A partial-occlusion clamp with interdigitating teeth is usually used on the aorta and one with serrations is used on the vena cava (Fig. 3.5).

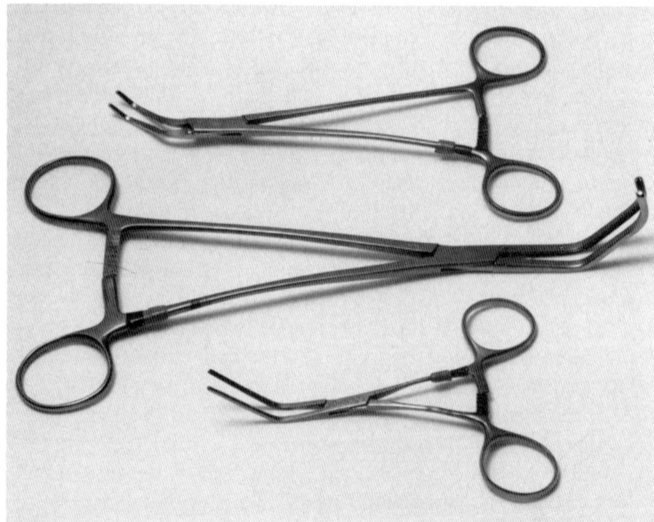

Figure 3.3. Vascular clamps are available in different sizes, shapes, and angles.

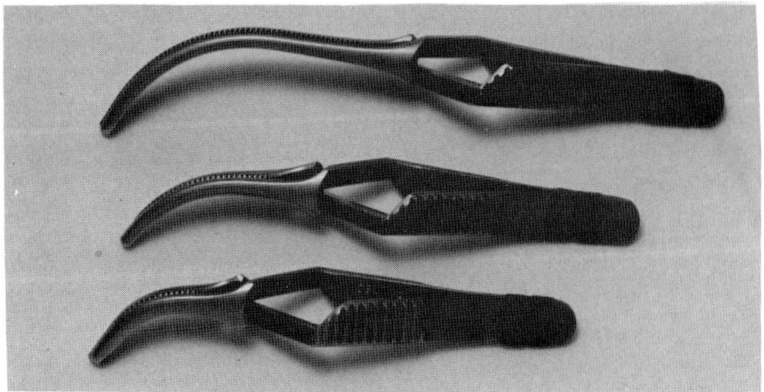

Figure 3.4. Bulldog clamps are very helpful for occluding small vessels.

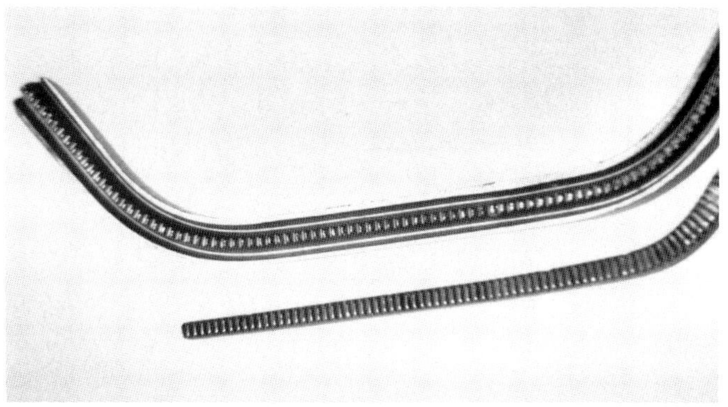

Figure 3.5. A close-up of the jaws of arterial and venous partial occlusion clamp. The clamp with teeth is for the aorta to avoid slippage with aortic pulsation.

Scissors

Fine Metzenbaum or Strulle scissors should be used to dissect arteries and veins. At times, very sharp Iris scissors are helpful in trimming the adventitia from the opening of a vessel before anastomosis. Pott's scissors with either a 45° angle or a 90° angle should be employed to extend incisions in vessel walls, spatulate vessels, or make elliptical openings in the sides of vessels (Fig. 3.6).

Suture Materials

Suture is available in a variety of materials and sizes, and with various needles. All needles should be swaged to the suture. A tapered, or slightly beveled, ½ to ⅜ circle needle is preferred. Vascular suture ranges in size from 2–0 to 7–0, with the larger sizes being reserved exclusively for suturing the aorta or vena cava. In suturing vessels the size of the renal artery or vein, 5–0 is the largest size used. For the renal vein, 5–0 is usually preferred; for the main renal artery, 6–0; for branches of the renal artery, 7–0.

Suture compositions include silk, Teflon-coated Dacron, monofilament polypropylene, etc. A synthetic suture should always be used when suturing a synthetic vascular graft. Because these anastomoses never heal, their integrity depends entirely on the tensile strength of the suture. Silk is more prone to suture fatigue and has a higher probability of disruption and pseudoaneurysm formation. For suturing an atherosclerotic vessel, synthetic monofilament sutures are preferred. These sutures slide more easily and are less likely to hang or tear the vessel wall. The author still prefers silk suture for the interrupted anastomosis of small autogenous vessels. Silk suture is less expensive, easier to handle, and requires, at most, three loops to form a secure knot. In the suturing of autogenous vessels, suture fatigue is not a factor.

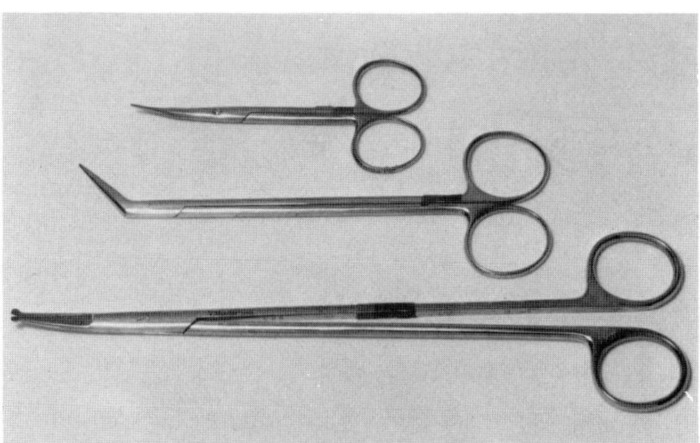

Figure 3.6. Three types of vascular scissors are helpful. Each type is particularly well suited for certain tasks.

GENERAL INFORMATION ON PHYSICAL FACTORS THAT INFLUENCE BLOOD FLOW THROUGH VASCULAR ANASTOMOSIS

When constructing a vascular anastomosis, the primary goals are to maximize anastomotic flow and promote laminar rather than turbulent flow of blood over the suture line. A brief review of the physical factors that increase or decrease flow and avoid the creation of turbulence will allow one to determine better the crucial technical steps in performing a vascular anastomosis.

General Information

Under normal conditions, blood resists coagulation. In physiologic low-flow states, the aggregation of erythrocytes is reversible. The vascular endothelium has fibrinolytic properties and entirely covers the subintimal collagen. A normal vessel with adequate flow can repair small injuries, such as a well-done vascular anastomosis, without the occurrence of coagulation. The crucial points are adequate approximation of the intima and maintenance of normal flow.

A technically well-done vascular anastomosis will be healed at approximately 2 weeks. Accurate approximation of the intima and the use of fine suture material produces a minimal insult to the vessel. Approximately 3 hr after completion of the anastomosis, platelet aggregates can be seen plugging the holes around the vascular suture. At 48 hr, a dense fibrin mesh covers the anastomosis. By 1 week, the endothelial cells have pushed pseudopods through the layer of fibrin and have begun covering the defect. Two weeks postoperatively, the defect and sutures are covered by a smooth unbroken endothelial layer.

Most vascular operations on the kidney, including renal allo- or autotransplantation, do not require systemic heparinization. However, although renal arterial blood flow can usually be safely interrupted for 30–60 min, using regional hypothermia with systemic or regional heparinization increases the margin of safety. In operations on the renal artery, regional or systemic heparinization is commonly used. For regional heparinization of the kidney, 10–20 ml of heparinized saline solution (aqueous sodium heparin diluted 1:1000 with sterile normal saline solution) are injected into the kidney after the arterial blood flow is interrupted.

When systemic heparinization is needed, aqueous sodium heparin should be given intravenously at a dose of 100 units/kg body weight. The effect of heparin is usually negligible after 3–4 hr and reversal with protamine sulfate frequently is unnecessary. If excessive bleeding necessitates the administration of protamine sulfate, it should be remembered that rapid intravenous injection can produce hypotension. Although protamine sulfate reverses heparin mg/mg, too large a dose will cause hypercoagulability. Because protamine sulfate is rarely given immediately after administration of heparin, it is customary to give one-half of the calculated dose of protamine sulfate over 5 min. Should the bleeding continue, additional 5-mg doses can be given every few minutes as needed.

Poiseuille's Law

Poiseuille (1799–1869) was a French physician interested in the dynamics of circulation. His initial studies of the mesenteric circulation were hampered by the unavailability of anticoagulants. After abandoning biologic systems, Poiseuille studied the characteristics of fluid flow through capillary tubes. His data allowed him to characterize the flow of liquids through cylindrical tubes, and could be expressed mathematically by the formula

$$Q = \frac{PR4}{8LN}$$

where Q represents flow, P the pressure gradient, R the radius of the vessel, L the length of the vessel, and N the viscosity of the fluid. The dominant force regulating flow was the diameter of the conduit because flow was a function of the fourth power of its radius. *This function is exponential—thus, minute changes in caliber will have a profound effect on flow.*

Flow Characteristics of End-to-End and End-to-Side Vascular Anastomoses

If flow through a vascular anastomosis is to be maximal and energy loss minimal, the anastomosis must be anatomically and hemodynamically correct. Anatomically, the vessels should be joined so that the lumen is not constricted and the intima is realigned accurately. Hemodynamically, conditions that favor the conversion of laminar flow to turbulent flow should be avoided. These conditions are: an irregular surface, a change in flow direction, a change in velocity, a sharp-edged ostium, and a change in tube diameter.

When possible, an end-to-end anastomosis is always the best way to join blood vessels. This anastomosis is technically easy and has excellent flow characteristics. Assuming the vessels are of relatively comparable sizes, virtually no energy is lost by the fluid as it crosses the anastomosis. An end-to-end union of vessels avoid dissipating energy through entrance or exit loss, as well as through a sudden change in direction of the fluid.

In many clinical situations, an end-to-end anastomosis is not feasible. The common alternative, an end-to-side anastomosis, is theoretically more inefficient than is an end-to-end anastomosis. Flow is reduced through an end-to-side anastomosis because the fluid suddenly changes direction, the vessels are frequently of different sizes, and the ostium may have sharp edges. All of these factors cause flow lines to converge and change from laminar to turbulent flow. However, the end-to-side anastomosis can be constructed so that its deficiencies assume no clinical importance.

Changes in direction of flow can be made to occur gradually by creating as small an angle as possible between the two vessels. If the angle is acute enough, the end-to-side anastomosis can approximate an end-to-end anastomosis (Fig. 3.7A and B). A sharp-edged ostium can be avoided by removing an ellipse from the recipient vessel. The resulting bell-shaped orifice causes less convergence of flow lines and decreases the turbulent flow (Fig. 3.8A and B). Because it is usually the end of a smaller vessel that is placed into the side of a

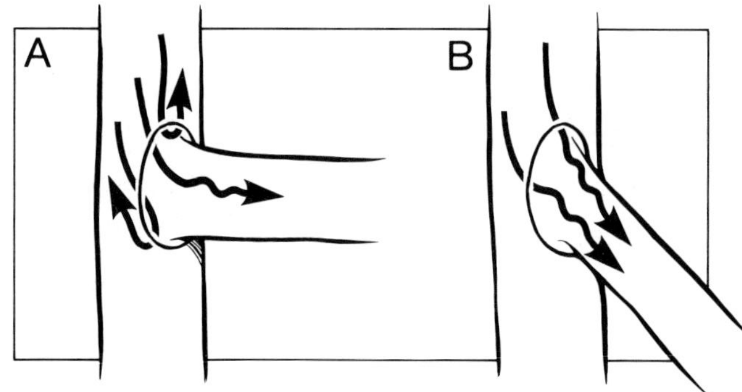

Figure 3.7. **A,** a right-angled end-to-side anastomosis causes convergence of flow lines and creates turbulence. Flow is decreased. **B,** by creating an acute angle of union, turbulence is decreased and flow increased.

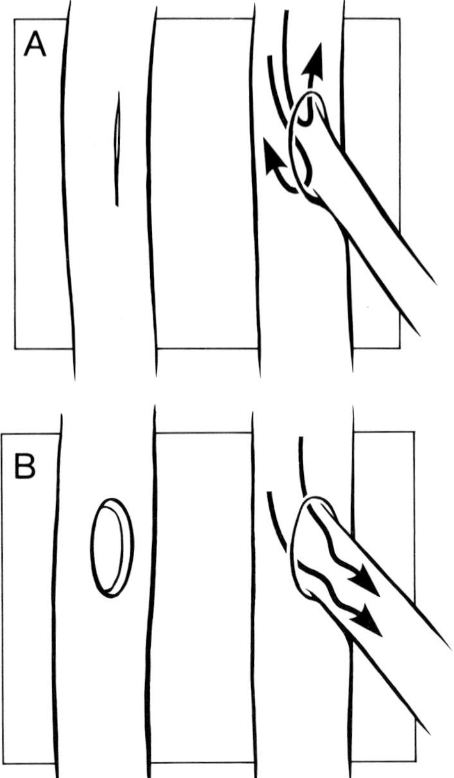

Figure 3.8. **A,** sharp-edged orifice creates turbulent flow. **B,** excision of an elliptical divot from the recipient vessel converts the sharp-edged orifice to a bell-shaped orifice and improves flow.

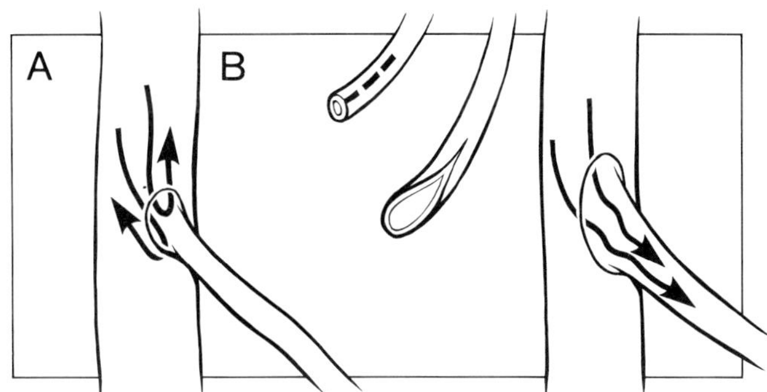

Figure 3.9. **A,** a rapid reduction in vessel size causes turbulent flow. **B,** spatulation of the smaller vessel allows for a more gradual change in vessel size and improves flow.

larger vessel, the difference in sizes can be minimized by spatulating the end of the smaller vessel (Fig. 3.9A and B).

Although all of the previously discussed elements of a vascular anastomosis are important, the most crucial points are avoidance of reduction of the lumen size (Poiseuille's law) and accurate realignment of the intima. Reducing the caliber of the vessel has an exaggerated effect on reducing flow because flow is a function of the fourth power of the vessel's radius. Failure to align the intima creates an irregular inner surface, which leads to turbulent flow, and allows blood to come in contact with the subendothelial collagen, which may activate the coagulation process. Both of these points assume progressively greater importance as the size of the vessel decreases.

GENERAL TECHNIQUES OF VASCULAR SURGERY

General techniques of vascular surgery are applicable to all surgical disciplines and focus upon the dissection, control, ligation, and repair of blood vessels.

Dissection and Control of Blood Vessels

Arteries and veins are surrounded by a fascial sheath. For a vessel to be ligated or repaired, a sufficient length must be circumferentially mobilized so that it can be controlled. Anatomic planes are highlighted by the use of traction and countertraction. Sharp and blunt dissection are used alternately to develop the planes thus exposed.

The fascial sheath covering the anterior vessel wall should be elevated and sharply incised. Because very few branches arise from a vessel's anterior surface, this portion of the dissection should be done first. Using a tonsil clamp, the lateral walls of the vessel are next freed from their fascial and loose connective tissue attachments. Posterior mobilization of the vessel is the most hazardous part of the dissection and should be done last. The danger can be minimized by placing vascular tapes under the vessel at either end of the anterior and lateral dissection. By applying gentle upward traction on the vessel and lateral or posterior traction on the surrounding fascial sheath, the posterior portion of the vessel can be removed safely from its bed. Using this maneuver, posterior branches can be identified easily and managed appropriately (Fig. 3.10).

To avoid perforation or tearing of the vessel wall, sharp-pointed forceps should not be employed for this dissection. When a right-angle clamp is passed under a vessel, its jaws may be spread, but they should not be closed until the clamp is removed. Repetitive opening and closing of the clamp when still under the vessel is bad technique and may tear the posterior wall or avulse small branches. As stated above, gentle traction is very helpful. Excessive traction is always to be avoided.

Ligation of Blood Vessels

As a general rule, an artery and a vein should be individually rather than jointly ligated. Joint ligation of large arteries and veins may be associated with the formation of arterio-

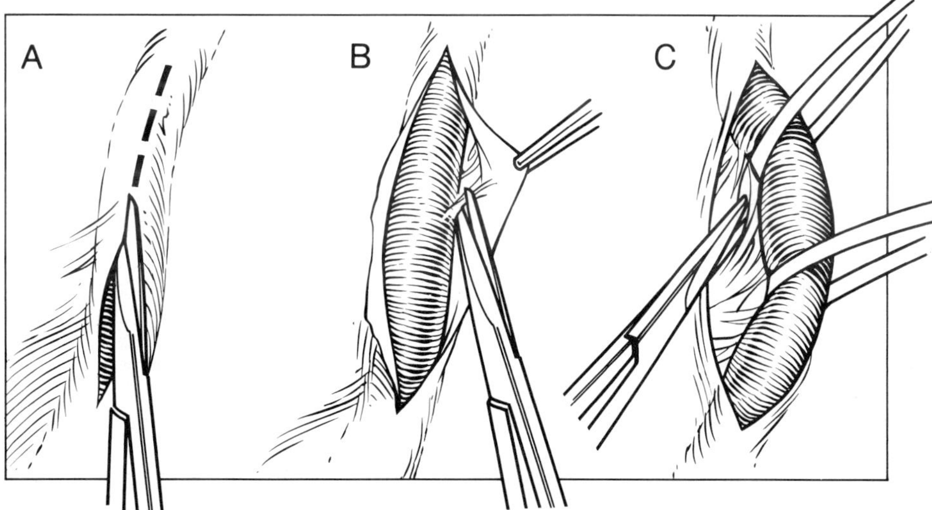

Figure 3.10. **A,** the surrounding fascial covering is incised, exposing the anterior surface of the vessel. **B,** using a tonsil clamp or Strule scissors, the fascial envelope is reflected from the lateral and medial walls of the vessel. **C,** vessel loops are around the vessel at its proximal and distal margins. Appropriate traction on the loops allows the posterior attachments to be divided, which completes circumferential mobilization.

venous fistulae. Arterial ligation poses problems slightly different from those of venous ligation. Venis tend to be thin-walled and too fine a ligature tied too vigorously can tear through the vessel. Veins should be ligated with generally heavier suture material and the ligatures tied to compress rather than tear the wall. Arterial ligation is complicated by the pulsatile pressure transmitted through the vessel and against the ligature. If inadequately secured, the ligature may be rolled off the vessel. A variety of techniques are used for arterial ligation (Fig. 3.11). Proper arterial interruption, regardless of the technique employed, always assumes that the vessel has been exposed sufficiently. Small arteries may be clamped, divided, and each end secured with a single ligature. Larger arteries should be doubly ligated. The first ligature occludes the lumen and decompresses the distal portion so that the distal tie is protected from the pulsatile force within the artery. For this technique to be effective, the ligatures must not be juxtapositioned but should be separated by as long an arterial segment as feasible. An equally effective method is to place a suture ligature distal to the first tie.

When interrupting flow in very large vessels such as the aorta or vena cava, it may be preferable to close the free ends formally with two layers of continuous vascular suture. The occasion may arise in which it is necessary to ligate a vessel in continuity, i.e., ligation without division. Ligatures are placed proximally and distally. Between these ties, a suture ligature should be placed to obliterate the lumen and prevent subsequent recanalization.

Repair of Vascular Lacerations

When repairing vascular lacerations, one has the dual objectives of stopping the bleeding and preserving the normal caliber of the vessel. The techniques used to achieve these objectives vary with the extent of injury and size of the injured vessel. If the injury is so extensive that repair would result in excessive construction of the vessel, the injured segment should be replaced with a bypass graft.

Simple lacerations may be closed in several ways (Fig. 3.12). Lacerations of the aorta or vena cava are closed with a continuous suture. When closing defects in smaller vessels, one must be certain that the closure does not result in a significant reduction in the vessel's diameter. Interrupted sutures should be used to close lacerations in medium-sized vessels. Closures of defects in small vessels, e.g., the renal artery, almost always must be augmented with vein patches.

Techniques of Anastomosis

The standard teaching regarding the interval between sutures in a vascular anastomosis is 1 mm apart and 1 mm from the edge. Whereas this spacing of sutures is adequate for larger vessels, smaller vessels joined with fine 6–0 or 7–0 vascular suture should have shorter distances between sutures.

It should be remembered that a vascular anastomosis involves suturing two arcs rather than two straight lines. Suture placement should have a radial configuration like the spokes on a wheel. This requires more conscious effort in an end-to-side anastomosis. The sutures adjacent to the apices should

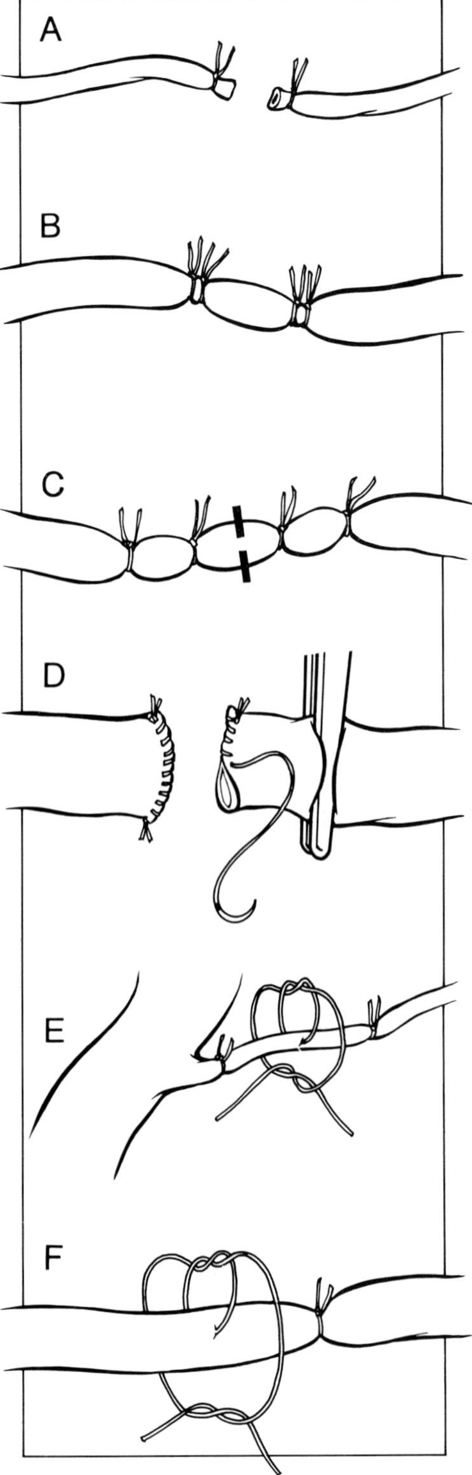

Figure 3.11. **A,** small vessels can be divided and the ends singly ligated. **B,** incorrect double ligation of a larger artery or vein. **C,** correct double ligation of a larger vessel. **D,** formal closure of the end of a large vessel with two layers of continuous suture. **E,** ligation of a vessel in continuity.

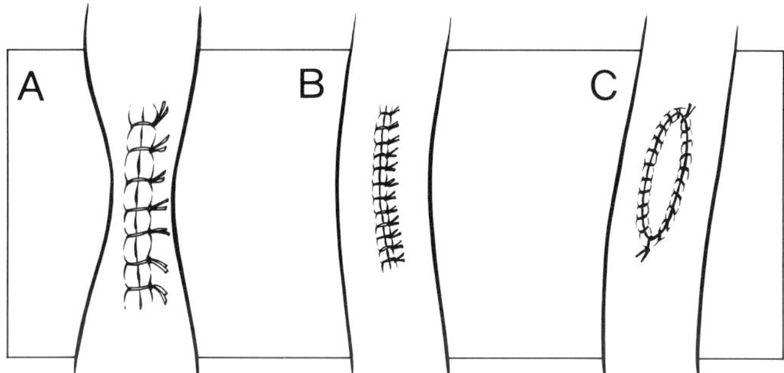

Figure 3.12. **A,** incorrect closure of a laceration. The diameter of the vessel has been compromised. **B,** interrupted closure of a vascular laceration. **C,** closure of a vascular laceration with a vein patch.

be almost parallel to the longitudinal axis of the recipient vessel. Subsequent sutures then progressively fan out until they become perpendicular in the midportion of the anastomosis (Fig. 3.13).

Satisfactory patency rates can be achieved consistently in small arterial anastomosis (<5 mm) by avoiding suture-line constriction and by accurately realigning the intima. This is best accomplished by using interrupted sutures rather than continuous sutures. With an interrupted-suture anastomosis there is no purse-string effect and the potential for growth of the anastomotic area still exists. If the sutures are placed but not tied, the surgeon can see inside the lumen of each vessel for the placement of all sutures. This decreases the possibility of incorporating the vessel's back wall and facilitates accurate alignment of the intima. Even more accurate suture placement is possible by the use of double-armed needles so that each stitch is started from within the lumen of each vessel.

Although a continuous suturing technique is fine for larger arteries, it should be remembered that its only advantage is speed. The extra 5–8 min necessary for an interrupted-suture anastomosis of a small artery is time well spent.

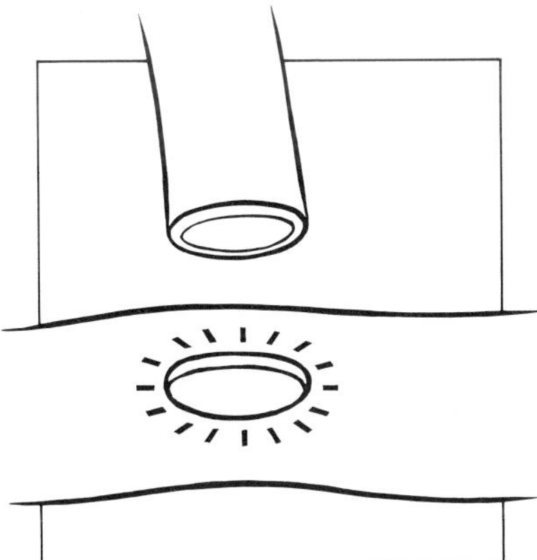

Figure 3.13. In joining two arcs, the sutures should have a radial configuration.

End-to-End Anastomosis

In performing an end-to-end arterial anastomosis, the two most common technical errors are related to vessel length and disparity in vessel sizes. Joining vessels under tension is the most obvious mistake associated with vessel length. Inadequate length makes the anastomosis technically difficult and predisposes to thrombosis or stenosis. Most surgeons are so aware of this problem that it infrequently occurs. To avoid doing the anastomosis under tension, vessels are commonly left too long. When flow is reestablished, the excessive length may cause twisting or severe angulation. This also can lead to stenosis or thrombosis and is a much more common mistake.

A 50% disparity in sizes can be easily overcome by spatulating the end of the smaller vessel. If there is more than 50% disparity, it becomes very difficult to join the two vessels precisely. The smaller vessel is frequently bunched and the resulting anastomosis is unusually prone to leakage and/or thrombosis. A reduction angioplasty of the larger vessel is usually not a good solution. The most prudent course in this situation is not to attempt the end-to-end anastomosis and instead to perform an end-to-side anastomosis.

After the vessels have been mobilized, controlled, and divided, their lumens are flushed with a dilute heparin solution. Using fine forceps and sharp scissors, the adventitia from around each vessel's ostium is pulled forward and divided. This "circumcision" of the adventitia allows it to retract away from the margin of the vessel wall. Failure to trim the adventitia adequately can result in sutures being entrapped in its substance. This either distorts the anastomosis or leads to incorporation of the adventitia in the suture line.

The first two sutures are placed 180° apart. These sutures are for alignment of the vessels and also provide traction. The anterior wall is sutured first. Beginning at each corner, sutures are alternately placed working toward the middle of the anastomosis (Fig. 3.14). The needle should be kept perpendicular rather than parallel to the vessel wall. This perpendicular orientation allows for accurate determination of the entrance and exit points of the needle (Fig. 3.15). By beginning at the corners, the most difficult portion of the anastomosis is done first. Any discrepancy that exists can then be more easily corrected in the middle of the suture line. Forceps are used to expose the lumen and stabilize the vessel wall. They are not used to grasp the vessel (Fig. 3.16). As the anastomosis of the anterior wall nears completion, a suitable number of sutures should be left untied so that no sutures are placed blindly. If the vessel is very small, all sutures on the anterior wall should be placed before any are tied.

Using the two original corner sutures, the vessel is rotated to expose the posterior wall. The posterior wall is joined in the same manner as was the anterior wall, beginning at each corner and working toward the middle of the vessel. Just before the last few sutures are tied, the vessels are flushed with a dilute heparin solution. After flow has been reestablished, bleeding from needle holes can be stopped by pressure. Gaps in the anastomosis should be closed by the placement of ad-

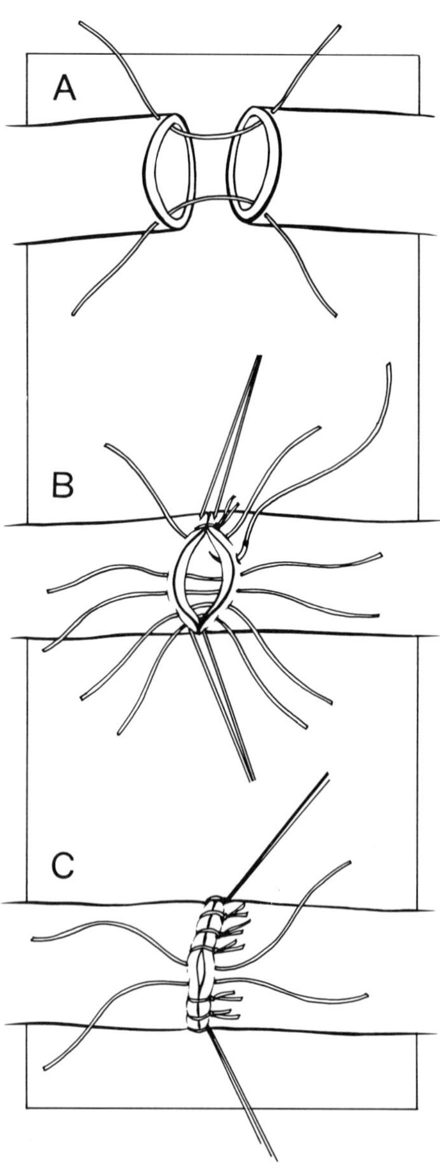

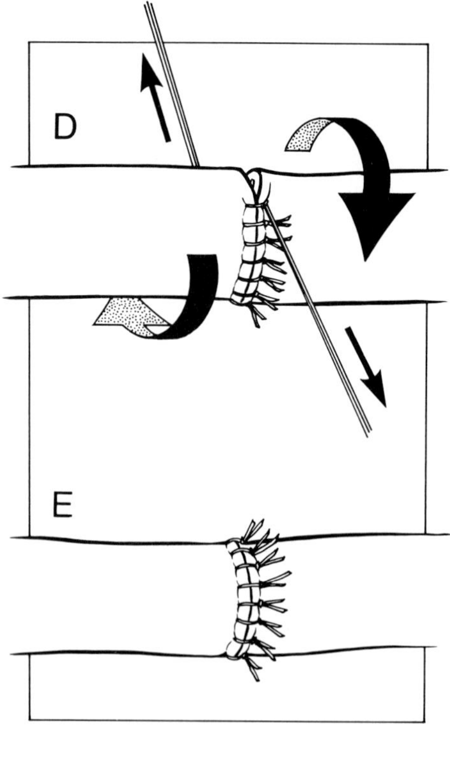

Figure 3.14. **A,** stay sutures are placed 180° apart. **B,** the anastomosis is begun at the corners. Sutures are alternately placed and the anastomosis continued toward the middle of the vessel. **C,** the last few sutures should be left untied until all anterior sutures have been placed. This eliminates the necessity for placing sutures blindly. **D,** using the stay sutures, the vessel is rotated so the posterior wall can be sutured. **E,** a completed end-to-end anastomosis.

ditional sutures. These sutures should include only the outer two layers of the vessel to avoid inadvertently incorporating the back wall. If the leak is substantial, sutures can be more accurately placed by partially occluding the vessel.

End-to-Side Anastomosis

An end-to-side anastomosis should be fashioned so that its flow characteristics are optimal. Unless the vessels are of comparable sizes, the end of the smaller vessel should be spatulated. This spatulation should be done so the two vessels form an acute angle. An elliptical divot should be excised from the wall of the recipient vessel. This is most easily and consistently done by using an aortic punch (Figs. 3.17 and 3.18). Apical sutures are then placed and tied (Fig. 3.19). Stay sutures should be used on the midportions of both walls of the arteriotomy to expose the lumen of the recipient vessel. The anastomosis is begun from each corner and sutures are alternately placed until the anastomosis of that wall has been completed (Fig. 3.20). Unless the smaller artery is more than 5 mm in diameter, interrupted sutures should be used. For larger vessels, double-arm needles can be used for both apical sutures. The arterial walls are approximated with continuous

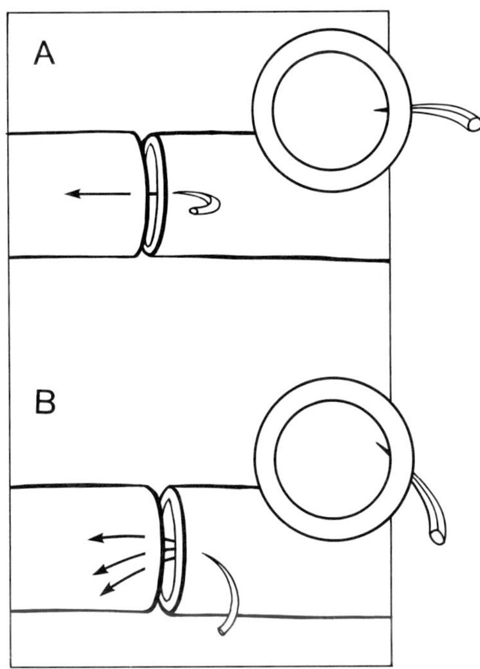

Figure 3.15. Suture placement is more accurate when the needle is kept perpendicular, (**A**), rather than parallel (**B**), to the vessel edge. The perpendicular placement allows one to be very exact in determining the needles' points of entrance and exit.

sutures that meet and are tied in the middle of the anastomosis. Starting at either corner, the identical process is repeated in the back wall. Upon completion of the anastomosis, the distal clamp should always be removed first so that any leak in the suture line can be repaired under low pressure.

Regardless of the type of anastomosis, the most reliable index of its adequacy is the surgeon's honest opinion at the end of the procedure. If sincere concern exists, the anastomosis should be taken down and redone.

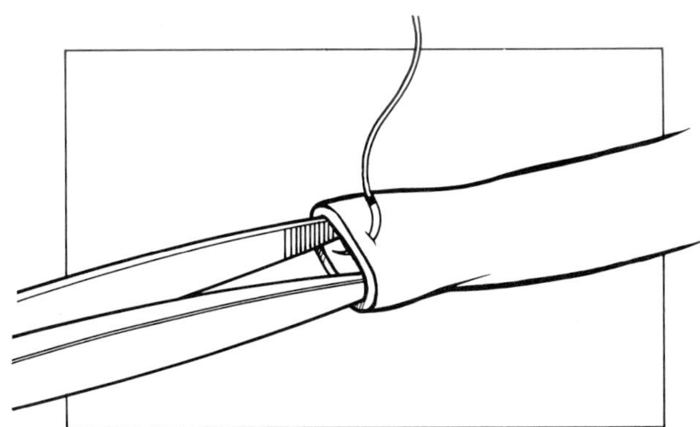

Figure 3.16. Forceps should be used to expose the lumen and stabilize the vessel wall.

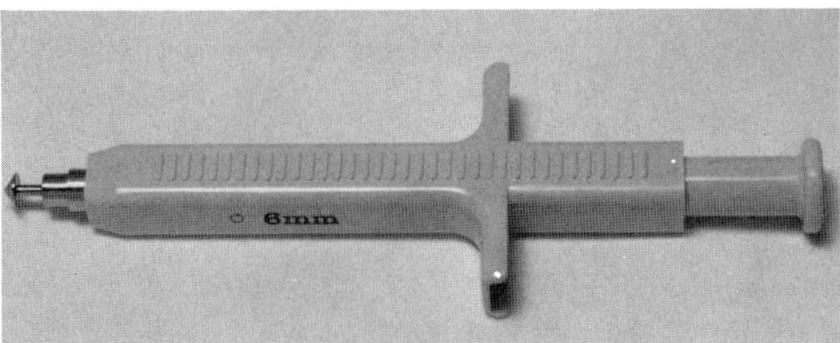

Figure 3.17. An aortic punch.

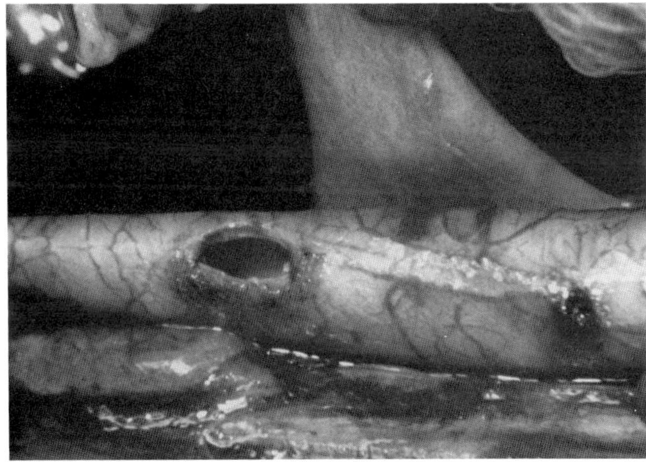

Figure 3.18. A smooth, bell-shaped arteriotomy created by the aortic punch.

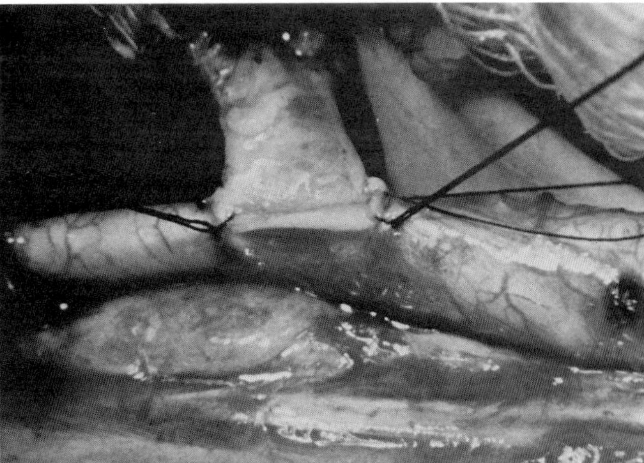

Figure 3.19. Both apical sutures have been placed.

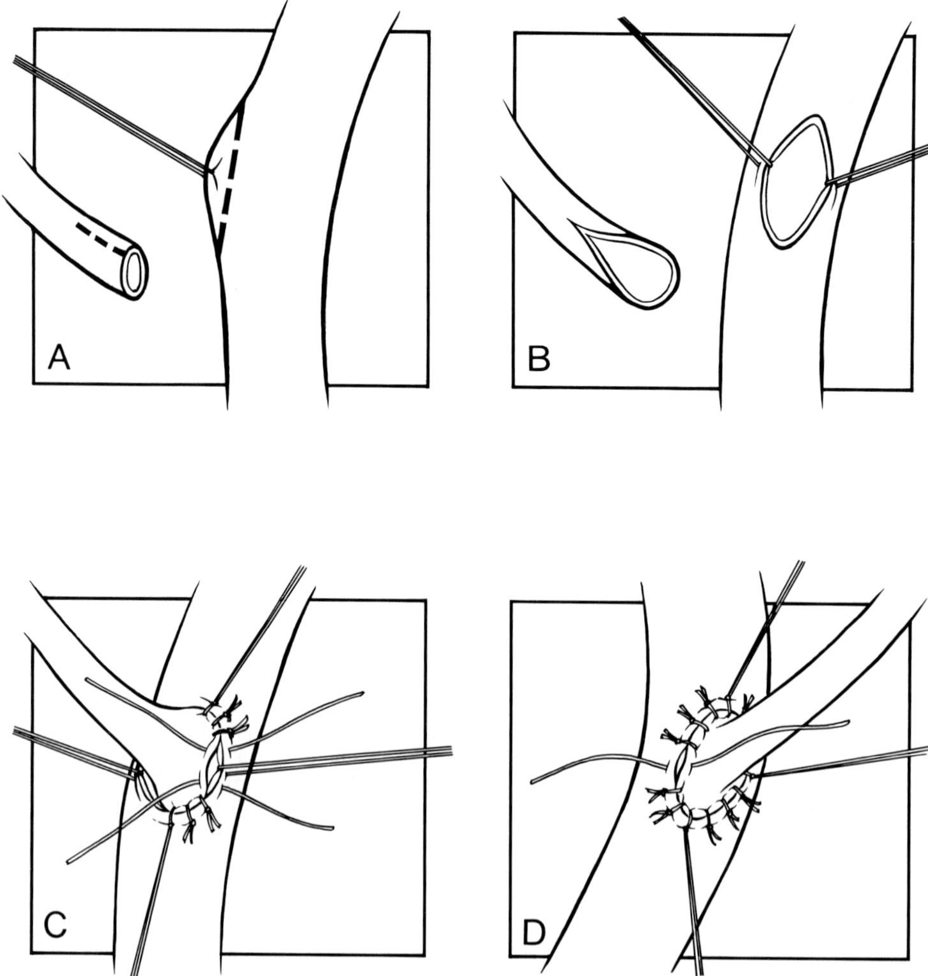

Figure 3.20. Technique of end-to-side anastomosis as described in text.

Suggested Readings

Banowsky L: Control of intraoperative renal and retroperitoneal hemorrhage. *Weekly Urology Update Series,* Vol. 1, Lesson 22. Princeton, N.Y., Biomedia, Inc. 1978, p. 3.

Banowsky L: A review of optical magnification in urological surgery. In Silber SJ (ed): *Microsurgery*. Baltimore, Williams & Wilkins, 1979.

Banowsky LH: Basic principles and techniques of vascular surgery. In: Novick AC, Straffon RA (eds): *Vascular Problems in Urologic Surgery*. Chap. 1. Philadelphia, WB Saunders, 1982.

Baxter TJ, O'Brien B, Henderson PN, et al: The histopathology of small vessels following microvascular repair. *Br J Surg* 59:617, 1972.

Goldstone J: Flow properties of blood in small vessels. In: Silber SJ (ed): *Microsurgery*. Baltimore, Williams & Wilkins, 1979.

Hurwitz A, Degenshein G: Hemostasis. In: *Milestones in Modern Surgery*. New York, Hoeber-Harper, 1958, p. 3.

Linton R: Special methods of securing blood vessels. In Linton R (ed): *Atlas of Vascular Surgery*. Philadelphia, WB Saunders, 1973, p. 34.

Rutherford RB: Basic vascular surgical techniques. In Rutherford RB, et al (ed): *Vascular Surgery*. Philadelphia, WB Saunders, 1977.

Szilagyi E, Whitcomb JF, Schenker W, et al: The laws of fluid flow and arterial grafting. *Surgery* 47:55–73, 1960.

CHAPTER 4

Renal Hypothermia In Situ

MICHAEL MARBERGER

In 1924 Avramovici stated "the tolerance of the canine kidney against anoxic damage is temperature dependent . . . and is improved considerably at lower temperatures." Using simple ice cooling, he was the first to successfully protect kidneys against the detrimental effects of temporary ischemia during renal transplantation. Today, after six decades of intensive research in the field, kidneys may be maintained viable outside the body for up to 1 week. Hypothermia, however, still remains the cornerstone of successful preservation.

In situ, with the kidney remaining in its normal position within the renal fossa, cooling is considerably more difficult to achieve than under ambiothermic conditions extracorporeally. The temperature of the surrounding tissue impedes effective cooling, and the integrity of the vascular pedicle prevents the use of the preservation techniques employed in transplant surgery. The limited space available and the need for surgical access to the kidney present further obstacles. Conversely, as compared to extracorporeal procedures, the duration of the ischemic insult rarely exceeds 3 hr in in situ surgery, so that the requirements on the quality of protection are less pronounced. A multitude of clinical methods that permit safe renal surgery in a bloodless field over an extended period of time has therefore become available.

HYPOTHERMIA AND KIDNEY FUNCTION

Lowering of the renal temperature rapidly reduces the energy-dependent metabolic activities of the kidney. Each decrease of 10°C decreases the metabolic rate by 2- to 3-fold (van't Hoff's law) and oxygen consumption drops in an exponential relationship to the renal temperature. The energy-intensive transport mechanism of the tubules, namely, sodium transport, comes to a complete standstill at approximately 18°C. Enzyme reactions at the cell membranes and in the organelles are reduced in a parallel fashion; in particular, ATP turnover, the Na^+-K^+-ATPase activity, and ion transport systems are reduced. With temporary cooling to a maximum of about 10°C, all function alterations are rapidly reversible; within 24 hr after rewarming, the kidney reaches its normal functional capacity again, and even with a long-term follow-up there is no functional loss.

The mechanisms of hypothermic protection against short-term ischemia, albeit well documented, are poorly understood. This is not surprising, as even the pathophysiology of acute renal failure after temporary ischemia is still being debated. Most authors consider the depression of renal metabolism, in particular of the energy-utilizing reactions, the decisive protective factor. A reduced production of metabolic waste products, which are not removed during ischemia and exert a detrimental influence at reperfusion, has been postulated by others. This hypothesis has received further support by the changing concept of the mechanisms involved in postischemic acute renal failure. The situation is mainly characterized by hemodynamic alterations during the reperfusions phase, in particular in the inner stripe of the outer zone of the medulla. Regional cooling during the ischemic insult completely prevents this malperfusion response.

Although renal metabolism is reduced most significantly at temperatures below 10°C, this does not necessarily imply this range of cooling to be the optimum range. Temperatures only slightly above the freezing point cause significant structural alterations of mitochondria and lysosomes, solidification of membrane lipids, and changes in membrane permeability. In contrast to kidneys preserved ex situ, the stagnant blood is usually not washed out of the vascular system of the ischemic kidney during in situ protection. Blood viscosity and the osmotic fragility of erythrocytes increase sharply at very low temperatures and may further contribute to regional postischemic malperfusion.

Various specific studies designed to define the optimum cooling temperature for in situ cooling resulted in suggestions ranging from 10 to 25°C. Only when ischemia was extended over 3 hr did more extensive cooling appear to be more effective. The issue was, however, conclusively cleared by the exhausting study of Ward, who clearly showed 15°C to be the optimum temperature for in situ renal hypothermia. In acute dog experiments, and based on precise parameters of glomerular and tubular function, he found no improved protection by cooling below this value. At 22 and 10°C, the protective effect was almost identical and was approximately 20% poorer than at 15°C. In situ cooling to 5°C resulted in severe

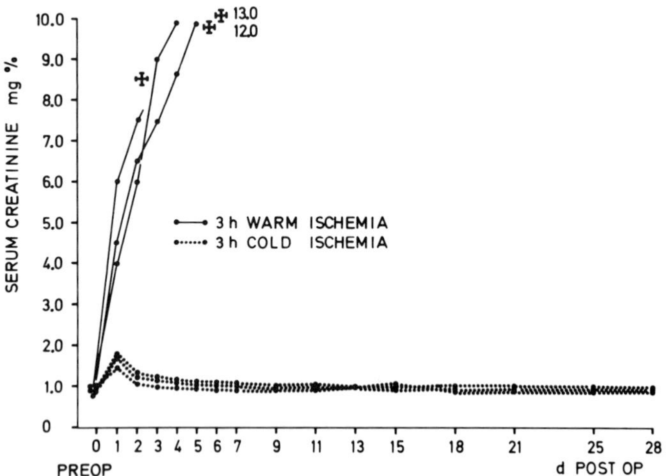

Figure 4.1. Serum creatinine of dogs with solitary kidney subjected to 3 hr of warm or cold ischemia in situ (balloon occlusion of renal artery, intermittent perfusion cooling with core temperatures of 18–25°C).

functional changes, and at 0° the damage was virtually identical to that caused by normothermic ischemia.

Optimum conditions, i.e., constant cooling of the entire kidney throughout the entire ischemic period, can only be achieved in an experimental setting. In clinical work the situation is complicated by the high temperature of the surrounding structures and the need for free surgical access to the organ. This results in the demand for adequate, although perhaps not optimum, cooling, as a compromise between technical feasibility, surgery, and protective effect. At 18–25°C, temporary ischemia of 2–3 hr, is tolerated without permanent impairment (Fig. 4.1) but this temperature is considerably easier to obtain in situ. As a guideline for clinical purposes, adequate protection is achieved for at least 2 hr of ischemia if the kidney is maintained at 15–25°C during this time. Predamaged kidneys are more vulnerable in toto, but the individual intact nephron is protected as effectively as the nephron of a normal kidney. With insufficient cooling, in particular inhomogenous cooling, the period of safe protection, however, is rapidly reduced to less than 60 min.

CLINICAL TECHNIQUES

The first clinical attempts to protect the human kidney against ischemic damage in situ utilized whole body cooling. Based on methods developed for cardiac and neural surgery, the body temperature was lowered by immersing the patient in an ice bath or by perfusion cooling via an extracorporeal cardiopulmonary circuit. Ischemic insults of up to 3 hr duration were managed with this approach, but as it is proved impossible to lower the body temperature below 27°C without severe cardiocirculatory side effects, the patients experienced transient, severe renal insufficiency. With the first reports on regional hypothermia, clinical interest rapidly turned to this safer and simpler concept. Although recent advances in cooling techniques have reduced the lethal limits of whole body hypothermia and humans have been shown to survive for 1–2 hr at body temperatures of only 4°C, today this approach has been abandoned totally.

The clinical techniques providing adequate in situ cooling may be subdivided into methods relying on surface cooling or on cooling by hypothermic perfusion via the vascular or collecting system. No single technique yet fulfills the postulates of an ideal method, i.e., homogenous cooling of the entire kidney to 15°C throughout the ischemic period, simplicity, low risk of complications, and no impediment to surgical exposure. If the specific limitations of each technique are respected, however, it should be no problem to successfully protect the kidney against the sequelae of 2–3 hr of ischemia, even in a hospital devoid of sophisticated technical facilities.

The essential prerequisite for successful cooling is complete interruption of the arterial circulation of the entire kidney. In view of the magnitude of renal blood flow, even a minor residual circulation, for example, via an unnoticed accessory artery, renders all cooling attempts futile. As successful cooling is the key to effective protection, the kidney core temperature should be monitored with an electric needle thermometer.

SURFACE COOLING

Direct contact of the kidney with a coolant is the simplest approach to regional hypothermia. The efficiency of cooling depends on the temperature of the coolant, the closeness of its contact with the kidney surface, the size of the kidney, and the time of cooling. The kidney is cooled inhomogenously, i.e., superficial parts will reach the optimum temperature earlier than the core but may also suffer from excessive cooling. Surface cooling naturally always impedes the surgical procedure per se and requires a compromise between continuous cooling and poor exposure, or intermittent cooling and intermittent surgery.

Ice Slush

By packing crushed ice around the ischemic kidney so that only the immediate field being operated on remains exposed and the rest of the kidney is covered by ice throughout the ischemic period, the kidney core temperature is sufficiently lowered for good short-term preservation. Crystalline "soft" ice or slush molds to the contours of the organ and seeps into parenchymal incisions for optimum cooling. In contrast, large chunks of ice may cool only the cortex in direct contact and may leave other parts of the kidney poorly protected. Likewise, the kidney is not cooled adequately by only placing bags of frozen saline around it; this may be used only as an adjunctive measure to sustain hypothermia after the kidney has been cooled initially by a more effective technique.

The method described by Metzer and Boyce is usually employed. Sterile ice slush is prepared by freezing an electrolyte solution packed in double-wrapped sterile vinyl bags. Solutions that freeze to a particularly soft and crystalline ice are commercially available and greatly facilitate the procedure, but any physiologic solution may be used. In case these are not provided in containers sterile inside and out, sterilization may be achieved by prepping with povidone-iodine, following a strict protocol, or the solution is supercooled in sterile, commercially available slush mugs. Sterilization with glutaraldehyde or gas sterilization with ethylene oxide may contaminate the solution and should be avoided. The slush may be formed by freezing the fluid in the freezing compartment of a conventional domestic refrigerator. A thermostat-controlled alcohol cooling bath situated in the operating room simplifies the procedure. Five to 10 bags of 500-ml solution are placed in the cooler approximately 30 min prior to the operation, and by the time ischemia becomes necessary, adequate slush is available. Vigorous shaking during the freezing process ensures the proper consistency of the ice, but larger chunks of ice may also be crushed under a sterile cloth with an orthopedic hammer on a side table.

The kidney is completely mobilized, the renal artery is occluded, and an 8 × 24-inch sterile latex rubber sheet is wrapped around the organ. The sheet has a 9-inch cut on one long border to accommodate the renal pedicle, and it is secured around the vessels along this slit with Allis clamps to form a more or less watertight dam around the kidney. Recently we have found the standard intestinal bags used for bowel surgery to provide an even better compartment for the ice around the kidney. The blind end of the bag is cut open, and the bag is placed over the kidney so that the original open end of the bag with a purse-string lace may be closed watertight around the pedicle. This dam is softer and less voluminous than the rubber sheet and confines the shush better to the perirenal space. In addition, the clamp on the renal artery remains visible for inspection through the transparent bag. The dam is filled with slush until only the operative field remains exposed (Fig. 4.2). Throughout the procedure, an assistant removes the dissolved slush with the sucker and replaces ice as needed to maintain the correct temperature.

The simplicity of this method and its universal applicability for all types of in situ kidney surgery have established it as the most commonly used technique for regional hypothermia. It is the only approach providing continuous cooling. Its main disadvantage, however, lies in the inhomogeneity of cooling. Core temperature falls slowly, and it may take 25–30 min until it reaches values around 15°C (Fig. 4.3). At the same time, the renal cortex and incised parenchyma are in continuous contact with the ice and may already approach temperatures around the freezing point. In addition, the ice impedes surgery by limiting the operative field and aggravating the maneuverability of the kidney. The ice must be removed for intraoperative roentgenography, as high sensitivity films also depict ice chunks, which are then difficult to differentiate from poorly opacifying calculous remnants. Even more annoying is the drenching of the operative field and subsequent general body cooling. Together with the jackknife position of the patient and the length of the procedures, body cooling appears to be mainly responsible for the high rate of pulmonary complications seen after this type of surgery.

Immersion Cooling

Continuous flushing of the surface of the ischemic kidney with ice-cold saline has some protective effect in emergency situations but is insufficient for formal kidney cooling. Effec-

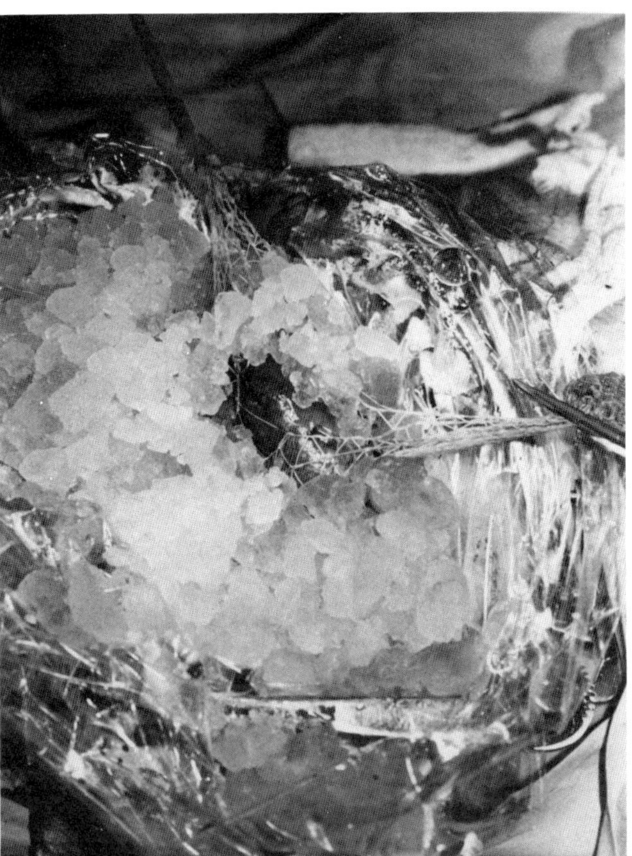

Figure 4.2. Surface cooling with soft ice; only the part of the kidney to be operated on is left uncovered.

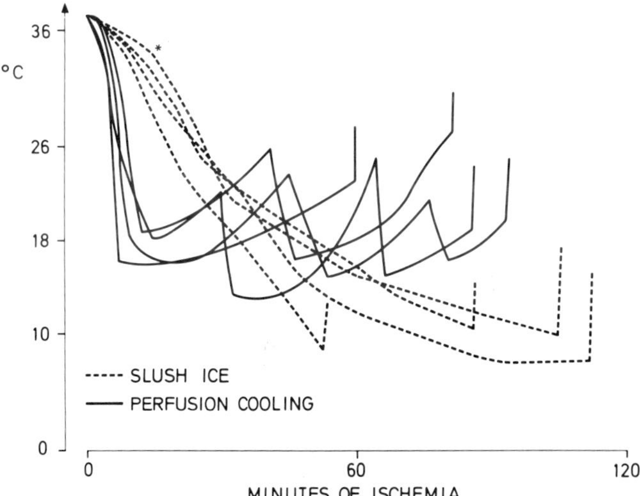

Figure 4.3. Core temperature of kidneys during extended nephrolithotomies in ischemia and hypothermia by surface cooling with soft ice or transarterial perfusion cooling. *accessory artery discovered and clamped.

tive hypothermia, however, may be obtained by encasing the kidney in a supple vinyl bag filled with a coolant.

The technique developed by Graves has found some acceptance. After occlusion of the renal artery, a standard polyvinyl bag is invaginated over the kidney, and the visceral layer of the bag is secured with a rubber band around the renal pedicle. The parietal layer of the bag is then turned back on itself and the ensuing dam is filled with a 30% glycerine-saline solution cooled to −10°C (Fig. 4.4). A thermometer probe is placed into the kidney through the barrel of a 20-ml syringe, which was inserted into the bottom of the bag to provide for a direct approach to the kidney. The kidney temperature is lowered to approximately 10°C. By exchanging the coolant once or twice, this temperature is usually achieved in about 10 min. The fluid is then suctioned off, the rubber band around the pedicle is cut, and the bag is removed. Surgery can now proceed in a dry field.

This method is simple, avoids the time-consuming preparation of sterile slush, and with a proper technique, does not drench the operative field. As a decisive disadvantage, however, it only provides temporary hypothermia. With removal of the coolant, the kidney rapidly rewarms and reaches core temperatures over 25°C within 20–30 min. To successfully cope with longer ischemic insults, the cooling procedure must be repeated, causing annoying interruptions of the surgical procedure.

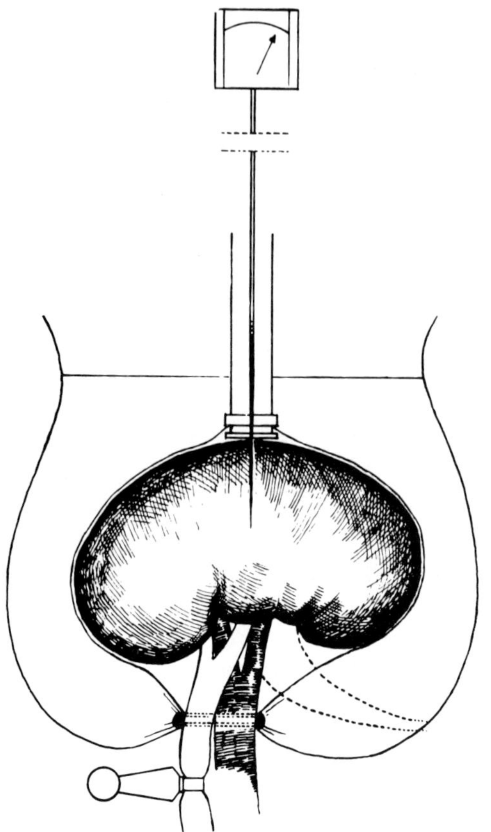

Figure 4.4. Technique of immersion cooling of kidney with invaginated vinyl bag filled with liquid coolant.

External Cooling Appliances

Saucer-shaped heat exchange coils made of rubber, metal, or vinyl may be placed around the kidney and perfused with cold solutions for effective surface cooling. Only since coolant fluids cooled to not less than 1–2°C have been in use has the problem of the heat exchanger freezing to the kidney been avoided.

The equipment and technique developed by Wickham et al. has found widespread clinical use. A commercially available cooling unit is used. It consists of disposable polyvinyl heat exchange coils, contoured to accommodate the kidney, and an external cooling source reservoir, which is filled with 2–3 pounds of ice cubes and approximately 10 liters of water (Fig. 4.5). The kidney is encased within the two cooling cups, and water cooled to 1–2°C is circulated through the coils at high speed. Renal core temperature, which is monitored with a built-in telethermometer, drops to 15–20°C in 8–10 min. The cups are then removed and the operation is continued.

The method provides a dry, clean operative field. Frostbite of renal tissue is impossible. Again, however, the kidney rapidly rewarms during surgery, and the procedure has to be interrupted every 20–25 min for recooling. Although the technical equipment needed is simple and moderately priced, it is available only in centers specializing in intrarenal surgery.

TRANSARTERIAL PERFUSION COOLING

Hypothermic perfusion via the renal artery rapidly and homogenously cools the kidney without any limitation to surgical access. Stagnant blood and waste products are removed from the vascular tree, further enhancing the postischemic normalization of renal hemodynamics. Therefore, transarterial hypothermic perfusion has become the routine cooling technique in ex situ kidney preservation both for renal allo- and autotransplantation. In in situ surgery, however, the intact renal pedicle limits the applicability of this approach and requires techniques, all of which have some inherent risk of vascular complications.

In extracorporeal preservation with initial flushing and hypothermic storage, the best long-term results were achieved with hyperosmolar perfusates resembling the intracellular electrolyte composition. Because of their high potassium content, these perfusates may not be administered sytemically. When used in situ, the renal vein must be clamped and the perfusate must be removed again via a venotomy or, on the left side, via the severed spermatic vein. For short-term preservation (up to 120 min of ischemia), however, similar protection is obtained with iso- and hyperosmolar perfusates of "extra-" or "intracellular" electrolyte content (Fig. 4.6); cooling appears to be the most important factor. Intracellular perfusates have been shown to be superior to Ringer's lactate only in ischemic insults exceeding 2 hr or with insufficient cooling. For in situ perfusion, the author therefore routinely uses Ringer's lactate, brought to an osmolarity of 430 mosm/liter by the addition of mannitol. This solution is nontoxic, stable, and simple to prepare and may be administered systematically.

To prevent vasospasm during manipulation of the renal ar-

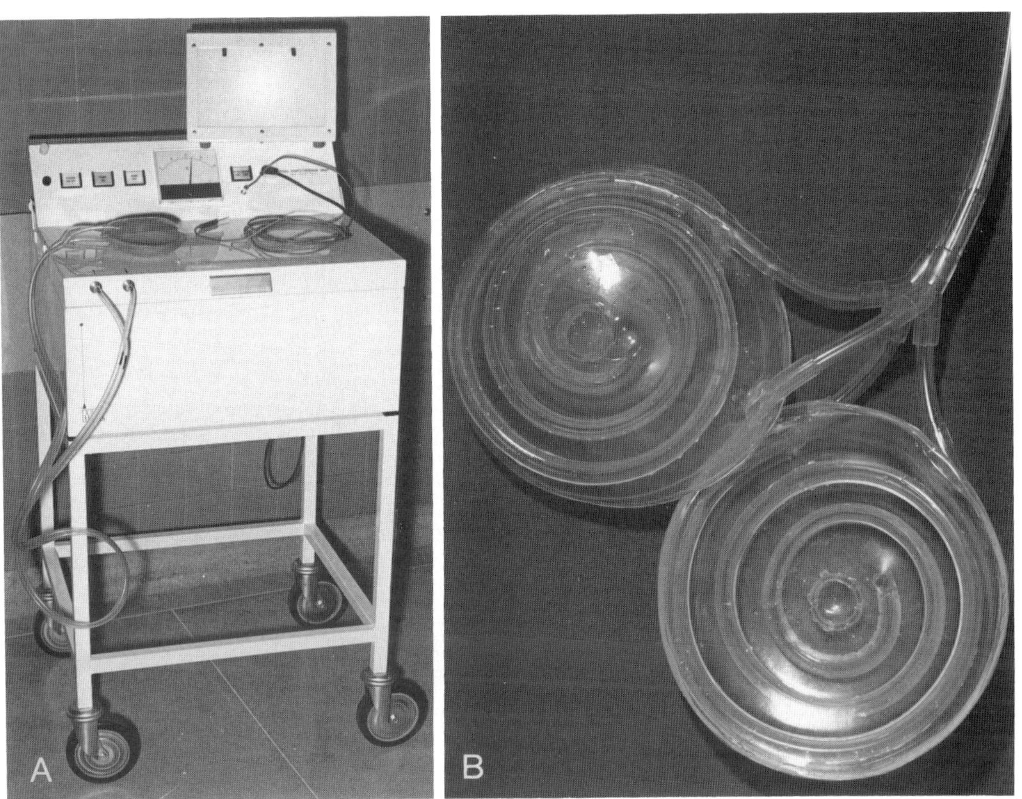

Figure 4.5. Renal hypothermia unit for surface cooling (Courtesy of J.E.A. Wickham, London).

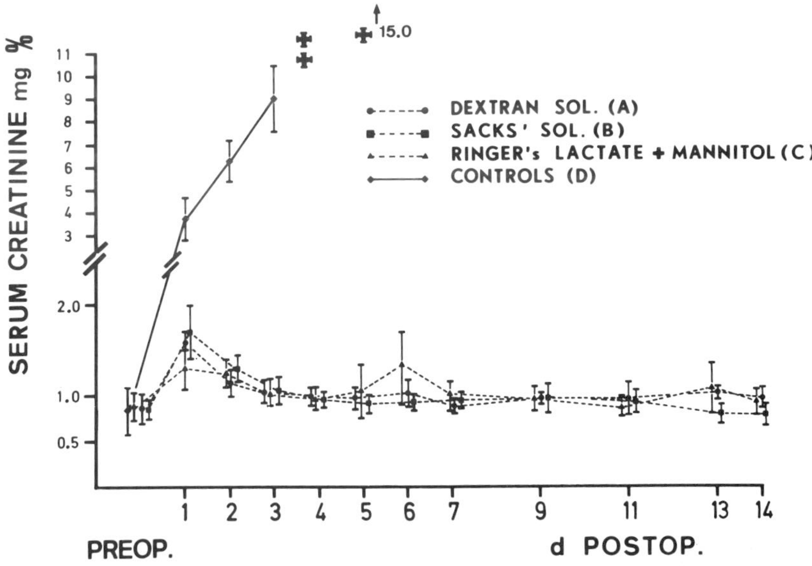

Figure 4.6. Serum creatinine of dogs with a solitary kidney subjected to 2 hr of warm ischemia or cold ischemia obtained by initial hypothermic perfusion with various cold perfusates (mean ± SD).

tery, 1 mg/kg body weight papaverine should be administered topically. The addition of vasodilators like procaine hydrochloride, phenoxybenzamine, or phentolamine to the perfusate does not improve the postischemic hemodynamic situation, probably because the tissue levels obtained with short-term perfusion are too low for a hemodynamic response.

The effectiveness of perfusion cooling depends on the temperature and flow rate of the perfusate, the temperature of the perirenal structures, the size of the kidney, and the completeness of ischemia. Ex situ flushing with a solution of 4°C at a flow rate of about 50 ml/min lowers the kidney core temperature to about 15°C within 5 min. In situ, with the kidney mobilized as usual for surgery, the temperature of the surrounding tissue slows the cooling process, and it may take up to 10 min to reach the optimum temperature range (Fig. 4.3).

Once a satisfactory temperature is reached, the kidney may be maintained at this range by continuous perfusion at a low flow rate ("trickle perfusion") or by intermittent bursts of high flow perfusion. The latter method offers the advantage of a periodically dry operative field. Renal temperature is maintained between 15 and 25°C. Although it is in this manner not continuously at the optimum range, the loss of protection is negligible in ischemia of up to 120 min duration. The dry periods can be expanded by generous exposure of the kidney, packing of the perirenal structures with sponges, and liberal use of cold saline for irrigation. Experimental data also suggests that with trickle perfusion the cortex may be perfused inhomogenously, resulting in endothelial damage and perfusate precipitation.

Cannulation of Renal Artery

In vascular operations requiring complete division of the renal artery, the severed vessel is freely accessible to cannulation with large caliber tubing. This permits rapid perfusion cooling at a low perfusion pressure either by gravity or with the help of a manometer-controlled air pressure cuff around the bag with the perfusate (Fig. 4.7). The perfusate may be allowed to drain systemically via the renal vein or may be retrieved through an incision in the renal or spermatic vein.

In the majority of kidney operations, however, the renal artery remains intact. In this event, kidneys can also successfully be perfusion-cooled via thin polyvinyl tubing inserted into the renal artery through an arteriotomy. In 1974, Farcon et al. reported on good clinical results with this technique. A no. 8 French tube is inserted into the renal artery through a formal arteriotomy distal to the occluding vascular clamp and is secured in place with umbilical tape. The large caliber of the tube permits gravity perfusion from a height of 100 cm above the kidney; the perfusate is cooled by passing it through heat exchange coils placed in an ice bath. Farcon et al. used Collins C_3 solution, which was drained from an incision in the renal vein. After removing the catheter, the vascular incisions are closed with interrupted sutures of 5–0 silk.

Wagenknecht et al. suggested a simpler technique. The renal artery is punctured with a fine needle, which serves as a guide for a rather rigid, beveled no. 15 polyethylene catheter advanced into the artery over the needle. After removing the stylet, the catheter is held in place with a Rumel-type tourniquet, which occludes the artery around the indwelling catheter. The thin tube requires rather high perfusion pressures of 150–250 cm of water, and for adequate cooling, the perfusate therefore has to be administered with a motor syringe or roller pump.

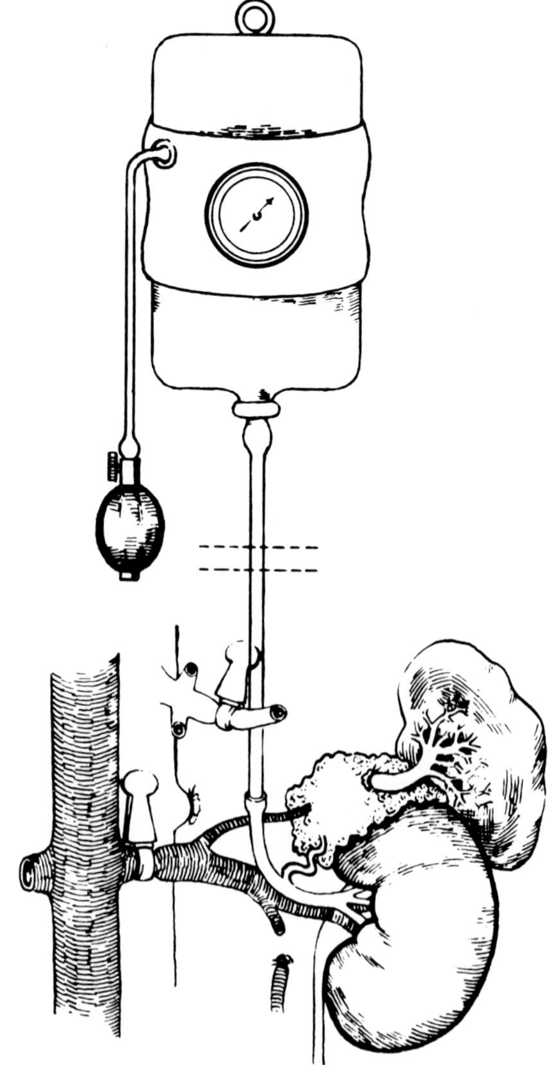

Figure 4.7. Gil-Vernet technique of in situ hypothermic perfusion if renal artery is severed.

The lesion in the renal artery is less significant if a needle rather than a catheter is inserted for perfusion. Gil-Vernet et al. designed a curved, beveled needle for this purpose (Fig. 4.8); by puncturing the artery in an oblique fashion in the direction of the blood stream, postocclusive leakage is further minimized. The thin lumen of the needle again requires high perfusion pressures and, therefore, machine perfusion. A safety valve interposed between needle and perfusor immediately stops perfusion, if the perfusion pressure rises excessively due to an incorrect position of the needle.

Direct cannulation of the renal artery in situ, however, may be extremely difficult, in particular with thin arteries of poor

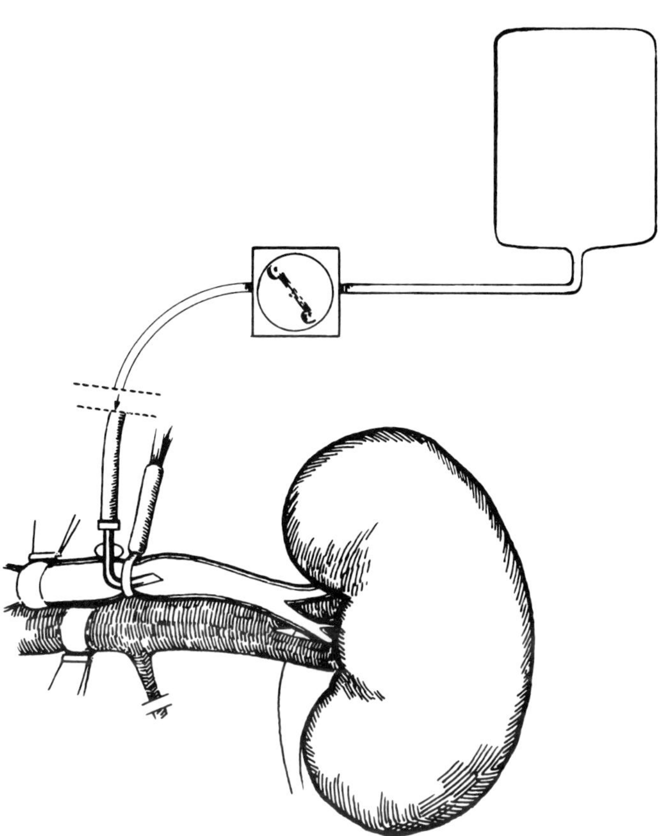

Figure 4.8. Gil-Vernet technique of in situ hypothermic perfusion of the ischemic kidney by cannulating the renal artery with a curved beveled needle.

kidneys or in secondary operations. Although vasospasm is less likely after the topical administration of papaverine, it occurs in particular when the vessel is overstretched for better exposure. In order not to pierce the endothelium of the contralateral wall or dissect it off, the artery has to be punctured before it is clamped; hemorrhage frequently complicates the procedure. The needles are difficult to secure within the artery, even when they have a special shape to facilitate their positioning, and tend to become dislocated. This may result in subendothelial hemorrhage or perfusate extravasation with the risk of thrombosis or late artery stenosis. Overall, these techniques are intricate, distract the surgeon's time and attention from the operation itself, and carry a high risk of vascular complications. Therefore, they have not found general acceptance.

Percutaneous Transcatheter Perfusion

Hazardous manipulations on the renal artery are avoided if the kidney is perfused via a catheter introduced percutaneously with angiography techniques prior to the operation. In the method developed by Eisenberger et al., a no. 7 Ducor angiography catheter is inserted into the renal artery via the femoral artery, using the Seldinger technique. The catheter remains in place and the kidney is exposed. To obtain ischemia a tourniquet is closed around the artery and the in-

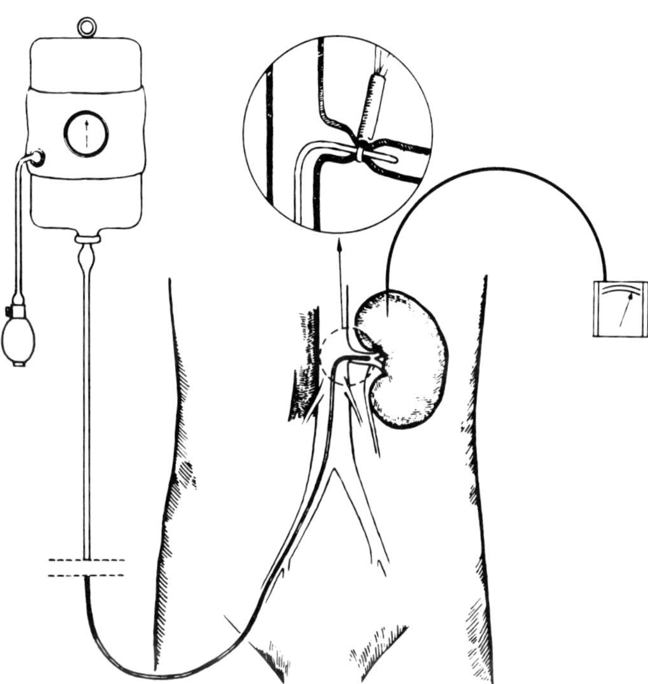

Figure 4.9. Eisenberger technique of transarterial hypothermic perfusion of the ischemic kidney.

dwelling catheter. Hypothermic perfusion is started simultaneously via the catheter, the large diameter of which permits adequate perfusion rates with a simple air pressure cuff perfusate system (Fig. 4.9). The technique is highly effective but requires dissection and direct manipulation of the renal artery. This is difficult in secondary operations and may induce vasospasm. Tourniquet occlusion of arteries around rather rigid catheters may also cause significant vascular damage.

The use of a double-lumen balloon catheter obviates the need for direct exposure of the renal vessels. Prior to the kidney operation, a no. 5 French Swan-Ganz balloon catheter is introduced into the femoral artery. After advancing it up the aorta under fluoroscopic control, its tip is floated into the renal artery with flow-directed technique and positioned proximal to all segmental arteries. The patient is then transported into the operating theater and the kidney is exposed as usual, but without dissecting the pedicle. As soon as ischemia is needed, the renal artery is occluded by simply inflating the balloon with 0.3–0.6 ml of saline. The precise inflation volume is determined during positioning of the catheter before the operation and depends on the caliber of the artery. To avoid overdistention, the ratio of arterial diameter (in millimeters) to inflation volume (in $\frac{1}{10}$ ml of saline) should never exceed 1. Under these circumstances, arteries 4–10 mm in diameter are reliably occluded without risk of significant vascular damage.

Hypothermic perfusion is started immediately, using a roller pump and a disposable perfusion system with heat exchange coils, which are immersed in an ice bath (Fig. 4.10). At a perfusate temperature of 4–6°C and a flow rate of 50 ml/min, renal core temperature usually drops to 15–20°C in 7–12 min.

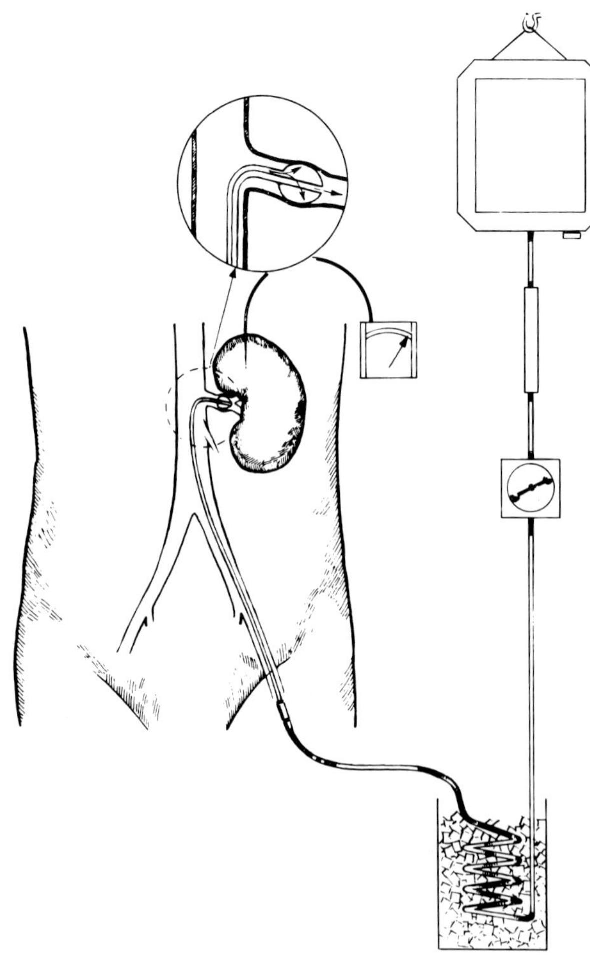

Figure 4.10. Technique of simultaneous balloon occlusion of the renal artery and hypothermic perfusion of the ischemic kidney with a double-lumen catheter.

Perfusion is then stopped and the operation is performed in a dry field. The core temperature is controlled continuously, and as soon as it reaches about 25°C, perfusion is restarted, usually now at a lower flow rate. The objective is to keep the kidney at 15–25°C. In general, about 1,500 ml of perfusate are needed per hour of ischemia for adequate cooling. The perfusate is administered systemically. If the fluid load appears precarious to the patient, the perfusate may be drained from the renal vein or perfusion cooling may be supplemented with surface cooling. To terminate ischemia, the balloon is deflated and the catheter is retracted into the aorta, from where it is removed after the operation.

Simultaneous balloon occlusion and hypothermic transcatheter perfusion ideally provide homogenous cooling of the entire kidney without impeding the surgeon. The protective effect is excellent and there is no need for dissection of the renal pedicle. In addition, perfusate squirting from any intrarenal vessel transsected during the nephrotomy facilitates that vessel's identification and precise hemostasis. Unfortunately, however, transcatheter perfusion techniques have an anatomical limitation: they cannot be employed in the presence of accessory renal arteries, which are found in about 21% of all kidneys. Theoretically, two balloon catheters could be used, but that is too complicated for a routine procedure. Although angiography facilities are usually available in most hospitals today, handling of the very pliable catheter requires some experience and extra concern by the radiologist. In addition, the catheter may slip from the renal artery during transport of the patient, especially if it could only be introduced into the artery for 1–2 cm due to early branching. Although experience and good cooperation between radiologist and urologist will reduce the failure rate, spontaneous catheter displacement results in an approximate failure rate of 10%. This remains without sequelae to the patient, who is only subjected to the discomfort and risks of an additional angiography, but it requires the availability of an alternative cooling technique. Finally, although transfemoral catheter angiography has a complication rate of less than 1%, there always remains some risk of iatrogenic vascular damage.

TRANSVENOUS PERFUSION

The kidney may also be cooled in situ by retrograde perfusion via the renal vein. Renal artery and vein are clamped, and the renal vein is intubated with a no. 18 polyvinyl tube or a special double-lumen irrigation cannula. Perfusion is performed by gravity from a height of 140 cm, with the perfusate draining from the kidney through the second lumen of the cannula, or only the nephrotomy.

The main advantage of the transvenous perfusion method lies in the fact that manipulation of the renal vein is simpler and less hazardous than that of the artery. Experience, however, has shown venous congestion to be particularly deleterious to postischemic renal function, and it seems unlikely that the low pressure venous system tolerates pressure of the magnitude of the arterial blood pressure without serious damage. Canine kidneys, at least, respond to a reversal of the direction of blood flow with rapid atrophy.

PERFUSION COOLING VIA THE COLLECTING SYSTEM

Jones and Politano originated a simple technique for in situ cooling via the collecting system. The kidney is exposed as usual, and the renal pelvis is punctured and intubated with a no. 7 polyvinyl tube. The tube is secured in place with a watertight purse-string suture and is connected to a standard transfusion system. The collecting system is then gravity flushed with saline precooled in a refrigerator; alternatively, heat exchange coils immersed in an ice bath may be interposed in the system between perfusate bag and kidney. The perfusate drains via the ureter and urethral catheter and cools the kidney to about 20°C in 7–12 min.

The method requires no elaborate equipment or preoperative preparation and is very simple. Unfortunately, the hypothermia achieved is rather inhomogenous. In kidneys with thick parenchyma and delicate calyces, which even may be occluded by calculi, the cortical temperatures are frequently insufficient. Once the collecting system is opened, reperfusion is difficult. Although possible, it requires particularly large caliber tubing and high flow rates and usually results in flooding of the operative field. The rather high irrigation pressure tends to dislodge smaller calculi, changing the situation documented on preoperative radiographs, and may flush calculous remnants unnoticed into the ureter.

SUMMARY

In conclusion, regional hypothermia is by far the most effective and reliable technique that is currently available for in situ protection of the kidney against temporary ischemia. Its safety has been demonstrated in numerous experimental and clinical studies over the last three decades. Albeit somewhat inconvenient, it must still be considered indispensable in any kidney operation requiring renal artery occlusion for longer than 60 min. Pharmacological protection has proven effective for less severe insults, but in clinical practice, it is often difficult to precisely predict the time of ischemia necessary for a certain surgical procedure. Although inosine protection, for example, may be combined with hypothermia in a sequential order, if extended ischemia becomes necessary unexpectedly, the quality and reliability of hypothermic protection are still unsurpassed, even for shorter bouts of ischemia.

The cooling technique chosen mainly depends on the experience of the surgeon, the equipment available, the operation to be performed, and the anatomical situation. At institutions specializing in intrarenal surgery, the entire spectrum of cooling techniques may be in use, with the individual choice depending on the surgeon's personal preference. In general, there is a trend toward the sophisticated methods, which provide better protection and surgical access at the cost of higher complexity. Daily routine may solve even difficult logistic problems, like cooperation with the radiologist, and may justify procuring expensive equipment. On the other hand, even in these centers the need for hypothermia may arise unexpectedly, such as in kidney trauma, so that a simple technique must always be available.

The author relies on transarterial perfusion cooling with a balloon catheter as the technique of choice and slush cooling as an alternative. With growing experience, the logistic difficulties of the former technique have been mastered; the advantages in the quality of protection and accessibility to the kidney are obvious. The technique is, however, not universally applicable and may fail due to catheter displacement. As this failure may not become apparent until ischemia is established, ice slush is also prepared. It is cheap and applicable in every situation requiring hypothermia and the surgeon needs no technical assistance. The main disadvantages, in homogenous cooling and drenching of the operative field, are, to a large extent, overcome by monitoring the kidney temperature, by continuous cooling, and by the use of an effective dam around the ice.

In the peripheral hospital only occasionally engaged in renal hypothermia, the selection of the technique is determined by the need for simplicity. This rules out transvascular perfusion as well as surface cooling with special equipment. As cooling via the collecting system is, in the author's opinion, unreliable, the spectrum is reduced to surface cooling with ice slush or immersion hypothermia. The former again merits simplicity and continuous cooling.

Suggested Readings

Avramovici A: Le transplantation due rein. *Lyon Chir* 21:734, 1924.

Cockett ATK: The kidney and regional hypothermia. *Surgery* 50:905, 1961.

Eisenberger F, Schmiedt E, Pfeifer KY, Chaussy G, Rother R, Klein V, Riedl P: In situ perfusion und kühlung der niere bei augussteinen. *Münch Med Wochenschr* 115:404, 1973.

Farcon EM, Morales P, Al-Askari S: In vivo hypothermic perfusion during renal surgery. *Urology* 3:416, 1974.

Gil-Vernet JM, Caralps A, Andrev J, Revert L, Tornos D: Now developments in surgical treatment of renovascular arterial hypertension. *Eur Urol* 3:362, 1977.

Graves FT: Regional hypothermia: An aid to partial nephrectomy. *Br J Surg* 50:362, 1963.

Jones WR, Politano V: The effects of renal artery occlusion on renal function under normothermic and regional hypothermia. *J Urol* 89:535, 1963.

Marberger M, Georgi M: Balloon occlusion of the renal artery in tumor nephrectomy. *J Urol* 114:360, 1975.

Marberger M, Piroth D, Günther R, Alken P, Scheiblich H: The impact of in situ balloon occlusion of the renal artery and hypothermic perfusion on renal blood flow. *Urol Res* 6:49, 1978.

Marberger M, Georgi M, Gunther R, Hohenfellner R: Simultaneous balloon occlusion of the renal artery and hypothermic perfusion on renal blood flow. *Urol Res* 6:49, 1978.

Marberger M, Eisenberger F: Regional hypothermia of the kidney: Surface or transarterial cooling? A functional study. *J Urol* 124:179, 1980.

Marberger M, Günther R, Alken P, Rumpf W, Ranc M: Inosine: Alternative or adjunct to regional hypothermia in the prevention of post ischemic renal failure. *Eur Urol* 6:95, 1980.

Metzer PJ, Boyce WH: Simplified renal hypothermia: An adjunct to conservative renal surgery. *Br J Urol* 44:76, 1972.

Novick AC, Magnusson MO: Extracorporeal and in situ renal preservation. In Novick AC, Straffon RA (eds): *Vascular Problems in Urologic Surgery*. Philadelphia, WB Saunders, 1982.

Pflüger H, Maier M, Wagner M, Binder R, Marberger M: Renal blood flow alterations after temporary ischemia: An experimental model in the rabbit. *Eur Urol* 9:113, 1983.

Wagenknecht LV, Hupe W, Bücheler E, Klosterhalfen H: Selective hypothermic perfusion of the kidney for intrarenal surgery. *Eur Urol* 3:62, 1977.

Ward JP: Determination of the optimum temperature for regional renal hypothermia during temporary renal ischemia. *Br J Urol* 47:17, 1975.

Wickham JEA, Coe N, Ward JP: One hundred cases of nephrolithotomy under hypothermia. *J Urol* 112:702, 1979.

CHAPTER 5

Omentum in Urologic Surgery

JAMES M. PIERCE, JR.

The greater omentum (Fig. 5.1) has always been recognized as having the ability to seal off areas of inflammation within the peritoneal cavity. It has been noted to have a very rich lymphatic supply that connects with the lymphatics of structures that it adheres to. This can occur within a few days (1). Omentum is quite mobile and has an excellent blood supply, primarily from the gastroepiploic blood vessels, right and left. Omentum has been used both with intact blood supply and as isolated pieces of tissue to seal off certain areas during operative procedures. An isolated piece of omentum disconnected from its blood supply obviously will die and be absorbed. It might seal off an area temporarily and allow healing of the local tissues without fistula development but certainly any longer term need for omentum requires that the blood supply be intact. This chapter will deal with the use of omentum with intact blood supply in solving certain problem areas in urologic surgery.

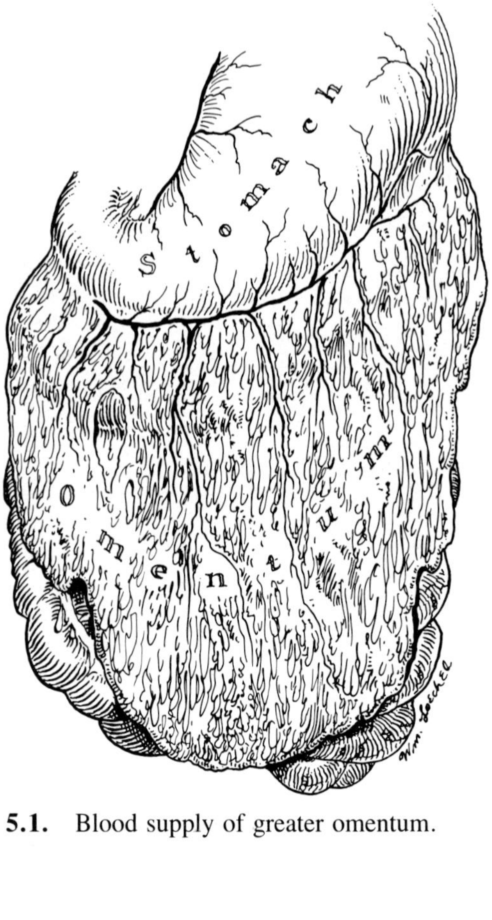

Figure 5.1. Blood supply of greater omentum.

OMENTUM WITH BLOOD SUPPLY NOT MOBILIZED OFF THE STOMACH AND TRANSVERSE COLON

Especially in people with a thin abdomen and nice thin omentum, one sometimes can split off a section of omentum or even divide it into two pieces, being careful to keep the blood supply intact. This can be used to wrap around a ureter and renal pelvis or both ureters.

This is especially useful in dealing with matters like retroperitoneal fibrosis in which the ureters have been freed from the surrounding sclerosing fibrous tissue. Frequently, with a well-developed, thin omentum, these two pieces can be run down into the pelvis (Fig. 5.2). In the individual with a very fat panniculus and extreme fat in the omentum, it is more difficult to use the omentum because of its extreme thickness and volume. In these situations, the surgeon must be careful not to occlude any bowel due to the volume and weight of any overlying omentum. Certain modifications of this type of procedure may be selectively available to the imaginative surgeon.

MAXIMUM MOBILIZATION OF OMENTUM

The normal omentum does not reach below the pelvic brim. Thus, in deep pelvic applications, it is necessary to mobilize the omentum so that it can reach the area being reconstructed but still maintain an intact blood supply.

Maximum mobilization of the omentum is for use in pelvic reconstructive procedures to seal off various areas and add blood supply and perhaps provide better lymphatic drainage. This involves mobilizing the omentum off the greater curvature of the stomach, keeping the gastroepiploic vessels on the

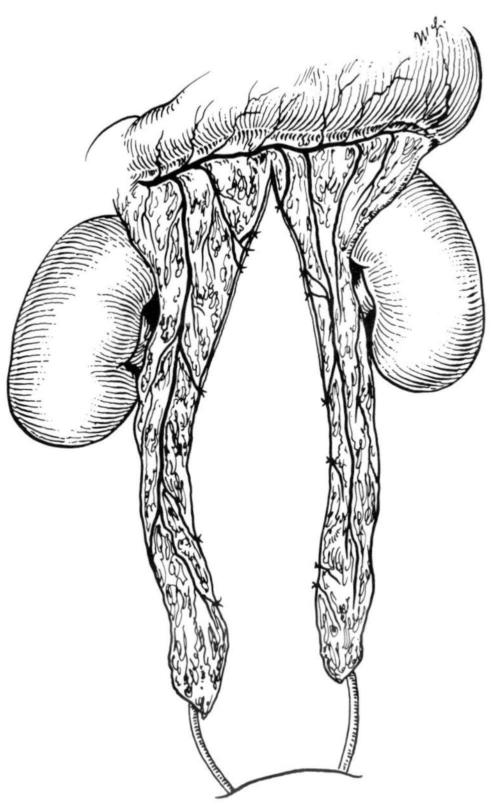

Figure 5.2. Bilateral ureteral omental wraps in severe retroperitioneal fibrosis.

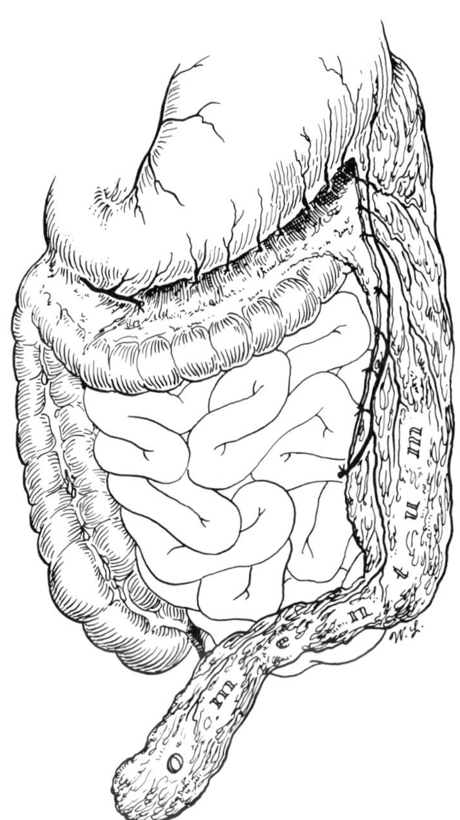

Figure 5.3. Mobilization from right to left as described by Kiricuta and Goldstein (2, 3).

omentum and, thus, using this for the blood supply. It can be mobilized from right to left or from left to right. One of the earliest references to this procedure was made by Kiricuta and Goldstein (2, 3). Kiricuta transected the right gastroepiploic artery just near the area of the pylorus and them mobilized this vessel with the omentum off the greater curvature over to the left side (Fig. 5.3). Then he mobilized the omentum off the colon and this totally mobilized omentum was run down the left gutter into the pelvis. Here it was used to seal off various fistulae that were difficult to close by ordinary techniques. Literally, the holes were plugged with omentum. Many of these cases were those in which the fistula was due to heavily irradiated tissue with poor blood supply. A significant number of these fistulae previously thought to be unrepairable seemed to close off successfully. The omentum in the pelvis was tacked to the fistula area covering it, thus, utilizing the blood supply and lymphatic drainage from the omentum to allow healing and closure of the fistula tract.

The mobilization can also be done from left to right as described by Richard Turner Warwick and associates (4, 5). This procedure is depicted in Figure 5.4. In this situation, the omentum is mobilized by cutting the gastroepiploic vessels on the left side leaving the short gastrics and several vessels from the gastroepiploic to provide blood supply to the stomach and the greater curvature. The omentum is also mobilized off the colon and freed up over to the pyloric end of the stomach. This big length of omentum can go down the right gutter but it can be extended even to a longer length by placing it posteriorly through a window in the right side of the transverse mesocolon, through the terminal portion of the mesentery, and then directly into the pelvis. It can be tacked posteriorly, thus, making it so that it cannot get bowel loops around it and the route to the pelvis is direct. Sometimes going down the right gutter allows a bulky omentum to compress the cecal area and may allow for loops of small bowel to get around it. Making the windows in the mesocolon and mesentery takes only a minute of time but leads to a neat application. It also gives the shortest distance, thus, greater length to the omentum. Sometimes, the omentum can be so long that it reaches below the knee. Sometimes, after exenterative procedures especially, if there has been a lot of radiation, one can use a mobilized omentum to fill the pelvis so that deep small bowel adhesions do not occur (Fig. 5.5). Another interesting use is when the lower abdominal wall cannot be closed because of multiple operations and/or radiation damage. In these cases, one can mobilize the omentum, pass it into the pelvis to fill the pelvis after the exenteration, and then roll it back on itself as in Figure 5.6. Thus, it can overlie the peritoneal cavity underneath the closure and be tacked under the sides of the open wound. That portion of the wound is left open and, frequently, there is enough blood supply and lymphatic drainage that the wound gradually will heal on its own.

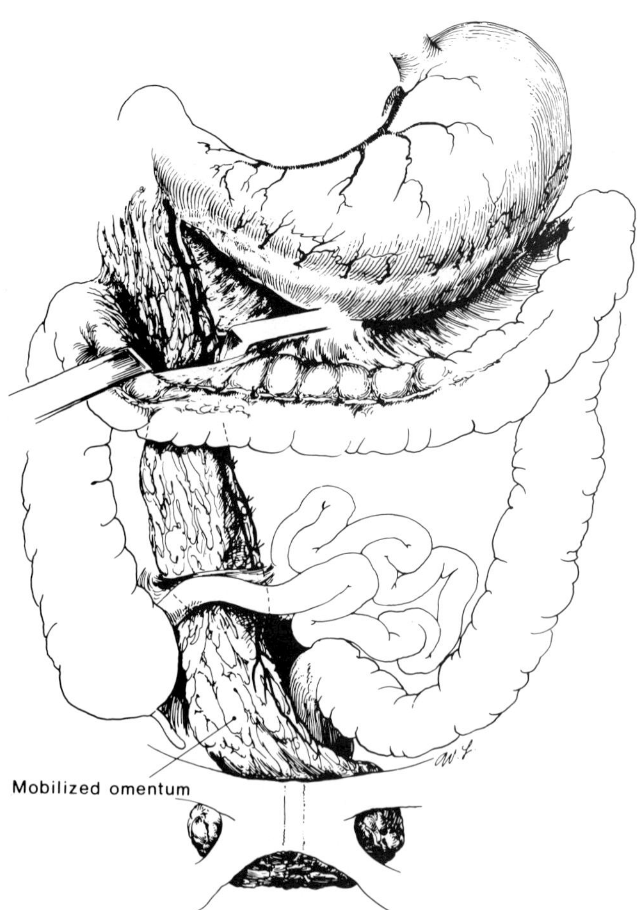

Figure 5.4. Mobilization from left to right as described by Turner-Warwick and associates (4, 5).

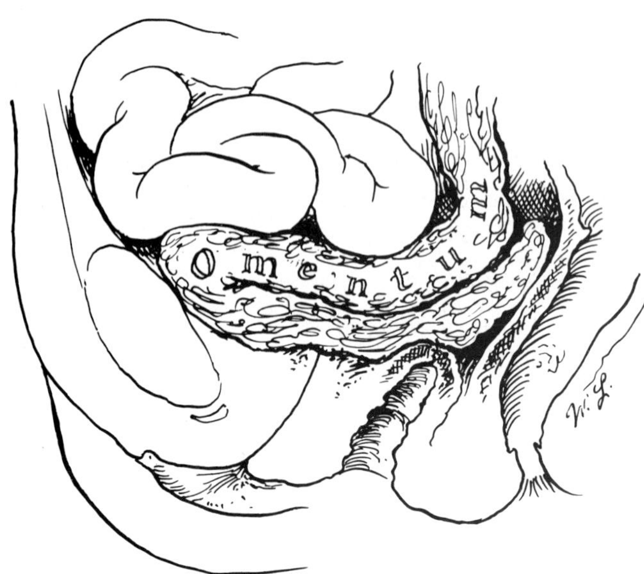

Figure 5.5. Omentum filling pelvic cavity after exenteration.

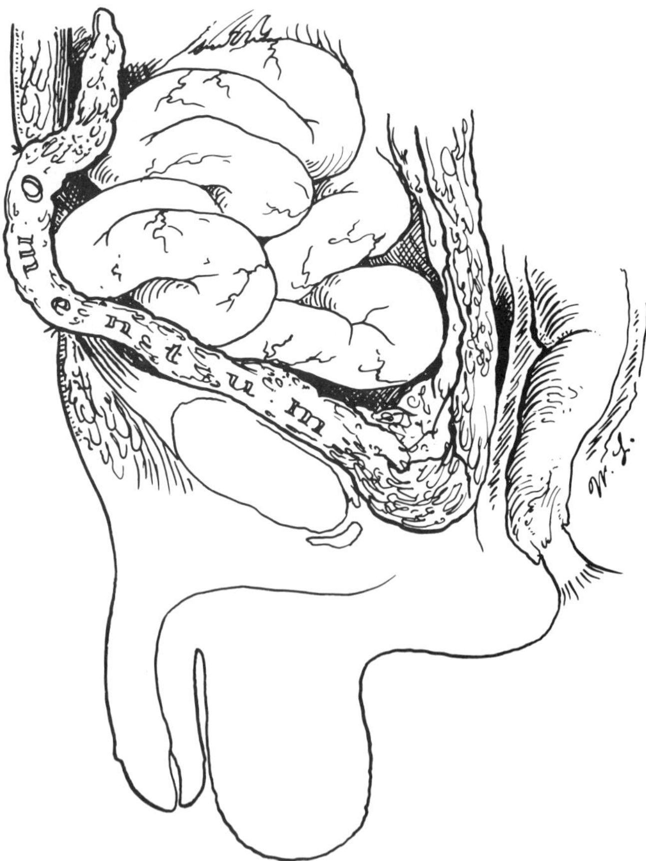

Figure 5.6. Omentum used to fill in space in an abdominal wall that is impossible to close after radical cystectomy and pelvic irradiation.

This can prove very useful in this difficult situation. Still another application is the occasional problem of difficult to close vesicovaginal fistulae. In some situations, it may be advisable to bring the mobilized omentum down between the closures of the vagina and the bladder (Fig. 5.7). this provides a layer that is viable and will prevent recurrence of the fistula. In very advanced cases, especially with severe radiation, one may not be able to close one or the other organs in vesicovaginal fistulae and one can mobilize omentum and, as suggested by Turner Warwick, actually bring it right through the fistula tract in the pelvis. Also, as shown in Figure 5.8, Kiricuta did not bring it through the fistulous tract but tacked the omentum to the edges of the fistula. However, bringing it through sometimes is a very good method and perhaps one can close the bladder and bring the omentum out through the fistula in the vagina, which may not close because it may be more heavily radiated. This does not always work but it does in a significant number of cases. The excessive omentum can be trimmed from the inside of the vagina at a later time. Figure 5.9 shows the application to a male vesical or urethral rectal fistula, which may be a problem especially in radiated tissues, and shows the omentum brought down between the two viscera. Figure 5.10 shows a worse situation in which the omen-

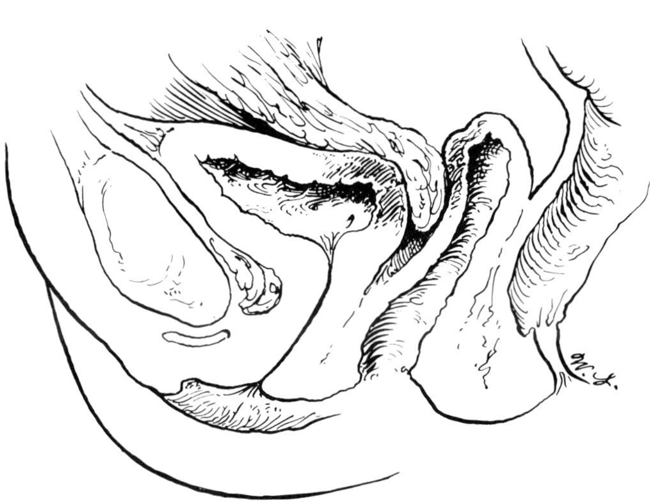

Figure 5.7. Omentum between vagina and bladder in vesicovaginal fistula repair.

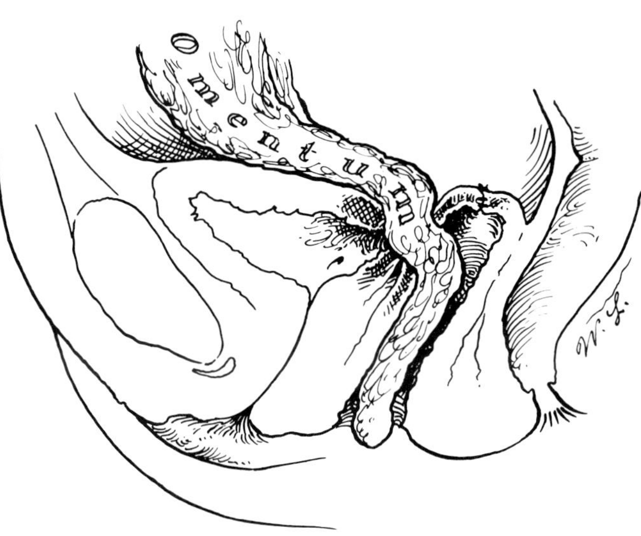

Figure 5.8. Omentum in repair of difficult vesicovaginal fistula with irradiation. Omentum comes out through the unclosable vagina.

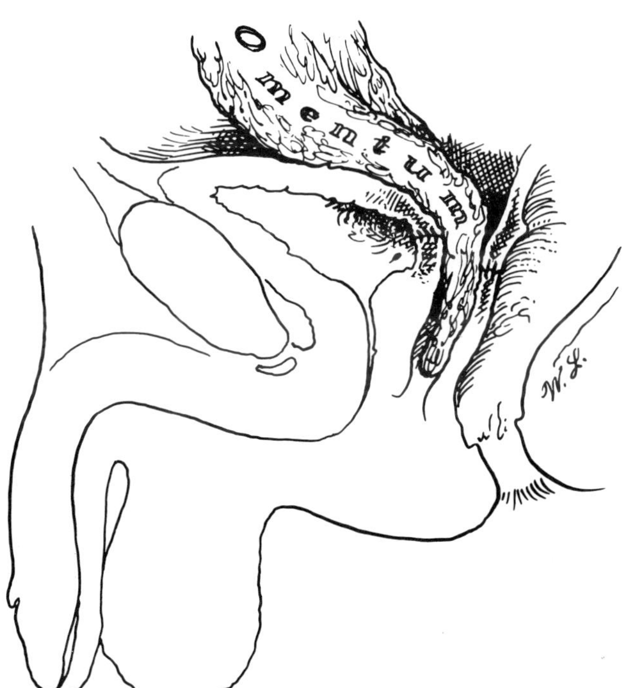

Figure 5.9. Severe vesicorectal fistulae with omentum separating them.

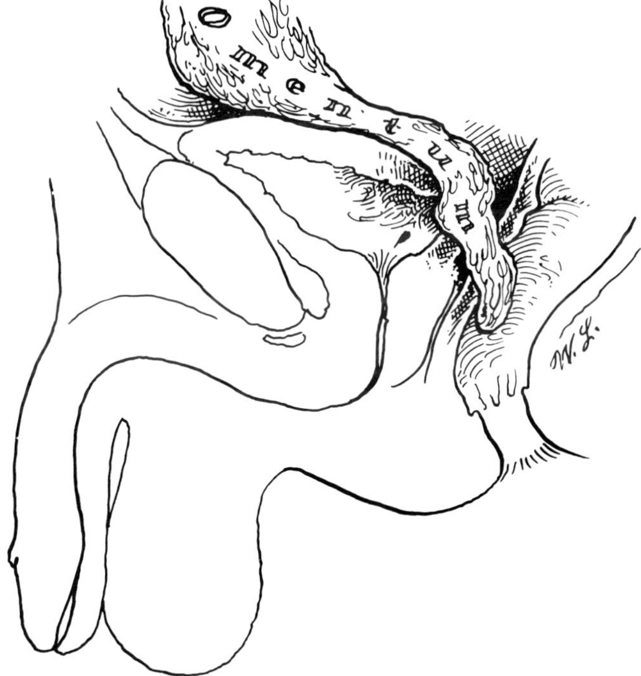

Figure 5.10. Severe vesicorectal fistula with omentum entering rectum.

tum is actually brought through the fistulous tract, thus, sealing off both the bladder and rectal portions of the fistula. In these more difficult radiation cases, sometimes one can close one viscus without the other and sometimes neither can be closed. Omentum does give the surgeon a chance perhaps to seal the fistulae.

Of course, one does not always have to mobilize the omentum maximally, as in the severe pelvic reconstructions. Sometimes, just a partial mobilization of a relatively small area of omentum may be done keeping the blood supply intact and using that in adjacent repairs. An omentum with its good blood supply and its very excellent lymphatic drainage that connects with structures to which it is adherent remains a very useful structure to remember when attacking some of these difficult reconstructive problems. It is useful in the surgeon's bag of tricks when he is required to improvise.

References

1. Simer PH, Webb RL: Lymphatics in omental adhesions. *Surg Gynecol Obstet* 64:872, 1937.
2. Kiricuta I, Goldstein AMB: Epiplooplastio vezicala, metoda de tratament curativ al fistulelor vezico-vaginale. *Obstetrica si ginecologica Bucuresti* 2:163, 1956.
3. Kiricuta I, Goldstein AMB: The repair of extensive vesicovaginal fistuals with pedicled omentum: A review 27 cases. *J Urol* 108:724, 1972.
4. Turner-Warwick RT, Wynne EJC, Handley-Ashken M: The use of the omental pedicle graft in the repair and reconstruction of the urinary tract. *Br J Surg* 54:849, 1967.
5. Turner-Warwick R: The use of the omental pedicle graft in urinary tract reconstruction. *J Urol* 116:341, 1976.

SECTION 2

Operations Upon the Adrenal Gland

Surgical approaches to the adrenal glands have varied greatly since Thornton first removed a large adrenal tumor en bloc with the left kidney in 1889. Considering the wide variety of diseases for which adrenal surgery is undertaken, the multiplicity of operative approaches is not surprising and, in most cases, is thoroughly justified. Although Charles Mayo successfully removed the first pheochromocytoma through a flank incision in 1927, it remained for Cahill to point out the wisdom of a bilateral transabdominal operation in patients with this disease. The fact that roughly 10% of these tumors are bilateral, extradrenal, or malignant makes this approach mandatory in patients with pheochromocytoma.

The desire to keep the operation retroperitoneal, and at the same time expose both glands simultaneously, has led many surgeons to adopt a posterior approach using two incisions with the patient in the prone position. Young first described this technique in 1936. Nesbit later used this approach in patients with primary aldosteronism and beautifully described the meticulous dissection necessary to expose tiny adenomas in glands rendered especially friable by this disease. This remains an excellent approach in patients requiring bilateral adrenalectomy for Cushing's syndrome or in patients undergoing unilateral adrenalectomy for a small benign adenoma.

Extremely wide exposure may be necessary in patients with large adrenal neoplasms, when radical extirpation of the tumor mass is anticipated. A modified flank incision, often combined with rib resection, was preferred by many earlier surgeons in this situation. Perhaps the widest exposure of all is possible through the thoracoabdominal approach, described by Chute and associates in 1949, for removal of large renal masses. Stewart recommended a combined flank and abdominal approach in 1965, resecting the ipsilateral 11th rib to gain maximum exposure and still keep the operation below the diaphragm..

There are valid merits and indications for most of the different techniques to gain exposure of the adrenal glands. In view of the variety of clinical conditions requiring adrenal surgery, this section will describe in detail those procedures felt best suited to each disease entity and with which the authors have had the greatest experience and the fewest complications.

SURGICAL ANATOMY

Regardless of the underlying adrenal disease process, operative approach, and skill of the attending surgeon, a knowledge of surgical anatomy is essential in the performance of safe and effective surgery upon the adrenal glands.

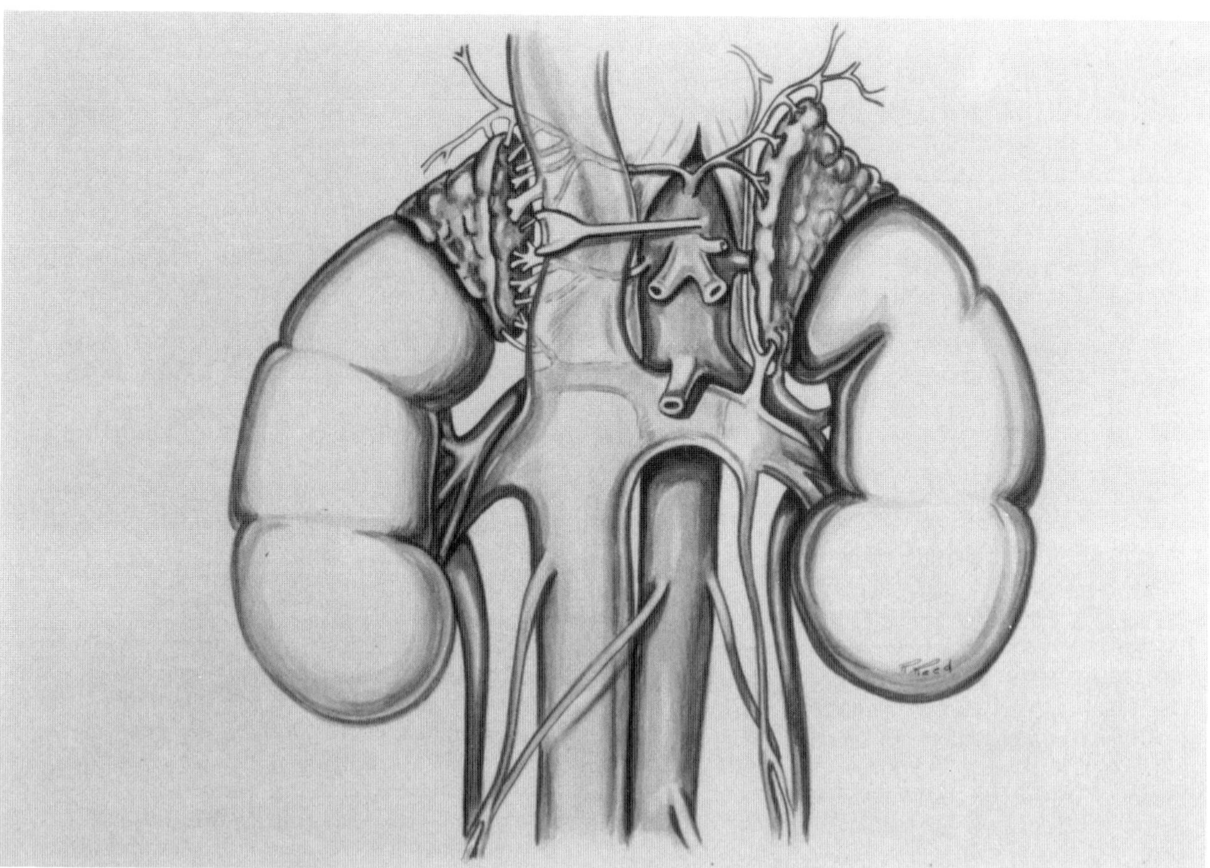

Figure 1. This figure provides a schematic representation of the surgical anatomy and blood supply to the adrenal glands. On the left side, the gland is supplied by multiple arteries which arise superiorly and enter the gland as branches of the inferior phrenic artery. Along the entire medial aspect of the gland, branches of multiple middle adrenal arteries arising directly from the aorta enter the substance of the gland after traversing through the periaortic lymph nodes and celiac ganglia. There is a rather constant inferior adrenal artery arising near the takeoff of the left renal artery, either just above it from the aorta or just distal to it from the proximal renal artery. Inadvertent transection of this vessel can cause troublesome bleeding when dissecting structures away from the renal artery near its takeoff. The venous drainage of the left adrenal gland is almost solely through the inferior adrenal vein, which begins as rather friable branches within the substance of the adrenal gland and coalesces into a single large vein entering the cephalic aspect of the left renal vein. Such entry occurs at a level near the lateral margin of the aorta, palpation of which can serve as a useful landmark when dissecting the renal vein to gain initial exposure of the adrenal vien. It should be noted that all of the blood supply enters the gland medially, inferiorly, and superiorly and that there is very little blood supply to the gland from its lateral aspect. There is a definite plane of dissection anteriorly between Gerota's fascia, overlying the anterior surface of the gland, and the posterior aspect of the pancreas, containing the friable splenic vein as well as the splenic artery. In gaining exposure of the adrenal gland through an anterior incision, the splenorenal ligaments must be divided and the colon reflected medially, after which this plane is entered and the pancreas and spleen can be gently elevated anteriorly and superiorly by blunt dissection to expose the anterior surface of the adrenal gland. Similarly, there is an avascular plane laterally and posteriorly between the posterior layer of Gerota's fascia and the paraspinous muscles, so that the entire gland can be gently mobilized away from surrounding structures without disturbing its major blood supply.

On the right side, the arterial supply arises again superiorly from branches of the inferior phrenic artery, which actually lies at a higher level than on the left, even though the kidney is lower in position on the right side. The presence of the overlying liver and the vena cava lying just medial to the superior vascular ligament can make the latter difficult to expose on the right side. The medial aspect of the gland is supplied by multiple middle adrenal arteries coursing from the aorta beneath the vena cava and through pericaval lymphatic and ganglionic structures to enter the gland medially. The inferior adrenal artery is rather constant in location and arises 1–2 cm distal to the origin of the right renal artery, where it courses upward into the lower aspect of the gland. The venous drainage of the gland is again by a single adrenal vein, this time rather short and friable and entering the vena cava directly at a level just below the hepatic venous branches. This vein is always higher and usually shorter than one might expect from reviewing standard anatomy texts. It is usually necessary to dissect away adjacent arterial and fascial structures to gain optimal exposure before securing this vein. As on the left side, there is a relatively avascular plane between Gerota's fascia covering the anterior surface of the gland and the undersurface of the liver. In gaining exposure of the gland through an anterior incision, the posterior peritoneum must be incised upward and all the way across, medially over the anterior surface of the vena cava, to allow complete reflection of the colon and duodenum medially and thereby expose the anterior surface of the adrenal gland. Likewise, there is a relatively avascular plane posteriorly between the posterior leaf of Gerota's fascia and the underlying paraspinous muscles. Thus, on the right side as well as on the left, complete mobilization of the anterior, posterior, and lateral aspects of the gland can be accomplished without disturbing its major blood supply, which enters medially, superiorly, and inferiorly. Occasionally, there are loose vascular attachments between the superior pole of the kidney and the inferior margin of the adrenal gland, lateral to the inferior adrenal artery, which can cause troublesome bleeding if inadvertently transected.

This basic anatomy must be kept in mind during the various operative procedures performed upon the adrenal glands, which are described in greater detail in the following chapters.

Suggested Readings

Cahill GF: Adrenalectomy for adrenal tumors. *J Urol* 71:123, 1954.

Chute R, Soutter L, Kerr WS: The value of the thoraco-abdominal incision in the removal of kidney tumors. *N Engl J Med* 241:951, 1949.

Edis AJ, Ayala LA, Egdahl RH: Surgery of the adrenals. *Manual Endocr Surg*. New York, Springer-Verlag, 123:207, 1975.

Glenn JF: Non-functioning adrenal tumors and aldosteronism. In Glenn JF (ed): *Urologic Surgery*, 3rd ed. Philadelphia, JB Lippincott, 1983.

Konnak JW, Cerny JC: The surgical treatment of Cushing's syndrome. *J Urol* 102:653–656, 1969.

Mayo CH: Paroxysmal hypertension with tumor of retroperitoneal nerve. *JAMA* 89:1047, 1927.

Stewart BH: Adrenal surgery: Current state of the art. *J Urol* 129:1, 1983.

Young HH: A technique for simultaneous exposure and operation on the adrenals. *Surg Gynecol Obstet* 54:179, 1936.

CHAPTER 6

Posterior Approach to the Adrenal Gland

ANDREW C. NOVICK

The posterior surgical approach to the adrenal gland was first described over 50 years ago and continues to find useful application in selected patients undergoing adrenalectomy. The advantages of this approach are that it is extraperitoneal, both adrenal glands can be exposed simultaneously, and adrenalectomy can be done with minimal disturbance of adjacent viscera. Anatomically, a posterior incision represents the most direct approach to the adrenal glands. Since no major muscles are transected with this incision, patient discomfort is generally minimal and early ambulation is possible.

The major disadvantage of the posterior approach is the relatively small operative field, which restricts visualization and exposure of the great vessels. Therefore, this approach should not be used to remove large adrenal lesions where wide exposure and major vascular control are necessary. This approach is also contraindicated in patients with a potentially malignant process, such as pheochromocytoma or a suspected adrenal cortical carcinoma, where an exploratory laparotomy must be done. In considering these limitations, the primary indications for posterior adrenalectomy are in patients with bilateral hyperplasia from Cushing's disease or those with a relatively small benign unilateral adenoma. The most common clinical diagnosis in the latter category is hyperaldosteronism, although such small adenomas may also cause Cushing's syndrome.

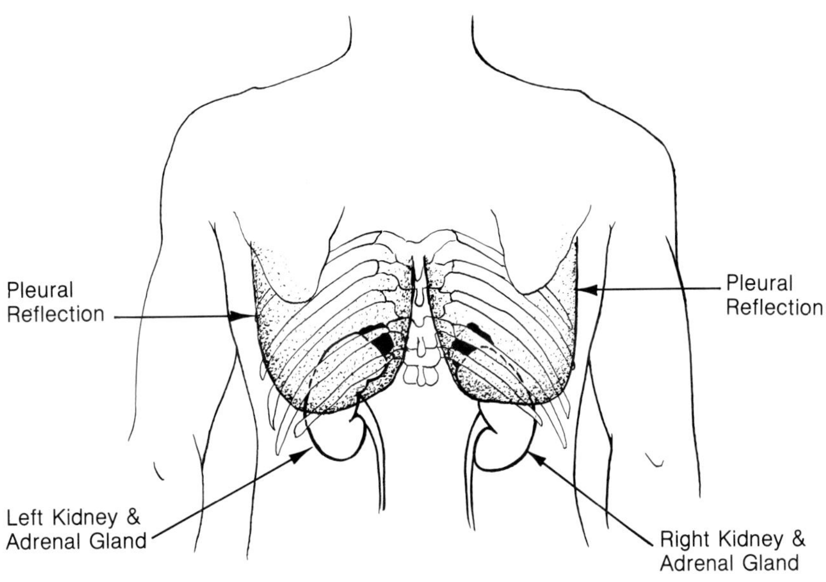

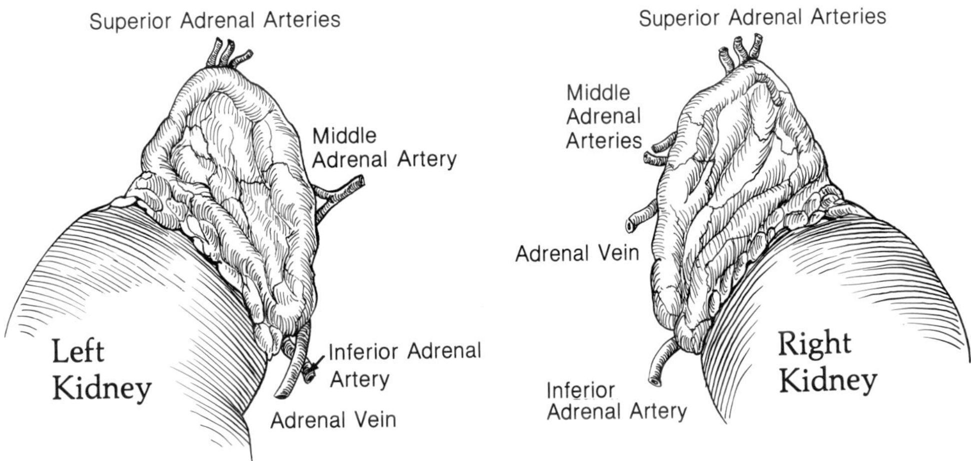

Figure 6.1. This figure depicts the posterior anatomical relationships of the adrenal glands. The pleural reflection extends below most of the 11th rib and a variable portion of the medial aspect of the 12th rib. In most cases, the location of the adrenal gland in relation to the ribs will be known from preoperative imaging studies. Occasionally, on the left side, adequate exposure can be obtained through an oblique incision made over the 12th rib, with upward mobilization and retraction of the pleura as described in chapter 2. Nevertheless, in most cases, the optimum incision is through the bed of the 11th rib, particularly on the right side where the adrenal gland often lies more superiorly. With an unusually high-lying adrenal gland, an incision through the bed of the 10th rib may be indicated. When operating through a posterior 11th rib incision, the pleura are directly adjacent to the periosteum in the depth of the wound and extend for a variable distance inferiorly and medially. In our experience, attempting to mobilize the pleura superiorly away from the incision is tedious and often leads to one or more inadvertent pleural entries. In such cases, we have found that simply opening the pleural and diaphragmatic layers of the thoracic cavity in line with the incision can be safely done and provides excellent direct exposure of the adrenal gland. This posterior transthoracic incision for adrenal surgery is illustrated below for the left side; however, the approach on the right side is essentially the same.

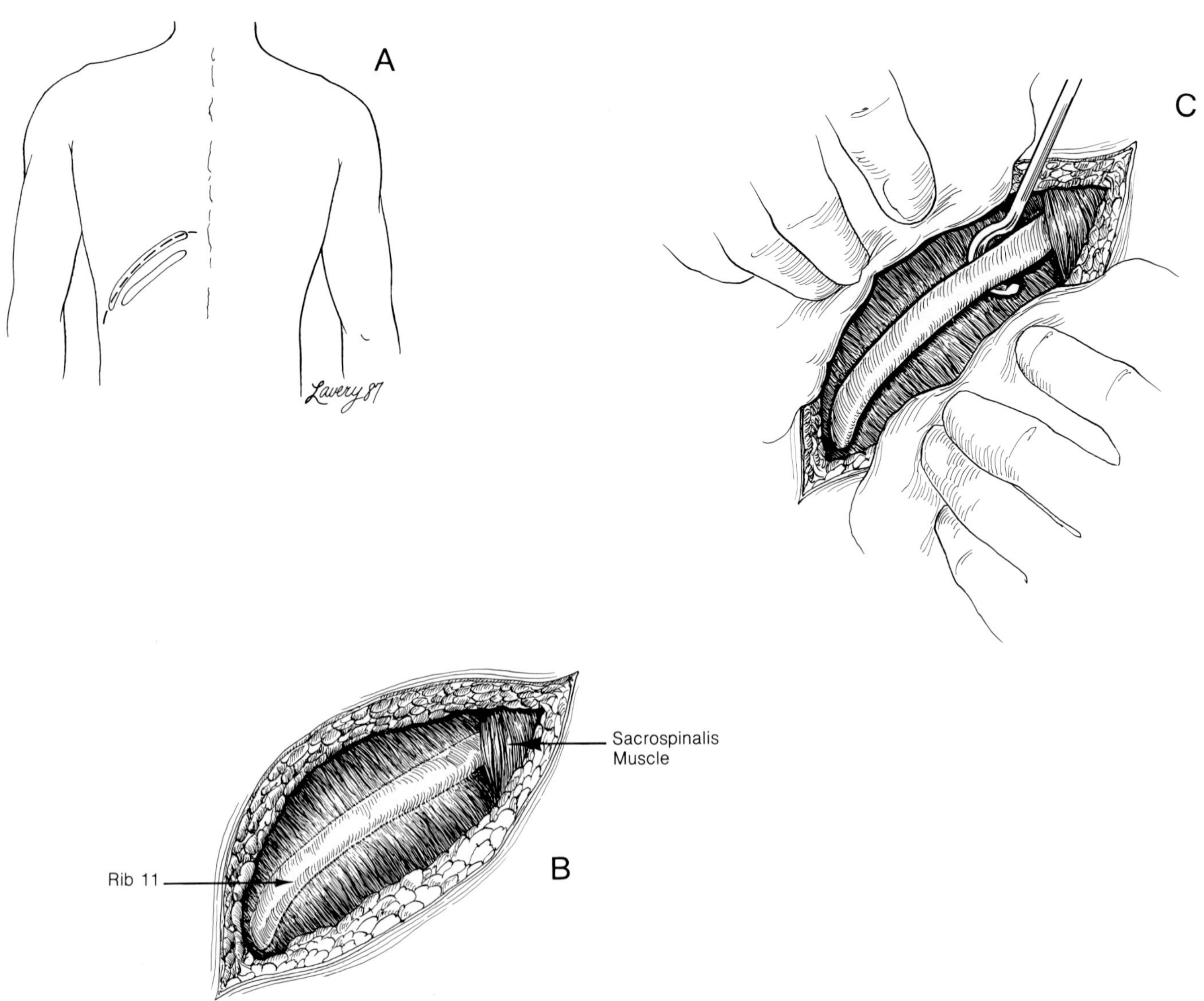

Figure 6.2. The patient is placed in the prone position on a laminectomy frame which provides flexion at the hips and allows gentle dorsal curvature of the spine from the midthoracic to the lower lumbar levels. When performing bilateral adrenalectomy for Cushing's disease, two surgical teams can operate simultaneously with the patient in this position. **A**, an oblique incision is made over the 11th rib with lateral extension almost to the midaxillary line. **B**, the incision is developed to expose the entire length of the rib as well as the sacrospinalis muscle medially. **C**, the rib is resected subperiosteally, including as much of its medial aspect as possible to optimize exposure of the adrenal gland; such exposure is also facilitated by medial retraction of the sacrospinalis muscle. **D**, the rib bed and subadjacent pleura are then divided in line with the incision, taking care not to injure the subcostal vessel and nerve. **E**, the thoracic cavity is entered exposing the diaphragm and the lung medially. **F**, the exposed lung is gently retracted medially with a padded curved retractor in preparation for incision of the diaphragm. **G**, a linear incision is then made in the diaphragm to enter the retroperitoneal space. **H**, upon exposing the retroperitoneum in this manner, the adrenal gland generally lies directly in the center of the operative field. When performing unilateral adrenalectomy a Finochietto retractor is inserted, as shown, to maintain exposure. If bilateral simultaneous posterior adrenalectomy is being done, a single Finochietto retractor is used for medial retraction of both incisions (see Fig. 6.3 below). Because of the distinct differences in anatomy on the right and left side, the operative technique for posterior removal of the adrenal gland is reviewed below, separately for the left and right sides.

D
Pleura
Diaphragm
F
Lung
Diaphragm
Lung
E
Diaphragm
Lavery 87
G
Pancreas
Adrenal Gland
Kidney
Peritoneum
H
Lavery 87

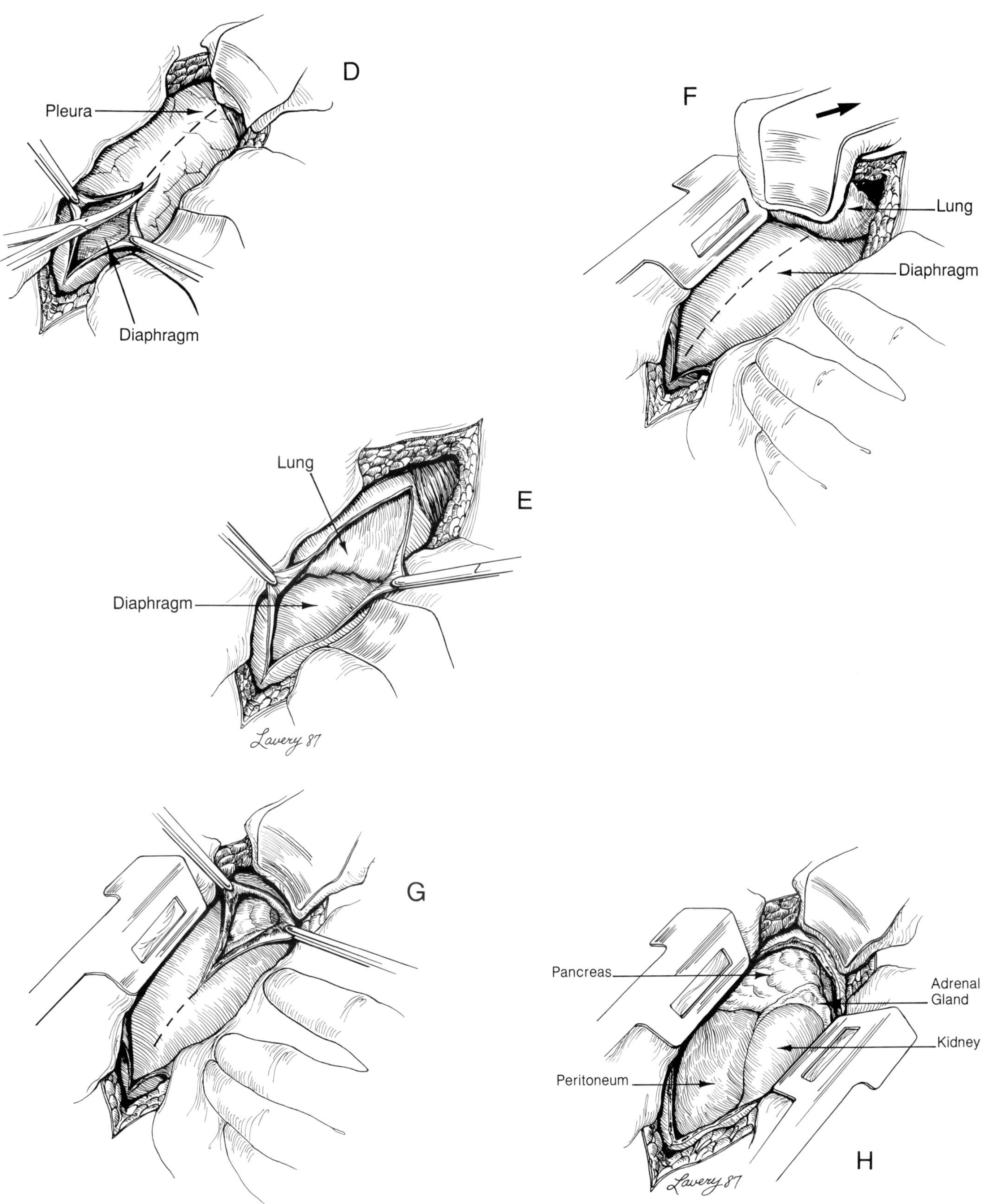

Figure 6.2. D–H

Figure 6.3. On the left side, after entering the retroperitoneal space, Gerota's fascia is incised and the posterior surface of the kidney and adrenal gland are exposed by sharp and blunt dissection. The attachment between the upper pole of the kidney and the inferior aspect of the adrenal gland should be kept intact, so that gentle downward traction upon the kidney can be done to enhance exposure. This is accomplished by placing a laparotomy pad over the upper surface of the kidney and using either the hand of the surgeon or a curved retractor held by an assistant. Once initial exposure has been gained, the apical vascular ligament is identified and transected between silver clips to deliver the gland more completely into the operative field.

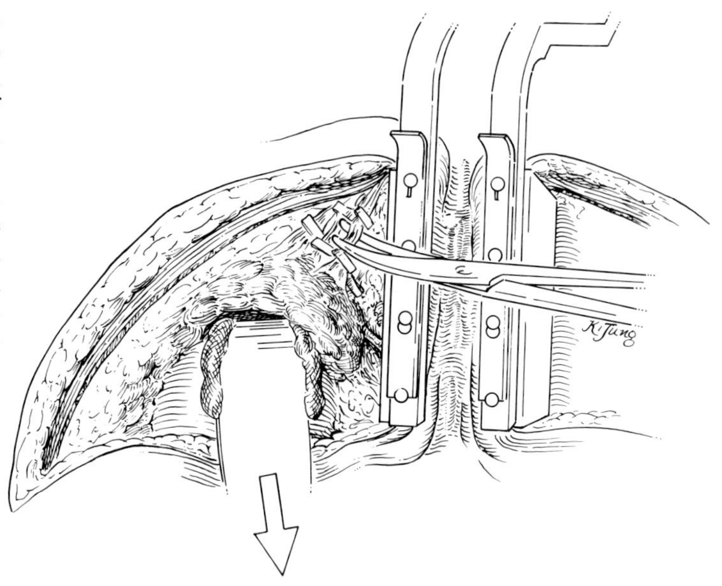

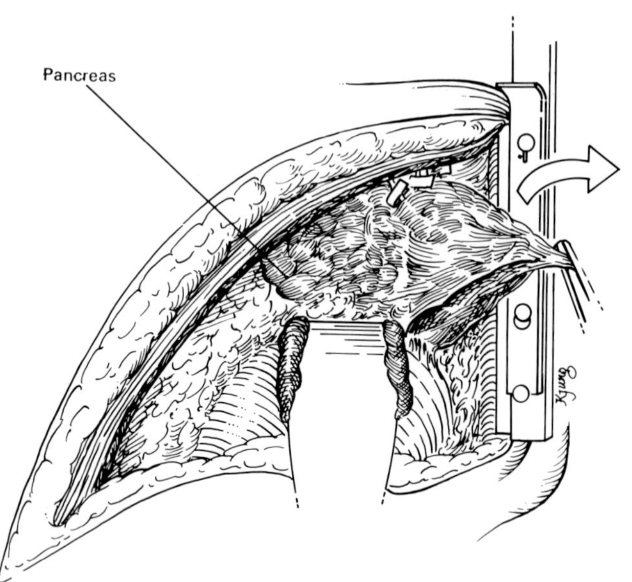

Figure 6.4. The lateral borders of the gland are then freed up and the gland is retracted medially to expose its anterior surface. Care must be taken not to injure the adjacent pancreas, which lies just beneath the adrenal gland when viewed from a posterior approach. The pancreas is firm in consistency, grayish in color, and is easily distinguishable from the bright orange-yellow color and softer consistency of the adrenal gland.

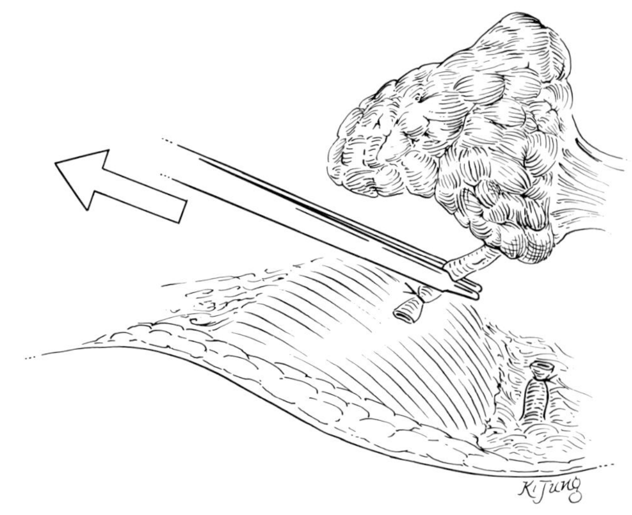

Figure 6.5. The left adrenal vein is exposed as it courses downward just medial and anterior to the upper pole of the kidney, to enter as a single vessel into the superior aspect of the left renal vein. The left adrenal vein is then ligated with 2–0 silk ligatures and divided. The upper stump of the vein can be left long and used as a handle for additional lateral traction upon the gland. The inferior adrenal artery is also secured individually at this stage as it courses upward from the proximal aspect of the renal artery.

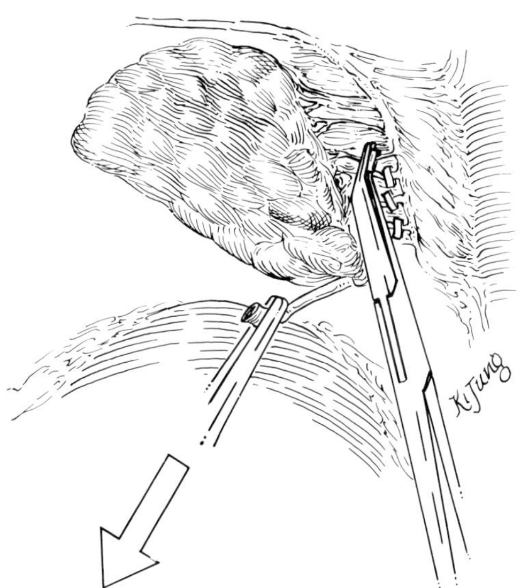

Figure 6.6. Utilizing lateral and upward traction upon the gland, the middle adrenal arteries are secured between silver clips as they course inward medially from the aorta. This completes removal of the left adrenal gland.

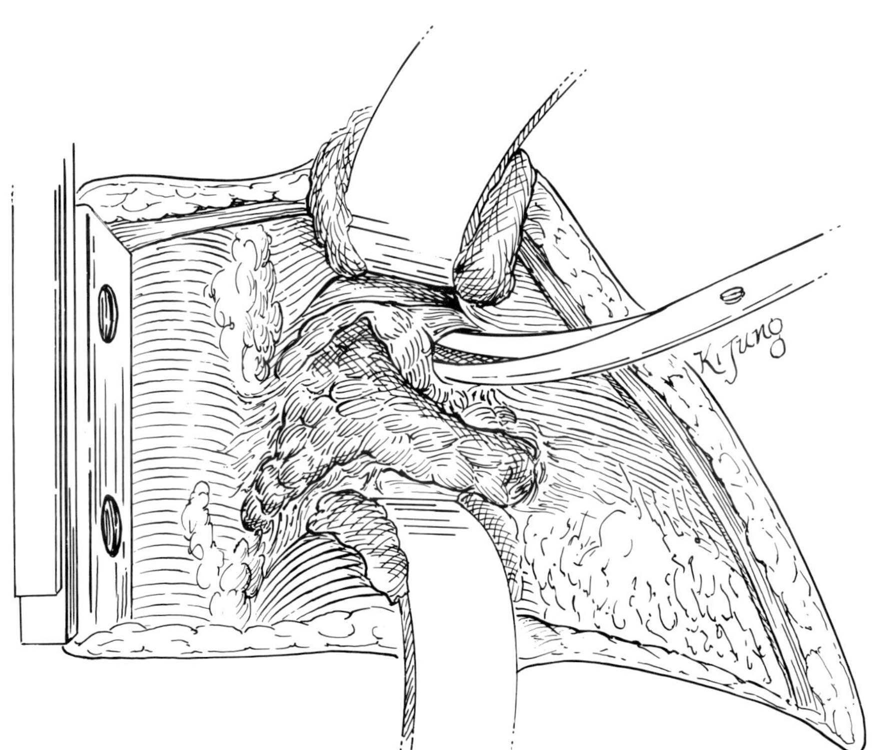

Figure 6.7. On the right side, the kidney is also gently retracted downward and the posterior surface of the adrenal gland is dissected free of fatty and areolar tissue. As the apex is approached, the liver is gently retracted upward to facilitate exposure. In some cases, the apex of the adrenal gland is quite adherent to the liver and must be dissected free with extreme care. The dissection is continued cephaled, and the apical vascular ligament is divided between silver clips.

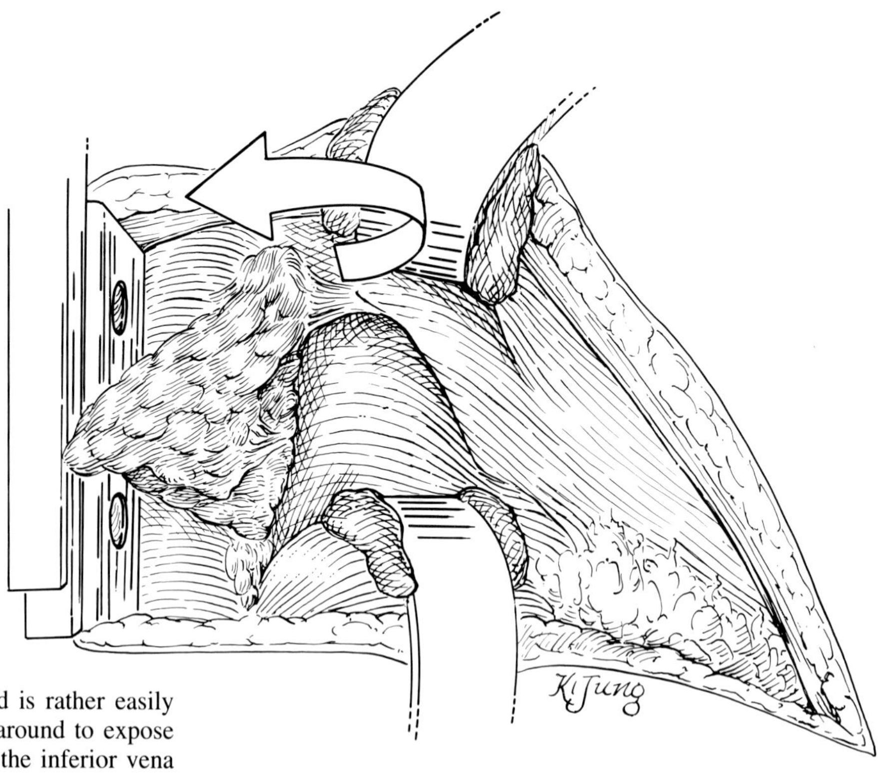

Figure 6.8. The lateral aspect of the gland is rather easily freed up, and the dissection is then carried around to expose the anterior surface medially to the level of the inferior vena cava. The inferior surface of the gland is separated from the upper pole of the kidney, keeping the dissection close to the renal capsule and fulgurating the small vessels that sometimes course between these two structures.

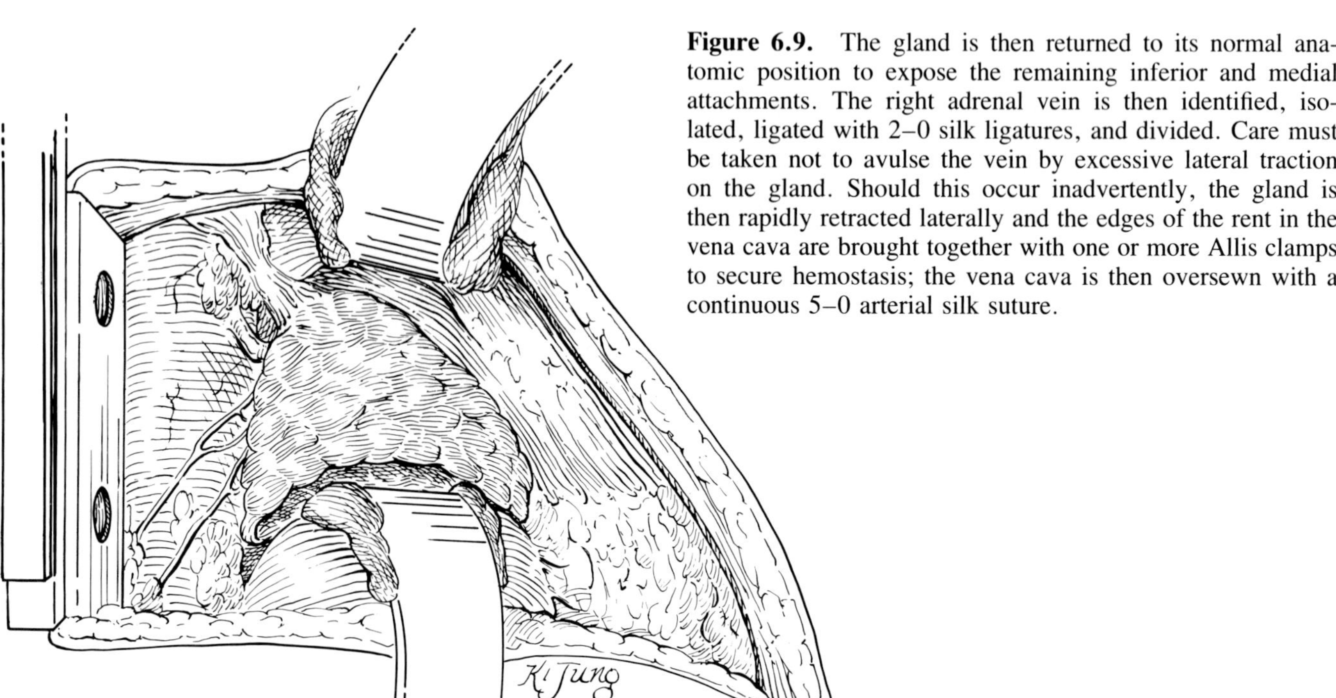

Figure 6.9. The gland is then returned to its normal anatomic position to expose the remaining inferior and medial attachments. The right adrenal vein is then identified, isolated, ligated with 2–0 silk ligatures, and divided. Care must be taken not to avulse the vein by excessive lateral traction on the gland. Should this occur inadvertently, the gland is then rapidly retracted laterally and the edges of the rent in the vena cava are brought together with one or more Allis clamps to secure hemostasis; the vena cava is then oversewn with a continuous 5–0 arterial silk suture.

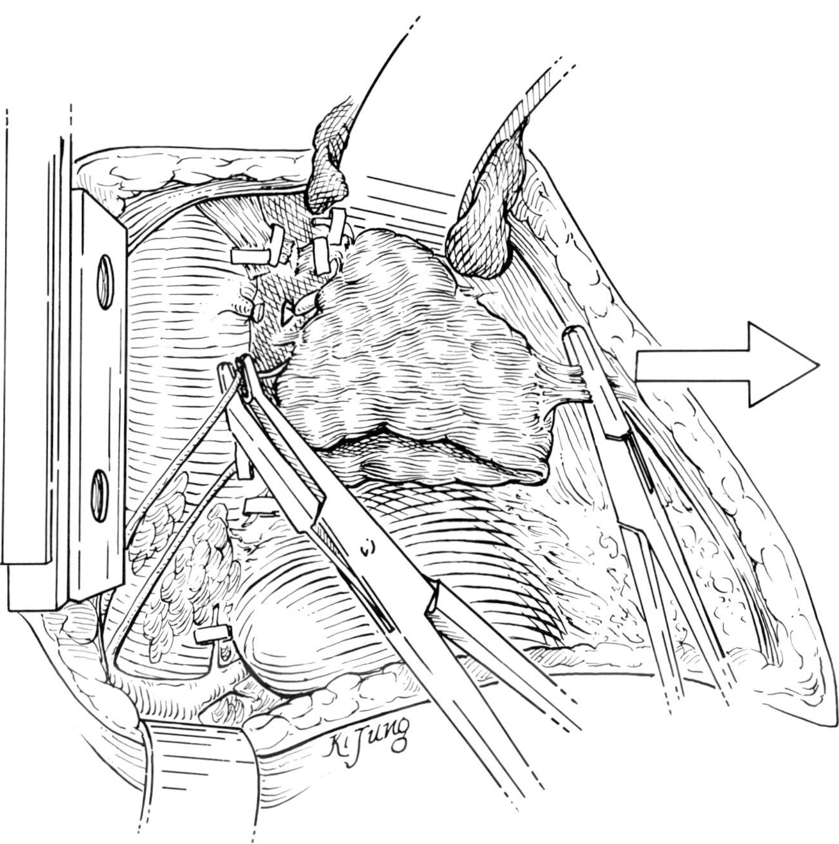

Figure 6.10. Following division of the adrenal vein, the gland is gently retracted laterally to expose the remaining inferior and medial arterial supply from the right renal artery and aorta, respectively. These remaining vascular attachments are divided between silver clips to complete removal of the right adrenal gland.

When adrenalectomy is completed, final hemostasis is achieved by electrocoagulation and the operative field is then irrigated with neomycin solution. To close the transthoracic incision, the diaphragm is reapproximated with interrupted 2–0 silk mattress sutures. Airtight closure of the plaura is achieved using 3–0 silk or chromic sutures with the lung under positive-pressure expansion. The pleural closure is facilitated by incorporation of the periosteum in the suture. Chest tube drainage is generally not necessary unless there has been difficulty in reapproximating the pleura; in this event, a multi-eyed catheter connected to water-sealed suction may be left indwelling for 24–48 hr postoperatively. No surgical drains are used. A chest x-ray is obtained several hours postoperatively in the recovery room to verify that the lung is fully expanded. Incisional discomfort with this approach is mild and ambulation is generally possible on the day after surgery.

Suggested Readings

Glenn JF: Current concepts of adrenal surgery. *Int Surg* 48:121, 1967.

Howards SS, Carey RM: The adrenals. In Gillenwater JY, Grayhack JT, Howards SS, Duckett JW (eds): *Adult and Pediatric Urology*. Chicago, Year Book, 1987.

Lachman E: A comparison of the posterior boundaries of lungs and pleura as demonstrated on the cadaver and on the roentgenogram of the living. *Anat Rec* 83:521, 1947.

McDougal WS: Surgery of the adrenal. In Dudley H, Carter D (eds): *Operative Surgery*. London, Butterworths, 1986.

Nesbit RM: Primary aldosteronism: Its diagnosis and surgical management. *J Urol* 97:404, 1967.

Rhamy RK: Cushing's syndrome. In Glenn JR (ed): *Urologic Surgery*. Philadelphia, JB Lippincott, 1983.

Young HH: A technique for simultaneous exposure and operation on the adrenals. *Surg Gynecol Obstet* 54:179, 1936.

CHAPTER 7

Anterior Approach to the Adrenal Gland

ANDREW C. NOVICK
BRUCE H. STEWART

In performing adrenal surgery, the anterior transperitoneal approach is preferable for adrenal lesions that are either large or potentially malignant. In such cases, wide exposure is necessary that cannot be achieved to the same extent through a posterior or flank incision. With potentially malignant adrenal masses, intraabdominal inspection of other organs for metastatic disease is required. An anterior approach is mandatory in patients with pheochromocytoma, where early vascular control is necessary and to allow exploration for bilateral or extraadrenal tumors. The optimum anterior approach is through a bilateral subcostal or ''Chevron'' incision, which provides much better exposure of the superior and lateral aspects of the adrenal gland than a midline incision. A vertical midline incision is used only if an extraadrenal pheochromocytoma is suspected in the retroperitoneal organs of Zuckerkandl or in the pelvis. The anterior approach is described below separately for the left and right adrenal glands.

ANTERIOR APPROACH TO LEFT ADRENAL GLAND

Figure 7.1. A bilateral or extended left subcostal incision is performed. After the peritoneal cavity is entered and explored, the posterior peritoneum lateral to the left colon is incised vertically and the incision is carried upward to divide the lienorenal ligament. Care must be taken to avoid tearing the delicate capsule of the spleen.

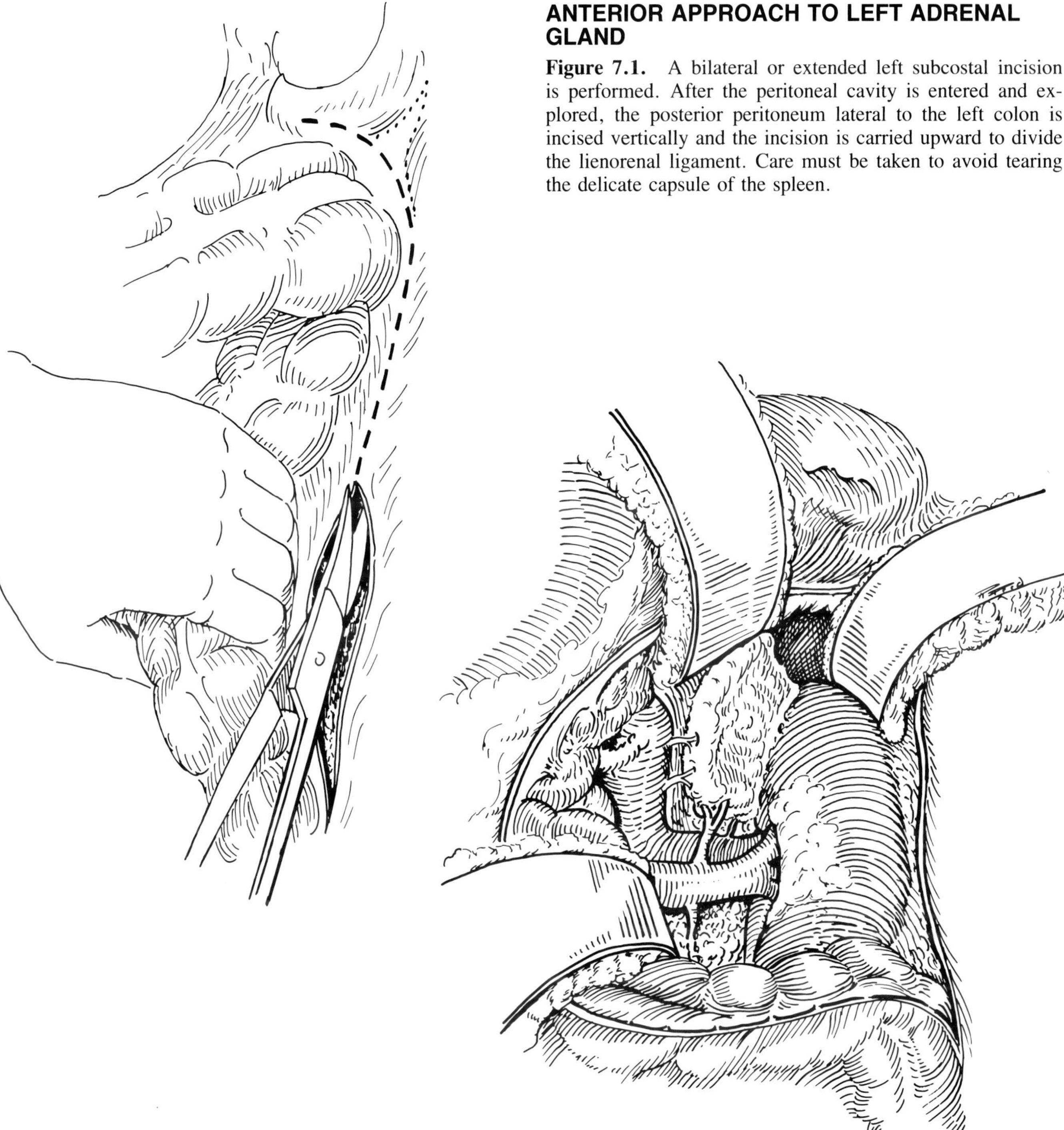

Figure 7.2. The plane between the kidney and adrenal gland posteriorly, and the pancreas and spleen anteriorly, is developed by blunt dissection. The left colon and duodenum are reflected medially, and the pancreas and spleen are reflected cephalad, with care taken not to injure the spleen or the pancreas. When adequate exposure of the adrenal gland has been obtained, a self-retaining ring retractor is inserted to maintain the operative field.

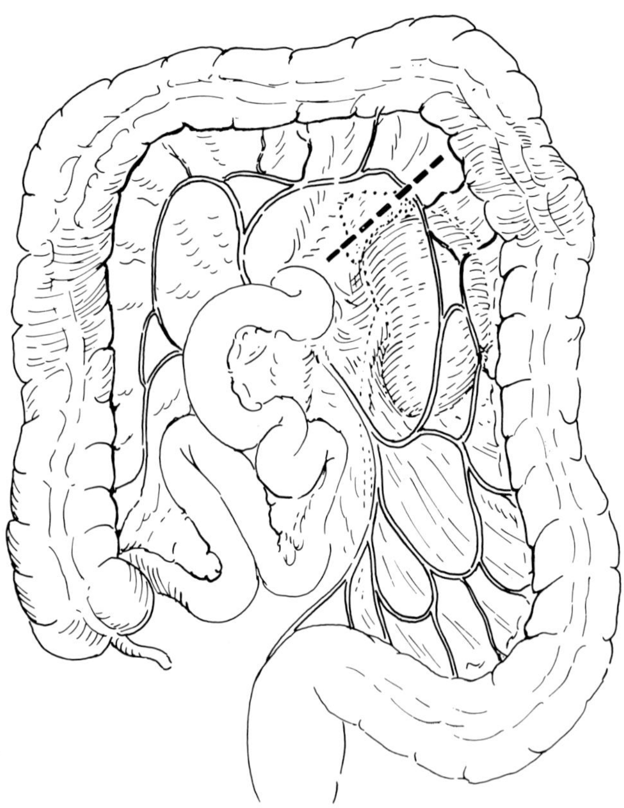

Figure 7.3. In slender patients and where the adrenal pathology is located anteriorly, the gland may be exposed by simple incision of the left mesocolon as shown. The small intestines are reflected to the right, and the stomach and spleen are reflected upward to expose the splenic flexure of the colon and its mesentery. The mesocolon is incised obliquely over the area of the left adrenal gland, transecting the arcuate vessels but preserving the major branches of the middle and left colic arteries.

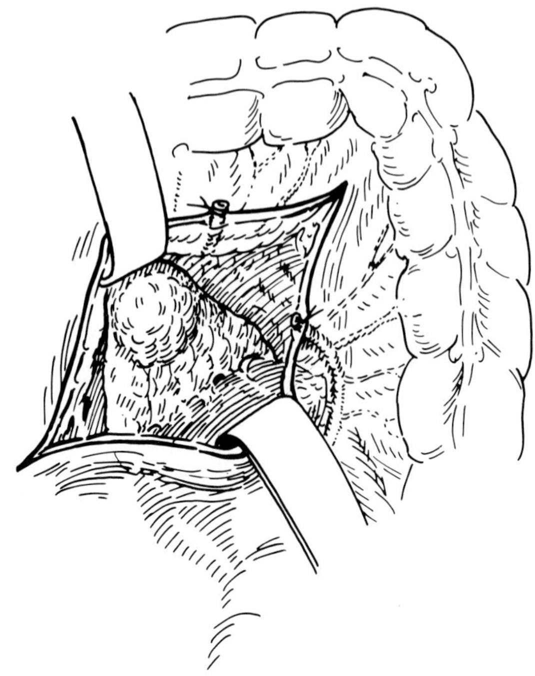

Figure 7.4. The leaves of the mesentery are retracted gently to expose the anterior surface of the adrenal gland, the upper pole of the left kidney, and the left renal and adrenal veins. Care must be taken not to extend the incision into the wall of the left colon or to injure it by excessive retraction. The exposure through this approach is quite limited and this should only be considered in a slender patient with a very small adrenal lesion.

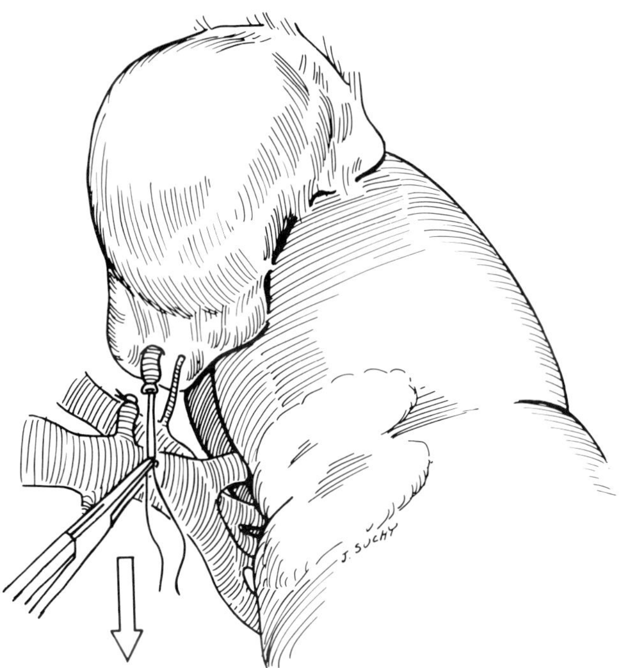

Figure 7.5. After gaining proper exposure of the left adrenal gland, the left adrenal vein is identified at its entry into the left renal vein. The adrenal vein is then ligated with 2–0 silk ligatures and divided. It is particularly important for this to be done initially in patients with pheochromocytoma to interrupt catecholamine release from the tumor into the systemic circulation. The ligature on the upper stump of the adrenal vein may be left long to serve as a retractor during subsequent dissection. The inferior adrenal artery is also secured and divided at this time.

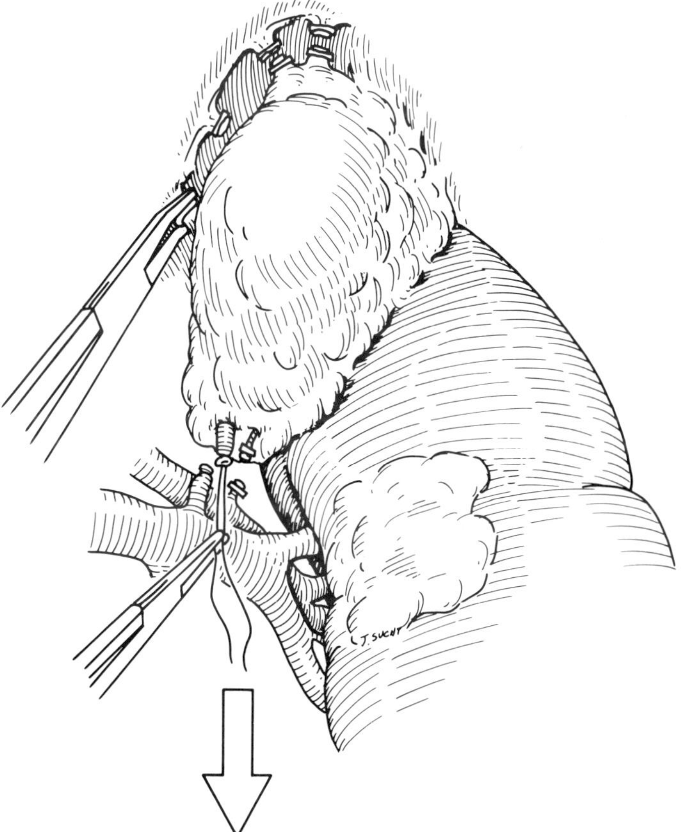

Figure 7.6. The adrenal gland is gently mobilized posteriorly and laterally by blunt dissection. The gland is then retracted downward to expose the superior vascular ligaments that are secured between silver clips and divided.

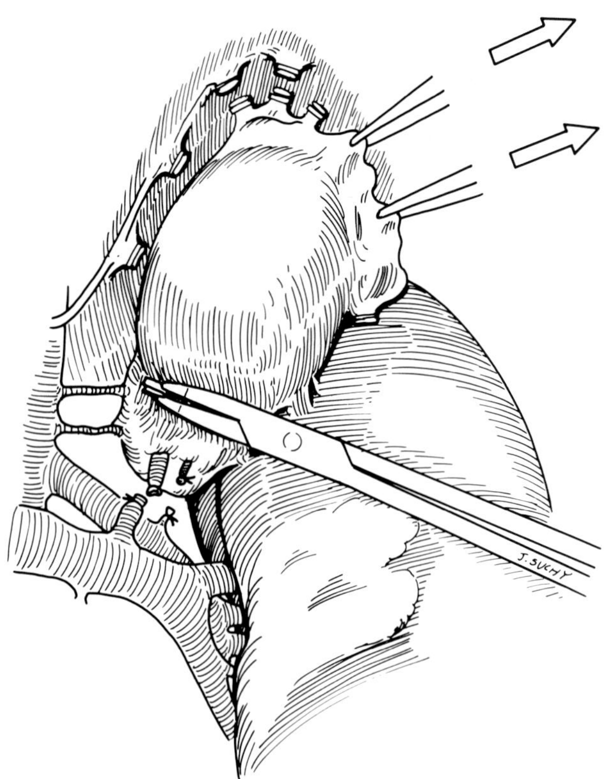

Figure 7.7. The gland is then retracted laterally to expose the remaining middle arterial blood supply and medial lymphatic vessels that are transected between silver clips. And residual attachments of the gland to the upper pole of the kidney are divided by sharp dissection, following the plane of the renal capsule and securing small perforating vessels by electrocautery.

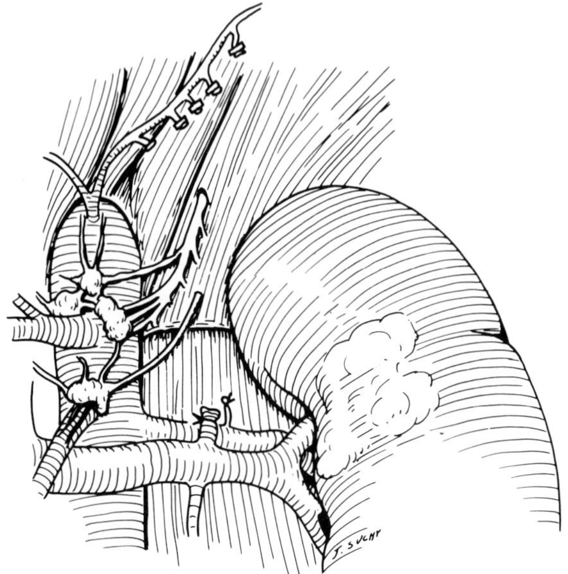

Figure 7.8. After removal of the left adrenal gland, if there is any suspicion of malignancy, a regional lymphadenectomy is performed from the level of the renal vessels up to the crus of the diaphragm. Celiac ganglia and splanchnic nerves are shown here preserved, but may be resected if anatomic circumstances require it.

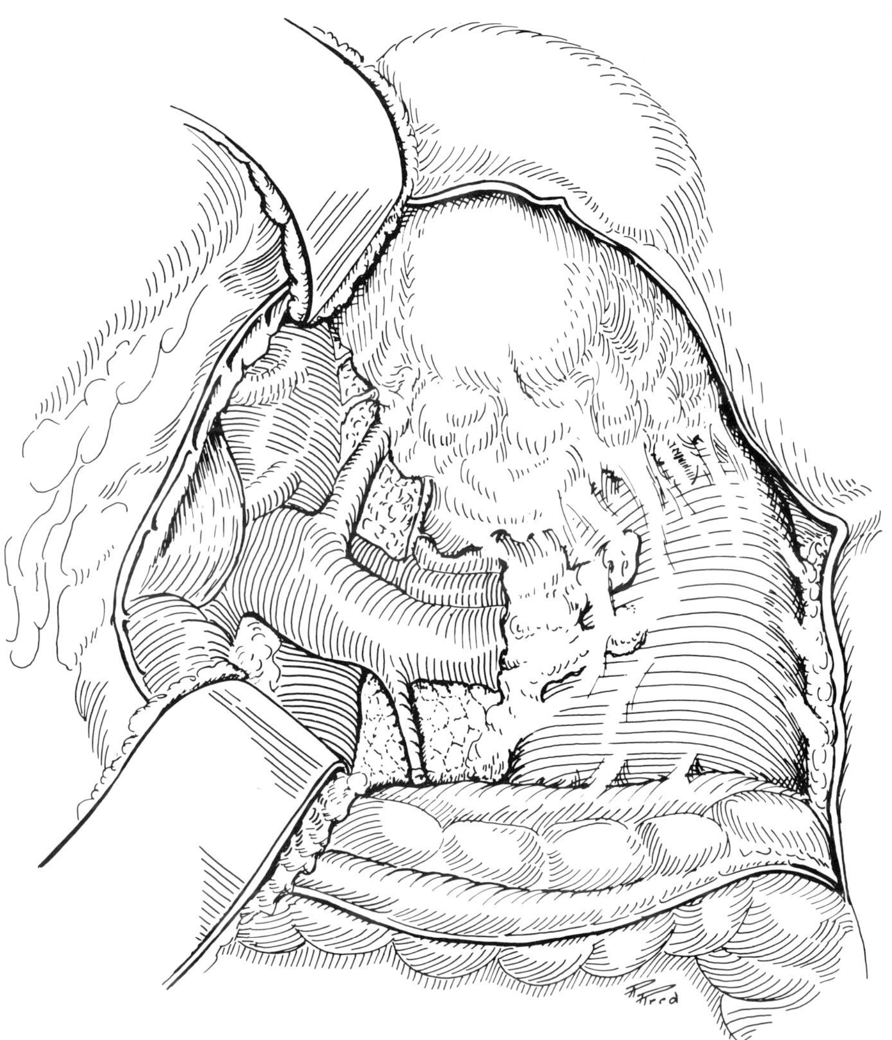

Figure 7.9. In some cases, an adrenal malignancy may actually invade the capsule of the upper pole of the kidney. In such patients, radical en bloc removal of both the kidney and adrenal gland within Gerota's fascia is the procedure of choice. The left colon is widely mobilized medially, as previously described, with the spleen and pancreas retracted upward to expose the mass. The spleen or tail of the pancreas may be involved by the mass and, if so, it may be necessary to perform splenectomy and/or distal pancreatectomy en bloc with the tumor mass.

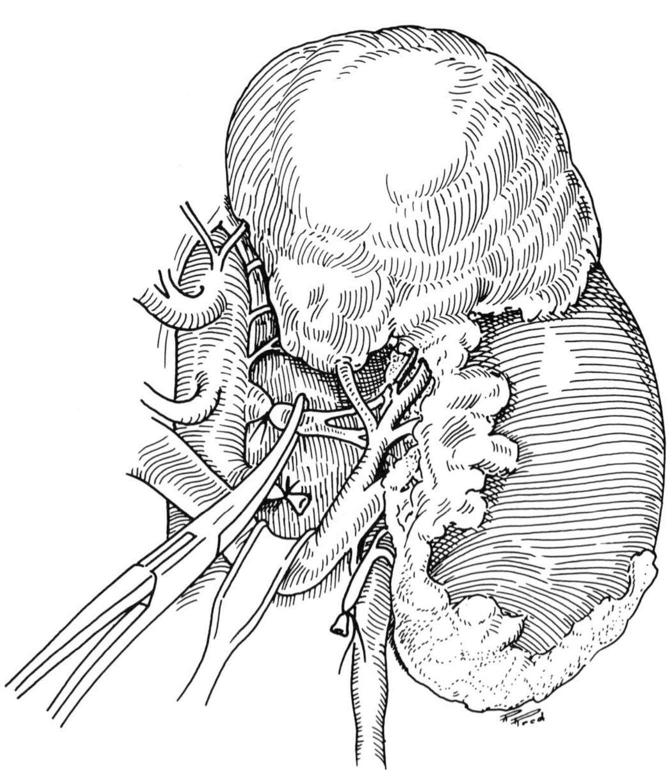

Figure 7.10. The aorta is first exposed just below the left renal vein and the dissection is carried upward to identify the origin of the renal artery. Occasionally, multiple renal arteries are present as shown here. The main renal arterial supply is secured with 0 silk ligatures and is then divided.

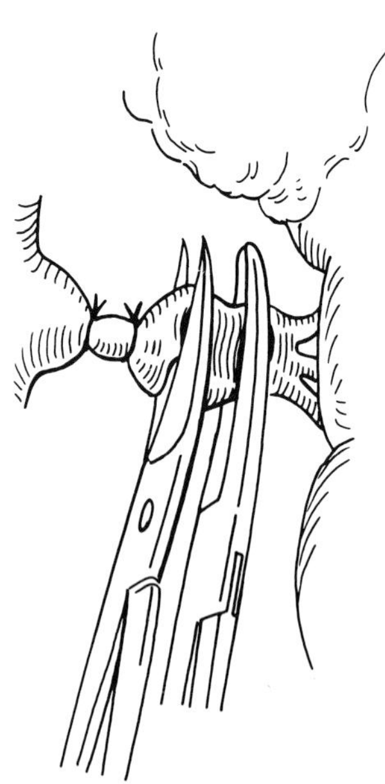

Figure 7.11. After division of the renal artery, the left renal vein is transected between hemostats and doubly ligated with 2–0 silk sutures. This must be done at a level medial to entry of the adrenal, gonadal, and lumbar veins into the main renal vein.

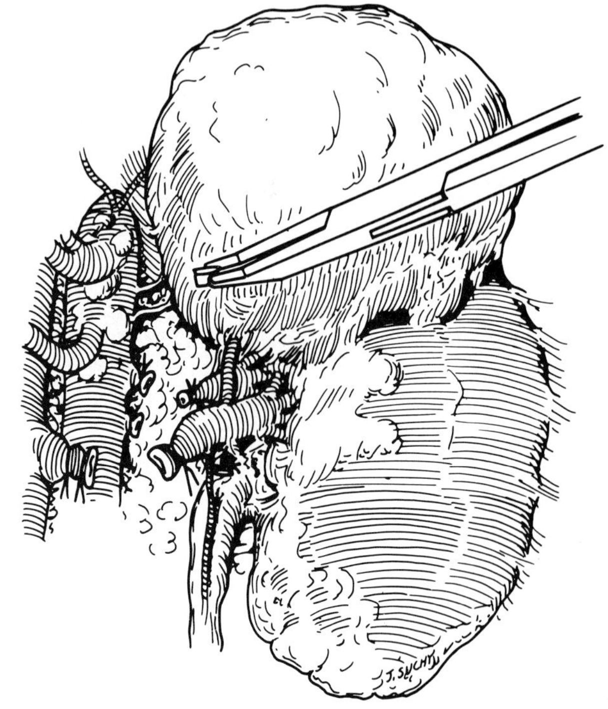

Figure 7.12. Utilizing the kidney as a handle, and exerting downward and lateral traction, the medial blood supply of the adrenal tumor can be better identified and secured as the vessels emerge from the lateral surface of the aorta. Larger arteries should be secured with ligatures or silver clips, whereas electrocautery is sufficient for smaller vessels. Care is taken to avoid injury to the superior mesenteric artery and pancreas.

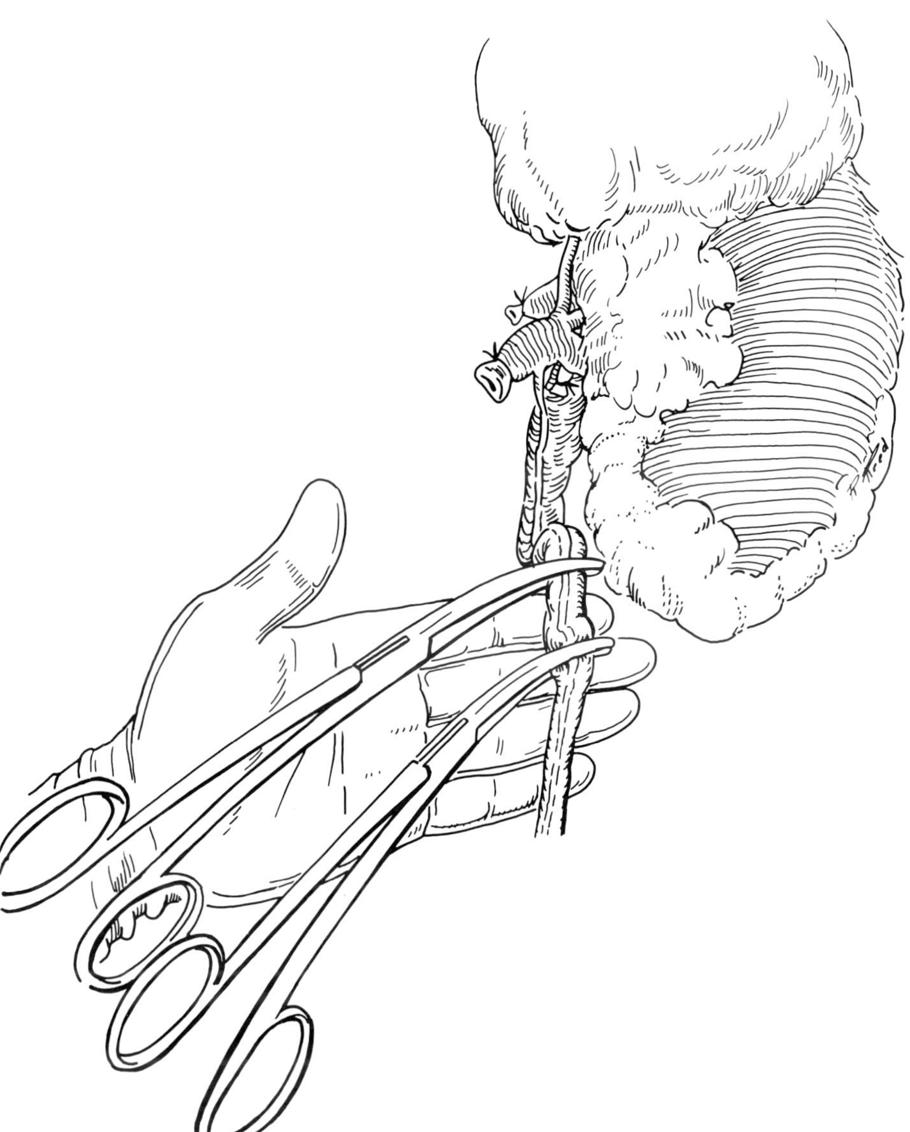

Figure 7.13. Attention is then redirected downward to expose the left ureter and gonadal vein, which are divided between hemostats and ligated. This maneuver can be done just as well as the initial step in the operation, at the discretion of the surgeon.

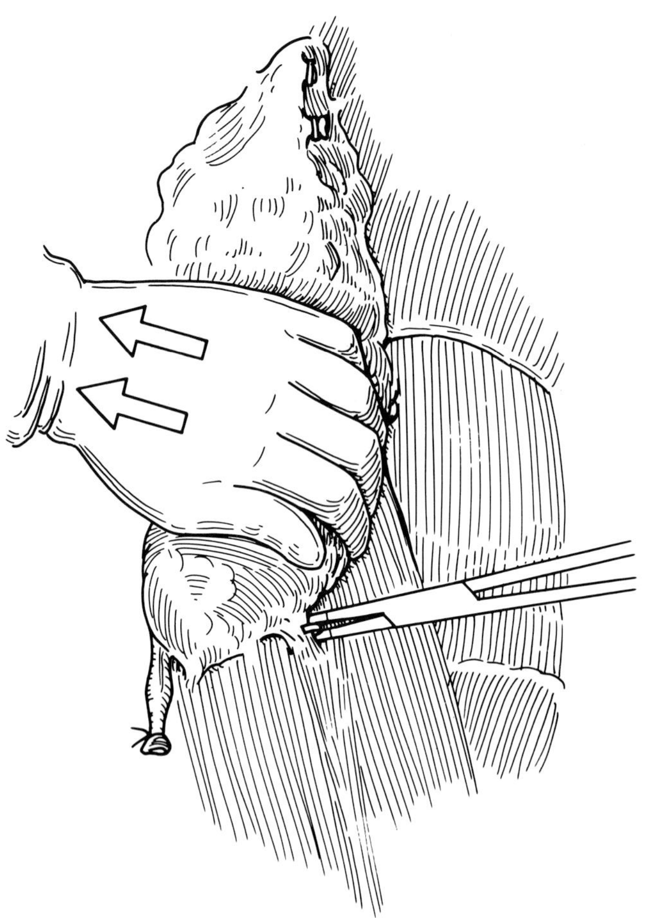

Figure 7.14. A plane is then developed posteriorly along the psoas fascia, bluntly mobilizing both the kidney and adrenal mass from behind and laterally, and dividing small collateral vessels between silver clips as they are encountered.

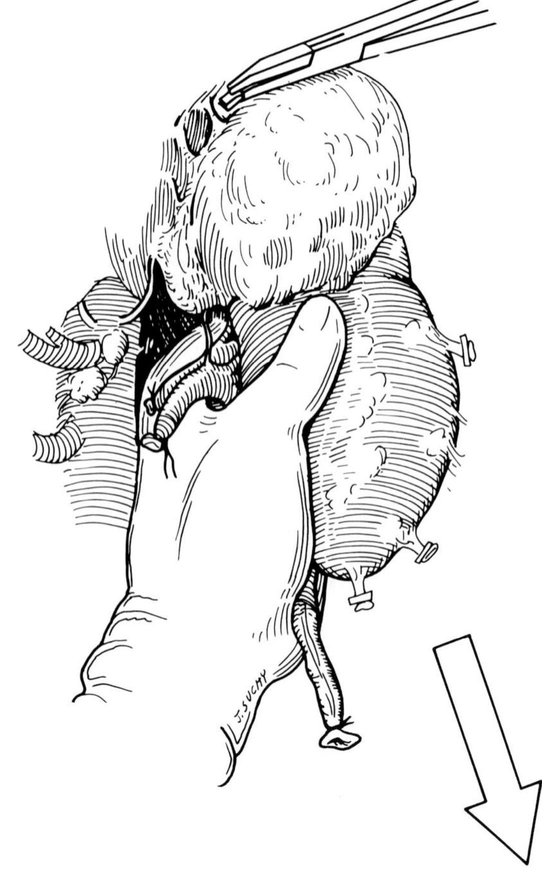

Figure 7.15. Using the ureter and kidney as a handle, the mass is retracted downward so that the upper vascular attachments may be visualized, secured, and divided. The mass is now attached by only a few vessels and lymphatics superiorly and medially, which are divided between silver clips to complete en bloc excision of the kidney and adrenal gland. A regional lymphadenectomy is then performed from the level of the inferior messenteric artery to the crus of the diaphragm. Splanchnic nerves and celiac ganglia may be sacrificed if adjacent nodes appear involved by neoplasm.

ANTERIOR APPROACH TO THE RIGHT ADRENAL GLAND

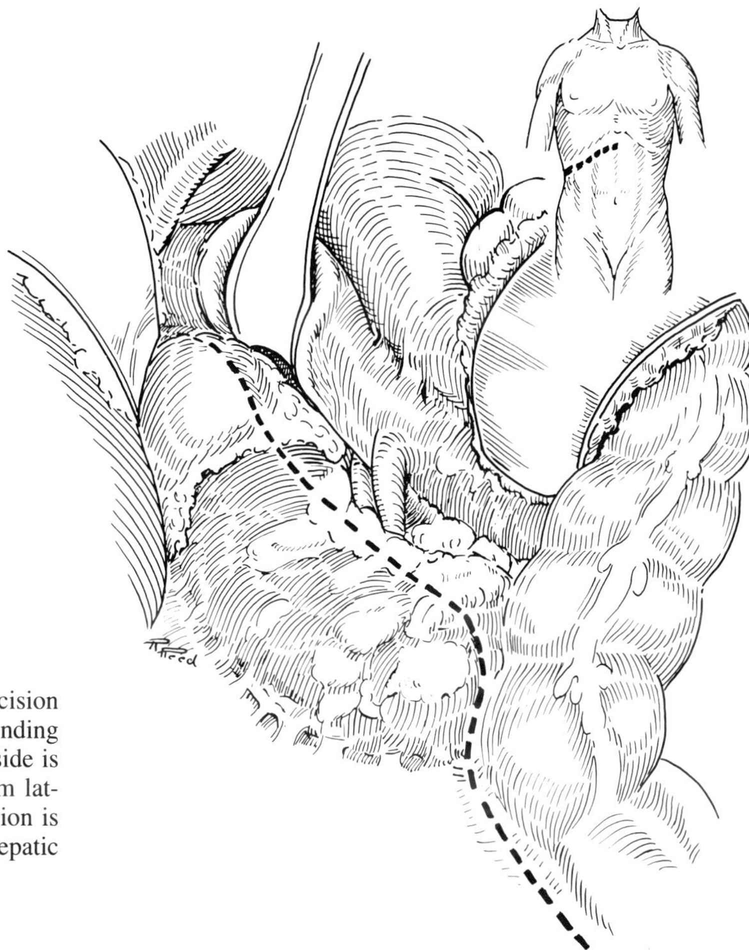

Figure 7.16. In a slender patient, a right subcostal incision is made as shown here. In most patients, however, extending the incision partially or completely across the opposite side is necessary for proper exposure. The posterior peritoneum lateral to the right colon is incised vertically and the incision is carried high up along the vena cava to the level of the hepatic veins.

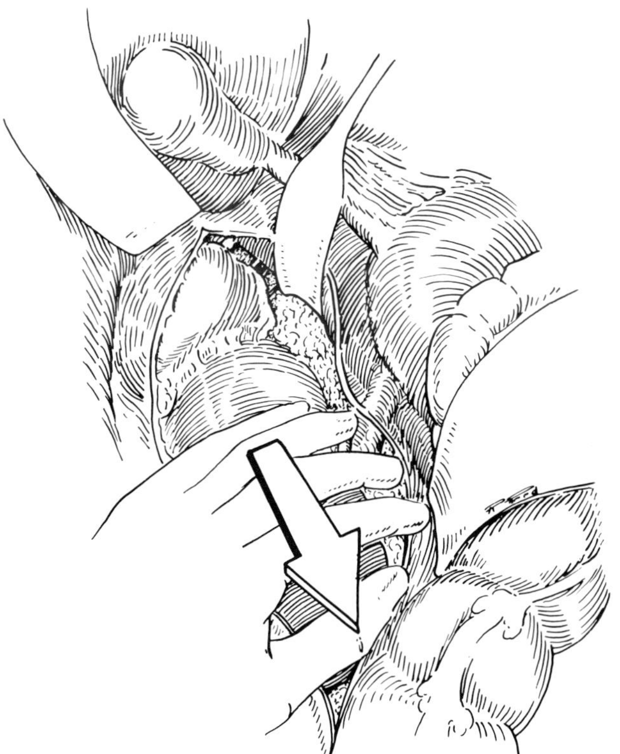

Figure 7.17. The right colon and duodenum are reflected medially, and the liver and gallbladder are retracted upward. The kidney is gently retracted downward to bring the anterior surface of the right adrenal gland into view. Care is taken to avoid trauma to the delicate hepatic veins, which may enter the vena cava at this level. When adequate exposure of the adrenal gland is obtained, a self-retaining ring retractor is inserted to maintain the operative field.

Figure 7.18. In cases of pheochromocytoma or suspected malignancy, it is best to isolate the blood supply first and carry out the lateral dissection later. Especially in cases of pheochromocytoma, it is important to secure the adrenal vein with silver clips or ligatures as soon as possible, before excessive manipulation of the gland. If the vein lies far cephalad, as it often does, rather extensive division of the arterial supply medially and inferiorly may be necessary before the vein can be exposed satisfactorily and safely. Surgical exposure is facilitated by medial retraction of the inferior vena cava. When the tumor is confined to the adrenal gland, after the blood supply has been secured, the remaining lateral and inferior attachments of the gland are readily mobilized and divided to complete the adrenalectomy.

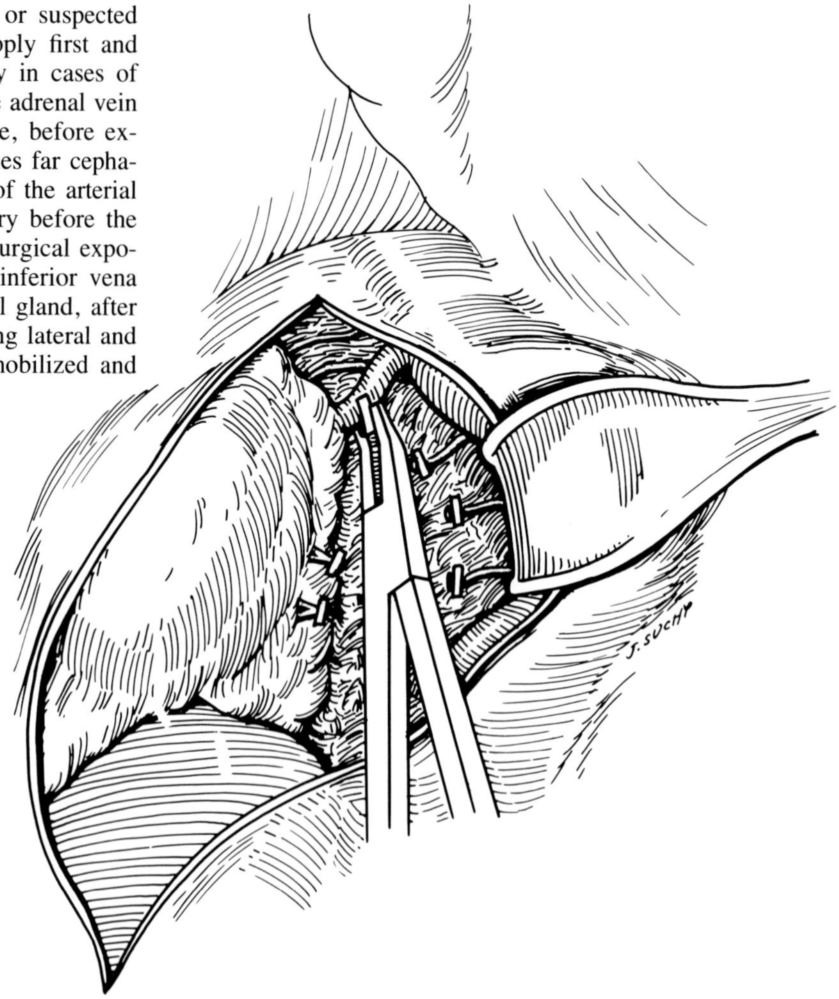

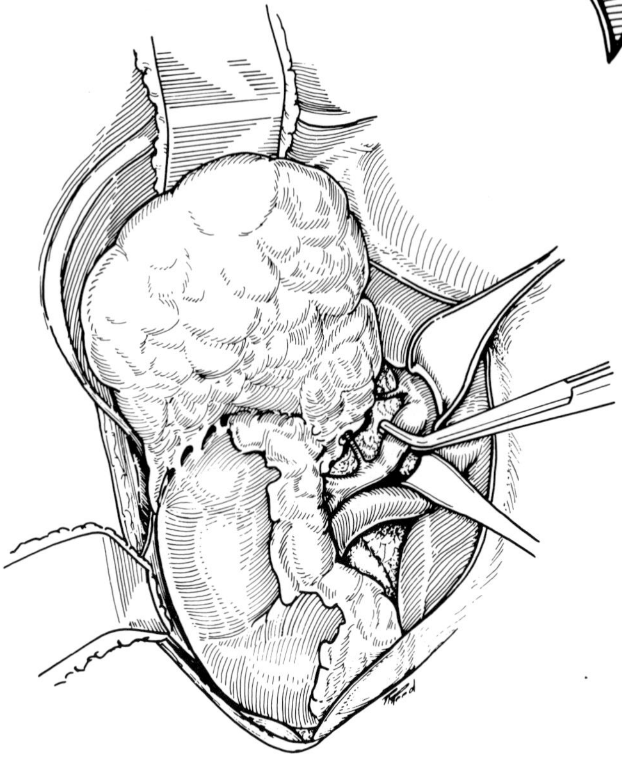

Figure 7.19 With malignant right adrenal tumors that invade the upper portion of the kidney, nephroadrenalectomy is the procedure of choice. Here, the right colon and duodenum have been retracted medially and the liver upward to gain maximum exposure of the tumor mass and right kidney. The vena cava and renal vein are retracted medially and downward to expose the right renal artery, which is transected between hemostats and doubly ligated with 0 silk as the first step in the procedure.

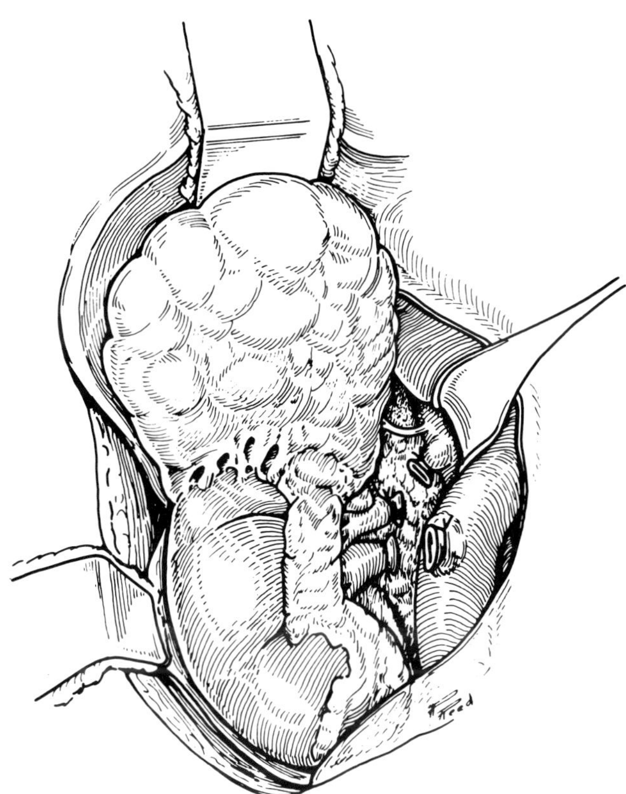

Figure 7.20. The right renal vein and ureter are next secured with 2–0 silk ligatures and divided. With downward and lateral retraction upon the kidney, the medial blood supply to the tumor mass can be better identified. The middle adrenal arteries are transected between silver clips or secured with electrocautery as they emerge from beneath the vena cava. Their exposure is faciliated by medial retraction of the vena cava.

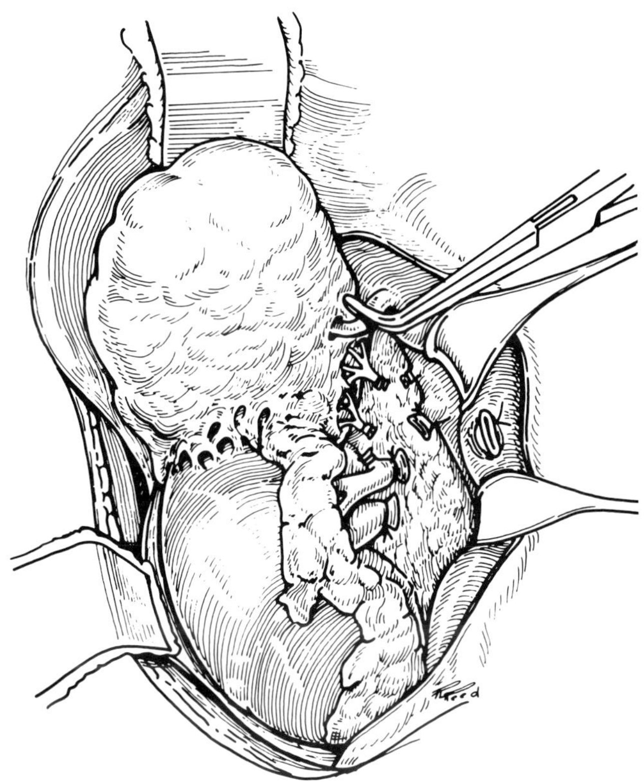

Figure 7.21. As the dissection proceeds upward, the adrenal vein is identified, secured with silver clips or hemostats, and divided. This vein is large, friable, frequently lies higher than the surgeon expects, and must be carefully dissected free from surrounding structures to avoid avulsion from the vena cava. Should such an avulsion occur, the caval entry is immediately secured with Allis clamps and the defect is oversewn with a continuous 5–0 arterial silk suture. After division of the adrenal vein, the dissection is carried upward and laterally to remove completely the tumor mass and kidney en bloc within Gerota's fascia.

Suggested Readings

Bodie B, Novick AC, Pontes JE, et al: The Cleveland Clinic experience with adrenal cortical carcinoma. *J Urol* (in press), 1989.

Cerny JC: Anatomy of the adrenal gland. *Urol Clin North Am* 4:169, 1977.

Dluhy RC, Gittes RF: The adrenals. In Walsh PC, Gittes RF, Perlmutter AD, Stamey TA (eds): *Campbell's Urology,* 5th ed. Philadelphia, WB Saunders, 1986.

Gonzalez-Serva L, Glenn JF: Adrenal surgical techniques. *Urol Clin North Am* 4:327, 1977.

Howards SS, Carey RM: The adrenals. In Gillenwater JY, Grayhack JT, Howards SS, Duckett JW (eds): *Adult and Pediatric Urology.* Chicago, Year Book, 1987.

McDougal WS: Surgery of the adrenal. In Dudley H, Carter D (eds): *Operative Surgery.* London, Butterworths, 1986.

Rhamy RK: Cushing's syndrome. In Glenn JF (ed): *Urologic Surgery,* 3rd ed. Philadelphia, JB Lippincott, 1983.

CHAPTER 8

Flank and Thoracoabdominal Approaches to the Adrenal Gland

ANDREW C. NOVICK
BRUCE H. STEWART

FLANK APPROACH TO THE ADRENAL GLAND

In our practice, unilateral exposure of the adrenal gland by the flank approach is rarely indicated. For patients with a relatively small benign tumor confined to one adrenal gland, we have found that the posterior surgical approach (described in chapter 6) is preferable. The latter is a more direct approach to the adrenal gland, provides superior exposure, and is better tolerated since no major muscles are transected. Nevertheless, in particularly obese patients, exposure of the adrenal gland through a posterior incision may be compromised. In such cases, the use of a generous flank incision may be preferable for performing adrenalectomy. Either the 12th or 11th rib is resected to enter the retroperitoneal space through a flank incision, as described in chapter 2.

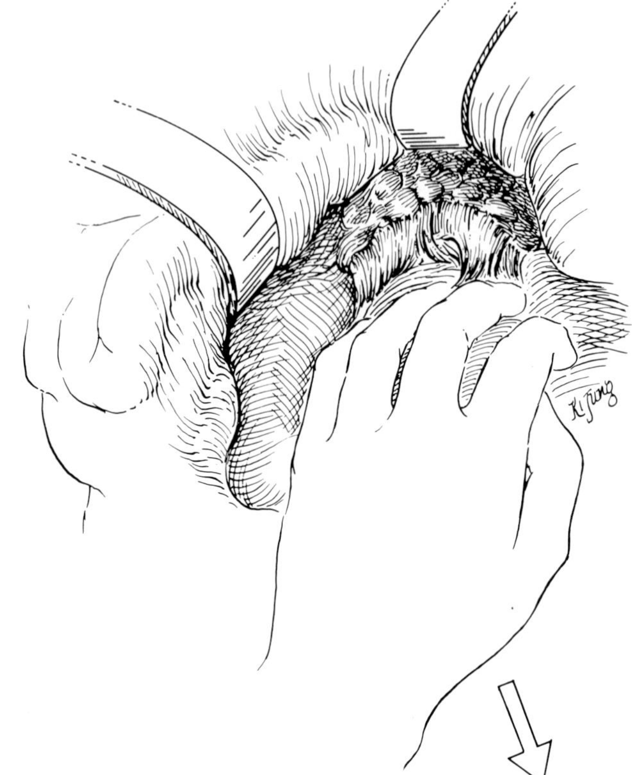

Figure 8.1. On the left side, the colon is reflected medially and the pancreas upward to expose the lateral and anterior surfaces of the kidney, which is then retracted downward to better expose the left adrenal gland.

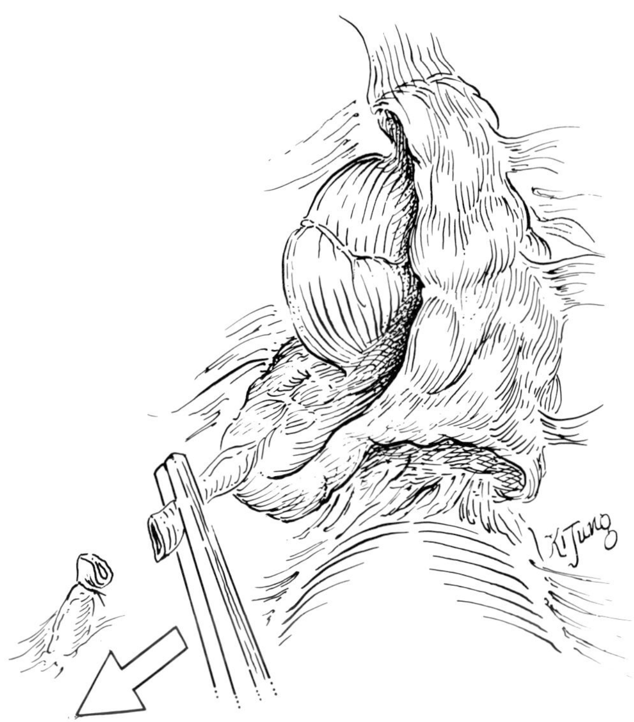

Figure 8.2. The adrenal gland is gently mobilized anteriorly and posteriorly in the avascular planes between the pancreas and paraspinous muscles, respectively. As the dissection is carried medially, the entry of the left adrenal vein into the renal vein is identified, at the level of the lateral aortic wall, which serves as a useful palpable landmark. The adrenal vein is then transected between hemostats and the proximal adrenal venous stump used as a handle to bring the adrenal gland further into the operative field.

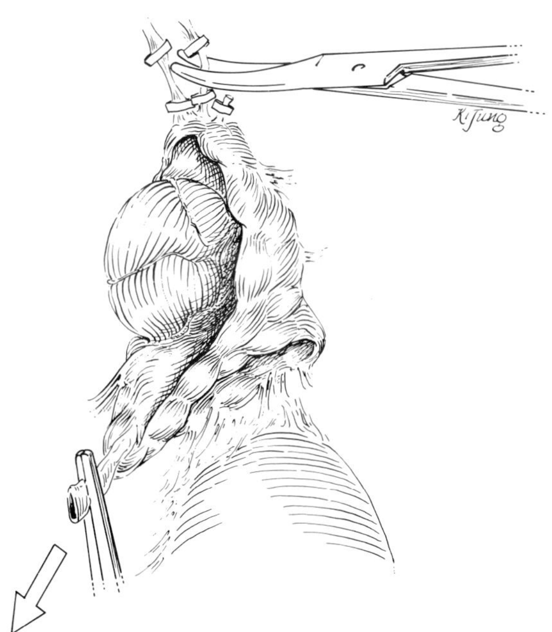

Figure 8.3. With downward traction, the apical vascular ligaments arising from the inferior phrenic artery are identified, secured with silver clips, and divided.

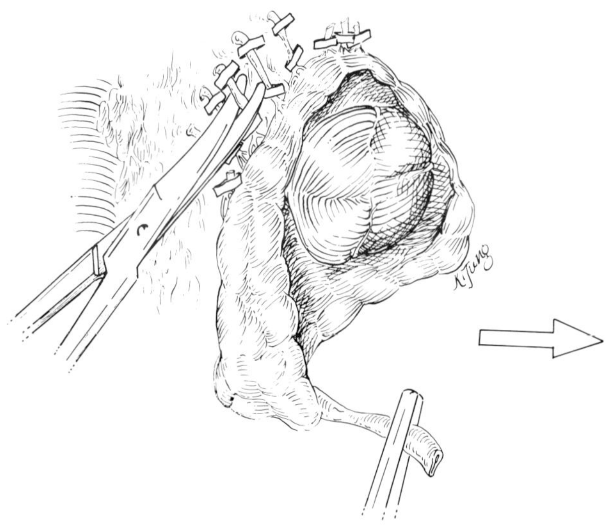

Figure 8.4. By further retracting the gland outward and laterally, arterial and lymphatic vessels arising medially from the aorta are identified and transected between silver clips to complete the adrenalectomy.

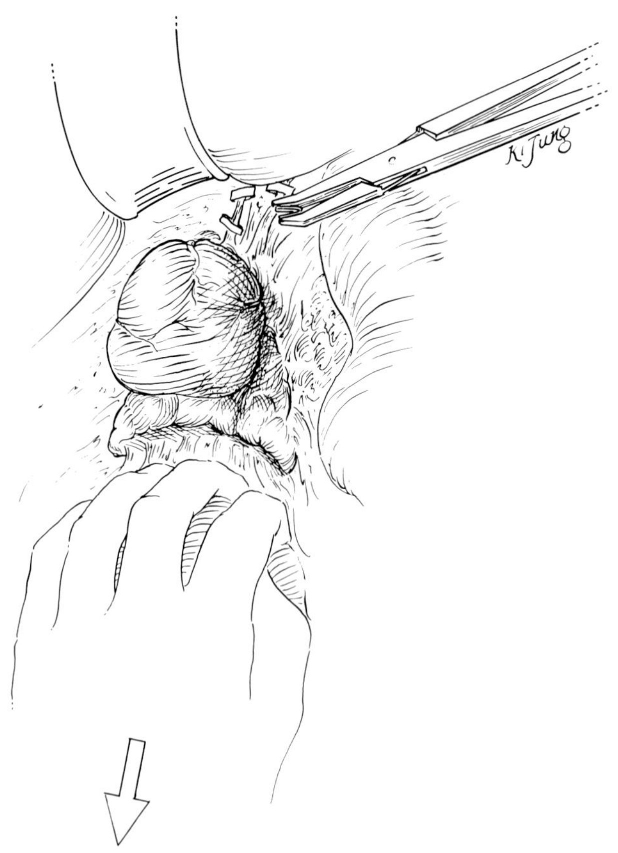

Figure 8.5. On the right side, the colon and duodenum are reflected medially and the liver is reflected upward to expose the kidney and adrenal gland. The kidney with its attached adrenal gland is retracted downward. The anterior, posterior, and apical aspects are obilized by blunt dissection from the undersurface of the liver posteriorly and from the duodenum and hepatic flexure of the colon anteriorly. The apical attachments of the gland are then divided between silver clips.

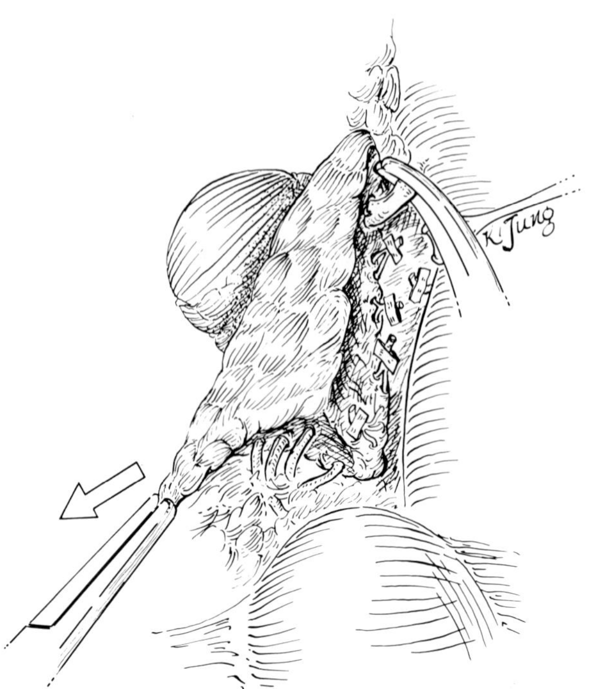

Figure 8.6. With the gland retracted laterally, small arterial branches entering the medial aspect of the gland are identified as they course beneath the vena cava. Branches of the inferior adrenal artery coursing upward from the proximal right renal artery are similarly identified. After securing and transecting these vessels, the right adrenal vein is brought into view. The adrenal vein is then clamped, divided, and secured with ligatures or clips. Any residual apical vascular branches are then similarly secured and transected to complete the adrenalectomy.

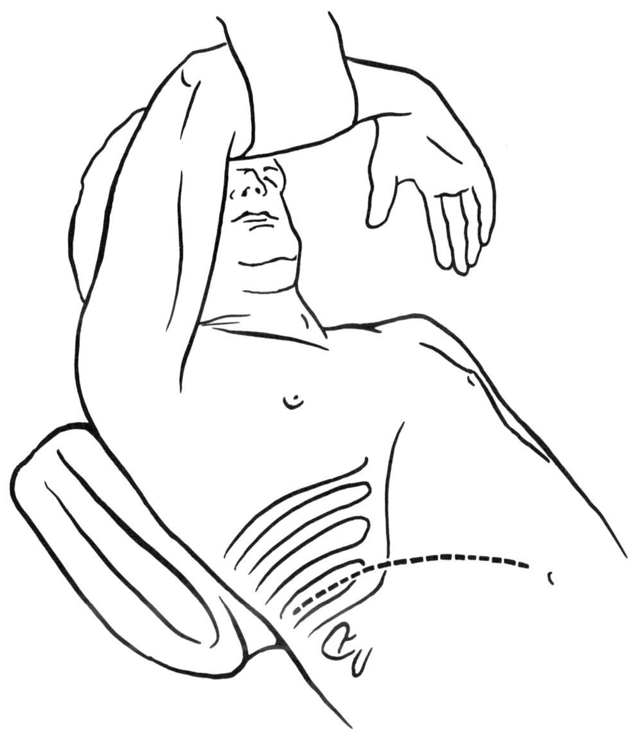

Figure 8.7. In this discussion, the thoracoabdominal incision is depicted on the right side; however, the approach is similar on the left side. The patient is placed in a semioblique position with a rolled sheet placed longitudinally beneath the flank and hemithorax. The incision is begun in the 8th or 9th intercostal space near the angle of the rib and is carried across the costal margin to the midpoint of the opposite rectus muscle above the umbilicus.

THORACOABDOMINAL APPROACH TO THE ADRENAL GLAND

The thoracoabdominal approach is desirable for very large adrenal tumors, particularly on the right side where the liver and its venous drainage into the upper vena cava can limit exposure and impair vascular control as the tumor mass is being removed. There is generally less need for thoracoabdominal exposure on the left side, since there is very little vascularity involving the superior, lateral, and posterior aspects of the tumor mass, and the spleen and pancreas can usually be elevated easily away from the tumor mass. The thoracoabdominal incision provides outstanding exposure of the suprarenal area. Nevertheless, since it involves additional operative time and perhaps greater potential pulmonary morbidity, this approach is reserved for patients in whom the additional exposure over that provided by an anterior subcostal incision is considered important to achieve complete tumor excision.

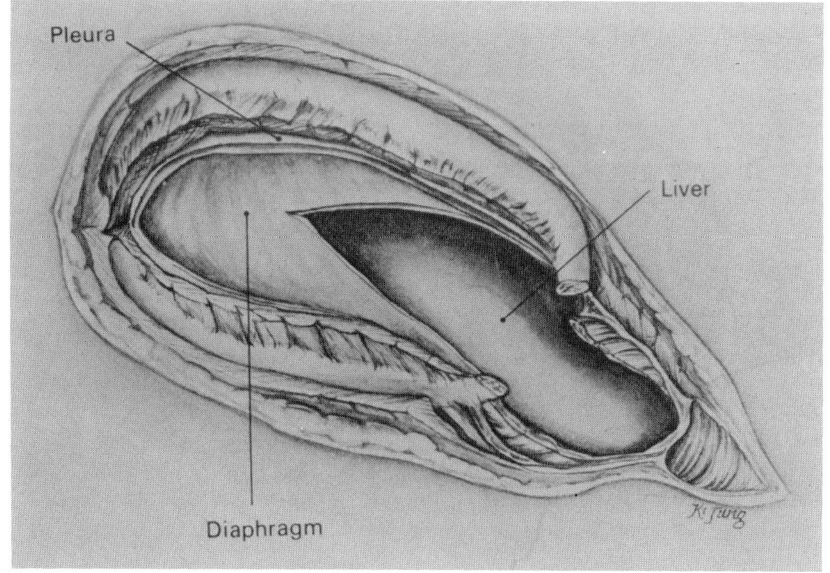

Figure 8.8. It is tempting at this point to incise longitudinally across the dome of the diaphragm to expose the liver, as depicted here. However, this diaphragmatic incision cuts across major branches of the phrenic nerve and can cause undesirable postoperative complications. This illustration demonstrates the *incorrect* method of incising the diaphragm when performing a thoracoabdominal incision.

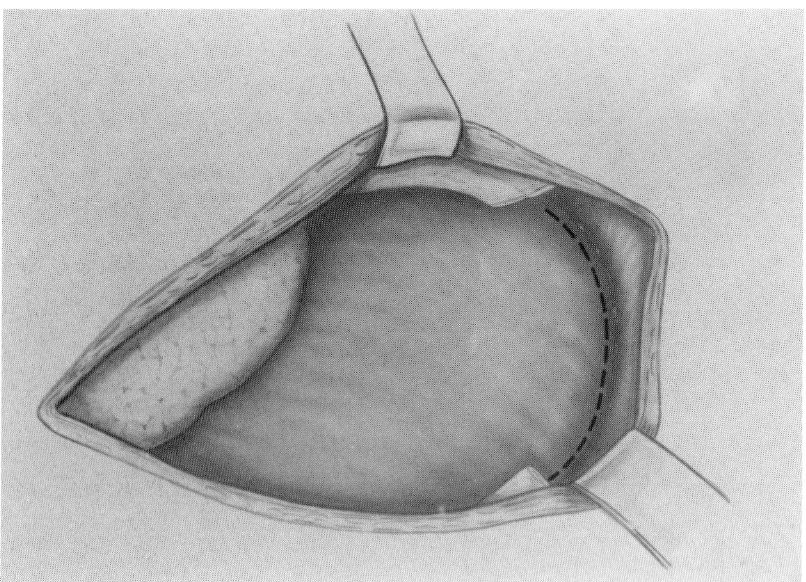

Figure 8.9. The preferred diaphragmatic incision is begun by incising the periphery of the diaphragm about 2 cm inside its attachment to the chest wall, with the incision then being carried around circumferentially to the posterior aspect of the diaphragm. In doing this, there must be at least 2 or 3 cm of diaphragm left attached to the rib cage to allow later reconstruction.

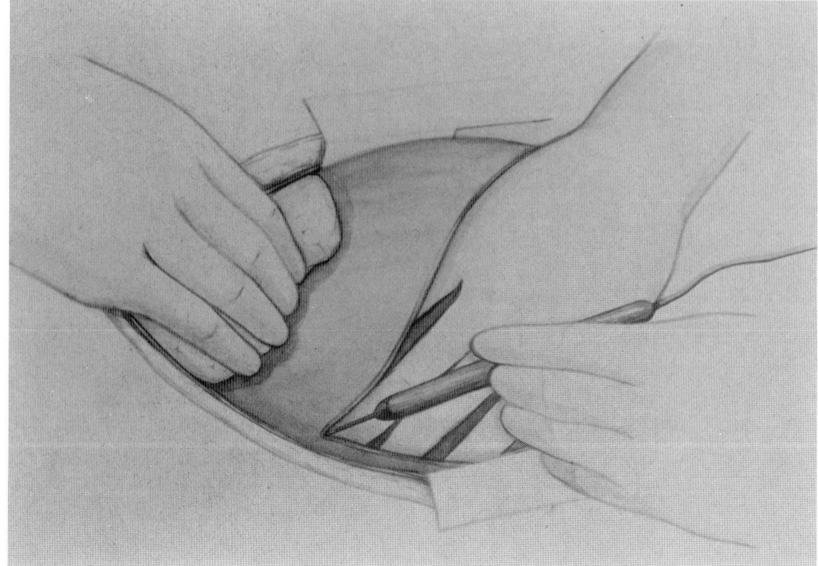

Figure 8.10. By dividing the diaphragm in a circumferential manner from anterior to posterior, damage to the phrenic nerve supply is avoided. This also creates a diaphragmatic flap, which can be pushed into the chest to provide complete exposure of the liver, which is then simply retracted upward. If further mobilization of the liver is needed, the right triangular ligament and coronary ligament can be incised to mobilize the entire right lobe of the liver upward. This provides excellent exposure of the suprarenal vena cava, including the site of entry of the right adrenal vein.

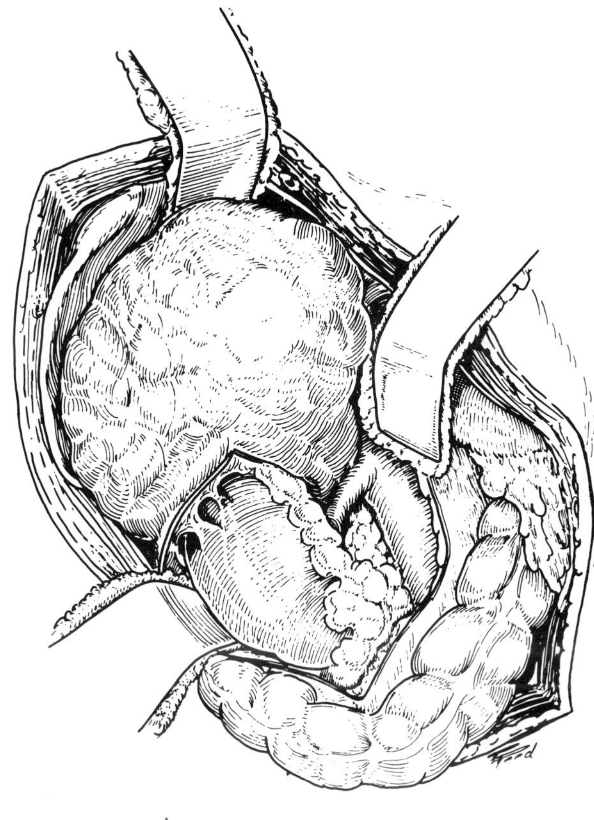

Figure 8.11. Once the liver has been retracted upward into the chest, the hepatic flexure of the colon and the duodenum are reflected medially to expose the anterior surface of the adrenal tumor, kidney, renal vein, and vena cava. A self-retaining ring retractor is then inserted to maintain exposure of the operative field. The illustrations that follow depict performance of nephroadrenalectomy for a large invasive adrenal malignancy.

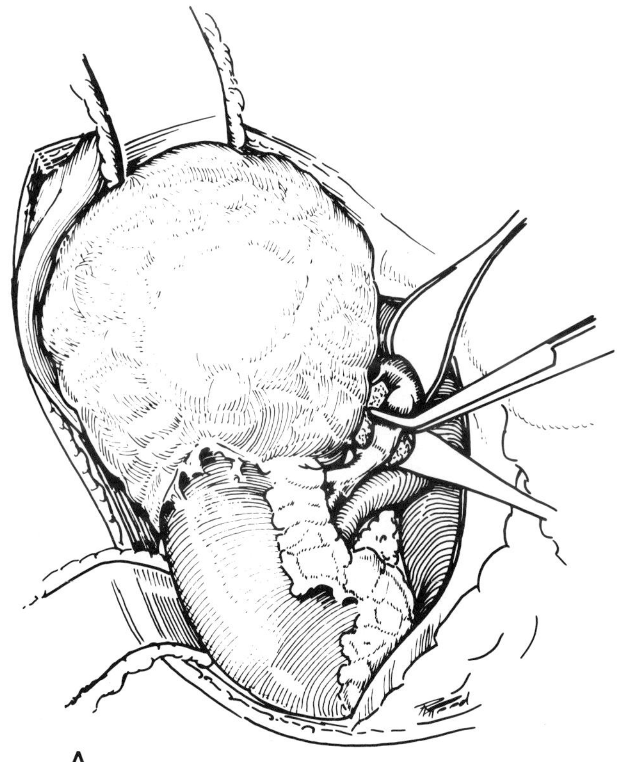

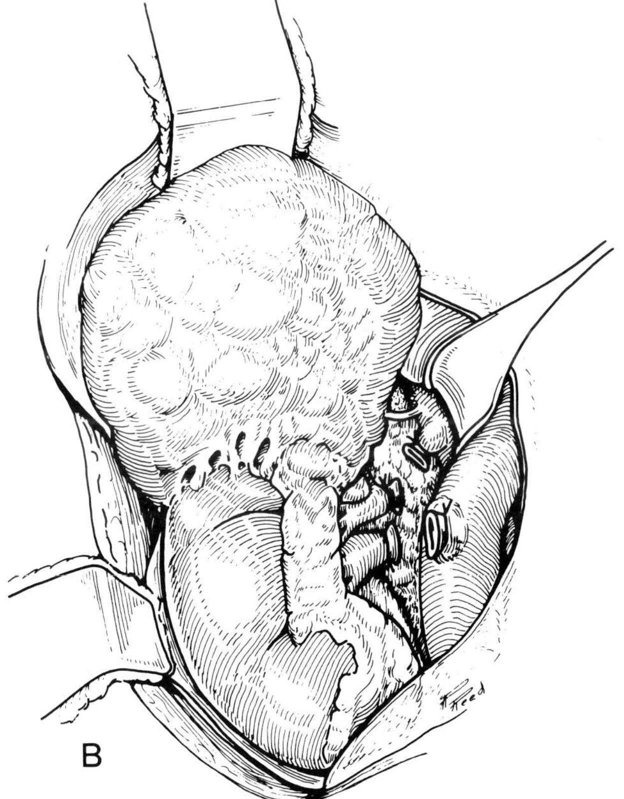

Figure 8.12. A and B, the renal artery is secured with silk ligatures and divided, and the renal vein is then similarly secured and transected. The ureter and right gonadal vein are ligated and divided, and the kidney is then mobilized outside Gerota's fascia.

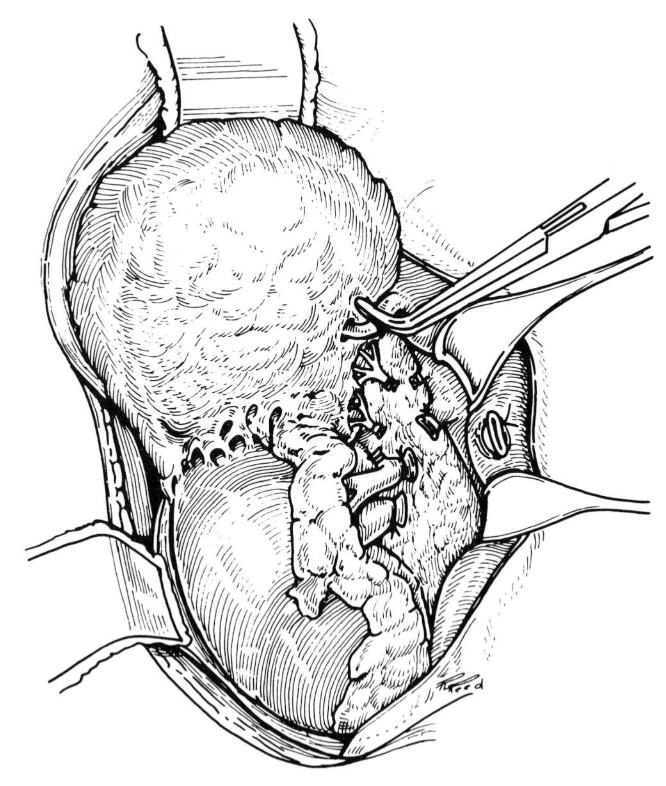

Figure 8.13. By downward and lateral retraction of the kidney and adrenal tumor mass, the dissection then can be carried upward to secure the middle adrenal arteries and the right adrenal vein. Exposure of these vessels is facilitated by medial retraction of the inferior vena cava. Further mobilization of the adrenal and division of remaining superior vascular attachments are performed as described in chapter 7. Care is taken to preserve small hepatic venous branches entering the vena cava at the superior margin of the mass. Retraction with upward elevation of the liver enhances exposure of this region and reduces the potential hazard of inadvertent avulsion of these vessels; should this occur, the excellent exposure provided by the thoracoabdominal approach facilitates appropriate measures for securing hemostasis.

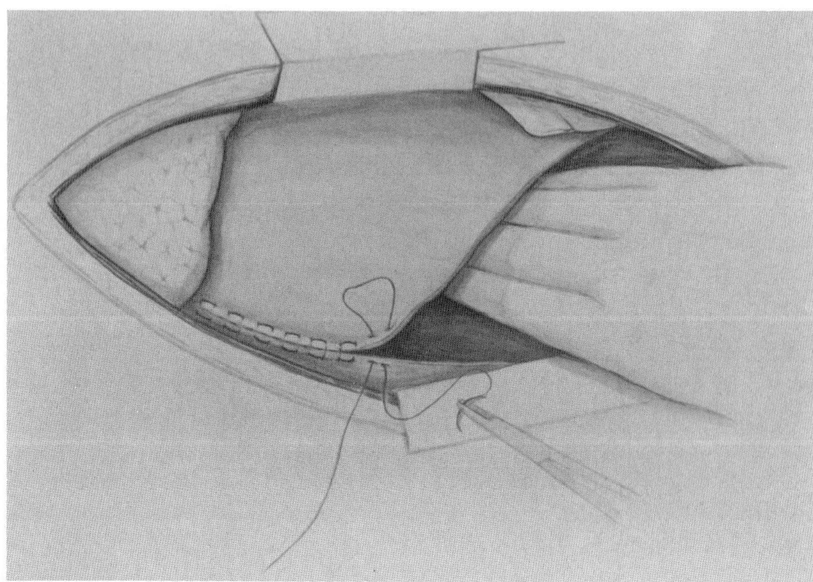

Figure 8.14. Proper closure of the thoracic aspect of the thoracoabdominal incision is important to prevent postoperative complications. The diaphragm is repaired, as shown, with interrupted 2–0 silk mattress sutures.

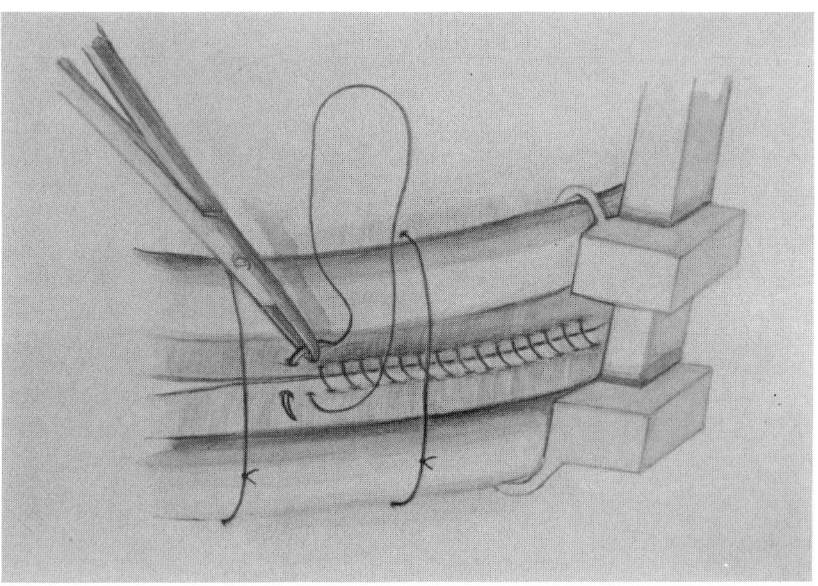

Figure 8.15 Retention sutures of 00 chromic catgut are passed around each rib above and below the intercostal incision. The intercostal muscles are then brought together with interrupted absorbable 0 chromic or Dexon sutures, taking care not to traumatize underlying lung tissue. Prior to completing closure of the thoracotomy incision, a chest tube is brought out through a lateral stab would and connected to water-sealed drainage. The abdominal portion of the incision is closed in standard fashion.

Suggested Readings

Barry JM, Hodges CV: The supracostal approach to the kidney and adrenal. *J Urol* 114:666, 1975.

Cerny JC: Anatomy of the adrenal gland. *Urol Clin North Am* 4:169, 1977.

Chute R, Soutter L, Kerr WS: The value of the thoraco-abdominal incision in the removal of kidney tumors. *N Engl J Med* 241:951, 1949.

Dluhy RG, Gittes RF: The adrenals. In Walsh PC, Gittes RF, Perlumtter AD, Stamey TA (eds): *Campbell's Urology,* 5th ed. Philadelphia, WB Saunders, 1986.

Glenn JF: Non-functional adrenal tumors and aldosteronism. In Glenn JF (ed): *Urologic Surgery,* 3rd ed. Philadelphia, JB Lippincott, 1983.

Rhamy RK: Cushing's syndrome. In Glenn JF (ed): *Urologic Surgery,* 3rd ed. Philadelphia, JB Lippincott, 1983.

Turner-Warwick RT: The supracostal approach to the renal area. *Br J Urol* 37:671, 1965.

SECTION 3

Surgery for Malignant Renal Disorders

CHAPTER 9

Radical Nephrectomy

J. EDSON PONTES

Radical nephrectomy is the standard treatment for patients with renal cell carcinoma. Nephroureterectomy is reserved for patients with transitional cell carcinoma of the renal pelvis or ureter. This chapter will deal with both radical nephrectomy and nephrouterectomy.

RADICAL NEPHRECTOMY

This operation for many years, has been accepted as the surgical treatment of choice for patients with renal cell carcinoma. Although in the last few years conservative surgery has been used for patients with renal cell carcinoma those cases should be individualized and selection should be made based on other factors rather than the disease proper.

The diagnostic workup of a patient with renal cell carcinoma has changed considerably within the last few years with the advent of new radiologic techniques, such as computed tomigraphy (CT) scan, digital subtraction angiography, and magnetic resonance imaging (MRI). Presently, in a large percentage of patients, the complete diagnostic workup can be done without the use of invasive means such as arteriography or venacavography. The use of these invasive procedures are selected for patients with larger tumors in whom suspicions of vena cava involvement exists or for cases with potential surgical difficulties.

Metastatic workup of patients with renal cell carcinoma should include a chest x-ray and, occasionally, a bone scan is used if suspicions of bony metastasis exist. CT and MRI have significantly improved our capabilities of diagnosing metastatic retroperitoneal lymph nodes or metastasis to other intraabdominal organs.

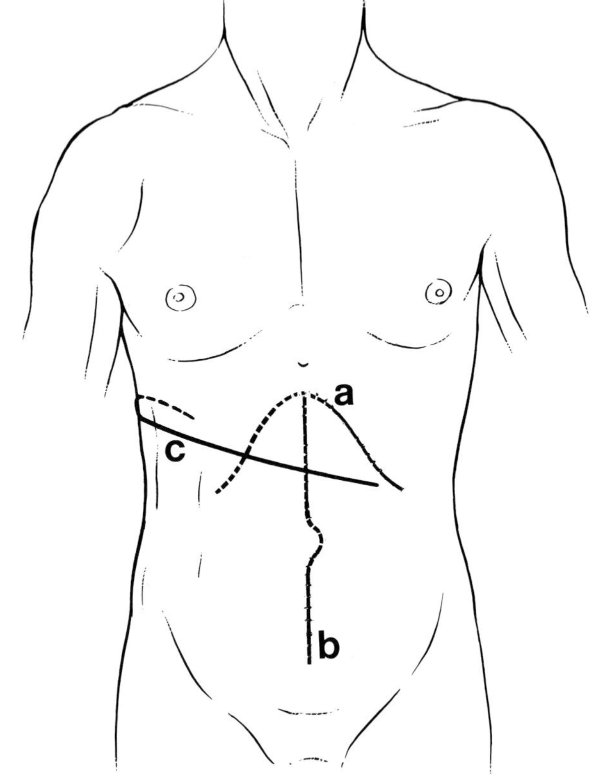

Figure 9.1. The choice of incision depends a great deal on the biotype of the patient as well as the size and location of the tumor. The operation is usually done transperitoneally to get access to the renal pedicle with minimal manipulation of tumor. This author prefers, in the majority of cases, a transverse (Chevron-type) incision although in patients with sharp xiphoid angle, an up-and-down incision is used. Thoracoabdominal incisions are selected for patients with large upper pole tumors.

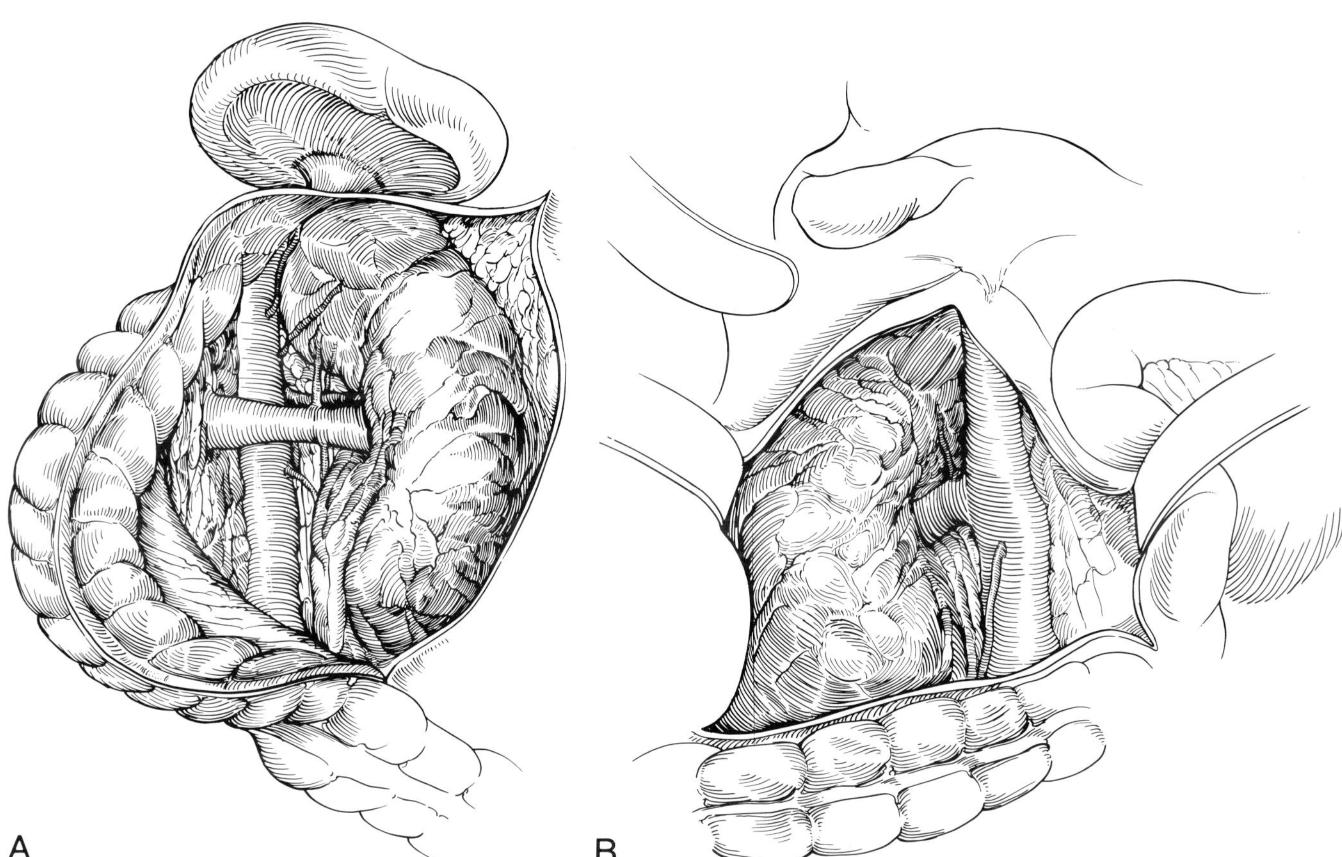

Figure 9.2. A and B, after opening the abdominal cavity, an exploration for metastatic disease is performed with visualization of any suspected areas. On the *left side,* the operation is started with a reflection of the left colon and liberation of the splenic colic ligaments. Failure to control and transect these ligaments often leads to splenic injury after the retractor is placed. The reflection of the colon will expose the great vessels medially. On the *right side,* the right colon together with the duodenum (Kocher maneuver) is reflected medially in order to expose the vena cava.

At this point, a self-retaining retractor is placed. For many years, the author has used a modification of the Smith ring called the Bookwalter retractor. Although this retractor is essential for good exposure care should be taken with regard to visceral injuries that can be caused by inappropriate position of the blades.

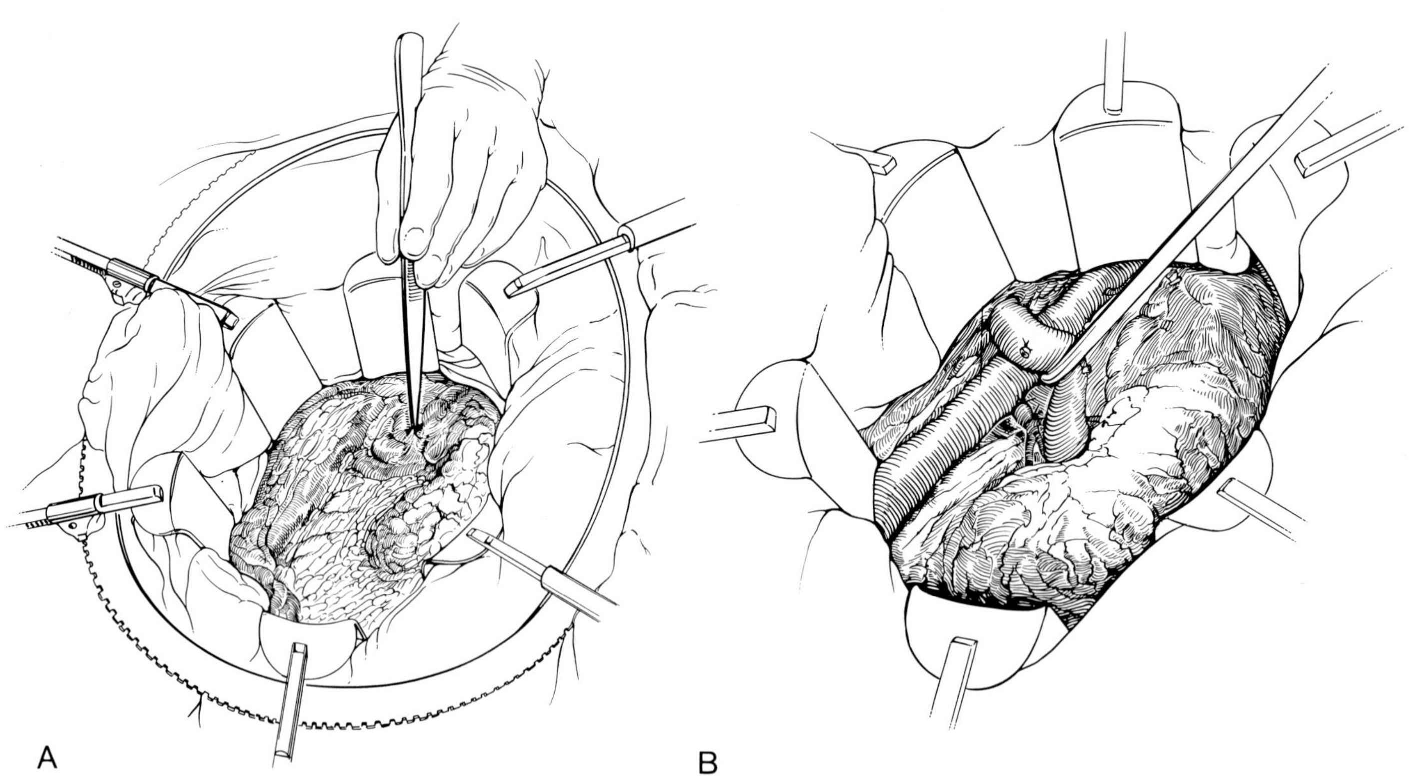

Figure 9.3. A and B, the operation on both sides is initiated with dissection of the renal pedicle. *Left Radical Nephrectomy.* The renal vein on this side is long as it stretches over the aorta. Dissection of the renal vein will lead to identification and ligation of the gonadal vein inferiorly and the adrenal vein superiorly. After the dissection and isolation of the renal vein with vessel loops, retraction of the renal vein is performed with the vein retractor in order to isolate the renal artery. Dissection of the artery is carried toward the aorta to get enough length for ligation and transection. A 0 silk is used for ligation of the renal artery and the vein. A double ligature is used proximally with a single ligature toward the specimen. **C,** *Right Radical Nephrectomy.* The renal vein on the right side is short. Care should be taken during its dissection not to injure the vena cava. After dissection and isolation of the renal vein with a vessel loop, of the renal artery is performed. The artery may be dissected laterally to the vena cava or in cases of early division, between the vena cava and the aorta as illustrated. Ligation of the renal artery and vein is performed as described for the left with 0 silk. Because the renal vein is short, ligation should take place at the level of its entrance to the vena cava.

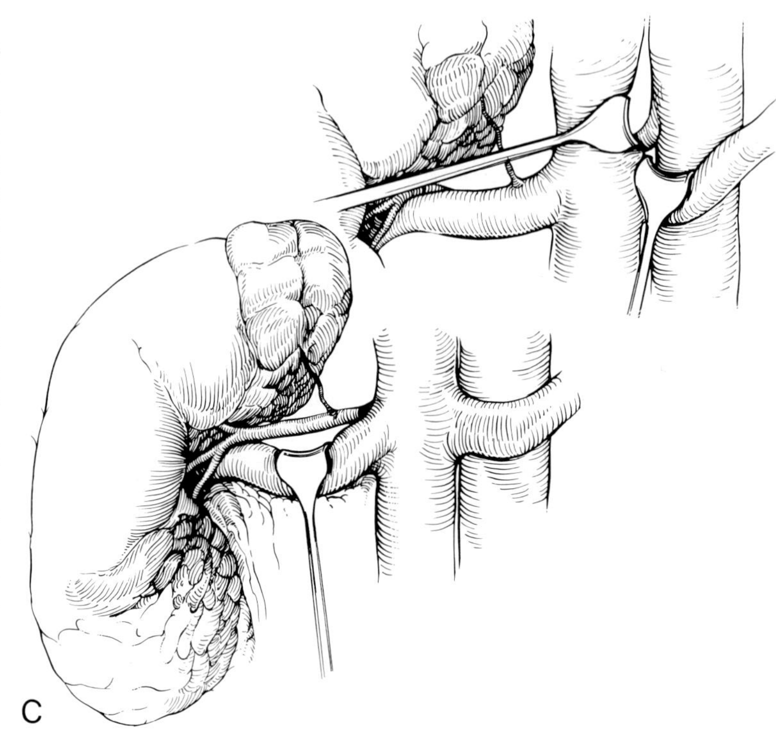

Figure 9.4. The procedure on both sides is continued with removal of all the perinephric tissue along the great vessels. This is accomplished by sharp dissection with ligatures of small vessels with nonabsorbable material or with metal clips. Dissection and removal of the adrenal glands is accomplished in the same manner.

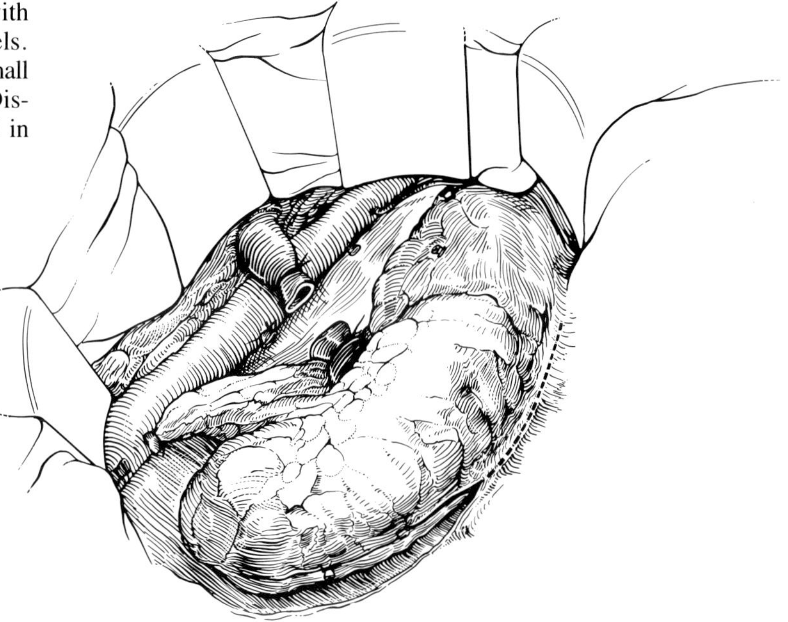

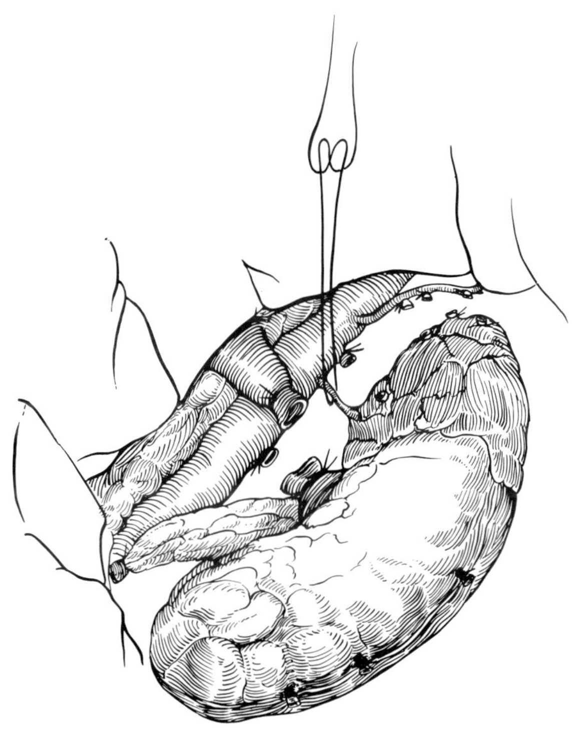

Figure 9.5. The remaining dissection of the lateral superior and lower pole of the kidney is done manually with ligation and transection of the ureter. The abdomen is closed in layers. No drains are left.

Postoperative Care

The postoperative care of patients undergoing radical nephrectomy is similar to any major surgical procedure. Because this operation is intraperitoneal and a postoperative ileus will develop, nasogastric decompression is needed for a few days. However, the majority of patients return to full oral intake within 3–4 days after surgery without need of parenteral nutrition.

Long-term follow-up of those patients is necessary because approximately 50% of patients with localized renal cell carcinoma will develop metastatic disease later. In the event of metastatic disease developing, patients may be candidates for clinical trials involving biologic response modifiers in view of the failure of the majority of chemo- or hormonal therapeutic agents to be effective in this disease.

NEPHROURETERECTOMY

Nephroureterectomy is the standard therapy for tumors of the renal pelvis and ureter. In recent years, a more conservative approach has been developed in which the renal unit may be preserved but such approach should be selected for special cases, i.e., solitary kidney, tumors with low biologic potential.

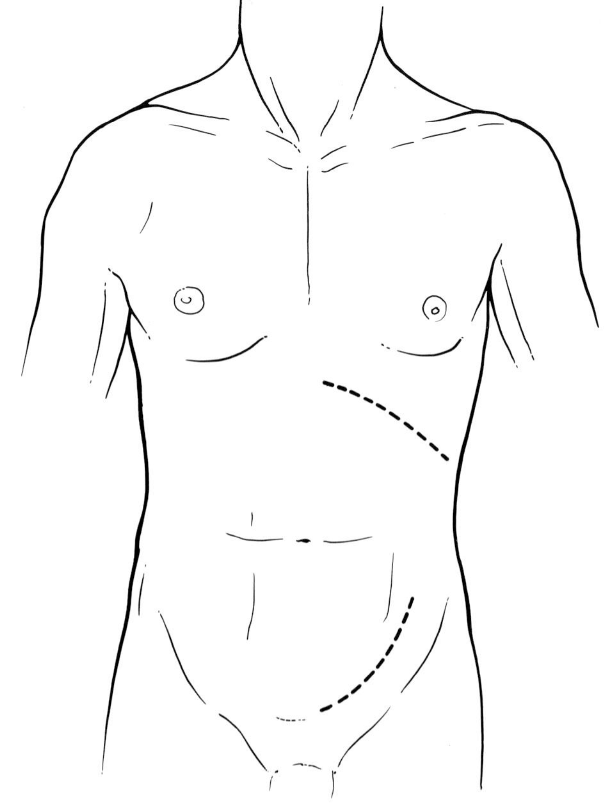

Figure 9.6. The choice of incision depends on individual preference and on the preoperative evaluation. The author usually prefers two incisions, one transverse upper abdominal and one lower abdominal (Gibson-type) incision. This approach obviates the need of changing the patient's position during the operation, which is necessary when one approaches the kidney through a flank position. Occasionally, in a slim patient, an extraperitoneal approach to the kidney can be used with those two incisions.

Alternative approaches are a modified flank incision that extends to the lower abdomen. In this case, the complete operation can be done extraperitoneally. The author believes that with this approach may be difficult to resect the lower ureter with a cuff of bladder. In using two incisions, the choice of starting at the kidney level or at the bladder must be individualized. Although, in general, the author starts with the nephrectomy, in some occasions in which there is a probability of more conservative surgery, such as in tumors in the lower ureter, one may elect to start with removal of the cuff of the bladder and the lower ureter in an attempt to decide at that point if distal ureterectomy is indicated.

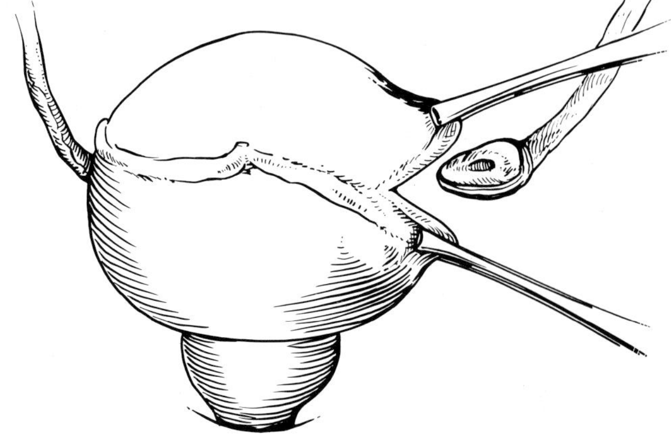

Figure 9.7. *Distal ureterectomy.* A Gibson-type incision is used. This portion of the operation can be done extraperitoneally. The ureter is identified and isolated as it crosses the common iliac artery. With blunt and sharp dissection the ureter and the periureteral tissues are freed toward the bladder. Dissection is carried out to the point of the intramural ureter. A cuff of urinary bladder is removed by applying the Ellis clamp to the bladder wall and excising a cuff around the ureter. This cuff must include the complete intramural ureter.

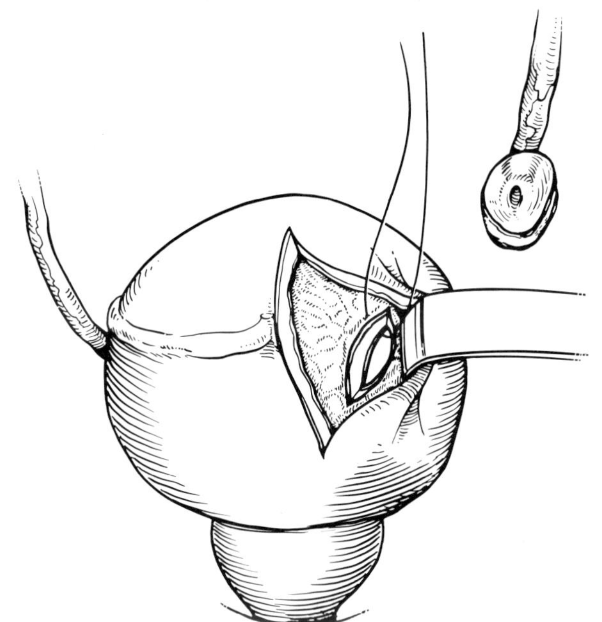

Figure 9.8. If for technical reasons it is not possible to remove a cuff of bladder through an extravesical approach, an open cystostomy is performed with removal of the cuff of the bladder intravesically. The bladder is closed using 4–0 and 3–0 polyglycolic sutures in two or three layers. Both incisions are closed by anatomic layers. The lower portion of the incision is drained using a closed drainage system. An indwelling Foley catheter no. 22 is left for 7–10 days.

The nephrectomy portion of this operation is similar to the one described in surgery for renal cell carcinoma (Fig. 9.1) with the exception that the ureter is not transected and that there is no good reason to include adrenal removal as part of this operation unless in extensive tumors. The ureter should be dissected as low as possible. The author prefers to leave the kidney and the ureter in situ to be removed as one anatomic piece to facilitate mapping of the specimen by the pathologist. If the specimen needs to be removed, ligation proximally and distally is necessary before transection to avoid the spillage and implantation of the tumor in the wound.

Postoperative Care

Postoperative care in these patients is similar to radical nephrectomy. The lower incision drain is removed after the removal of the Foley catheter to assure that there is no urinary leak. Because there is an incidence of approximately 30% of bladder tumors in patients with transitional cell carcinoma of the upper tract, those patients must be followed with cystoscopic examination at 6-month intervals.

Suggested Readings

Montie JE: Management of Stages I, II and III Renal Adenocarcinoma. In Javadpour N (ed.) *Principles and Management of Urologic Cancer.* Baltimore, Williams & Wilkins 1983, pp. 492.

Robson CJ, Churchill BM, Anderson W: The results of radical nephrectomy for renal cell carcinoma. *J Urol* 101:297, 1964.

Ziegelbaum M, Novick AC, Streem S, Montie J, Pontes JE, Straffon RA: Conservative surgery for transitional cell carcinoma of the renal pelvis. *J Urol* 138:1146, 1987.

CHAPTER **10**

Surgery for Renal Cell Carcinoma Involving the Inferior Vena Cava

ANDREW C. NOVICK
JAMES E. MONTIE

One of the unique features of renal cell carcinoma is the frequent pattern of growth intraluminally into the renal venous circulation. In extreme cases, this growth may extend into the inferior vena cava (IVC) with cephalad migration as far as the heart. The absence of metastases in some patients with renal cell carcinoma and a vena caval tumor thrombus is an intriguing aspect of this cancer's biological behavior.

Involvement of the IVC with renal cell carcinoma occurs in 3–7% of cases and renders the task of complete surgical excision more complicated. Yet, operative removal remains the only curative treatment for this disease. In patients with renal cell carcinoma extending into the IVC, an aggressive approach is justified when metastases are absent. In this setting, 5-year survival rates of 20–50% have been reported after complete surgical excision. The best results have been achieved in patients whose tumor did not involve the perinephric fat and regional lymph nodes.

Interestingly, the surgical principles involved in removing such tumors were first established more than 60 years ago. In 1913, Berg used a transverse abdominal incision to perform inferior vena cavotomy and tumor thrombectomy, whereas in 1922, Rehn actually reimplanted the contralateral renal vein after resecting the vena cava. Notwithstanding the sophistication of modern surgical techniques and instrumentation, radical operations in such patients still involve the ever-present dangers of intraoperative hypotension, pulmonary embolism, as well as postoperative hepatic and renal insufficiency. The diagnosis of vena caval involvement from renal cell carcinoma is dependent upon a high degree of clinical suspicion and thorough roentgenographic evaluation. This possibility should be considered in patients who have lower extremity edema, a varicocele, dilated superficial abdominal veins, albuminuria, pulmonary embolism, a right atrial mass, or nonfunction of the involved kidney. Inferior vena cavography remains the definitive diagnostic study for demonstrating the presence and extent of caval involvement; however, such involvement may also be demonstrated with computed tomography (CT) scanning, ultrasonography, or magnetic resonance imaging. If there is complete occlusion of the inferior vena cava, superior cavography or a formal heart catheterization study, or both are indicated.

In planning the appropriate operative approach for tumor removal, it is essential for preoperative radiographic studies to define accurately the distal limits of a vena caval tumor thrombus. There are four levels of vena caval involvement, which are categorized and depicted in Figure 10.1.

PREVENTION AND CONTROL OF VENA CAVAL HEMORRHAGE

A knowledge of potential bleeding sites, familiarity with vascular techniques, and the availability of proper illumination and vascular instruments are all necessary prerequisites for performing major surgery on the inferior vena cava. Intraoperative hemorrhage from the vena cava may be significant and the surgeon must be familiar with methods for preventing and/or controlling this problem. In most cases, vena caval hemorrhage is caused by the laceration or avulsion of large yet fragile veins entering the vena cava at predictable locations.

Lumbar veins enter the posterolateral aspect of the vena cava at each vertebral level and undue traction on the cava can result in their avulsion with troublesome bleeding. To prevent this, care should be taken to retract the vena cava very gently with curved vein retractors during its dissection; if additional mobilization is necessary, these veins should be dissected free from surrounding structures, doubly clamped, and securely ligated. In ligating venous tributaries entering the vena cava, 3–0 to 4–0 suture material should be used, and the ligatures should not be tied too tightly, as this can cause shearing through the fragile venous wall with further

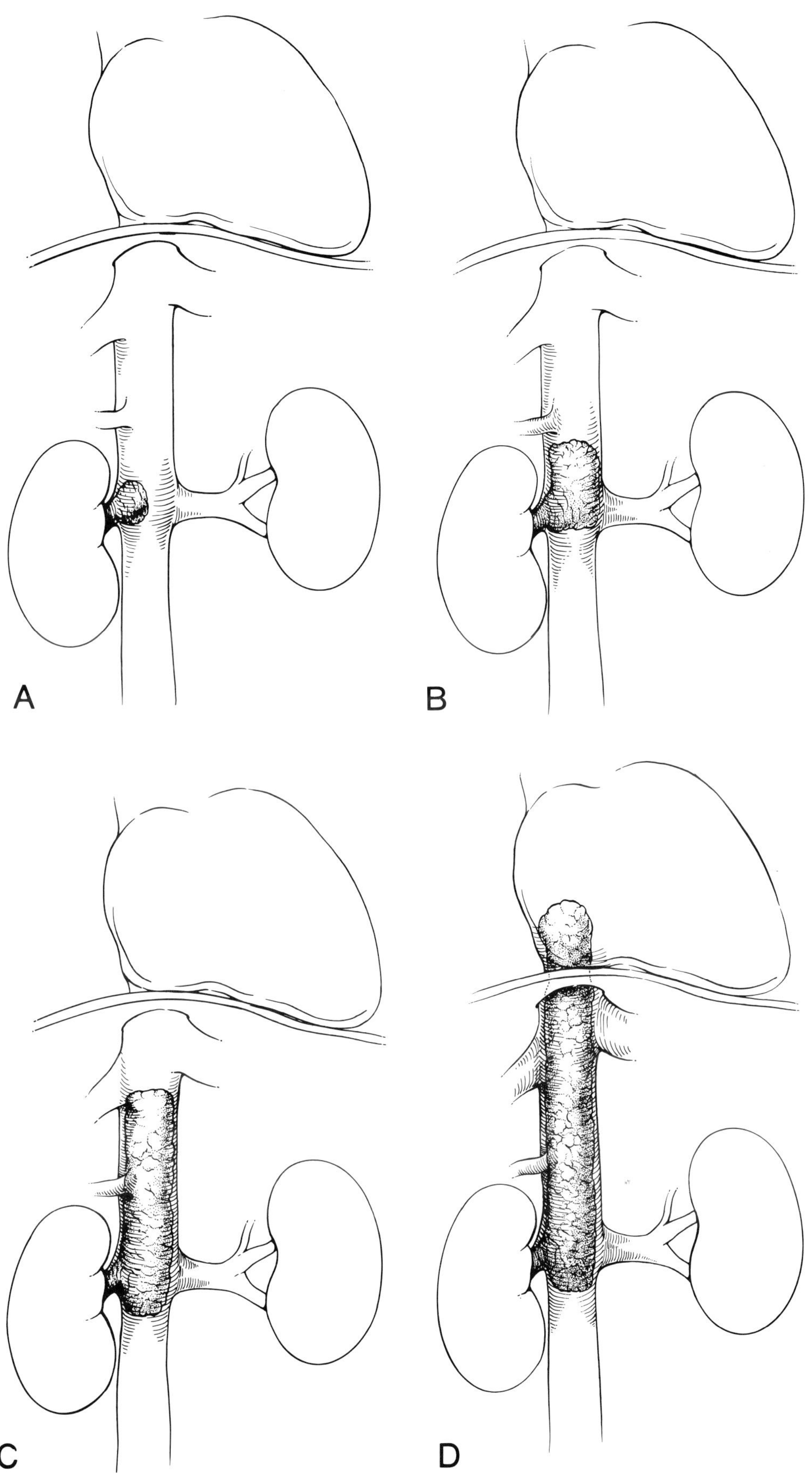

Figure 10.1. A, level 1 refers to tumor thrombus at the entry of the renal vein with <2 cm extension into the vena cava. **B,** level 2 refers to tumor thrombus within the lumen of the vena cava but below the entry of the most inferior hepatic vein (i.e., infrahepatic). **C,** level 3 refers to tumor thrombus extending into the intrahepatic vena cava but below the diaphragm. **D,** level 4 refers to tumor thrombus extending above the diaphragm or into the right atrium.

hemorrhage. After the ligature has been applied, it should not be pulled too tightly before the ends of the ligature are cut, again for fear of avulsing the entrance of the vein into the vena cava.

A second predictable bleeding site is the entry of the right gonadal vein into the anterolateral surface of the vena cava. This is an extremely thin-walled vein and excessive traction or mobilization of the cava at this level can lead to its avulsion, with resulting hemorrhage.

The third predictable site of bleeding lies at the level of the renal veins, where large lumbar veins will often course posteriorly from the left renal vein just lateral to the aorta, or from the posterior aspect of the vena cava close to the entry of the right renal vein into the vena cava itself. Injudicious mobilization of the renal veins, without consideration of these fragile and often large-caliber veins, can result in severe hemorrhage that is difficult to control, because of their posterior entry into the vena cava or renal veins.

Finally, excessive vena caval hemorrhage can be prevented by careful dissection in proper tissue planes along the vena cava. This may be difficult when tumor involves the vena cava, but usually a plane can be established along the vena caval wall which, if followed, can allow safe and relatively bloodless exposure. One should follow the general principle of isolating a relatively normal area of vena cava and working upward or downward from that level to expose the diseased portion.

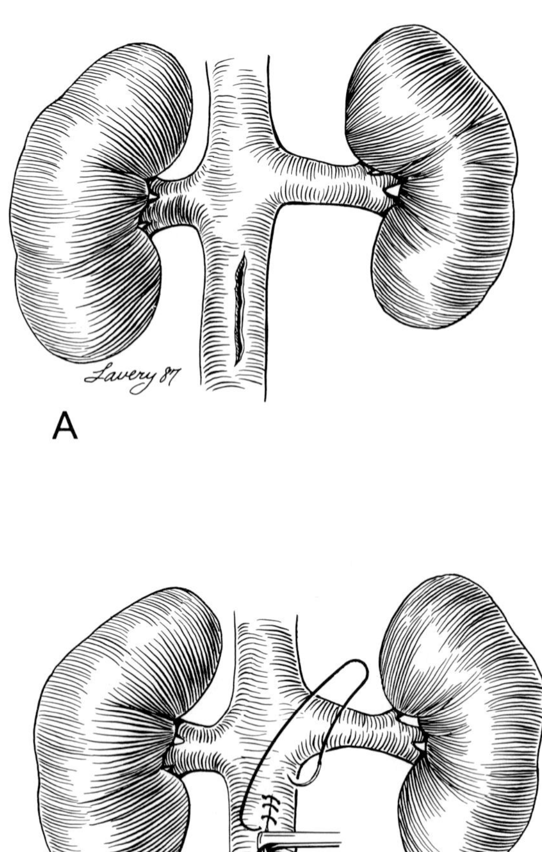

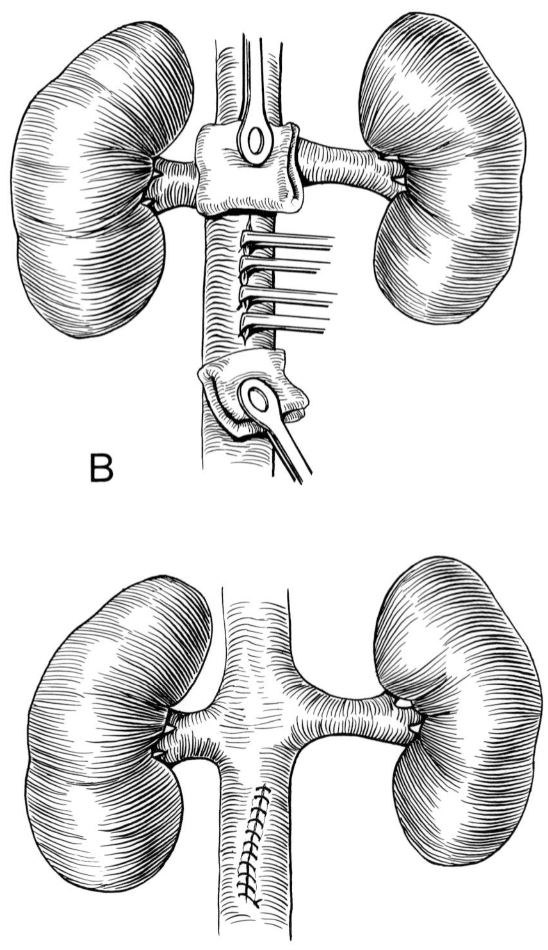

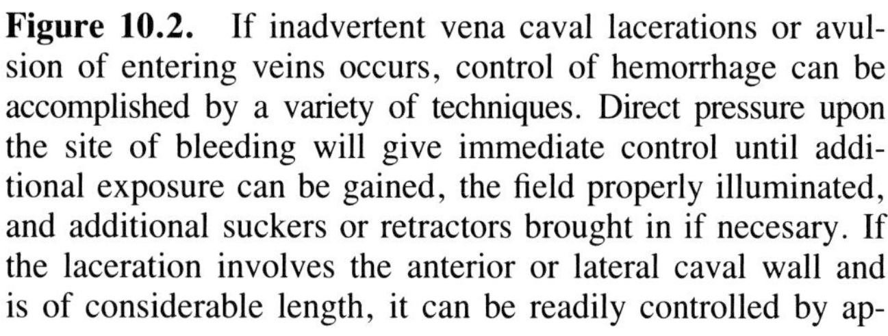

Figure 10.2. If inadvertent vena caval lacerations or avulsion of entering veins occurs, control of hemorrhage can be accomplished by a variety of techniques. Direct pressure upon the site of bleeding will give immediate control until additional exposure can be gained, the field properly illuminated, and additional suckers or retractors brought in if necesary. If the laceration involves the anterior or lateral caval wall and is of considerable length, it can be readily controlled by applying a series of Allis clamps over the edges of the laceration in serial fashion. The edges of the laceration are then oversewn with running vascular suture material, the clamps released, and the suture run back along the laceration to the original point of entry to further control bleeding. Additional interrupted sutures may be necessary if the laceration is extensive.

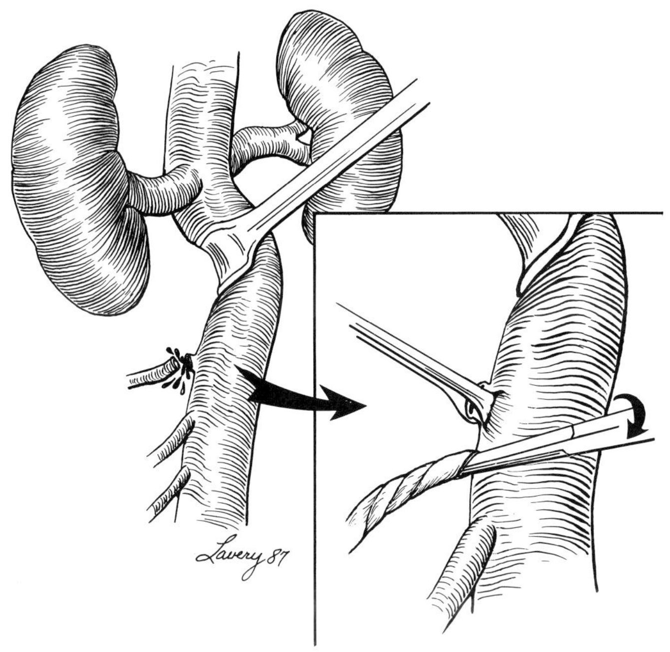

Figure 10.3. If avulsion of an entering lumbar vein is the cause of bleeding, the vena cava should be rolled medially, with digital compression above and below the site of bleeding, until the posterolateral entry of the avulsed vein is exposed. This is then grasped with one or two Allis forceps, which can be used as tractors to bring the avulsion into better view for oversewing with vascular suture material. Persistent bleeding can occur from the proximal end of the avulsed lumbar vein, which may retract into the psoas muscle and be difficult to secure. This can be controlled in some cases by grasping the end of the vein with a hemostat, then twisitng the hemostat, bringing the end of the vein into better view for suture ligation. If this is not possible, bleeding can be controlled by inserting a figure-eight 2–0 silk suture through the muscle overlying the vein.

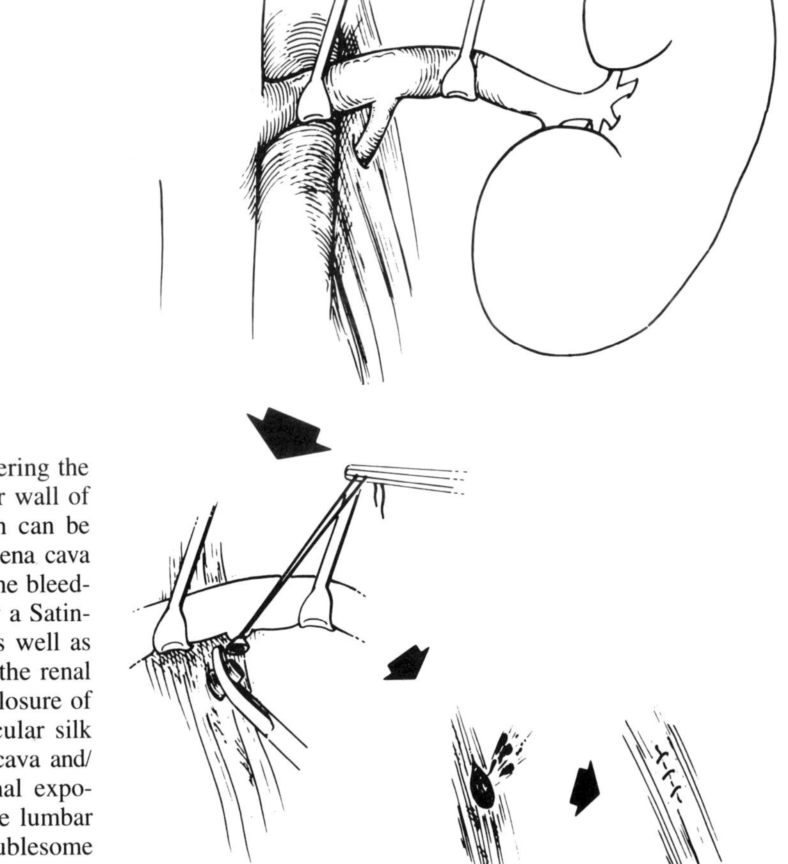

Figure 10.4. Bleeding from large lumbar veins entering the posterior aspect of the left renal vein or the posterior wall of the vena cava near the entry of the right renal vein can be particularly troublesome. Further mobilization of the vena cava and renal veins while compression is maintained on the bleeding site is often needed. It may be necessary to apply a Satinsky side-clamp across the entry of the renal vein, as well as a distal bulldog clamp beyond the bleeding point in the renal vein, in order to control the hemorrhage and allow closure of the venous defect with interrupted 5–0 or 6–0 vascular silk sutures. Mobilization and gentle rotation of the vena cava and/or renal veins may also be necessary to gain optimal exposure. In this situation, as well, the distal entry of the lumbar vein into the posterior musculature can cause troublesome bleeding and must be controlled as described above.

SURGICAL REMOVAL OF RENAL CELL CARCINOMA WITH INFRAHEPATIC VENA CAVAL INVOLVEMENT

It has been our experience that an anterior surgical approach through a bilateral subcostal transperitoneal incision provides excellent exposure for performing radical nephrectomy and removal of level 1 or 2 thrombi from the infrahepatic vena cava. For extremely large tumors involving the upper pole of the kidney, a thoracoabdominal approach, alternatively, may be employed.

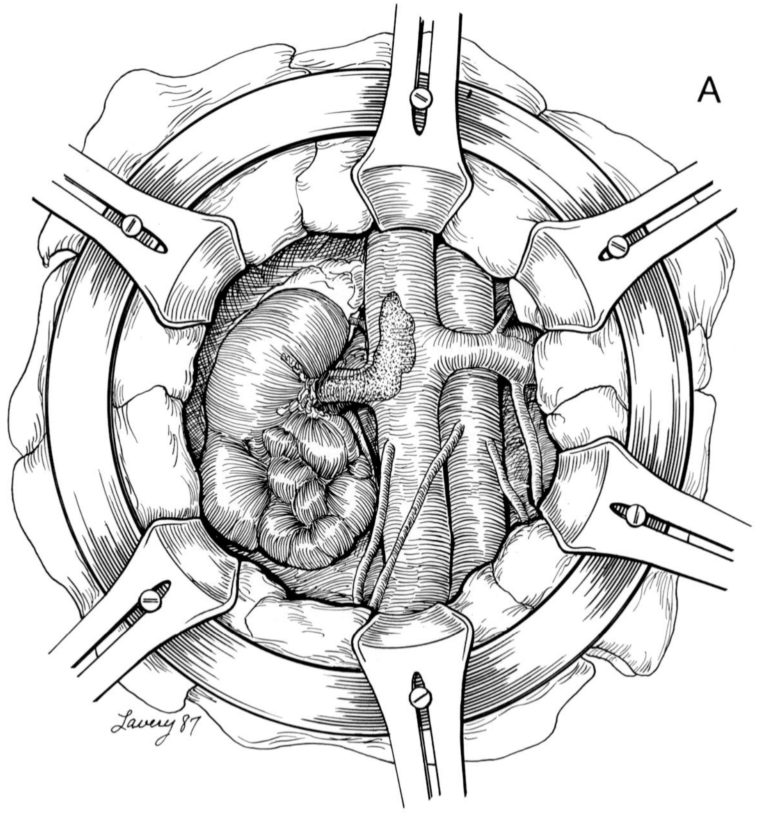

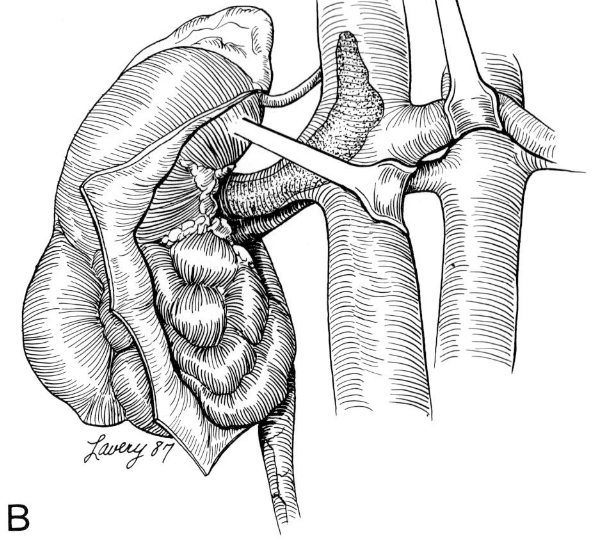

Figure 10.5. A, after the abdomen has been entered, the colon is reflected medially and a self-retaining ring retractor is inserted to maintain exposure of the retroperitoneum. The renal arterial suply and the ureter are ligated and divided, and the entire kidney is mobilized outside Gerota's fascia before any attempt is made to transect the renal vein. **B,** it may be easiest to expose the right renal artery by dissecting between the aorta and the vena cava. During the initial dissection, care is taken to avoid unnecessary manipulation of the renal vein and vena cava.

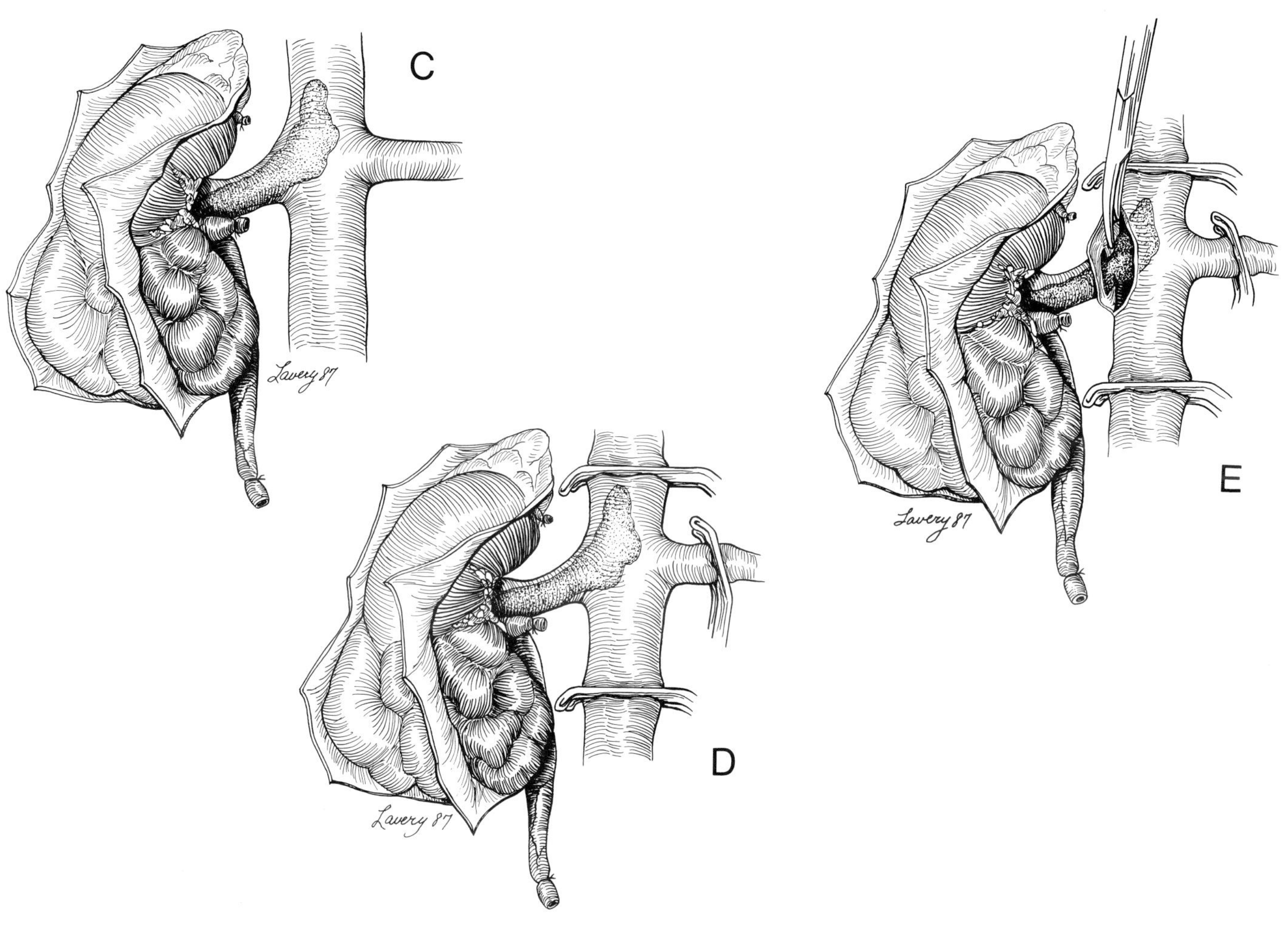

Figure 10.5. C, the vena cava is then completely dissected from surrounding structures above and below the renal vein, and the opposite renal vein is also mobilized. A level 1 tumor thrombus (not illustrated here) can be managed by simply placing a curved Satinsky clamp around the perirenal vena cava, incising the renal vein, extracting the thrombus, and repairing the vena cava. The illustrations here demonstrate the technique for removing a level 2 infrahepatic tumor thrombus. **D,** with a level 2 infrahepatic tumor thrombus, it is essential to obtain exposure of the suprarenal vena cava above the level of the tumor thrombus. If necessary, perforating veins to the caudate lobe of the liver are secured and divided to allow separation of the caudate lobe from the vena cava. This maneuver can allow an additional 2- to 3-cm length of vena cava to be exposed. The infrarenal vena cava is then occluded distally with a Satinsky venous clamp, and the opposite renal vein is gently secured with a small bulldog vascular clamp. Finally, in preparation for tumor thrombectomy, a curved Satinsky vascular clamp is placed around the suprarenal vena cava above the level of the tumor thrombus and the clamp is then closed. **E,** the anterior surface of the renal vein is then incised over the tumor thrombus and the incision is continued posteriorly with scissors, passing just beneath the tumor thrombus. In most cases, there is no attachment of the thrombus to the wall of the vena cava.

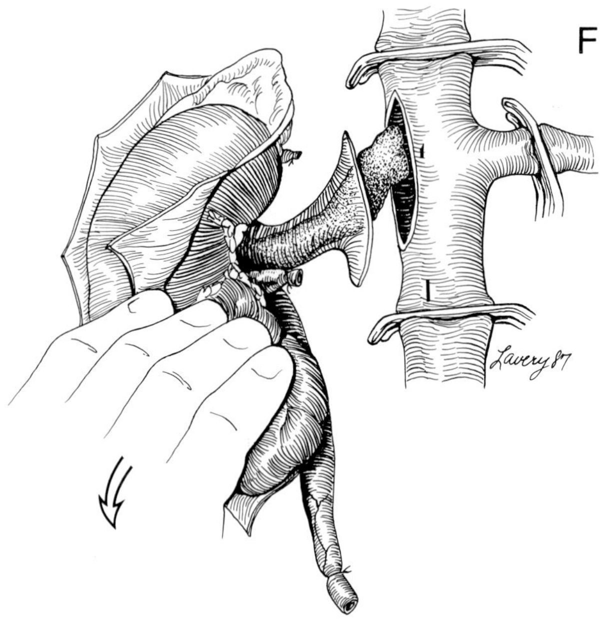

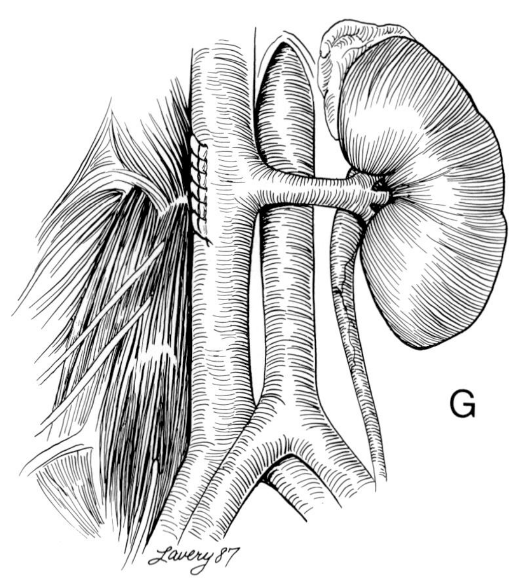

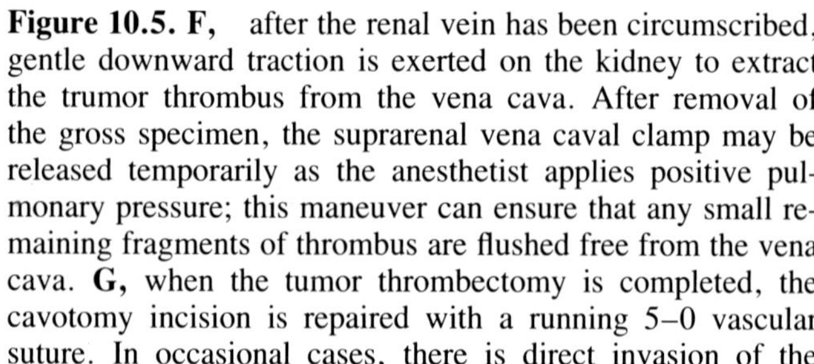

Figure 10.5. F, after the renal vein has been circumscribed, gentle downward traction is exerted on the kidney to extract the trumor thrombus from the vena cava. After removal of the gross specimen, the suprarenal vena caval clamp may be released temporarily as the anesthetist applies positive pulmonary pressure; this maneuver can ensure that any small remaining fragments of thrombus are flushed free from the vena cava. **G,** when the tumor thrombectomy is completed, the cavotomy incision is repaired with a running 5–0 vascular suture. In occasional cases, there is direct invasion of the tumor at the level of the entrance of the renal vein and for varying distances. In patients with complete occlusion of the cava evident preoperatively, there is minimal risk in resecting the cava because adequate collaterals have been established. In patients without preexisting collateral circulation, every effort should be made to reconstruct the cava. Narrowing of the caval lumen by 50% does not appear to have appreciable adverse effect in our experience. After repair of the vena cava, the vascular clamps are released. Further bleeding points may be secured with additional interrupted 5–0 vascular sutures.

The entire retroperitoneal space then is carefully inspected for lymphatic or vascular leakage, which can be controlled with electrocautery, silver clips, or ligatures. Whenever possible, the colon and duodenum are replaced over the right upper quadrant, and retroperitonealization is accomplished with interrupted 3–0 silk sutures.

In most cases, involvement of the vena cava from renal carcinoma is in the form of a tumor thrombus that can be extracted utilizing the technique described above. In some patients, direct growth of tumor into the wall of the vena cava obviates performance of thrombectomy and necessitates resection of the involved portion of the vena cava to achieve complete tumor removal. The prognosis for patients with extensive tumor growth into the vena caval wall is generally poor, particularly when hepatic venous tributaries are also involved. Surgical extirpation may be indicated for patients with either significant associated symptoms or with localized infrahepatic vena caval involvement.

Several important principles must be kept in mind when undertaking vena caval resection. Resection of the infrarenal portion of the vena cava usually can be done safely, because an extensive collateral venous supply will have developed in most cases. With right-sided kidney tumors, resection of the suprarenal vena cava is also possible provided the left renal vein is ligated distal to the gonadal and adrenal tributaries, which then provide collateral venous drainage from the left kidney.

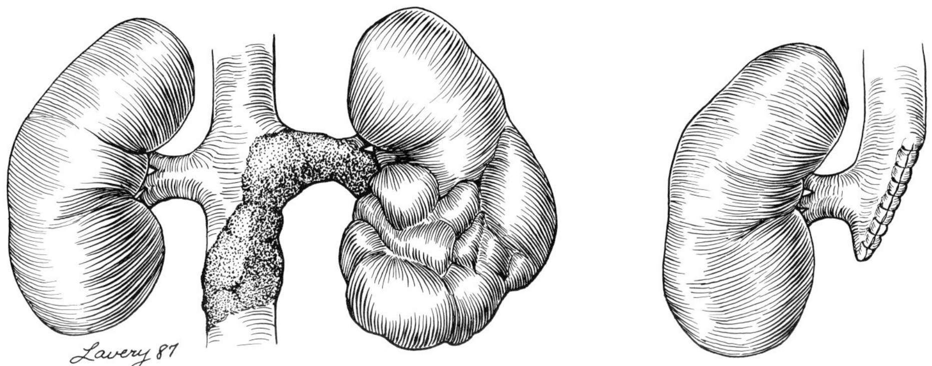

Figure 10.6. With left-sided kidney tumors, the suprarenal vena cava cannot be resected safely owing to the paucity of collateral venous drainage from the right kidney. In such cases, an attempt can be made to preserve a tumor-free strip of vena cava to provide right renal venous drainage; alternatively, the right kidney can be autotransplanted to the pelvis or an interposition graft of saphenous vein may be placed from the right renal vein to the splenic, inferior mesenteric, or portal vein.

SURGICAL REMOVAL OF RENAL CELL CARCINOMA WITH INTRAHEPATIC OR SUPRADIAPHRAGMATIC VENA CAVAL INVOLVEMENT

In patients with renal cell carcinoma and a level 3 or 4 tumor thrombus, the hazards and difficulties of surgical extirpation are significantly increased. In such cases, the operative technique must be modified because it is not possible to obtain subdiaphragmatic control of the vena cava above the tumor thrombus. Several different surgical maneuvers have been used to provide exposure, prevent uncontrolled bleeding, and achieve complete tumor removal in this setting.

In patients with an intrahepatic (level 3) vena caval tumor thrombus, one described technique for obtaining vascular control involves temporary occlusion of the intrathoracic vena cava. To reduce hepatic venous congestion and troublesome backbleeding, the porta hepatis and superior mesenteric artery are also temporarily occluded. It should be stressed that temporary occlusion of the porta hepatis may be safely tolerated for only 20 minutes. Although we consider this technique an effective approach for removing a level 3 tumor thrombus, we have thus far elected to employ cardiac bypass with circulatory arrest for patients with levels 3 and 4 tumor thrombi. Our experience with this approach has been quite favorable and the relevant technique aspects are described below.

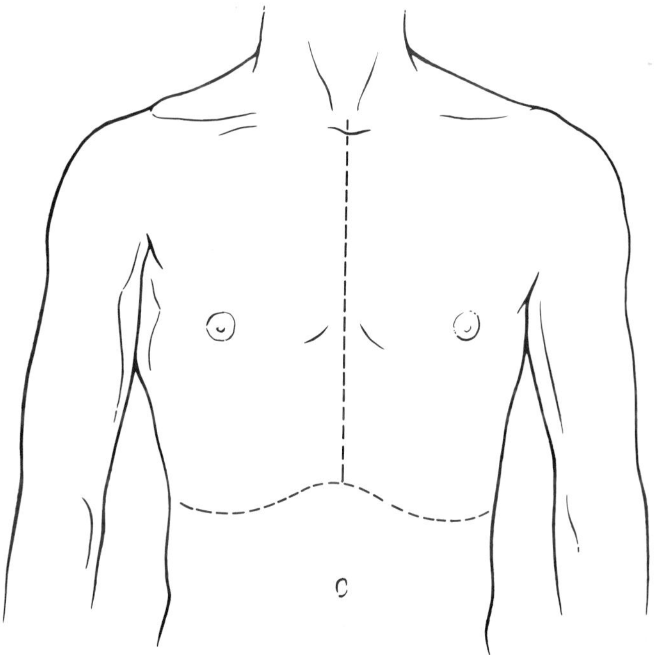

Figure 10.7. A bilateral subcostal incision is used for the abdominal portion of the operation. The kidney is completely mobilized outside Gerota's fascia with division of the renal artery, such that the kidney is left attached only by the renal vein. Precise retroperitoneal hemostasis is essential before proceeding with cardiopulmonary bypass due to the risk of bleeding associated with systemic heparinization. A median sternotomy is performed, the patient is heparinized, and the ascending aortic and right arterial venous cannulae are placed. Cardiopulmonary bypass is initiated. When deep hypothermic circulatory arrest is used, cooling is initiated by reducing arterial inflow blood temperature as low as 10°C. With the onset of ventricular fibrillation, the aorta is cross-clamped and a cooled cardioplegia solution is infused. Cooling is continued until a nasopharyngeal temperature of 18°C is obtained. The head and abdomen are packed in ice during the cooling process. When circulatory arrest is used, 95% of the blood volume is drained into the pump and there is essentially no flow to any organ in the body.

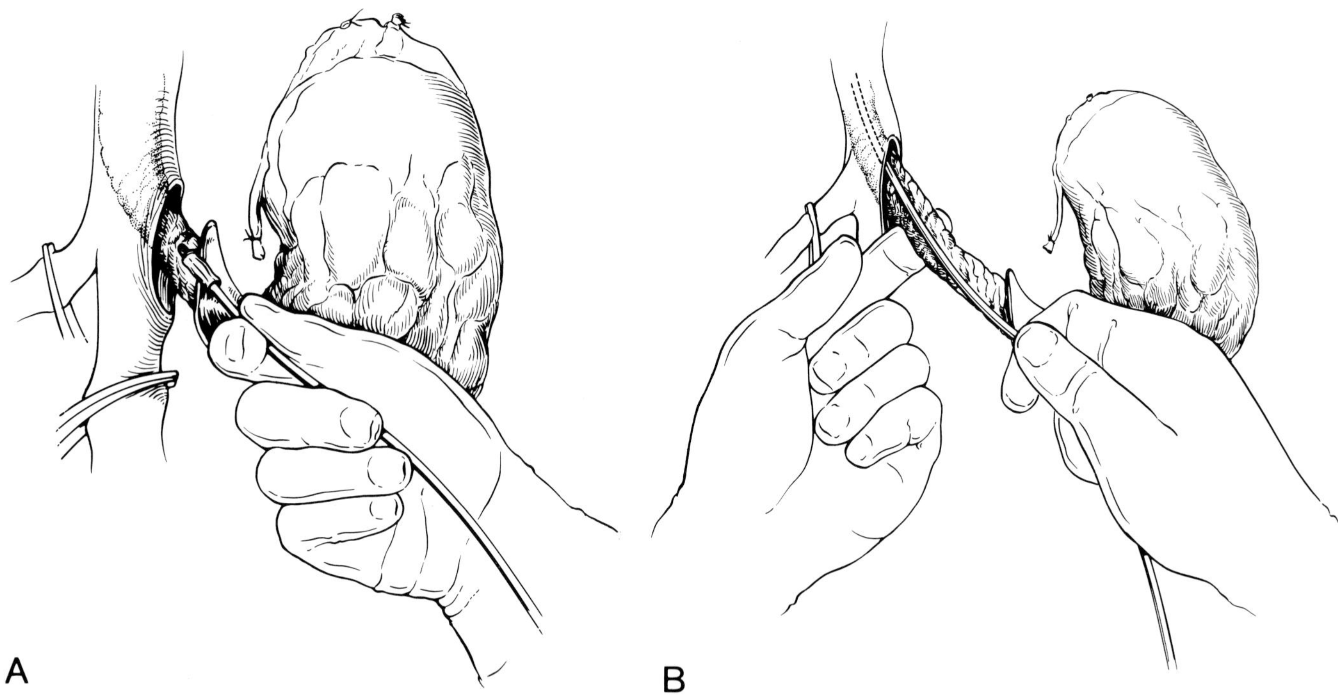

Figure 10.8. A and B, an incision is made at the ostium of the involved renal vein where it enters the vena cava and this is carried circumferentially around the vena cava. When the vena cava is markedly enlarged from a tumor thrombus, a cavotomy as long as 10–15 cm may be necessary. The tumor thrombus is gently teased from the vena caval wall with an endarterectomy knife or blunt forceps. If the thrombus appears to be mobile, a 45-ml venous Fogarty catheter can be inserted in the vena cava to assist in extraction.

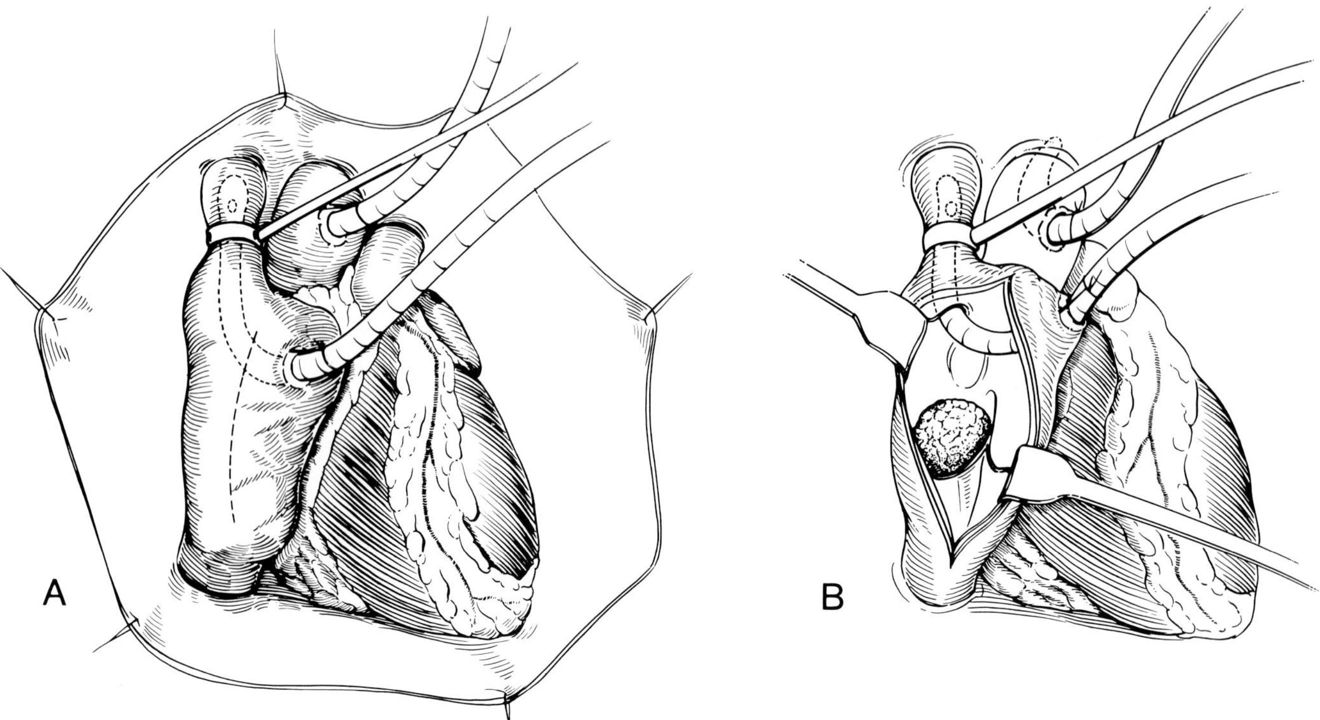

Figure 10.9. A and B, when the tumor thrombus extends into the right atrium, a vertical atriotomy incision is made to inspect the lumen.

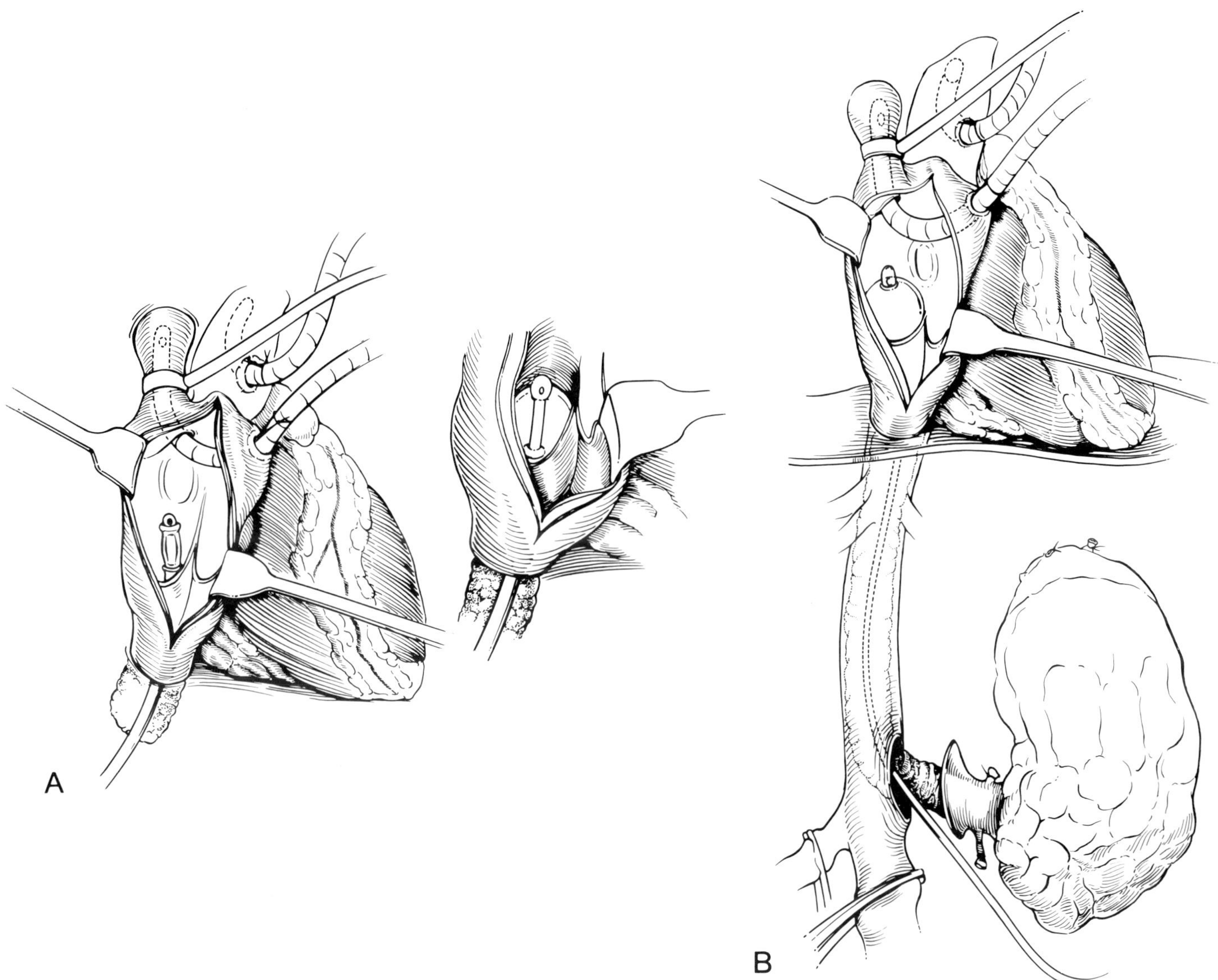

Figure 10.10. A and B, it may be possible to deliver the tumor thrombus through the vena cavotomy incision with downward pressure from above in the atrium. Occasionally, a dumbbell-shaped thrombus is present and it is necessary to remove a portion of the thrombus from above directly through the atrium. In many situations, the tumor thrombus is adherent to the inner lumen of the vena cava. After the bulk of the thrombus has been excised, the inner lumen of the cava can be inspected and small fragments removed ''piecemeal'' or stripped from the lumen. After all fragments have been excised, the vena cava is thoroughly irrigated and closed with a running 5–0 vascular suture.

As soon as the cavotomy has been closed, rewarming of the patient is initiated. Rewarming takes 40–50 min and is continued until a nasopharyngeal temperature of approximately 38°C is obtained. Cardiopulmonary bypass is then terminated. The patient is decannulated and heparinization is reversed. Platelets, fresh frozen plasma, desmopression acetate or aminoprocic acid, or a combination of the above may be used when a coagulopathy is suspected. Mediastinal chest tubes are used but the abdomen is not drained unless there is concern relative to intraabdominal hemostasis.

The technique of cardiopulmonary bypass, hypothermia, cardiac arrest, and exsanguination is an important advance that has improved the safety and efficacy of removing level 3 or 4 tumor thrombi associated with renal cell carcinoma. This approach allows such thrombi to be removed completely in a controlled operative setting that provides excellent exposure and reduces the potential for massive blood loss or major vascular injury.

Suggested Readings

Cherrie RJ, Goldman DG, Lindner A, deKernion JB: Prognostic implications of vena caval extension of renal cell carcinoma. *J Urol* 128:910, 1982.

Marshall FF, Reitz BA: Technique for removal of renal carcinoma with suprahepatic vena caval tumor thrombus. *Urol Clin North Am* 13:551, 1986.

Montie JE, Jackson CL, Cosgrove DM, Streem SB, Novick AC, Pontes JE: Resection of large inferior vena caval thrombi from renal cell carcinoma with the use of circulatory arrest. *J Urol* 139:25, 1988.

Neves RJ, Zincke H; Surgical treatment of renal cancel with vena cava extension. *Br J Urol* 59:390, 1987.

Novick AC, Cosgrove DM: Surgical approach for removal of renal cell carcinoma extending into the vena cava and the right atrium. *J Urol* 123:947, 1980.

Pritchett TR, Lieskovsky G, Skinner DG: Extension of renal cell carcinoma into the vena cava: Clinical review and surgical approach. *J Urol* 135:460, 1986.

Schefft P, Novick AC, Straffon RA, Stewart BH: Surgery for renal cell carcinoma extending into the inferior vena cava. *J Urol* 120:28, 1978.

Sosa RE, Muecke EC, Vaughn ED Jr, McCarron JP Jr: Renal cell extending into the vena cava: The prognostic significance of the level of vena caval involvement. *J Urol* 132:1097, 1984.

CHAPTER 11

Partial Nephrectomy for Renal Cell Carcinoma

ANDREW C. NOVICK

The first partial nephrectomy was performed in 1884 by Wells for removal of a perirenal fibrolipoma. In 1887, Czerny was the first to use partial nephrectomy for excision of a renal neoplasm when he successfully removed an angiosarcoma from the upper third of the right kidney in a 30-year-old gardener. This approach was received initially with enthusiasm, but it was soon abandoned owing to an excessive postoperative morbidity. Interest in the application of partial nephrectomy to the treatment of renal tumors was revived in 1950 by Vermooten. He suggested that partial nephrectomy could be performed for peripheral clear-cell renal carcinoma even in the presence of a normal contralateral kidney. However, Robson and associates later demonstrated that nephrectomy for carcinoma performed outside Gerota's fascia yielded improved survival over pericapsular nephrectomy.

Although radical nephrectomy must still be considered optimum curative therapy for patients with localized renal cell carcinoma, partial nephrectomy is the treatment of choice for localized carcinomas present bilaterally or in a solitary functioning kidney. In such patients, partial nephrectomy allows complete surgical excision of the primary tumor while preserving sufficient renal parenchyma to avoid the need for renal replacement therapy. This approach is gaining acceptance and popularity due to surgical advances that have extended its technical feasibility to include patients with large complex tumors, and because of accumulating data indicating that long-term cancer-free survival can be accomplished in a high percentage of patients. We reported an actuarial 5-year patient survival rate of 60% in 23 patients who underwent partial nephrectomy for localized renal cell carcinoma before 1980 with a mean follow-up of 65 months. This is comparable to corresponding rates that have been reported after radical nephrectomy for stage I renal cell carcinoma. As a result of studies such as this, the indications for partial nephrectomy have been expanded to include patients with localized renal cell carcinoma and a functioning opposite kidney when that kidney is involved with a disorder (such as calculi, diabetes, pyelonephritis, nephrosclerosis, etc.) that might cause progressive renal functional impairment in the future. Some groups, including ours, are also using this approach to remove small, confined peripheral tumors with a completely normal opposite kidney.

A variety of surgical techniques are available for performing partial nephrectomy in patients with renal cell carcinoma. These include: *(a)* simple enucleation; *(b)* polar segmental nephrectomy with preliminary ligation of the appropriate renal arterial branch; *(c)* wedge resection; *(d)* major transverse resection; and *(e)* extracorporeal partial nephrectomy and renal autotransplantation. All of these techniques require adherence to basic principles of early vascular control, avoidance of ischemic renal damage, complete tumor excision with free margins, precise closure of the collecting system, careful hemostasis, and closure or coverage of the renal defect with adjacent fat, fascia, peritoneum, or oxycel. The following description of these parenchyma-sparing techniques is based on our experience with over 100 of these operations in patients with renal cell carcinoma at the Cleveland Clinic.

GENERAL CONSIDERATIONS

Patients undergoing partial nephrectomy for renal cell carcinoma should be studied preoperatively with standard catheter renal arteriography to delineate the main renal artery and its branches. Knowledge of the number and location of these vessels helps greatly in removing the tumor with minimal blood loss and injury to adjacent parenchyma. In most patients, intravenous digital subtraction angiography does not provide satisfactory visualization of the renal artery branches.

There are important distinctions between the arterial and venous blood supply of the kidney that must be kept in mind when performing these operations. All segmental renal arteries are end-arteries with no collateral circulation; therefore, all branches supplying tumor-free parenchyma must be preserved to avoid devitalization of functioning renal tissue. The renal venous drainage system differs significantly from the arterial blood supply in that the intrarenal venous branches intercommunicate freely between the various renal segments. Ligation of a branch of the renal vein, therefore, will not result in segmental infarction of the kidney because collateral venous blood supply will provide adequate drainage. This is important clinically because it enables one to obtain surgical access safely to tumors in the renal hilus by ligating and dividing small adjacent or overlying venous branches. This allows major venous branches to be mobilized completely and retracted freely in either direction to expose the tumor with no vascular compromise of uninvolved parenchyma.

In the vast majority of patients undergoing conservative surgery for renal cell carcinoma, partial nephrectomy can be done in situ. Extracorporeal partial nephrectomy and autotransplantation are only required in the patient with an exceptionally large central tumor. Whichever approach is used, every attempt should be made to minimize intraoperative ischemic renal damage. In all cases, administration of 200 ml/hr of intravenous fluid is initiated the evening before operation to ensure optimal renal perfusion in the operating room. Important general intraoperative measures include prevention of hypotension during anesthesia, administration of mannitol, and avoidance of traction and/or excessive manipulation of the renal vessels. When the renal circulation is interrupted temporarily, additional specific protective measures are indicated, as outlined in the following sections of this chapter.

Patients with localized synchronous bilateral renal carcinoma present an interesting dilemma in terms of the approach to partial nephrectomy. Most of these patients are in the fifth or sixth decade, are otherwise healthy, and have a life expectancy of 10–20 years if they remain free of malignancy. In general, operative therapy should be oriented toward preserving as much tumor-free renal parenchyma as possible to guard against either a renal-threatening surgical complication or the development later in life of a disorder that impairs renal function. Therefore, our present approach is to perform bilateral partial nephrectomies if these are technically feasible. In most cases, it is more prudent to stage these operations, although bilateral simultaneous renal surgery may be done if both kidneys are involved with relatively small tumors. When one of the involved kidneys is extensively replaced by tumor, then a radical nephrectomy on that side and a contralateral partial nephrectomy are indicated. Again, unless partial nephrectomy is being done for a small tumor, it is more prudent to stage these operations. In this situation, the partial nephrectomy is done first and, when a good surgical result is assured, the contralateral radical nephrectomy is done. This sequence obviates the need for temporary dialysis if acute tubular necrosis occurs after the partial nephrectomy.

IN SITU PARTIAL NEPHRECTOMY

As mentioned previously, it is usually possible to perform partial nephrectomy for renal cell carcinoma in situ by using an operative approach that optimizes exposure of the kidney and by combining meticulous surgical technique with an understanding of the renal vascular anatomy in relation to the tumor. We employ an extraperitoneal flank incision through the bed of the 11th or 12th rib for all of these operations. This incision allows the surgeon to operate on the mobilized kidney almost at skin level and provides excellent exposure of the peripheral renal vessels. With an anterior incision, the kidney is invariably located in the depth of the wound, and the surgical exposure is simply not as good.

When performing in situ partial nephrectomy for renal cell carcinoma, the kidney is mobilized inside Gerota's fascia; however, the perirenal fat around the tumor is left undisturbed. For small encapsulated renal tumors, it may not be necessary to occlude the renal artery temporarily. In most cases, however, partial nephrectomy is performed most effectively after temporary renal arterial occlusion. The latter measure not only limits intraoperative bleeding but, by reducing renal tissue turgor, also improves access to intrarenal structures. In general, normothermic renal ischemia may not exceed 30 minutes if permanent damage to the kidney is to be avoided. Because the anticipated period of arterial occlusion in patients undergoing partial nephrectomy for renal cell carcinoma usually is longer than 30 minutes, additional protection from postischemic renal injury is necessary, and local hypothermia currently offers the most effective technique. The most popular methods of in situ renal hypothermia have involved surface cooling with ice slush packed around the kidney, various kinds of bags with cold saline solution and ice, a plastic pouch perfusion system, and advanced cooling coils. All of these techniques allow safe tolerance of at lest 3 hr of renal arterial occlusion with no resulting permanent kidney damage.

When performing partial nephrectomy with renal arterial occlusion, we use ice slush cooling for surface renal hypothermia because of its relative ease and simplicity. An important caveat with this method is to keep the entire kidney covered with ice slush for 10–15 minutes immediately after occluding the renal artery and before commencing the partial nephrectomy. This amount of time is needed to obtain core renal cooling to a temperature (15–20°C) that optimizes in situ renal preservation. During excision of the tumor, invariably large portions of the kidney are no longer covered with ice slush and, in the absence of adequate prior core renal cooling, rapid rewarming and ischemic renal injury can occur.

Another issue that arises in these cases is the need for systemic or regional anticoagulation before temporary renal arterial occlusion to prevent intrarenal vascular thrombosis. In our experience, these measures are not necessary unless there is existing small vessel or parenchymal disease involving the tumor-free portion of the kidney. Finally, we emphasize that intermittent clamping of the renal artery with short periods of recirculation should be avoided because this is more damaging to the kidney than continuous arterial occlusion for an equivalent interval of time.

When performing partial nephrectomy for renal cell carcinoma after excision of all gross tumor, the surgeon should verify absence of malignancy in the remaining portion of the kidney intraoperatively by frozen section examinations of biopsies obtained at random from the renal margin of excision. It is unusual for such biopsies to demonstrate residual tumor but, if so, additional renal tissue must be excised. After completing the partial nephrectomy, the surgeon may remove a few lymph nodes along the perirenal aorta or vena cava for prognostic purposes.

Simple Enucleation

Many renal carcinomas are completely enveloped by a distinct pseudocapsule of fibrous tissue that can allow relatively avascular tumor removal by enucleation with maximal conservation of renal tissue. These are generally small and low-grade lesions. The technique of enucleation involves circumferential incision of the parenchyma around the tumor, identifying the plane between the pseudocapsule and adjacent uninvolved parenchyma, and then bluntly shelling out the lesion with the butt end of a scalpel (Fig. 11.1). For in situ enucleation of peripheral tumors, it is generally unnecessary to occlude the renal artery, and the few transected blood vessels at the base of the enucleation can simply be ligated with 4–0 chromic sutures. While these ligatures are being inserted, the surgeon can control surface bleeding by gentle digital compression of the parenchyma. Fat or oxycel can be placed into the cavity and the margins of the parenchyma can be sutured together to be further assured of complete hemostasis.

In situ enucleation also can be done for small or medium-sized centrally located tumors that are accessible in the renal sinus. Tumors in this location often are vascularized directly from major segmental renal arterial or venous branches. Therefore, such enucleations are done best under surface hypothermia after temporary occlusion of the renal artery.

The technique of enucleation should be used only for tumors that are surrounded completely by a distinct pseudocapsule. The presence of such tumor encapsulation can be established preoperatively with a high degree of accuracy by combined arteriography and CT scanning. Our current practice is to remove a surrounding margin of normal parenchyma when this can be done readily, as in most peripheral tumors. We reserve enucleation primarily for encapsulated centrally located tumors, which otherwise may be impossible to excise, and for patients with von Hippel-Lindau disease who generally present with multiple encapsulated tumors. When enucleation is employed, the advantages of this technique are that it is simple and rapid to perform, renal arterial occlusion is often not necessary, maximal functioning renal parenchyma is preserved, and multiple tumors can be removed with this method.

Segmental Polar Nephrectomy

In patients with cancer confined to the upper or lower pole of the kidney, partial nephrectomy can be performed by isolating and ligating the segmental apical or basilar arterial branch while allowing unimpaired perfusion to the remainder of the kidney from the main renal artery. This is illustrated in Figure 11.2 for a tumor confined to the apical vascular segment. The apical artery is dissected away from adjacent structures, ligated, and divided. Often, a corresponding venous branch is present, which is similarly ligated and divided. An ischemic line of demarcation will then generally appear on the surface of the kidney and outlines the segment to be excised. If this is not obvious, a few milliliters of methylene blue can be directly injected distally into the ligated apical artery to outline the limits of the involved renal segment better. An incision is then made in the renal cortex at the line of demarcation, which should be at least 1–2 cm away from the visible edge of the cancer. The parenchyma is divided by sharp and blunt dissection, and the polar segment is removed. It is generally not possible to preserve a strip of capsule beyond the parenchymal line of resection for use in closing the renal defect.

Often, a portion of the collecting system will have been removed with the cancer during a segmental polar nephrectomy. The collecting system is carefully closed with interrupted or continuous 4–0 chromic sutures to ensure a watertight closure. Small transected blood vessels on the renal surface are identified and ligated with shallow figure-eight 4–0 chromic sutures. The edges of the kidney are then reapproximated as an added hemostatic measure. This is done with simple interrupted 2–0 or 3–0 chromic sutures inserted through the capsule and a small amount of parenchyma. Before these sutures are tied, one can insert perirenal fat or oxycel into the defect for inclusion in the renal closure. If the collecting system has been entered, a Penrose drain is left in the perinephric space.

Wedge Resection

Wedge resection is an appropriate technique for removing peripheral tumors on the surface of the kidney, particularly ones that are larger, not well encapsulated, or both. Because these lesions often encompass more than one renal segment and because this technique is generally associated with heavier bleeding, it is best to perform wedge resection with temporary renal arterial occlusion and surface hypothermia (Fig. 11.3).

In performing a wedge resection, the physician removes the tumor with a 1- to 2-cm surrounding margin of grossly normal renal parenchyma. Again, the parenchyma is divided by a combination of sharp and blunt dissection. Invariably, the tumor extends deeply into the kidney and the collecting system is entered. Often, prominent intrarenal vessels are identified as the parenchyma is being incised; if so, these may be directly suture-ligated at that time when they are most visible.

With wedge resections involving removal of a significant amount of parenchyma, an internal ureteral stent is passed distally into the bladder through an opening in the renal collecting system, with the proximal end positioned in the renal pelvis. The collecting system is closed with interrupted or continuous 4–0 chromic sutures. Remaining transected blood vessels on the renal surface are secured with figure-eight 4–0 chromic sutures. Bleeding at this point is usually minimal, and the operative field can be kept satisfactorily clear by gentle suction during placement of hemostatic sutures.

The renal defect can be closed in one of two ways. The kidney may be closed upon itself by approximating the transected cortical margins with simple interrupted 2–0 or 3–0 chromic sutures, after placing a small piece of oxycel at the base of the defect. If this is done, there must be no tension on the suture line and no significant distortion (angulation or

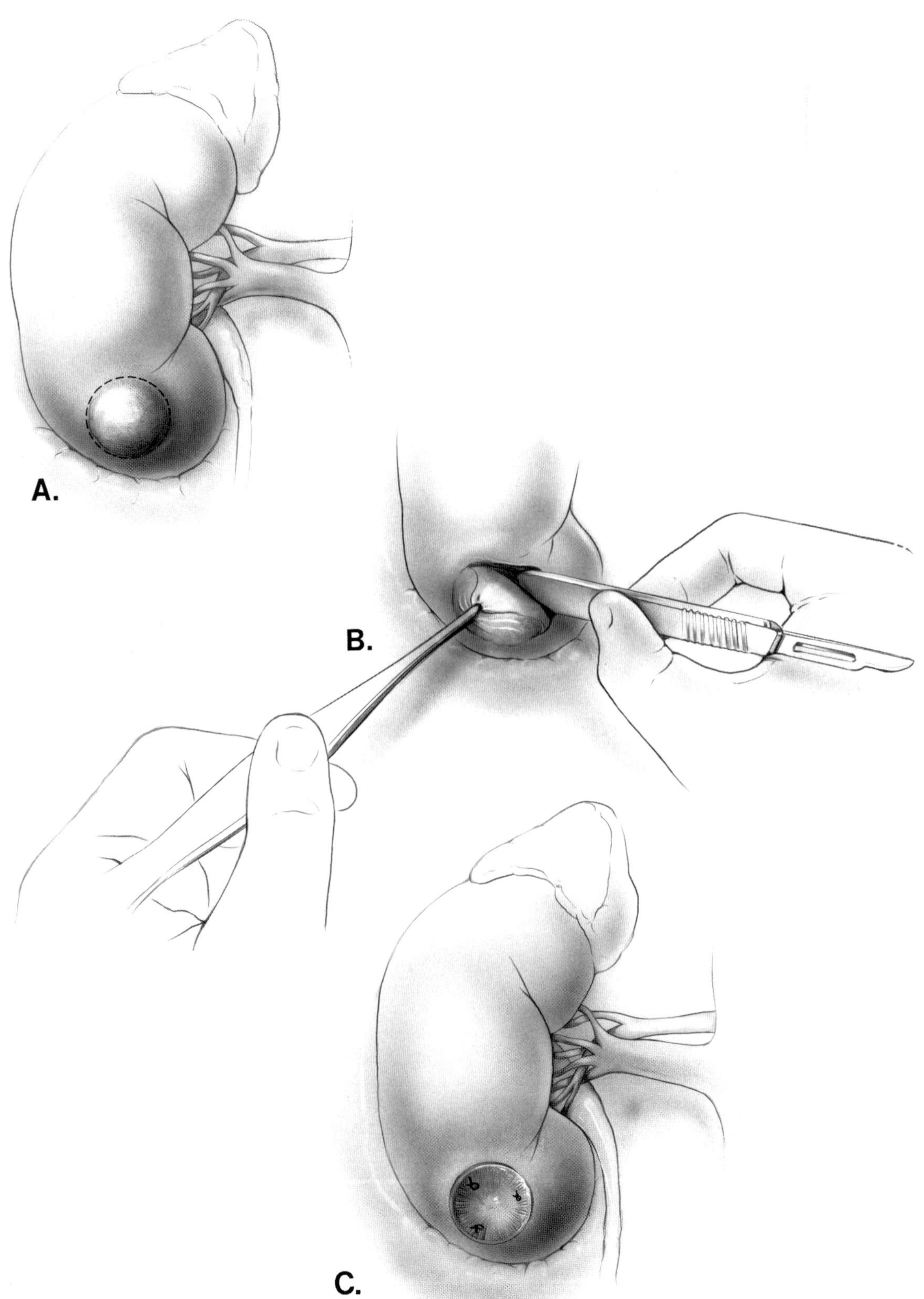

Figure 11.1. Technique of enucleation for tumors with a surrounding pseudocapsule. This can often be done without temporary renal arterial occlusion. (From Novick AC: Partial nephrectomy for renal cell carcinoma. *Urol Clin North Am* 14:419, 1987.)

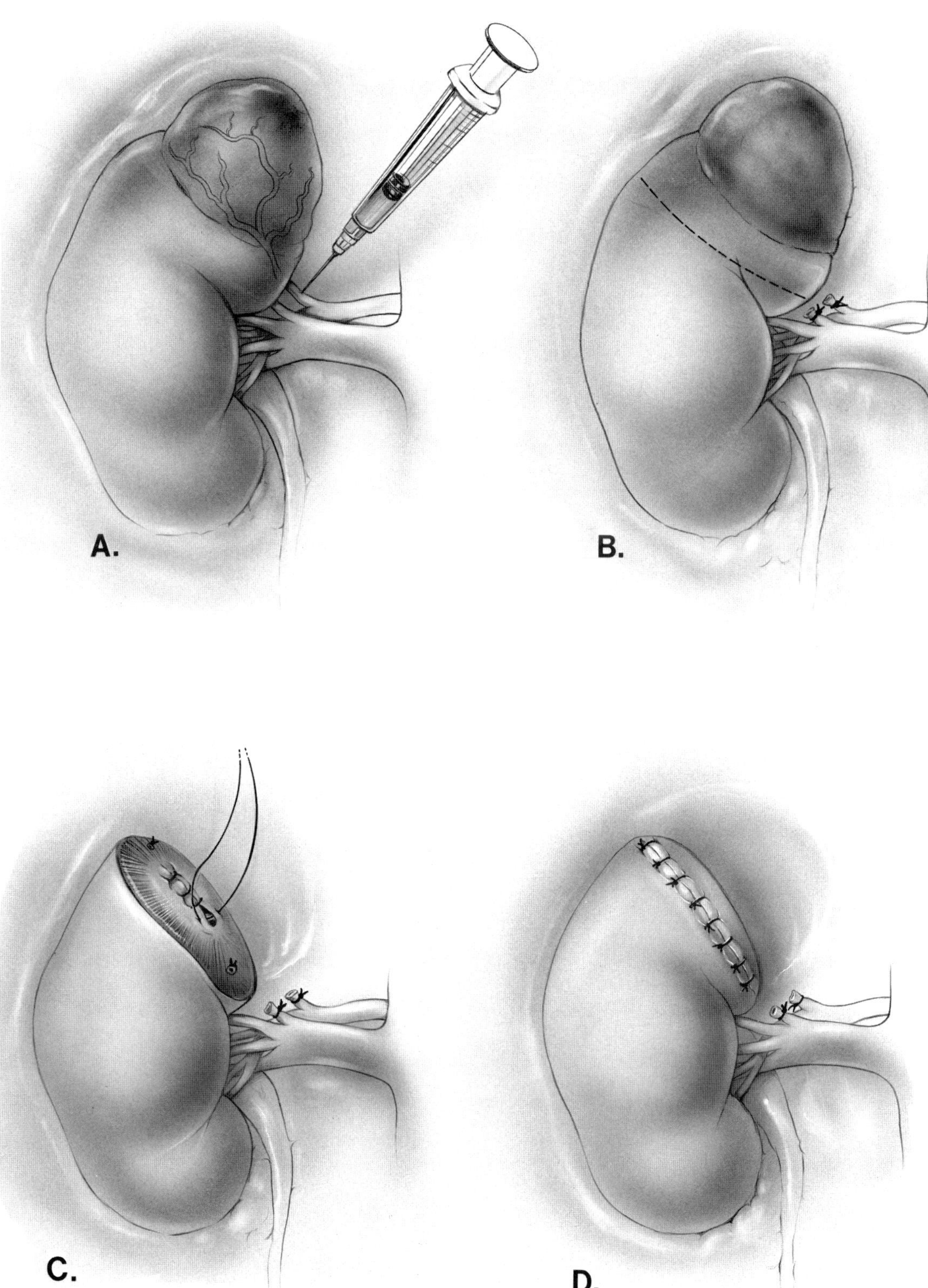

Figure 11.2. Technique of segmental (apical) polar nephrectomy with preliminary ligation of apical arterial and venous branches. Methylene blue can be injected into the arterial branch to delineate the line of demarcation. (From Novick AC: Partial nephrectomy for renal cell carcinoma. *Urol Clin North Am* 14:419, 1987.)

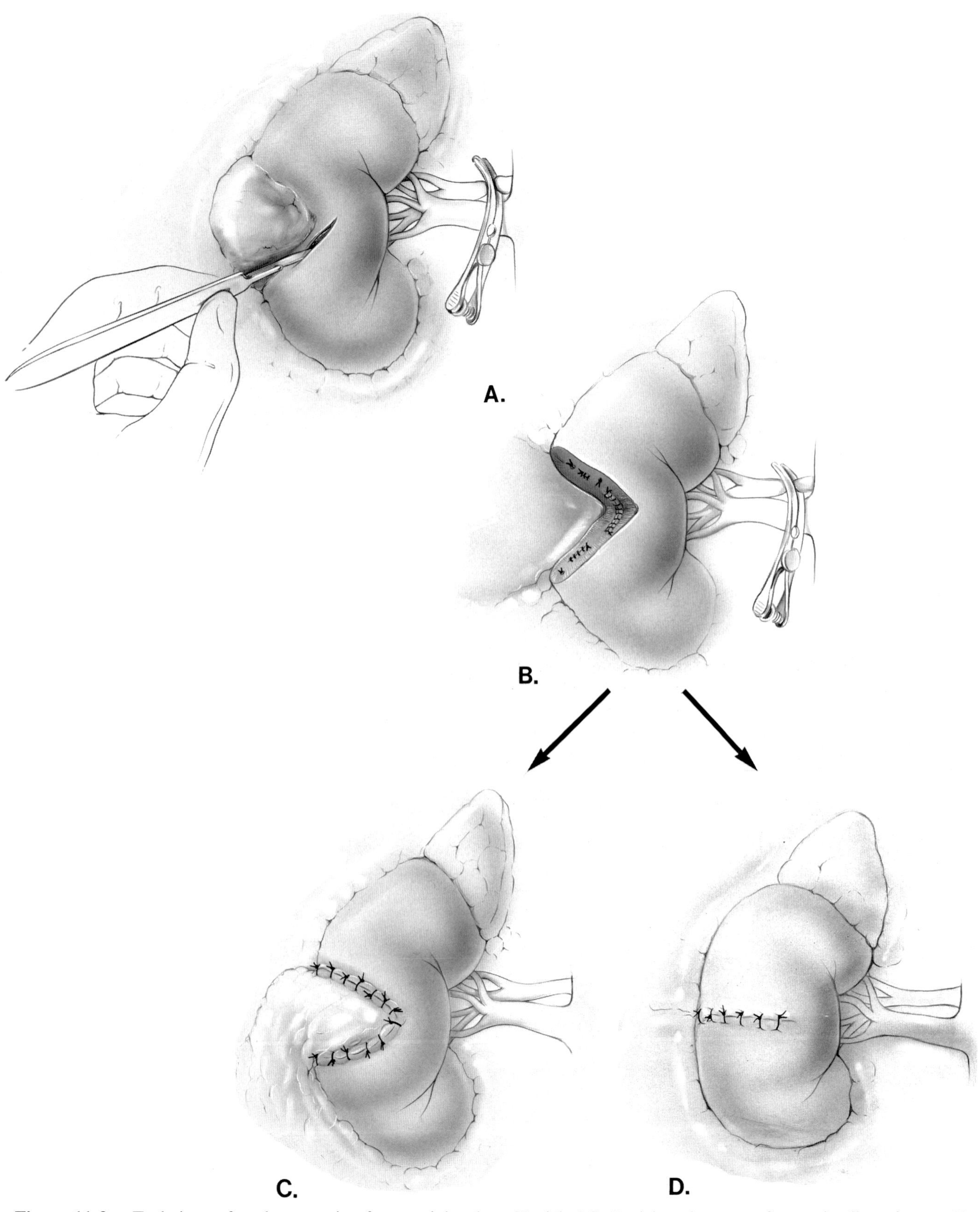

Figure 11.3. Technique of wedge resection for a peripheral tumor on the surface of the kidney. The renal defect may be closed upon itself, **D,** or covered with perirenal fat, **C.** (From Novick AC: Partial nephrectomy for renal cell carcinoma. *Urol Clin North Am* 14:419, 1987.)

kinking) of blood vessels supplying the kidney. Alternatively, a portion of perirenal fat may simply be inserted into the base of the renal defect as a hemostatic measure and sutured to the pharenchymal margins with interrupted 4–0 chromic sutures. After closure or coverage of the renal defect, the renal artery is unclamped and circulation to the kidney is restored. A Penrose drain is left in the perinephric space.

Major Transverse Resection

A transverse resection is done to remove large tumors that extensively involve the upper or lower portion of the kidney (Fig. 11.4). This technique is performed under surface hypothermia after temporary occlusion of the renal artery. Major branches of the renal artery and vein supplying the tumor-bearing portion of the kidney are identified in the renal hilus, ligated, and divided. If possible, this should be done before temporarily occluding the renal artery to minimize the overall period of renal ischemia.

After occluding the renal artery, the physician divides the parenchyma by blunt and sharp dissection, leaving a 1- to 2-cm margin of grossly normal tissue around the tumor. Transected blood vessels on the renal surface are secured as previously described and the hilus is inspected carefully for remaining unligated segmental vessels. The collecting system is closed after placement of an internal ureteral stent. If possible, the renal defect is sutured together with one of the techniques just described. If this cannot be done without tension or without distorting the renal vessels, then a piece of peritoneum or perirenal fat is sutured in place to cover the defect. Circulation to the kidney is then restored and a Penrose drain is left in the perirenal space.

EXTRACORPOREAL PARTIAL NEPHRECTOMY AND AUTOTRANSPLANTATION

Extracorporeal partial nephrectomy enables removal of complex renal tumors previously considered inoperable. This

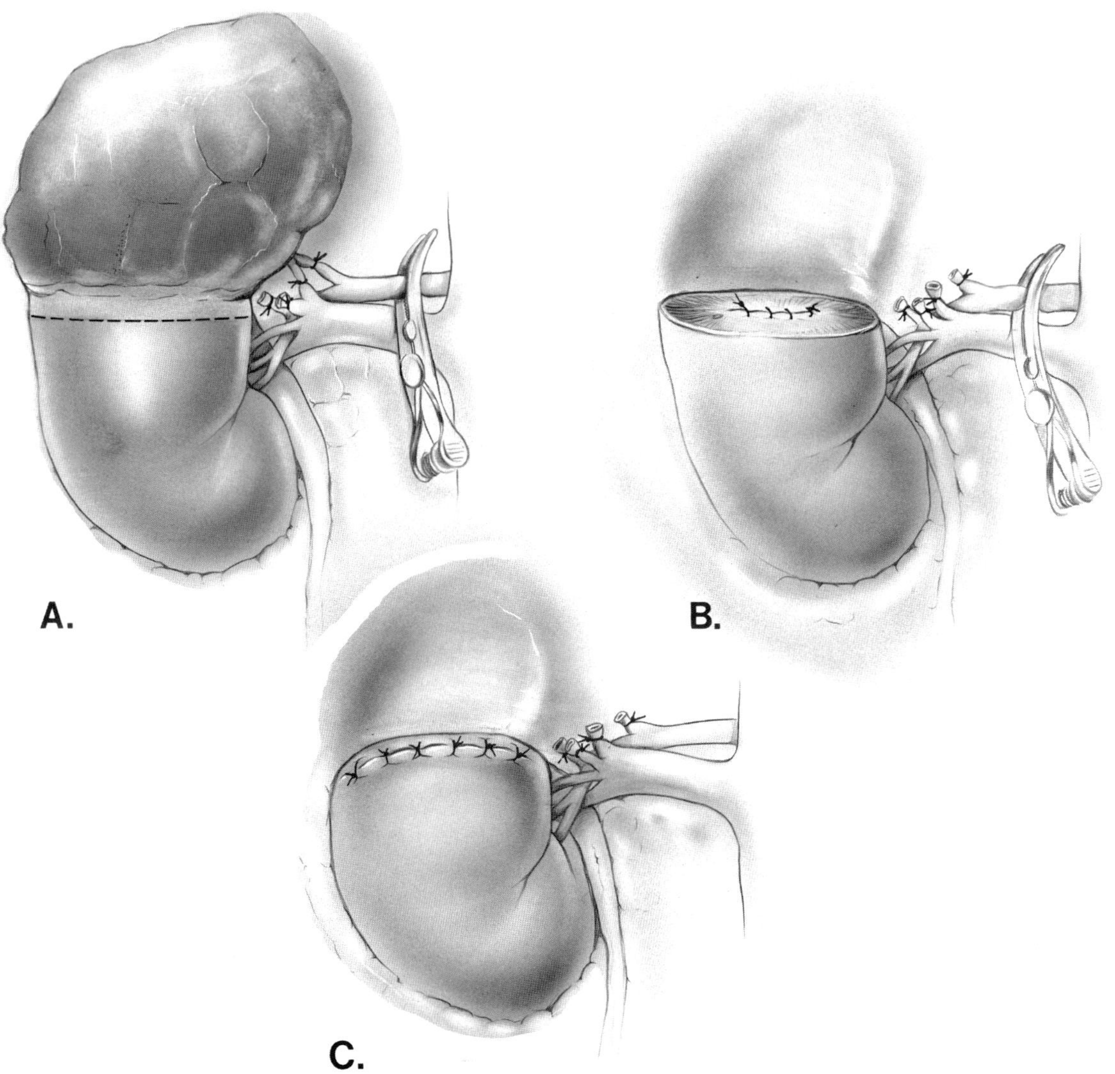

Figure 11.4. Technique of transverse resection for a tumor involving the upper half of the kidney. (From Novick AC: Partial nephrectomy for renal cell carcinoma. *Urol Clin North Am* 14:419, 1987.)

technique involves increased operative time with greater potential morbidity and, therefore, should be reserved for the relatively small number of patients with large, hypervascular central tumors that are not amenable to in situ excision. The advantages of an extracorporeal approach in such cases include optimum exposure, a bloodless surgical field, the ability to perform a more precise operation with maximal conservation of renal parenchyma, and greater protection of the kidney from prolonged ischemia. Some data also suggest that postoperative local tumor recurrence is less common with this approach than when partial nephrectomy is done in situ.

Extracorporeal partial nephrectomy and renal autotransplantation are generally performed through a single midline incision. In heavy-set or obese patients, an anterior subcostal transperitoneal incision is combined with a separate lower quadrant transverse semilunar incision. The kidney is mobilized and removed outside Gerota's fascia with ligation and division of the renal artery and vein as the last steps in the operation. A regional lymphadenectomy may then be done. Immediately after dividing the renal vessels, the removed kidney is flushed with 500 ml of chilled Collins' solution and is then submerged in a basin of ice slush saline solution to maintain hypothermia. Under these conditions, if warm renal ischemia has been minimal, the kidney can safely be preserved outside the body for as much time as needed to perform extracorporeal partial nephrectomy.

If possible, it is best to leave the ureter attached in such cases to preserve its distal collateral vascular supply, particularly with large hilar or lower renal tumors where complex excision may unavoidably compromise the blood supply to the pelvis, ureter, or both. When this is done, the extracorporeal operation is done on the abdominal wall of the patient. If the ureter is left attached, it must be occluded temporarily to prevent retrograde blood flow to the kidney when it is outside the body. Often, unless the patient is thin, working on the abdominal wall with the ureter attached is cumbersome because of the tethering and restricted movement of the kidney. If this is observed, the ureter should be divided and the kidney placed on a separate workbench. This will provide better exposure for the extracorporeal operation and, as this is being done, a second surgical team simultaneously can be preparing the iliac fossa for autotransplantation. If concern exists about the adequacy of ureteral blood supply, the risk of postoperative urinary extravasation can be diminished by restoring urinary continuity through direct anastomosis of the renal pelvis to the retained distal ureter.

Extracorporeal partial nephrectomy is done with the flushed kidney preserved under surface hypothermia (Fig. 11.5). The kidney is first divested of all perinephric fat to appreciate the full extent of the neoplasm. Because such tumors are usually centrally located, dissection is generally begun in the renal hilus with identification of major segmental arterial and venous branches. Vessels clearly directed toward the neoplasm are secured and divided; those vessels supplying uninvolved renal parenchyma are preserved. The tumor is then removed by incising the capsule and parenchyma to preserve a 1- to 2-cm surrounding margin of normal renal tissue. Transected blood vessels visible on the renal surface are secured and the collecting system is closed as described for in situ partial nephrectomy.

After completing the resection, the surgeon verifies tumor-free margins by frozen section histopathology. There is little indication for extracorporeal arteriography; however, if this is done, iothalamate rather than diatrizoate contrast material should be used because the latter may crystallize at low temperatures. Also, the kidney should be immediately reflushed to prevent contrast-induced toxicity.

At this point, the renal remnant is placed on the pulsatile perfusion unit primarily to facilitate identification and suture ligation of remaining potential bleeding points. The kidney is alternately perfused through the renal artery and vein to ensure both arterial and venous hemostasis. Because the perfusate lacks clotting ability, there may continue to be some parenchymal oozing, which can safely be ignored. If possible, the defect created by the partial nephrectomy is closed by suturing the kidney upon itself to further ensure a watertight repair.

Autotransplantation into the iliac fossa is then done using the same vascular technique as in renal allotransplantation. Urinary continuity may be restored with ureteroneocystostomy or pyeloureterostomy, leaving an internal ureteral stent in place. When removal of the neoplasm has necessitated extensive hilar dissection of vessels supplying the renal pelvis, a nephrostomy tube is also left indwelling for postoperative drainage. After autotransplantation, a Penrose drain is positioned extraperitoneally in the iliac fossa away from the vascular anastomotic sites.

RENAL CARCINOMA IN PATIENTS WITH VON HIPPEL-LINDAU DISEASE

Renal cell carcinoma is known to be present in 35–40% of patients with von Hippel-Lindau disease. There are several distinctive features associated with renal cell carcinoma in this setting. These tumors are found in younger patients more often than sporadically occurring renal cell carcinoma, and they are generally multiple and bilateral. Although such tumors may be solid, it is more common for renal cell carcinoma to be present within the wall of one or more renal cysts. The latter are generally low-grade papillary renal cell carcinomas with a hypovascular appearance on arteriography.

There is no way to determine the nature of a cystic renal mass in such patients other than through surgical excision and histopathologic examination. Therefore, in patients with von Hippel-Lindau disease who undergo partial nephrectomy for renal cell carcinoma, all solid and cystic renal lesions must be excised to ensure complete tumor removal (Fig. 11.6). Some of these lesions may be quite small, and their number and location are established by a combination of preoperative CT scanning and direct intraoperative inspection of the renal surface. Partial nephrectomy technically may be more complicated in patients with von Hippel-Lindau disease but can be done using the techniques described in this article.

POSTOPERATIVE FOLLOW-UP

Patients who undergo partial nephrectomy as curative treatment for renal carcinoma must be followed closely for local

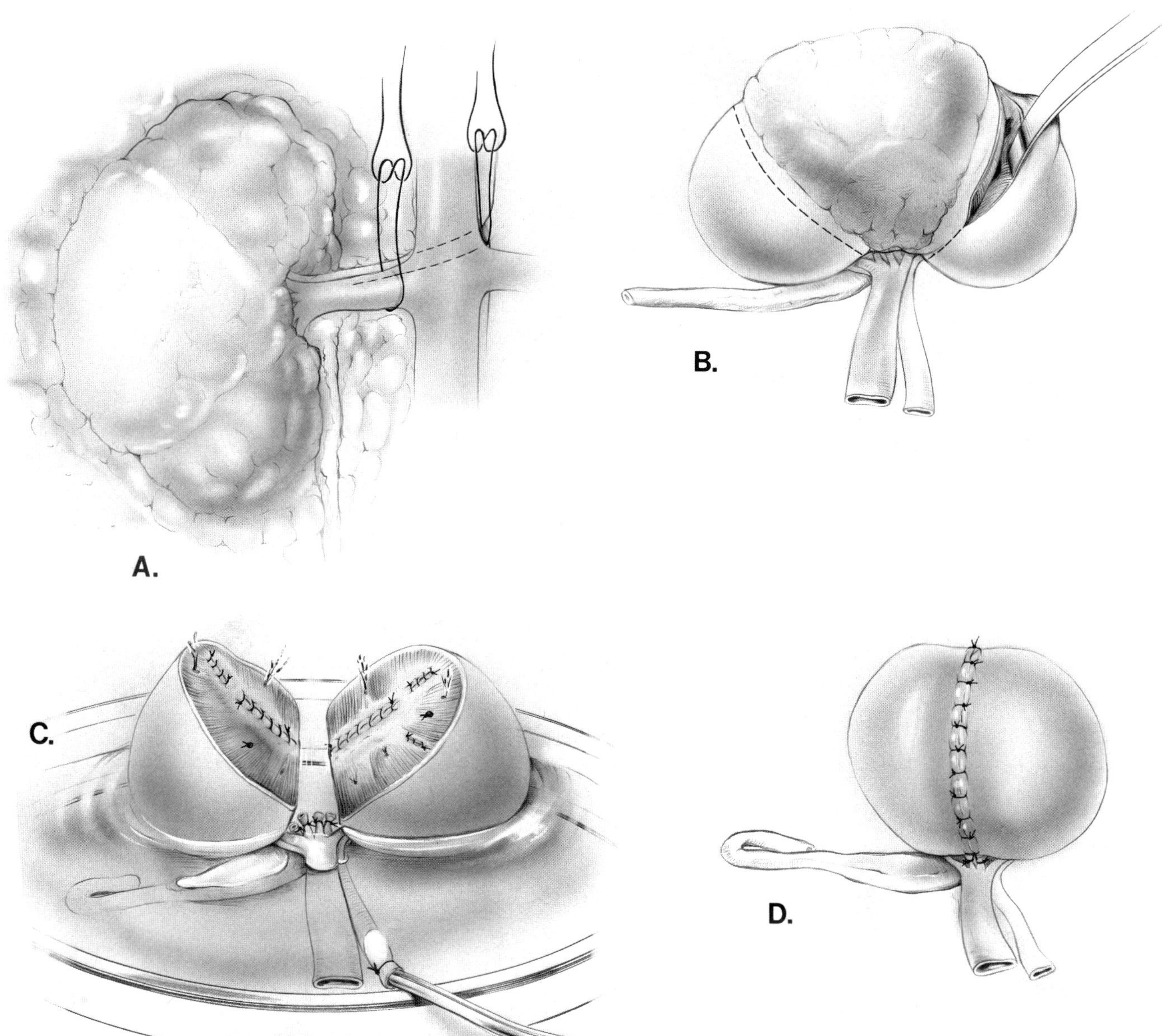

Figure 11.5. Technique of extracorporeal partial nephrectomy for a large central tumor. **A,** the kidney is removed outside Gerota's fascia. **B,** the tumor is excised extracorporeally while preserving the vascular branches to uninvolved parenchyma. **C,** pulsatile perfusion is used to identify transected blood vessels. **D,** the kidney is closed upon itself. (From Novick AC: Partial nephrectomy for renal cell carcinoma. *Urol Clin North Am* 14:419, 1987.)

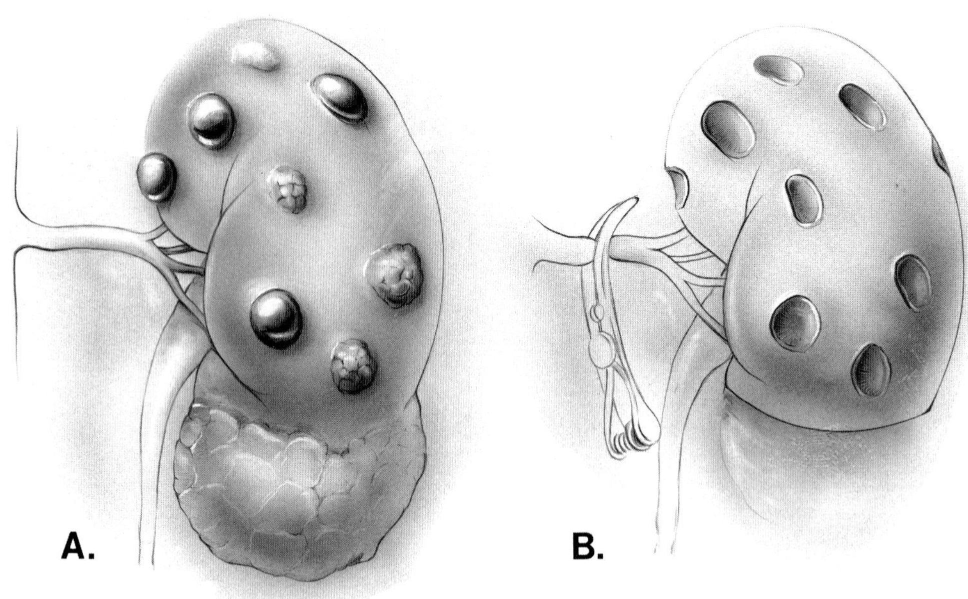

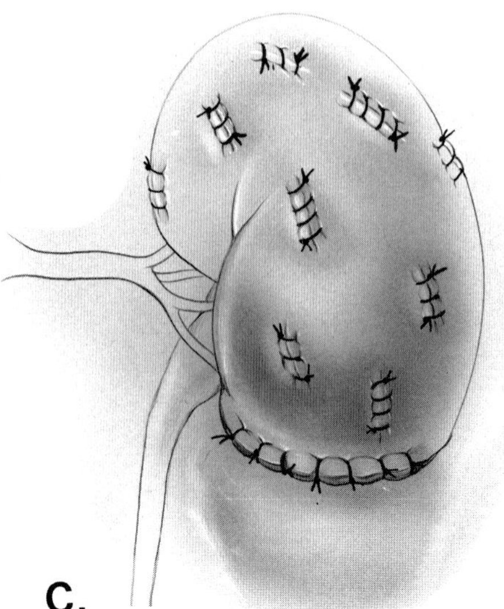

Figure 11.6. These sketches illustrate the typical excision of multiple cystic and solid tumors from the kidney in patients with von Hippel-Lindau disease. (From Novick AC: Partial nephrectomy for renal cell carcinoma. *Urol Clin North Am* 14:419, 1987.)

and/or metastatic recurrence of their malignancy. Local tumor recurrence in the treated kidney is a potential disadvantage of partial nephrectomy and this has been reported in 9–13% of patients. Computed tomography scanning is presently the most accurate diagnostic method for detecting such recurrence, and this should be done at least every 6 months postoperatively to ensure an early diagnosis. Patients who develop a local recurrence with no signs of metastasis may be considered for secondary surgical treatment. In some cases, another partial nephrectomy can be done with complete tumor excision and preservation of renal function. If this is not technically possible, total nephrectomy with initiation of chronic dialysis and subsequent renal allotransplantation is an available option that can achieve extended cancer-free survival with restored renal function.

Suggested Readings

Czerny HE: Cited by Herczel E: Ueber Nierenextirpation Beitr. 2. *Klin Chir* 6:485, 1980.

Gittes RF, Blute RD Jr: Repeat bench surgery on a solitary kidney. *J Urol* 127:530, 1982.

Jacobs SC, Berg SI, Lawson RK: Synchronous bilateral renal cell carcinoma: Total surgical excision. *Cancer* 46:2341, 1980.

Marberger M, Pugh RCB, Auvert J, et al: Conservative surgery of renal carcinoma: The EIRSS Experience. *Br J Urol* 53:528, 1981.

Novick AC: Renal hypothermia: In vivo and ex vivo. *Urol Clin North Am* 10:637, 1983.

Novick AC, Stewart BH, Straffon RA: Partial nephrectomy in the treatment of renal adenocarcinoma. *J Urol* 118:932, 1977.

Novick AC, Straffon RA: Management of locally recurrent renal carcinoma following partial nephrectomy. *J Urol* 138:603, 1987.

Novick AC, Zincke H, Neves RJ, et al: Surgical enucleation for renal cell carcinoma. *J Urol* 135:235, 1986.

Penn I: Transplantation in patients with primary renal malignancies. *Transplantation* 24:424, 1977.

Robson CJ, Churchill BM, Anderson W: The results of radical nephrectomy for renal cell carcinoma. *J Urol* 101:297, 1969.

Skinner DG, Colvin RB, Vermillion CD, et al: Diagnosis and management of renal cell carcinoma: A clinical and pathologic study of 309 cases. *Cancer* 28:1165, 1971.

Smith RB, DeKernion JB, Ehrlich RM, et al: Bilateral renal cell carcinoma and renal cell carcinoma in the solitary kidney. *J Urol* 132: 450, 1984.

Spencer W, Novick AC, Montie JE, Streem SB: Surgical treatment of renal cell carcinoma in von Hippel-Lindau disease. *J Urol* 139:507, 1988.

Topley M, Novick AC, Montie JE: Long-term results following partial nephrectomy for localized renal adenocarcinoma. *J Urol* 131:1050, 1984.

Vermooten V: Indications for conservative surgery in certain renal tumors: A study based on the growth pattern of clear cell carcinoma. *J Urol* 64:200, 1950.

Wells S: Successful removal of two solid circum-renal tumors. *Br Med J* 1:758, 1884.

Zabbo A, Novick AC: Digital subtraction angiography for non-invasive imaging of the renal artery. *Urol Clin North Am* 11:409, 1984.

Zincke H, Swanson SK: Bilateral renal cell carcinoma: Influence of synchronous and asynchronous occurrence on patient survival. *J Urol* 128:913, 1982.

CHAPTER 12

Conservative Surgery for Renal Pelvic Transitional Cell Carcinoma

ANDREW C. NOVICK
STEVAN B. STREEM

Transitional cell carcinoma (TCC) of the renal pelvis comprises 5–7% of all renal malignancies and the incidence of bilaterality is 2–4%. In patients with localized renal pelvic TCC, nephroureterectomy with a bladder cuff has been the standard approach to treatment for several reasons. These include the multifocal nature of this malignancy, the high attendant risk of ipsilateral recurrence, the low incidence of contralateral renal involvement, and the anatomically thin wall of the upper urinary tract, which may favor local invasion and metastatic spread at an early stage.

A conservative surgical approach to renal pelvic TCC with local tumor excision and preservation of the involved kidney was first suggested 40 years ago by Vest. At the present time, this approach is primarily reserved for selected patients with low grade, noninvasive malignancy present bilaterally or in a solitary kidney to avoid the need for dialytic renal replacement therapy.

A variety of conservative treatment approaches are available for patients with renal pelvic TCC. The most commonly performed operations in these patients have been partial nephrectomy and open pyelotomy with tumor excision and fulguration. Recently, endourologic techniques have been used to treat these patients. Topical use of chemotherapeutic agents directly instilled into the upper urinary tract is another alternative that may prove to be efficacious in the conservative management of renal pelvic TCC.

We describe below those techniques which have proven most useful at our center when a nephron-sparing approach is indicated for renal pelvic TCC.

OPEN PYELOTOMY AND TUMOR EXCISION

Open pyelotomy and tumor excision may be employed in patients with noninvasive TCC confined to a portion of the renal pelvis. Occasionally, small lesions involving an infundibulum may be accessible for this approach. This operation is performed through an extraperitoneal flank incision with mobilization of the entire kidney within Gerota's fascia.

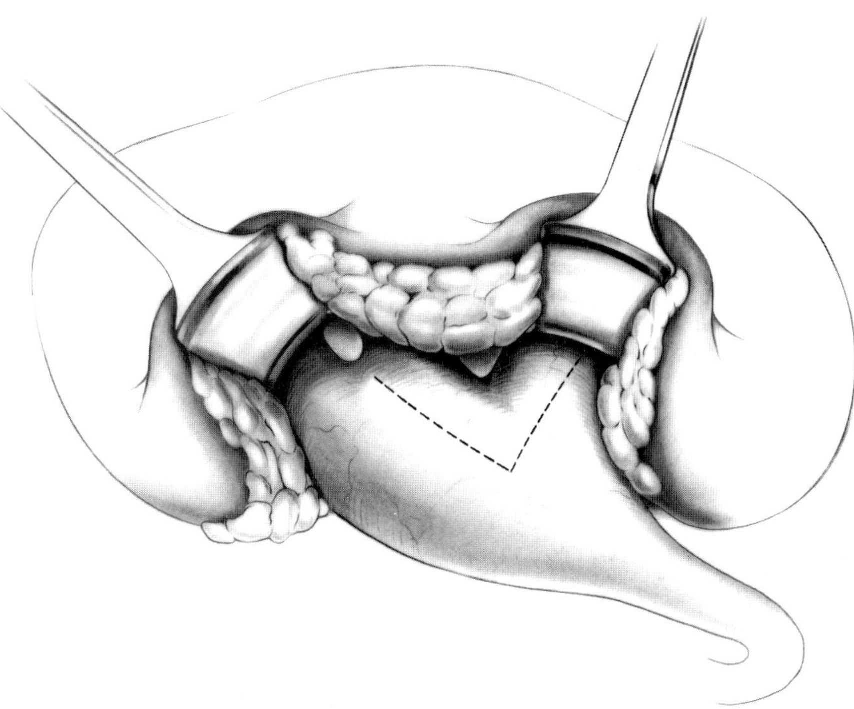

Figure 12.1. The upper ureter and renal pelvis are mobilized along the posterior renal aspect. The renal pelvic dissection is carried into the renal sinus, which often also exposes one or more infundibula. Small vein or Gil-Vernet retractors are used to maintain this operative exposure. The planned incision into the renal pelvis is shown. This incision may be extended into an infundibulum if necessary.

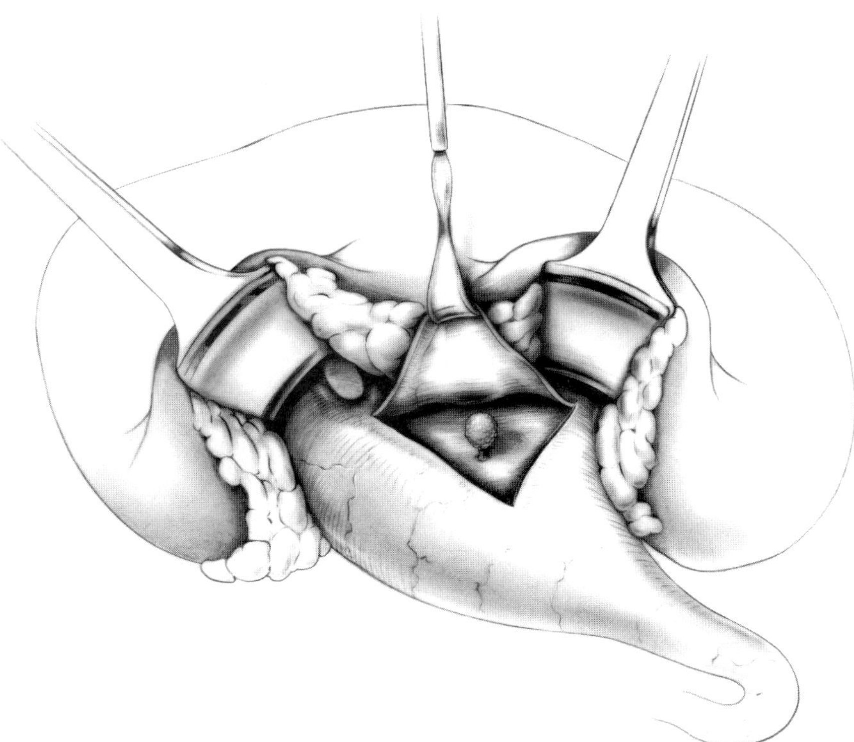

Figure 12.2. The renal pelvic incision is made to expose the tumor-bearing portion of the renal pelvis.

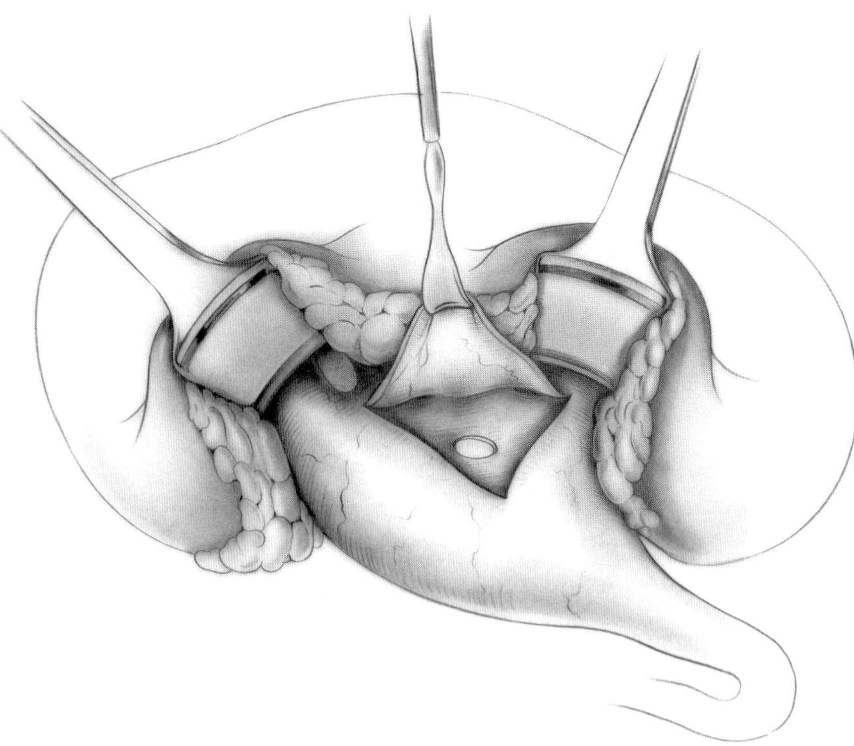

Figure 12.3. We prefer, when possible, to excise a full-thickness segment of the renal pelvis encompassing the tumor, as shown here. Frozen sections are prepared to ensure that the resected margins are free of disease. An alternative approach is to sharply excise the tumor at its base, while preserving the integrity of the renal pelvic wall, and then to fulgurate the base and surrounding area extensively.

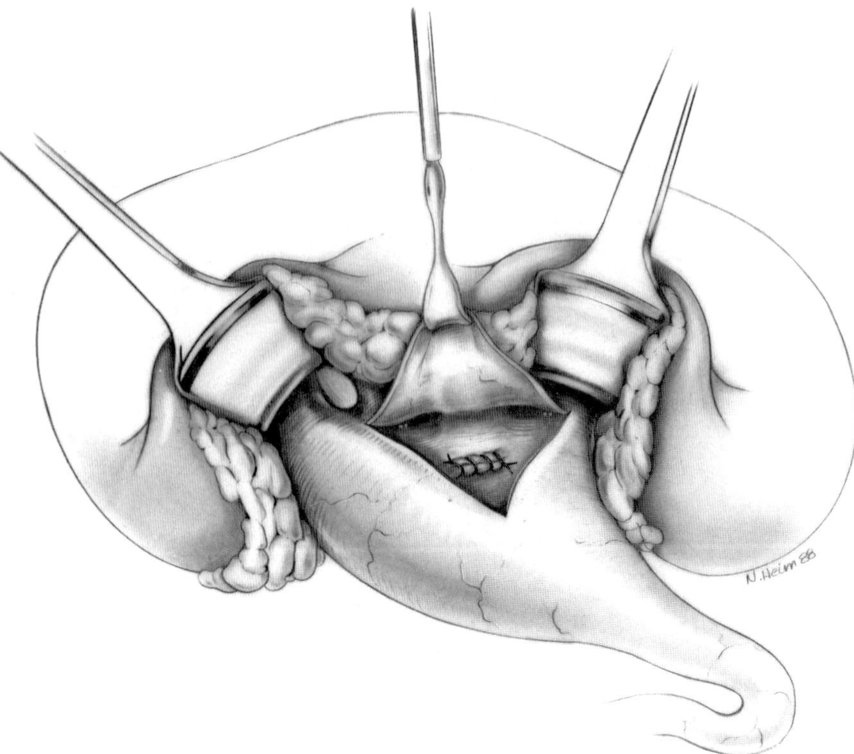

Figure 12.4. Following excision of all gross tumor, operative pyeloscopy is used to examine the intrarenal collecting system for any remaining lesions. The site of renal pelvic tumor excision is repaired with 4–0 chromic suture and the pyelotomy incision is then similarly closed.

PARTIAL NEPHRECTOMY

In selected patients, partial nephrectomy may be performed. This approach is indicated when the lesion involves an infundibulum or calyx rather than the renal pelvis. At times, partial nephrectomy may be combined with open pyelotomy (described above) for lesions involving both areas of the collecting system. The various techniques for performing partial nephrectomy are described in detail in chapter 11.

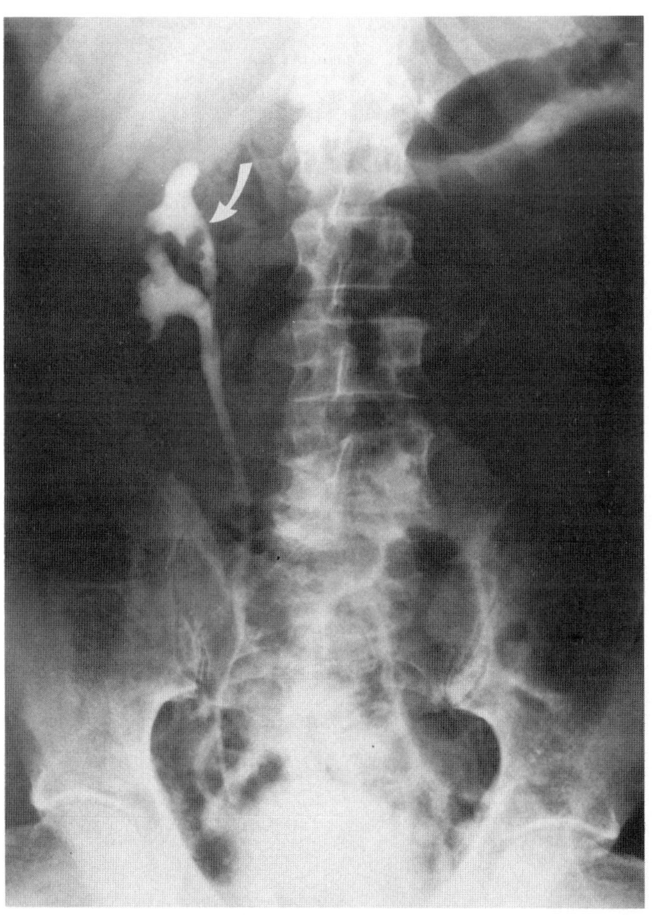

Figure 12.5. This patient had undergone left nephroureterectomy for multifocal transitional cell carcinoma of the left renal pelvis and ureter. Intravenous urography now suggested a lesion in the upper infundibulum of the remaining right kidney. This was confirmed at the time of retrograde pyelography *(arrow)*.

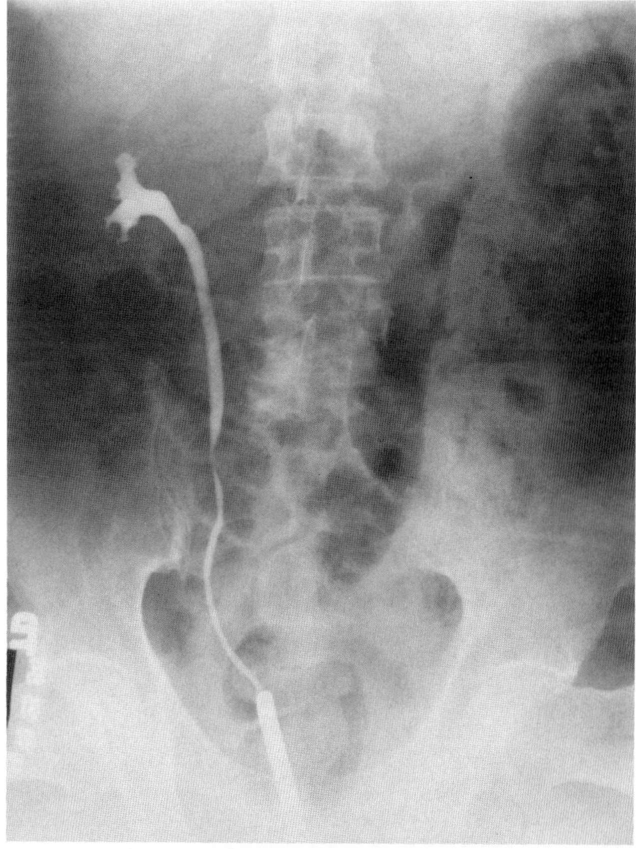

Figure 12.6. Upper pole partial nephrectomy was performed, leaving the pelvis and lower infundibulocalyceal system intact, as demonstrated on this postoperative retrograde pyelogram.

PERCUTANEOUS MANAGEMENT

Some patients who are candidates for conservative treatment of renal pelvic TCC may be considered for percutaneous management. The site for percutaneous access is chosen as it would be for a stone in a similar location. That is, lesions in the mid or lower infundibula or calyces are approached directly through the involved area. Renal pelvic lesions may be approached through the lower or mid infundibulocalyceal system. Upper infundibulocalyceal lesions are difficult to access but may be reached through a lower infundibulocalyceal approach. The access, dilatation, and resection of the lesion should be performed as a single stage procedure whenever possible to minimize the risk of tumor seeding in the tract.

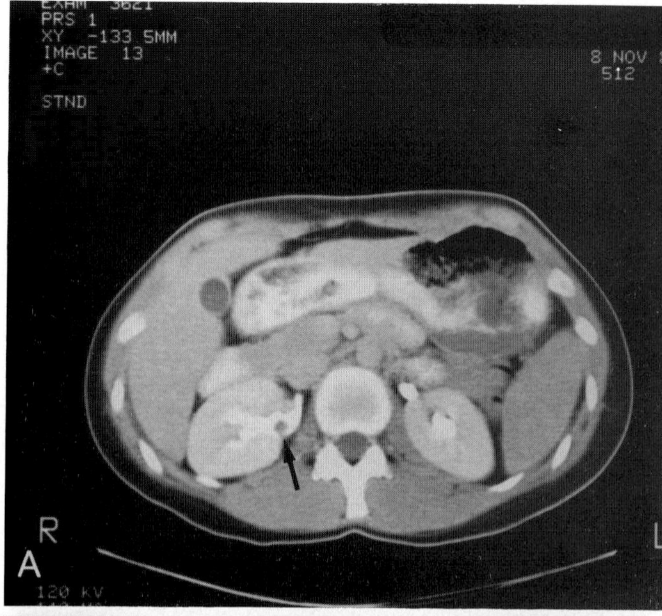

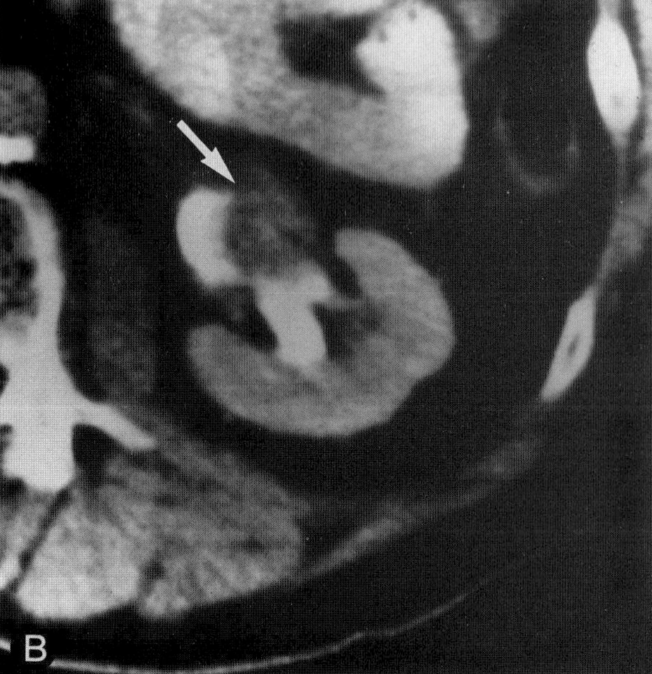

Figure 12.7. Computed tomography (CT) is performed routinely in these patients to exclude those with deeply invasive lesions. **A,** this CT scan suggests a superficial lesion in the right renal pelvis *(arrow)*. **B,** this CT scan, in another patient, suggests an invasive lesion of the left renal pelvis *(arrow)*. As such, this patient would not be considered for a percutaneous approach.

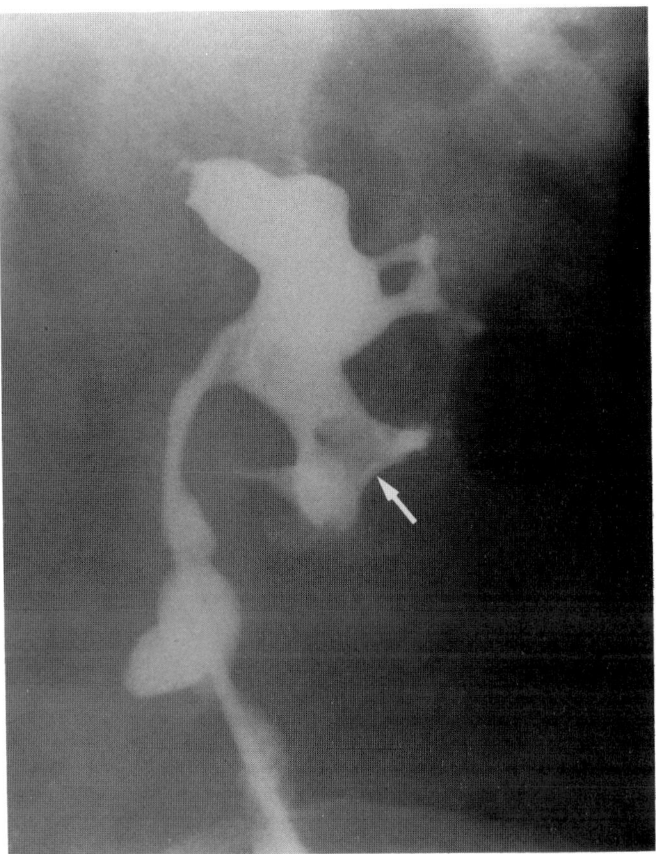

Figure 12.8. This patient has undergone cystectomy, right nephroureterectomy, and subtotal left ureterectomy with ileoconduit diversion for multifocal transitional cell carcinoma. He now presented with hematuria and was found to have a lesion in the lower infundibulocalyx of the remaining left kidney *(arrow)*.

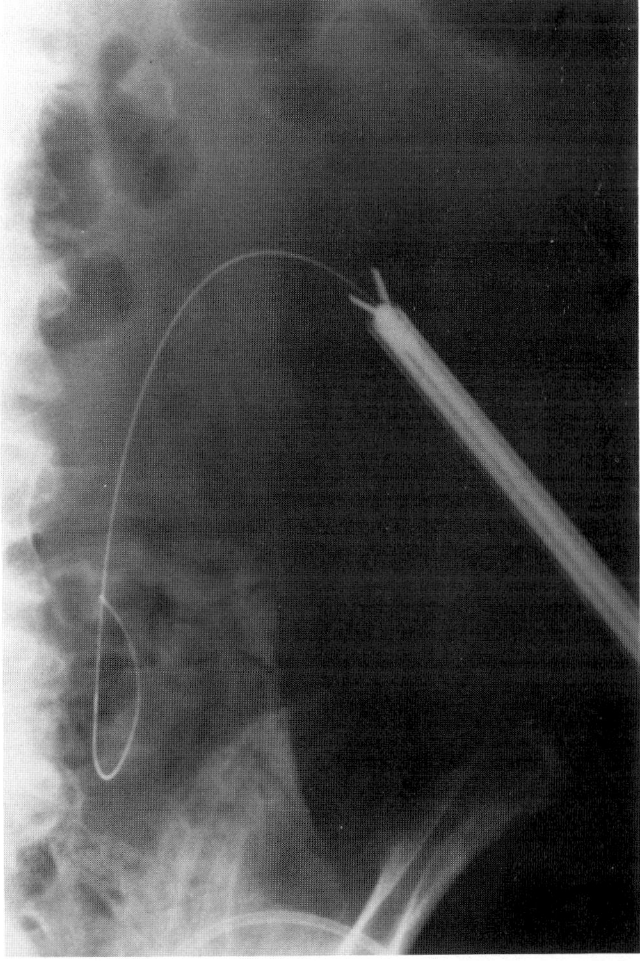

Figure 12.9. Percutaneous access is obtained through the involved portion of the collecting system. The tract is dilated and nephroscopy performed. The lesion is then biopsied.

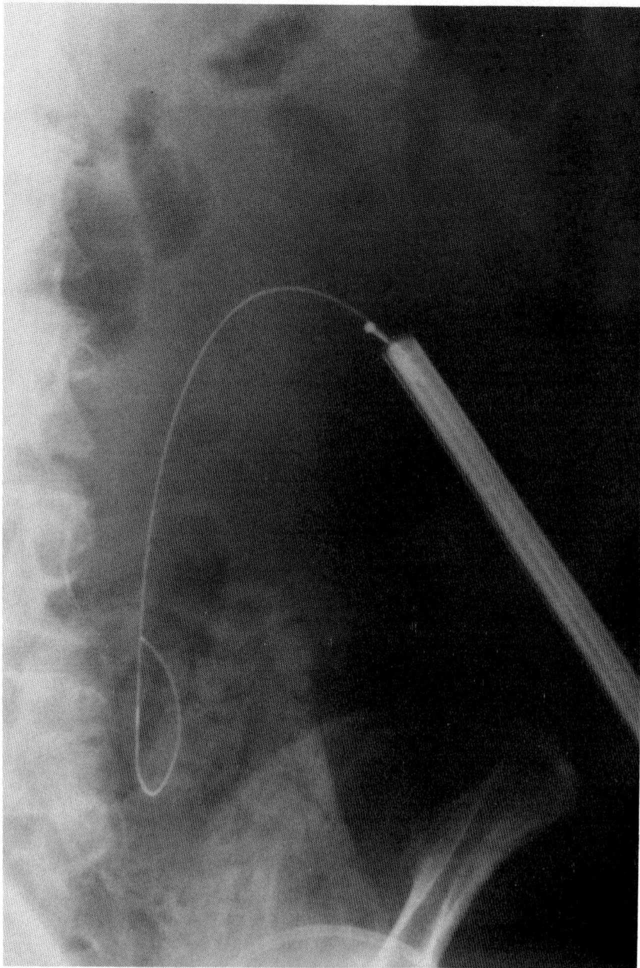

Figure 12.10. The base of the lesion is fulgurated with the Bugbee electrode. 1.5% glycine should be used as the irrigant. Alternatively, laser may be utilized at this point.

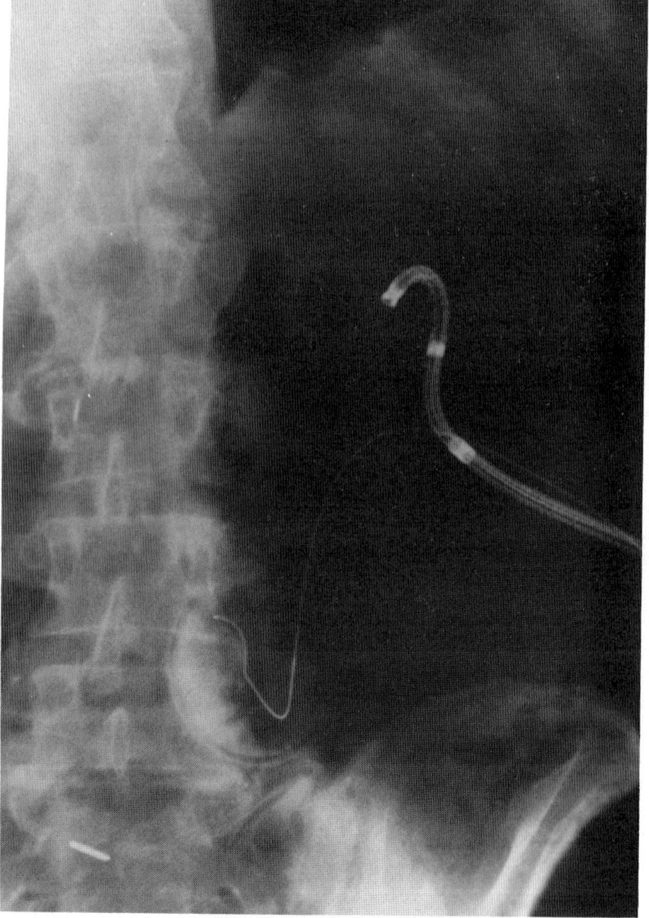

Figure 12.11. Flexible nephroscopy is routinely performed 48–72 hr later for a ''second look'' through the mature tract, as these lesions may be multifocal. Any remaining suspicious areas are biopsied and fulgurated at this time.

Conservative Surgery for Renal Pelvic Transitional Cell Carcinoma

Conservative surgical techniques can provide satisfactory treatment for selected patients with low grade, low stage, renal pelvic TCC. Patients managed in this fashion are at risk for developing recurrent urinary tract TCC and must be followed closely to allow early detection and treatment of such recurrence. This approach should be reserved for patients in whom preservation of functioning renal parenchyma is necessary to avoid kidney failure.

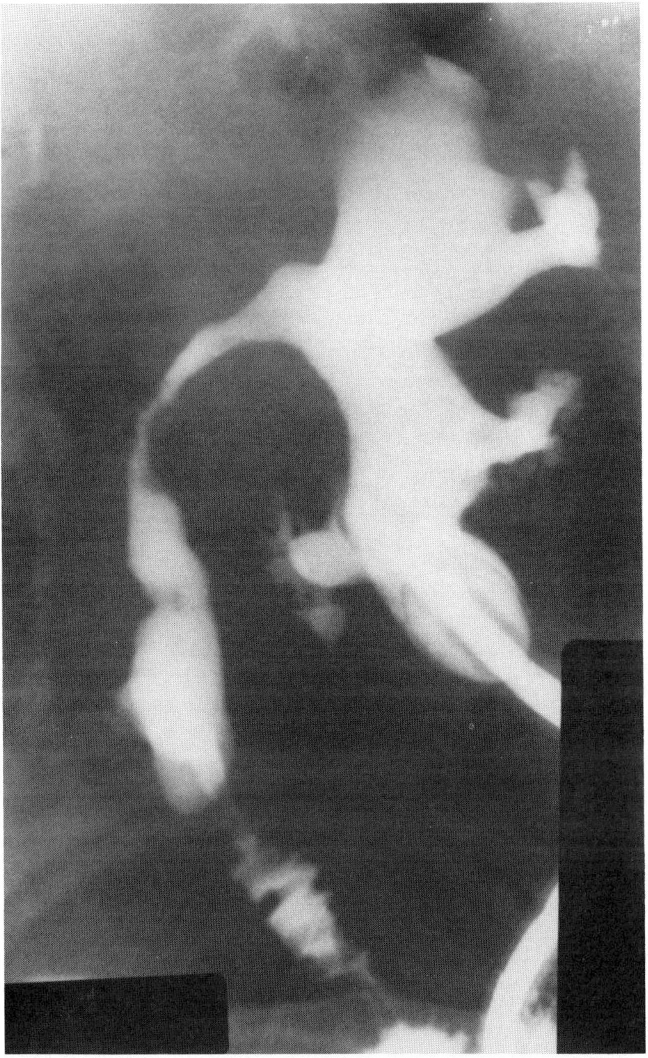

Figure 12.12. A nephrostogram is performed 1 or 2 days later. If there is no obstruction or extravasation, the nephrostomy tube is clamped for 12–24 hr and removed if tolerated. Alternatively, the nephrostomy tube may be utilized for antegrade instillation of chemotherapeutic agents prior to its removal.

Suggested Readings

Bagley DH: Flexible endoscopy in the urinary tract. *Semin Urol* 4:198, 1986.

Huffman JL, Bagley DH, Lyon ES, Morse MJ, Herr HW, Whitmore WF: Endoscopic diagnosis and treatment of upper-tract urothelial tumors. *Cancer* 55:1422, 1985.

Marshall FF, Walsh PC: In situ management of renal tumors: Renal cell carcinoma and transitional cell carcinoma. *J Urol* 131:1045, 1984.

Mazeman E: Tumors of the upper tract calyces, renal pelvis and ureter. *Eur Urol* 2:120, 1976.

Smith AD, Orihaela E, Crowley AR: Percutaneous management of renal pelvic tumors: A treatment option in selected cases. *J Urol* 137:852, 1987.

Streem SB, Pontes EJ: Percutaneous management of upper tract transitional cell carcinoma. *J Urol* 135:773, 1986.

Tomera KM, Leary FJ, Zincke H: Pyeloscopy in urothelial tumors. *J Urol* 127:1088, 1982.

Vest SA: Conservative surgery in certain benign tumors of the ureter. *J Urol* 53:97, 1945.

Wallace DMA, Wallace DM, Whitfield HN, Hendry WF, Wickham JEA: The late results of conservative surgery for upper tract urothelial carcinomas. *Br J Urol* 53:537, 1981.

Ziegelbaum M, Novick AC, Streem SB, et al: Conservative surgery for transitional cell carcinoma of the renal pelvis. *J Urol* 138:1146, 1987.

Zincke H, Neves RJ: Feasibility of conservative surgery for transitional cell cancer of the upper urinary tract. *Urol Clin North Am* 11:717, 1984.

SECTION 4

Surgery for Renal Calculous Disease

CHAPTER 13

Insertion of Percutaneous Nephrostomy and Related Procedures

MICHAEL A. GEISINGER

During the early 1970s, percutaneous nephrostomy gained acceptance as a method for drainage of an obstructed upper urinary tract. It proved particularly helpful in cases where the obstruction resulted in urosepsis, often with dramatic resolution of the septicemia. Since that time, the role of percutaneous nephrostomy has expanded considerably and is now employed as an initial step in a wide variety of interventional procedures. Renal calculi can be extracted percutaneously through a nephrostomy tract utilizing an ultrasonic lithotripser, Dormia basket, or forceps. Some renal calculi can be dissolved by irrigation of solvents through a nephrostomy catheter. A percutaneous nephrostomy can also serve as an access route for balloon dilatation of a ureteral stricture or for placement of a ureteral stent across an area of ureteral obstruction or leakage. Each of these procedures, however, begins with a basic percutaneous nephrostomy, with a few minor modifications depending on the secondary procedure to be performed.

PATIENT PREPARATION

As with any interventional procedure, the first step is careful explanation to the patient of the procedure and its possible complications. Once informed consent is secured, the appropriate laboratory data is obtained. Prothrombin time, partial thromboplastin time, and platelet count should be checked and corrected for any abnormalities in order to reduce the risk of significant bleeding. Patients at high risk for bleeding should be typed and screened for blood products. Renal function (blood urea nitrogen and serum creatinine) is also assessed to determine the safety and efficacy of contrast administration for opacification of the collecting system. The patient is placed on a clear liquid diet beginning the midnight before the procedure. If general anesthesia is expected (as in cases of nephroscopic stone extractions), the patient is given nothing by mouth after midnight. An intravenous line is started either the night before or the morning of the procedure in order to provide for adequate hydration and to serve as an access route for intravenous antibiotics and sedation. If the patient is not already on an antibiotic for a concomitant urinary tract infection, a prophylactic antibiotic is administered intravenously, usually a cephalosporin. Patients are not sedated until they arrive in the fluoroscopy suite. At that time, a narcotic (fentanyl) and an anxiolytic (diazepam) are administered intravenously, generally beginning with 1 ml of fentanyl and 5 mg of diazepam (although large patients will require more). Repeat doses are administered as needed during the procedure to ensure patient comfort.

BASIC TECHNIQUE OF PERCUTANEOUS NEPHROSTOMY

The patient is placed on a fluoroscopic table in the prone position. A C-arm fluoroscopy unit is preferable because it permits multiple angle viewing without the need to turn the patient manually. The patient is prepped and draped in a sterile fashion.

Opacifying the Collecting System

Because it is preferable to place the nephrostomy catheter through a calyx or infundibulum rather than directly into the renal pelvis, it is important to have adequate visualization of the collecting system. If the patient's serum creatinine is <2 mg/ml, opacification can usually be achieved by intravenous contrast administration.

In cases where contrast administration would be either unsafe (a history of serious adverse reaction to contrast) or useless (a serum creatinine >3 mg/dl), ultrasound can be used to localize the collecting system. It is usually easier to use ultrasound to guide a thin 22-gauge needle into the renal pelvis (a relatively large target) rather than to attempt puncturing directly the appropriate calyx (a relatively small target). Contrast can then be injected through the 22-gauge needle. When a collecting system is obstructed, it is important to remember to remove an amount of urine equal to or greater than the amount of contrast to be instilled. This prevents overdistention of the collecting system that can lead to extravasation of contrast or to pyelovenous backflow, possibly resulting in septicemia. Once the collecting system has been adequately opacified with contrast via the 22-gauge needle, a percutaneous nephrostomy can be performed in the standard fashion.

Another method to opacify the collecting system is through a cystoscopically placed ureteral catheter. This method is particularly useful when the nephrostomy is being performed for a staghorn calculus or for ureteral stone removal, as will be discussed later.

Selecting the Entry Site

Most percutaneous nephrostomies are placed from a posterolateral approach. The justification for this approach is based primarily on considerations aimed at keeping complications to a minimum. The anterior renal arterial branches typically supply the anterolateral two-thirds of the renal parenchyma, whereas the posterior branches supply the remaining posterior one-third of the kidney. As a result, the posterolateral margin of the kidney tends to be devoid of large arteries, thus decreasing the risks for significant hemorrhage and arteriovenous fistula formation.

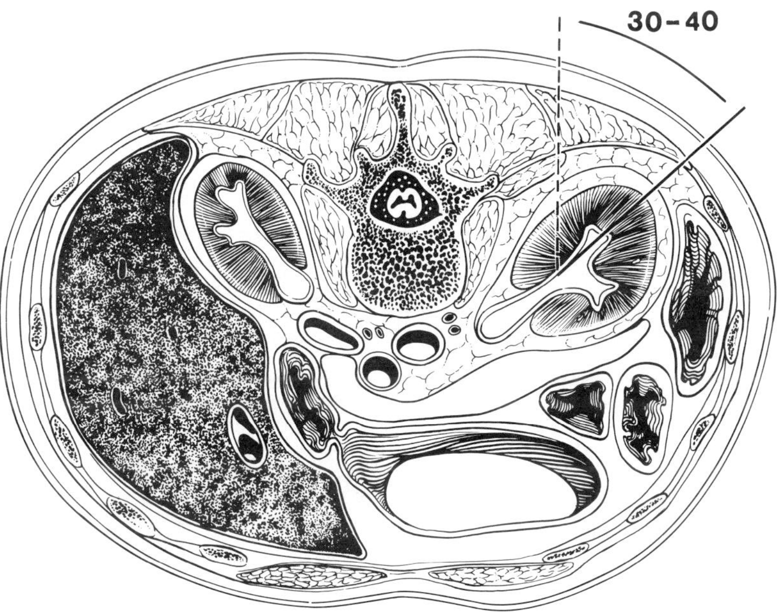

Figure 13.1. The standard technique for percutaneous nephrostomy is to puncture a posterior calyx in the lower pole or midportion of the kidney from a posterolateral approach (30–40° from the vertical). An approach too posterior would traverse the paraspinal muscles and an approach too lateral may traverse the colon, spleen, or liver. A posterolateral approach also helps to keep the operator's hands outside of the x-ray beam; this is not possible when a direct posterior route is used.

For the average-sized patient, the cutaneous entry site is approximately 15 cm from midline, just below the 12th rib. Percutaneous punctures above the 12th rib are avoided when possible in order to prevent violation of the pleural space and the potential risk of subsequent pneumothorax, hydrothorax, or hemothorax.

Once the entry site has been selected, local anesthesia (lidocaine or the longer lasting anesthetic, bupivacaine) is generously instilled to the level of the kidney.

Entering the Collecting System

There are many commercially prepared percutaneous nephrostomy kits now available from a number of manufacturers, but most are based on the following system.

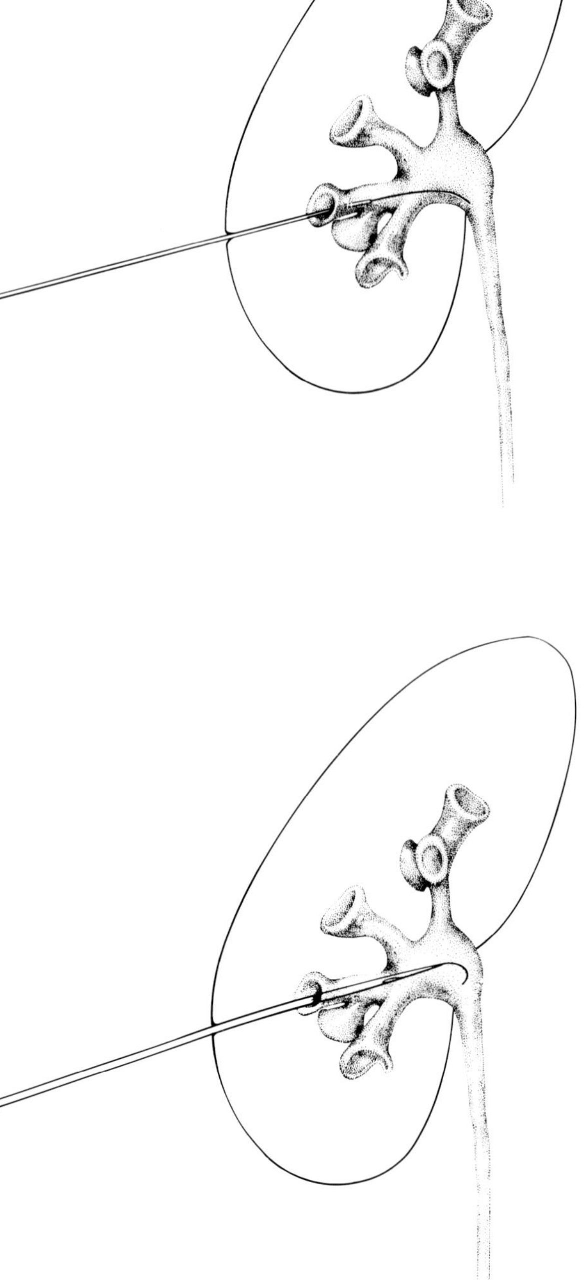

Figure 13.2. A 21-gauge needle is fluoroscopically advanced into one of the posterior calices or infundibula of the lower pole or midportion of the kidney. Once position in the collecting system has been confirmed by flow of urine from the needle hub, a thin (0.018-inch diameter) stainless steel wire with a flexible tip is advanced into the needle and then directed through the caliceal infundibulum and into the renal pelvis. The needle is then removed, taking care to keep the tip of the wire within the renal pelvis.

Figure 13.3. A no. 6 French dilator is placed over the 0.018-inch guidewire and is advanced into the renal pelvis. This dilator has a sidehole to permit passage of a larger J wire.

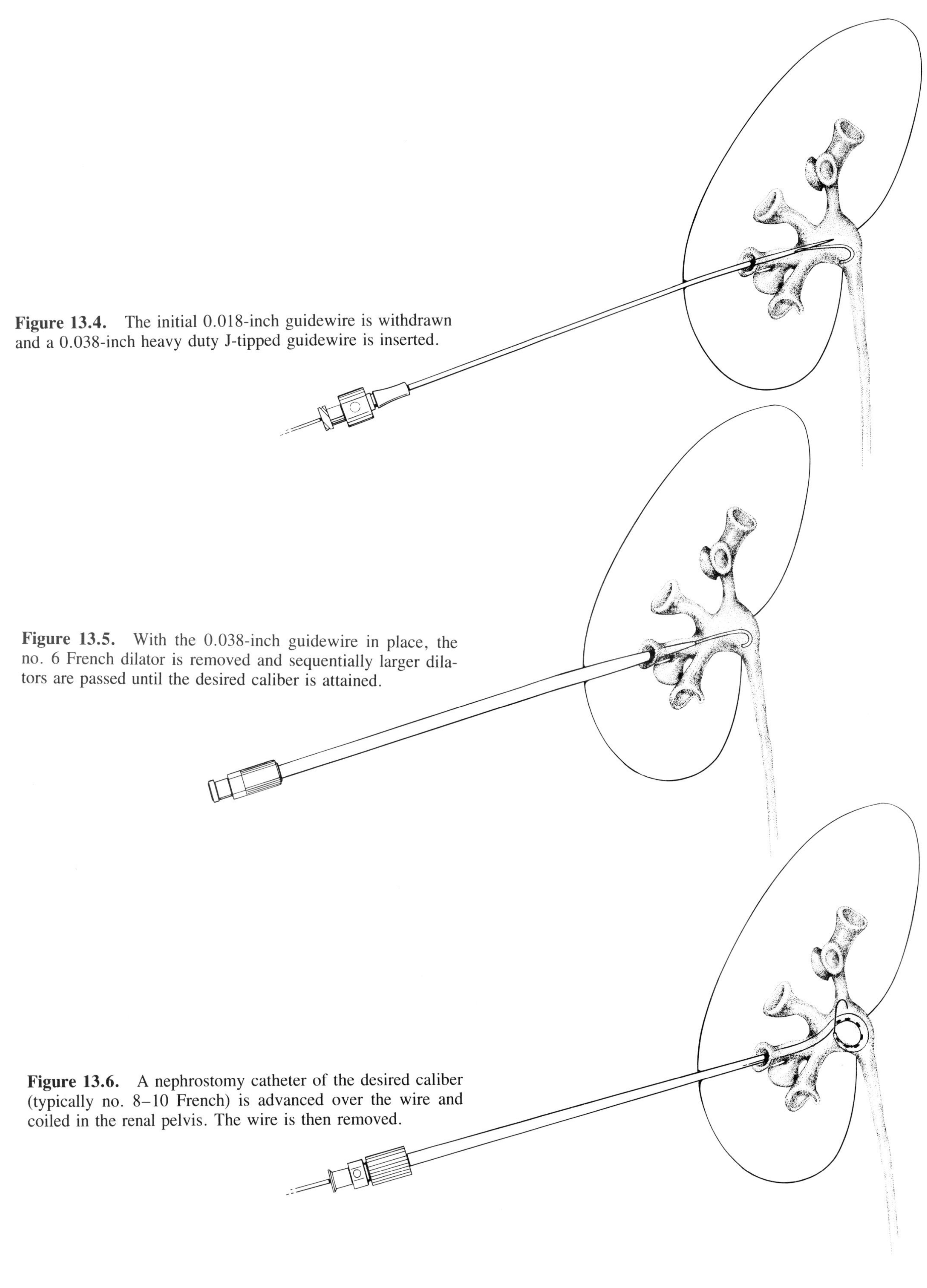

Figure 13.4. The initial 0.018-inch guidewire is withdrawn and a 0.038-inch heavy duty J-tipped guidewire is inserted.

Figure 13.5. With the 0.038-inch guidewire in place, the no. 6 French dilator is removed and sequentially larger dilators are passed until the desired caliber is attained.

Figure 13.6. A nephrostomy catheter of the desired caliber (typically no. 8–10 French) is advanced over the wire and coiled in the renal pelvis. The wire is then removed.

Choosing a Nephrostomy Catheter

When a percutaneous nephrostomy is performed for decompression of an obstructed collecting system, a no. 8 or 10 French Cope loop nephrostomy catheter is a good choice and is available from several different manufacturers.

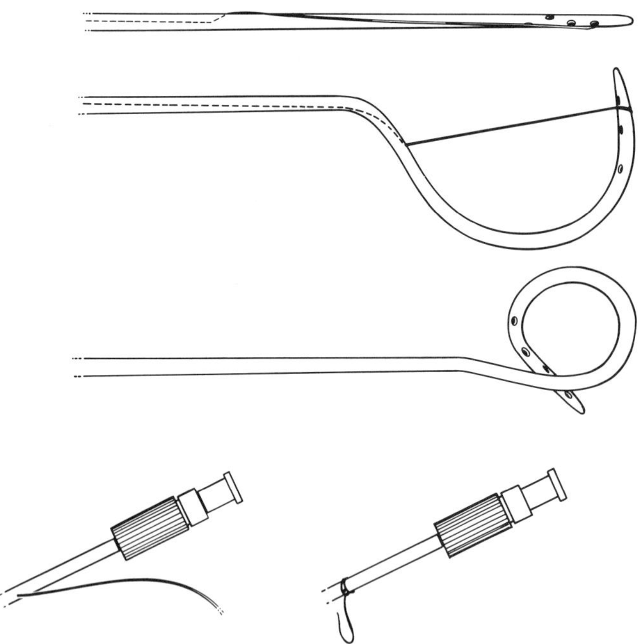

Figure 13.7. A Cope loop nephrostomy catheter contains a long piece of suture material that is fixed to the end of the catheter in such a fashion that when tension is applied to the suture, a loop of catheter is formed in the renal pelvis. This helps to secure the catheter within the renal pelvis and to prevent its inadvertent withdrawal.

Alternatively, a simple no. 8 or 10 French pigtail nephrostomy catheter can be positioned within the renal pelvis and sutured to the skin at the entry site. At a later date, the nephrostomy track can be dilated under local anesthesia to no. 12 or 14 French. The choice of catheters at no. 14 French is wider than at no. 8 French and includes not only simple pigtail and Cope loop catheters but also Malecot catheters and Foley catheters.

NEPHROSTOMY MODIFICATIONS FOR NEPHROSCOPIC STONE REMOVAL

When the percutaneous nephrostomy is performed in preparation for stone removal via the nephroscope, the selection of the caliceal entry site becomes critical. Because the principal instrument for this procedure is a rigid nephroscope that cannot turn corners, the placement of the nephrostomy tract must be well planned and precisely executed.

Selecting an Entry Site

Renal pelvic calculi can be approached from either a lower pole calyx or midcalyx, as either permits a fairly good range of view of the renal pelvis and, usually, the ureteropelvic junction. For caliceal calculi, there is often only one possible route.

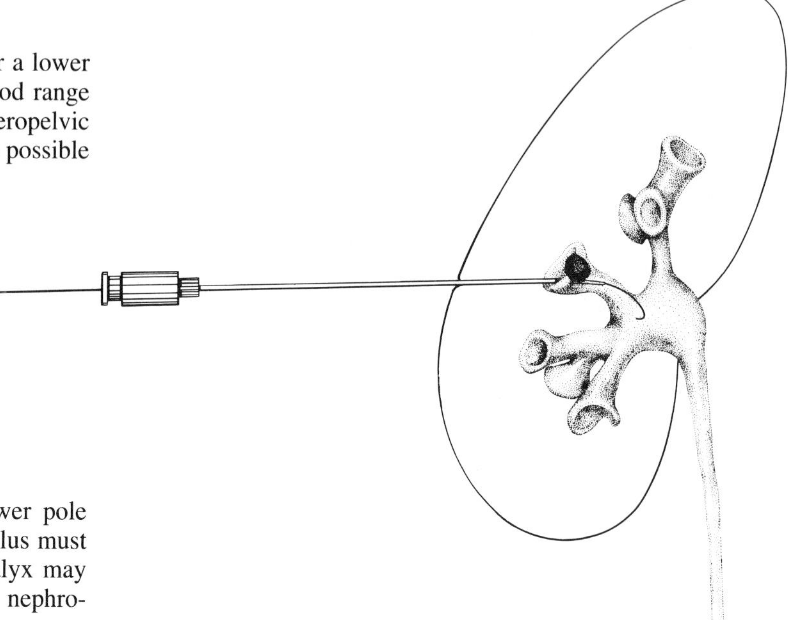

Figure 13.8. When the stone resides within a lower pole calyx or a midcalyx, the calyx that contains the calculus must be punctured directly. Failure to enter the correct calyx may result in failure to visualize the calculus when the nephroscope is inserted.

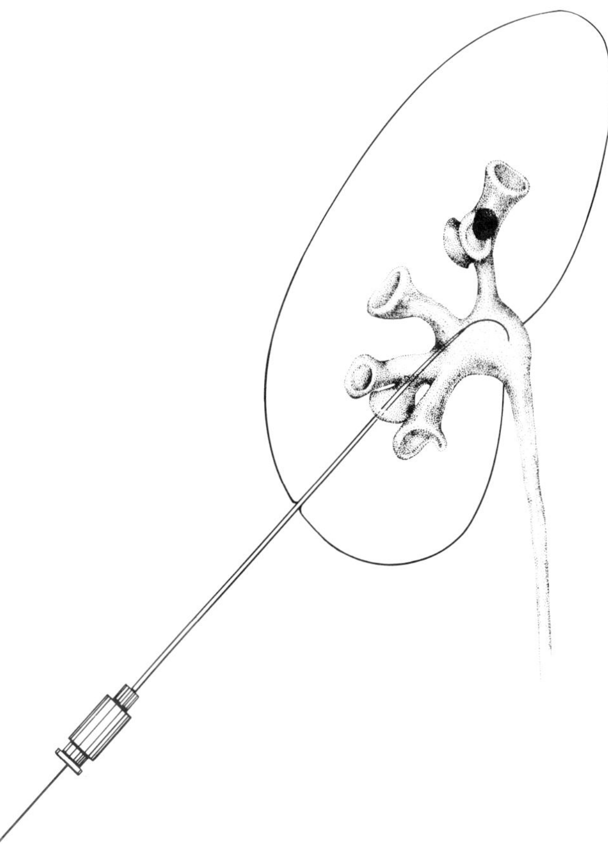

Figure 13.9. If the calculus resides within an upper pole calyx, a lower pole entry site usually will permit visualization of the upper caliceal system.

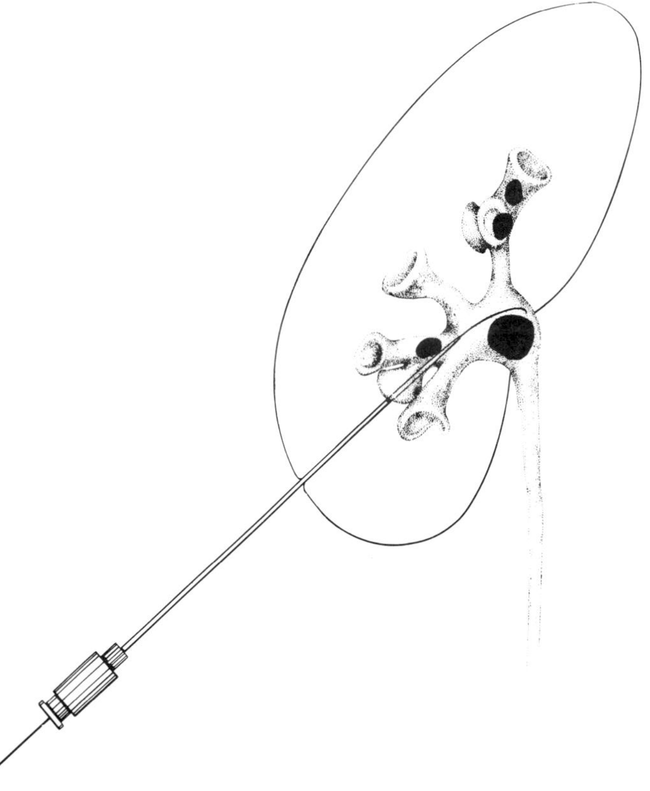

Figure 13.10. In cases where multiple caliceal stones are present, a lower pole entry site usually will afford access to the greatest number of calices.

Occasionally, a second nephrostomy tract will be necessary to gain access to all of the calices containing calculi. Rarely, an intercostal route above the 12th rib will be necessary, usually in cases of high-lying kidneys or when direct puncture of an upper pole calyx is required. When such an intercostal approach is used, the operator should be prepared to deal with possible complications that may arise should the pleural space be violated.

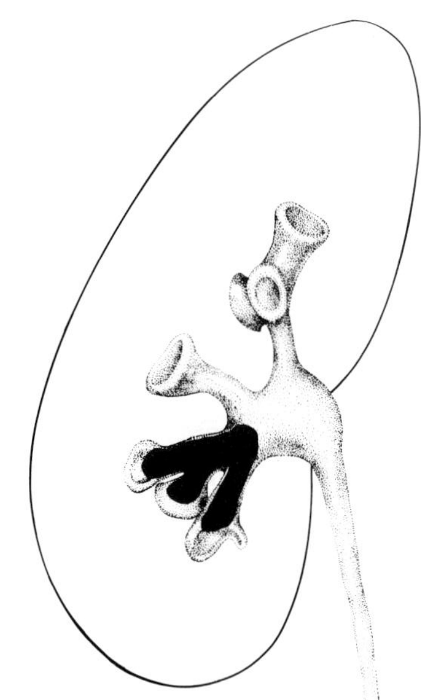

Figure 13.11. Staghorn or branch calculi can present a special problem. These calculi lie in close proximity to the wall of the collecting system, leaving very little room for wire insertion and maneuverability.

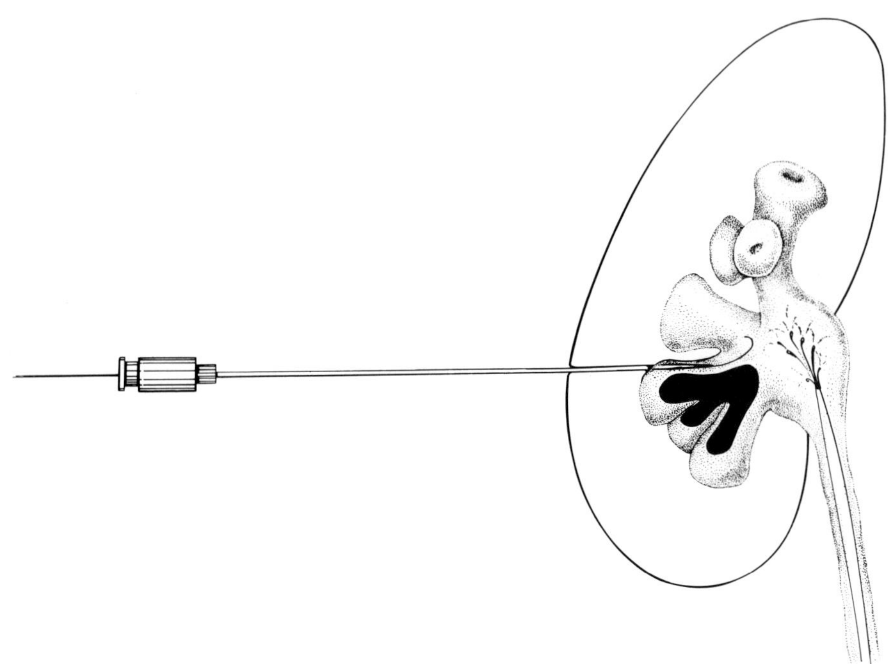

Figure 13.12. Often the problem can be surmounted by cystoscopically placing a ureteral catheter in the proximal ureter beforehand. Then, at the time of needle insertion, the collecting system can be distended with contrast via the ureteral catheter, providing the room necessary for the wire and catheter manipulation. Better distention of the collecting system sometimes can be obtained if the ureteral catheter has an occlusion balloon on it.

Placing a Pyeloureteral Catheter

Once percutaneous access is gained through the appropriate calyx and the 0.038 wire is in the renal pelvis, an attempt is made to place a pyeloureteral catheter rather than a looped catheter in the renal pelvis. This pyeloureteral catheter will enable placement of the relatively stiff Lunderquist wire down the ureter at the time of nephrostomy tract dilatation in the operating room, greatly facilitating the dilatation process.

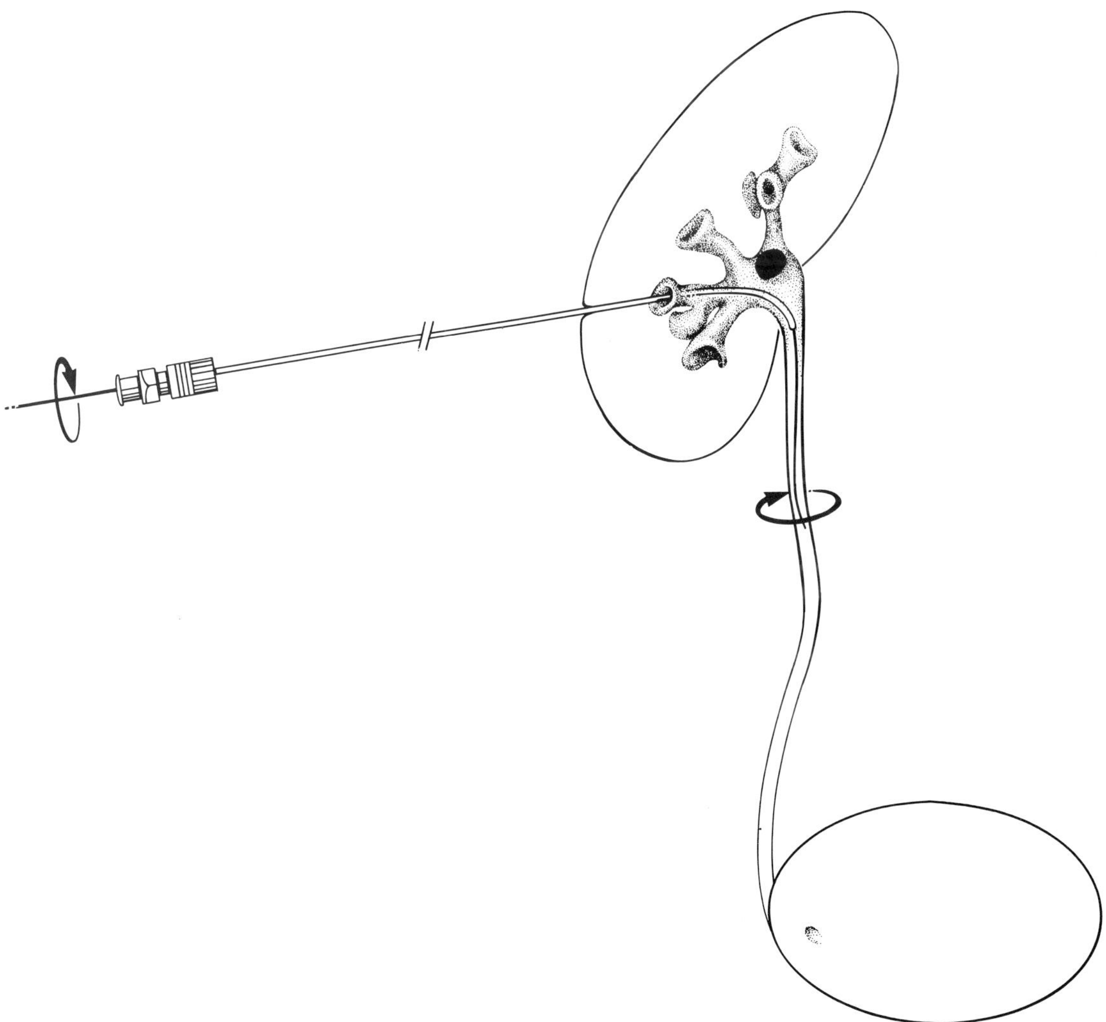

Figure 13.13. To place a pyeloureteral catheter, a pre-curved no. 6 French angiography catheter is placed over the heavy duty wire and positioned at the ureteropelvic junction. A steerable torque wire is then placed through the catheter and carefully maneuvered down the ureter.

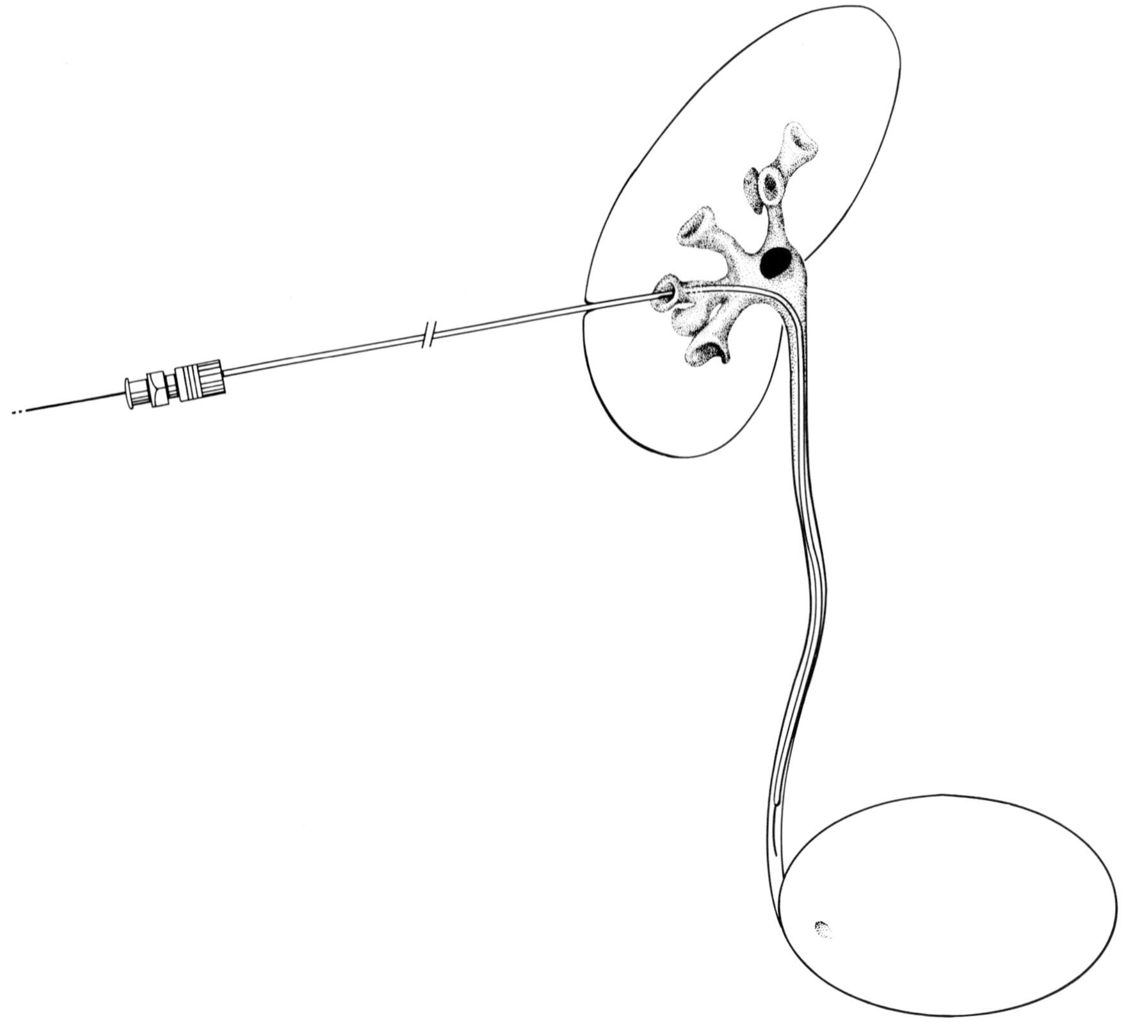

Figure 13.14. Once the tip of the torque wire is in the distal ureter, the curved catheter is removed and a straight no. 6.5 French Teflon pyeloureteral catheter with multiple sideholes is passed over the wire. The wire is removed and the catheter is placed to gravity drainage while the patient awaits the trip to the operating room for tract dilatation and nephrostomy insertion (chapter 15).

PERCUTANEOUS URETERAL PROCEDURES

A number of ureteral problems can also be dealt with through a percutaneous nephrostomy tract: specifically, retrieval of ureteral stones, balloon dilatation of ureteral strictures, and placement of ureteral stents for obstructions or leaks. For these ureteral procedures, the initial percutaneous nephrostomy should be placed through a posterior calyx in the midportion of the kidney as this offers the best approach to the ureteropelvic junction and the most stable configuration for the passage of various wires and catheters down the ureter.

Retrieving Ureteral Calculi

When a ureteral calculus has not passed spontaneously and retrograde cystoscopic techniques at stone removal have failed or are not feasible, an antegrade attempt at stone retrieval can be made. Access to the ureter is gained in the manner described previously for pyeloureteral catheter placement.

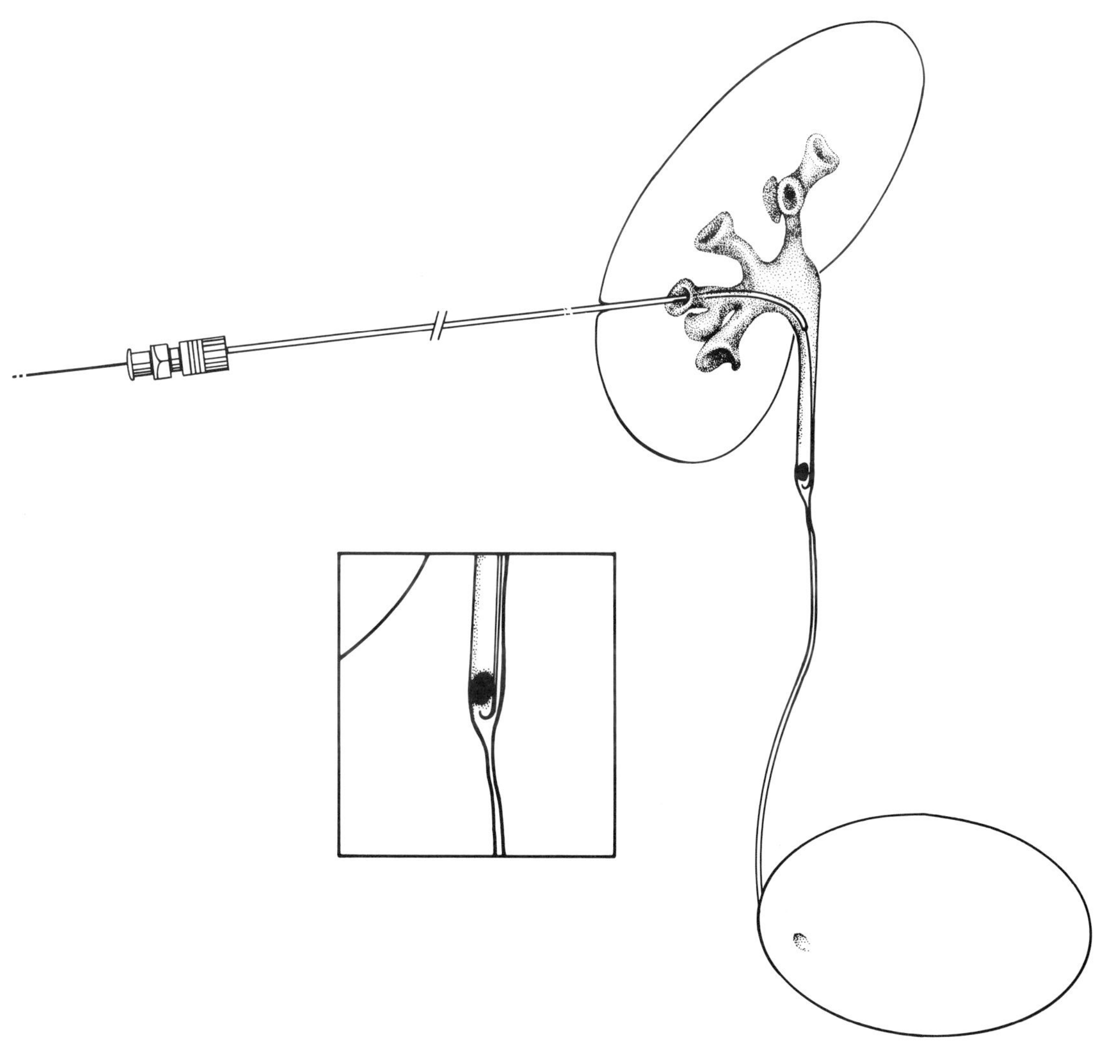

Figure 13.15. The 0.038-inch torque wire is carefully steered beyond the calculus. This is accomplished by slowly turning the wire and cautiously probing for a passageway around the calculus.

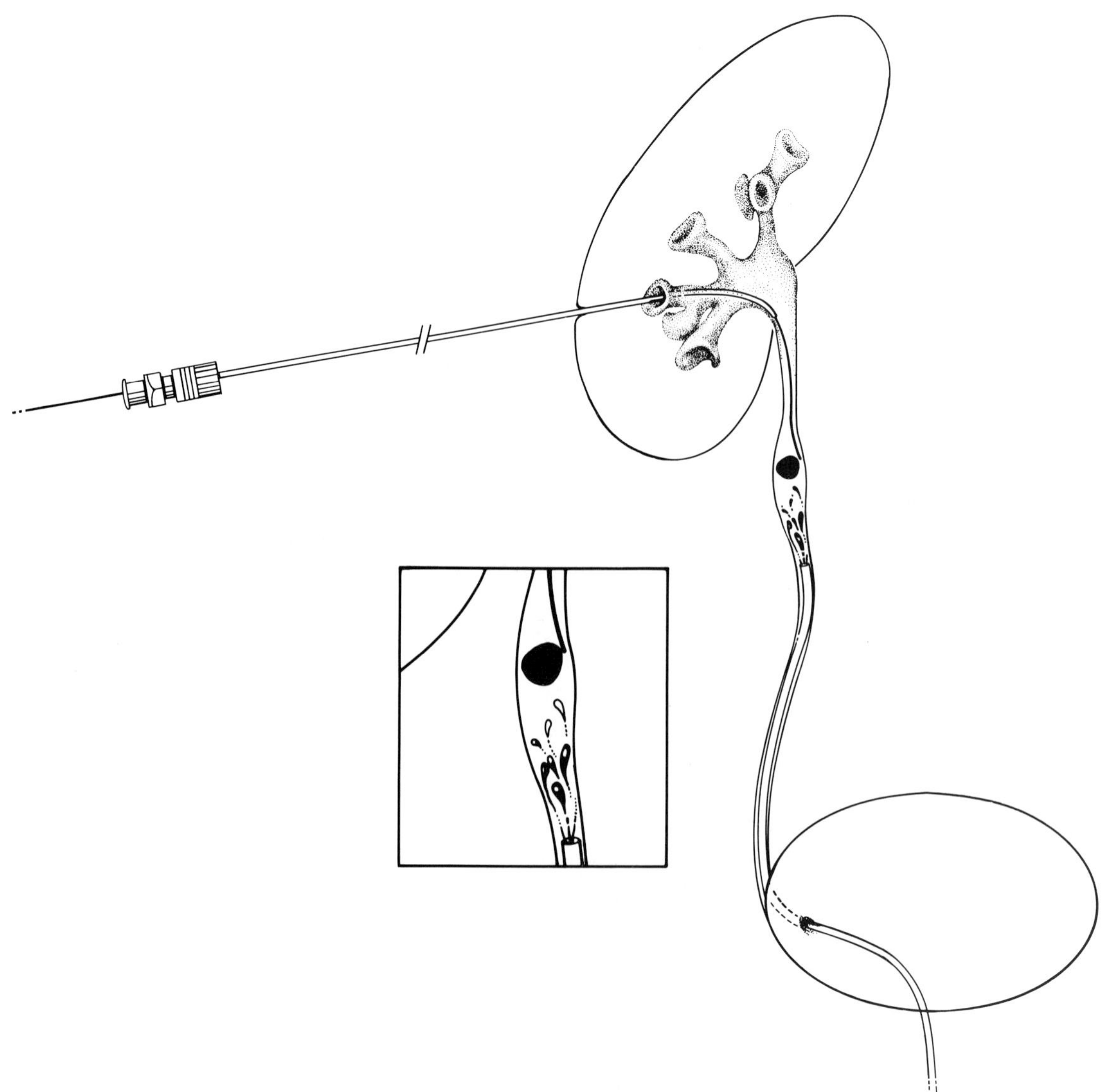

Figure 13.16. A ureteral catheter cystoscopically placed from below can often aid in traversing the ureter at the level of the calculus. Contrast is injected through the retrograde catheter, resulting in distention of the ureter and of any potential channel around the calculus.

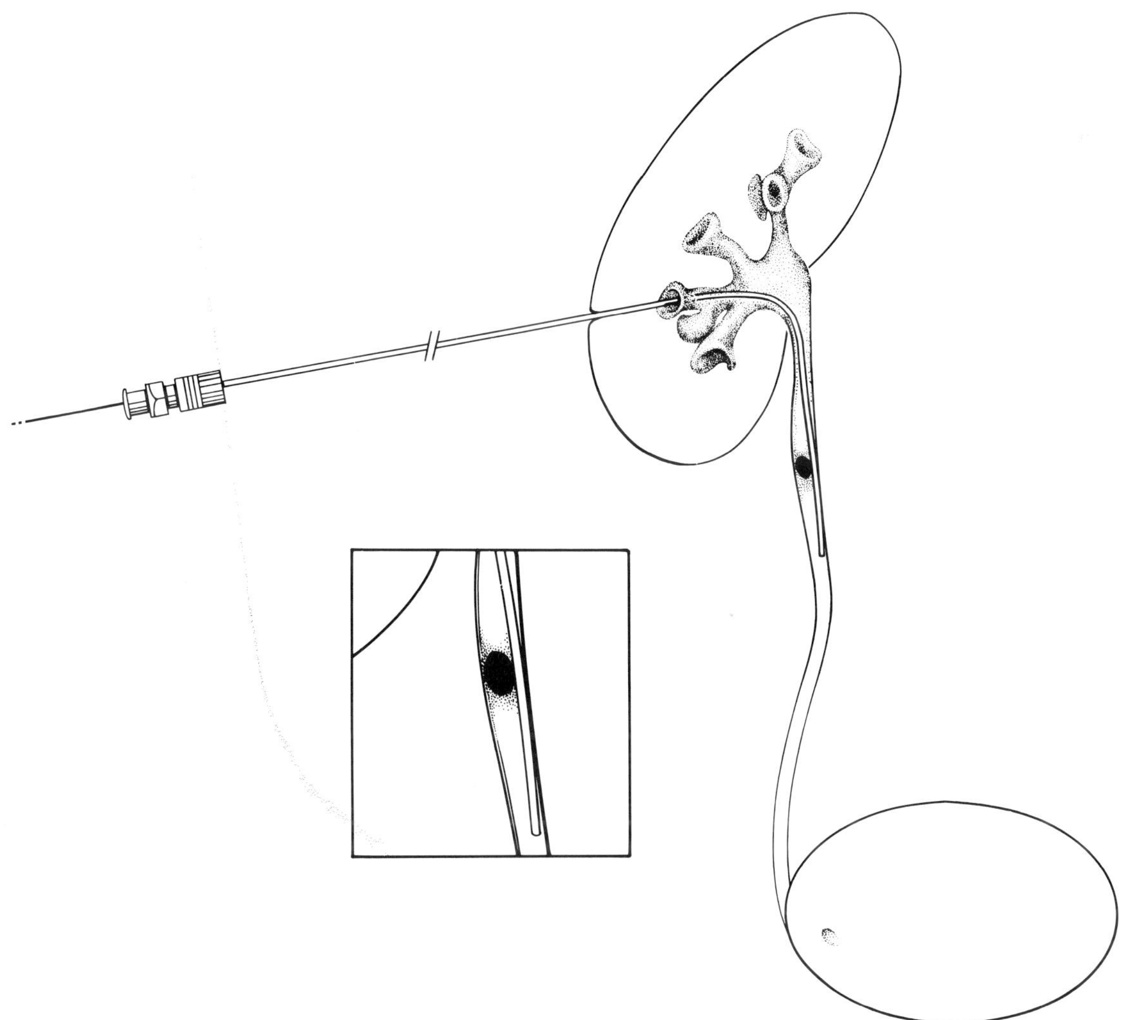

Figure 13.17. Once the wire is beyond the calculus, the catheter is advanced over the wire. The wire is then removed and the catheter is injected with contrast in order to confirm its location within the ureter.

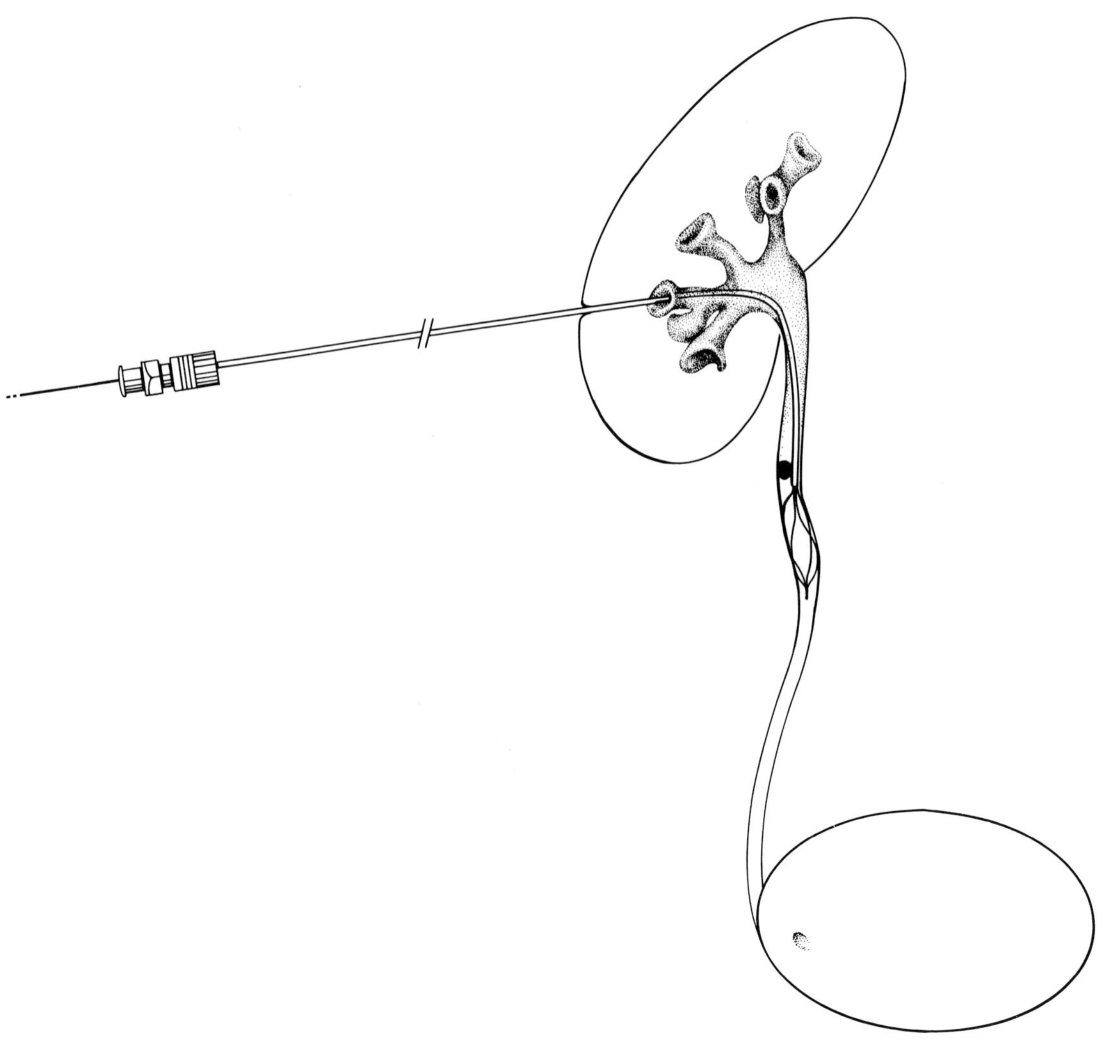

Figure 13.18. A Dormia retrieval basket is then placed through the catheter and unsheathed beyond the stone. An attempt is made to engage the stone within the basket. If successful, the stone is withdrawn into the renal pelvis and removed nephroscopically. Small calculi (4 mm or less) can be removed directly through the nephrostomy tract in the retrieval basket, provided a no. 14 French working sheath has been placed in the nephrostomy tract beforehand.

Dilating Ureteral Strictures

The development and successful usage of angioplasty balloon catheters for vascular stenoses has led to trials of balloon dilatation for benign ureteral strictures. Although large series are not available, balloon dilatation of ureteral stenoses appears to be successful in approximately 50% of cases. As a general rule of thumb, strictures secondary to fairly recent surgery have the best rate of success. Ischemic or densely fibrotic strictures tend to be less amenable to dilatation. The technique consists of advancing a 0.038-inch torque wire across the stricture in the same manner as described for passing the wire beyond a ureteral calculus.

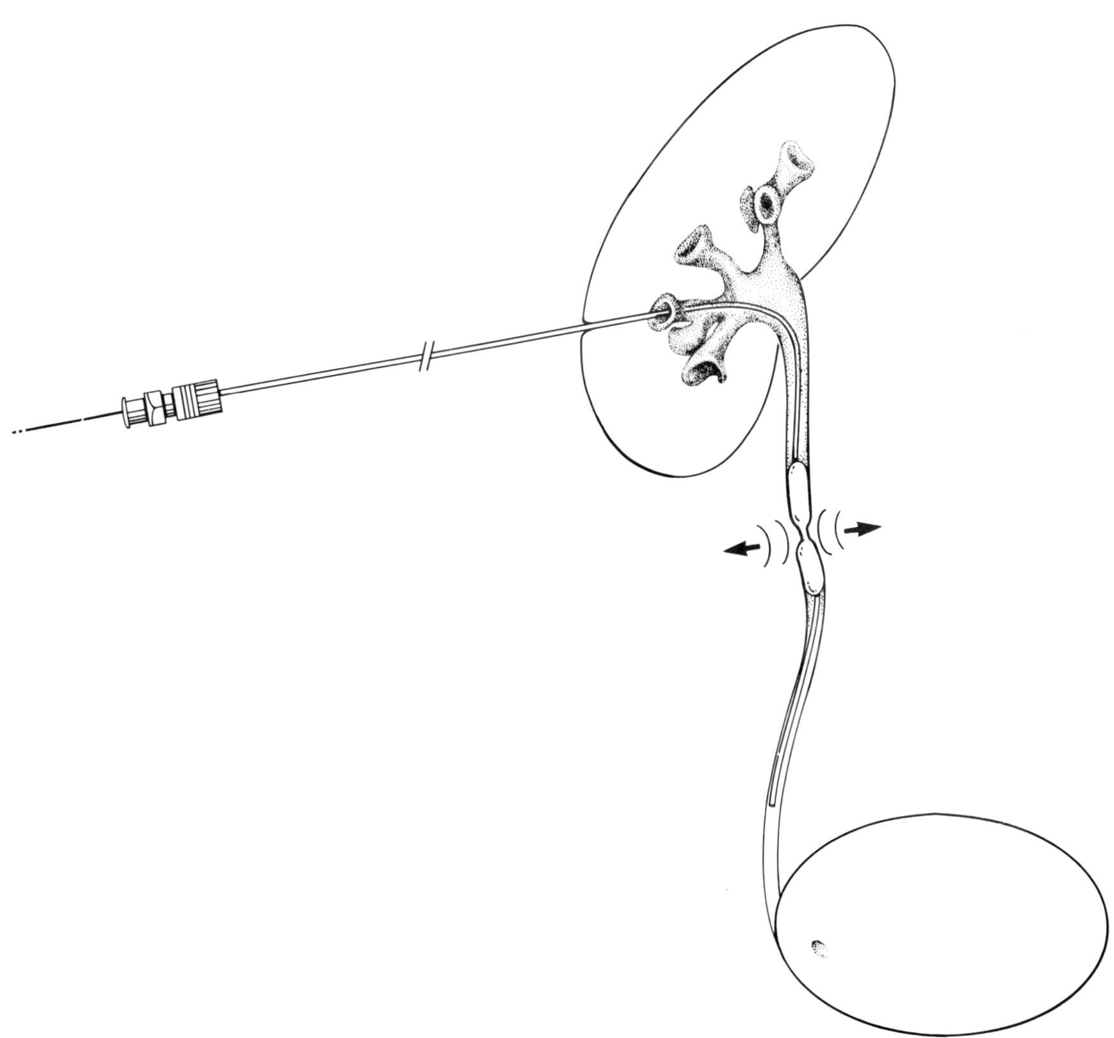

Figure 13.19. A 6- or 8-mm diameter angioplasty balloon catheter is passed over the wire and the balloon is centered across the stricture. The balloon is inflated with dilute contrast material and constant pressure is maintained on the inflating syringe for 45–60 sec. The balloon is then deflated. The balloon inflation procedure is repeated one or two additional times until there is either no residual deformity remaining or no further dilatation occurs. The ureter is then stented with either an internal double-J ureteral stent or a percutaneous pyeloureteral catheter for 2–6 weeks.

Placing Double-J Ureteral Stents

Double-J ureteral stents have become popular for managing a number of ureteral problems. They have proved particularly useful in patients requiring long-term decompression and in patients with malignant obstructions or ureteral leaks. In most cases, these stents can be passed via cystoscopic approach. When a cystoscopic approach is unsuccessful, however, an antegrade approach via a percutaneous nephrostomy tract will be successful many times. This is probably secondary to the greater degree of maneuverability and stability afforded by the nephrostomy tract.

This technique utilizes a no. 7 or 8 French double-J ureteral stent that has been modified for an antegrade approach and is now readily commercially available. The modifications consist of placement of endholes (which enable the stent to be placed over a wire) and the attachment of a monofilament to the cephalad end (which assists in optimal placement of the stent). A relatively stiff pusher catheter is also provided.

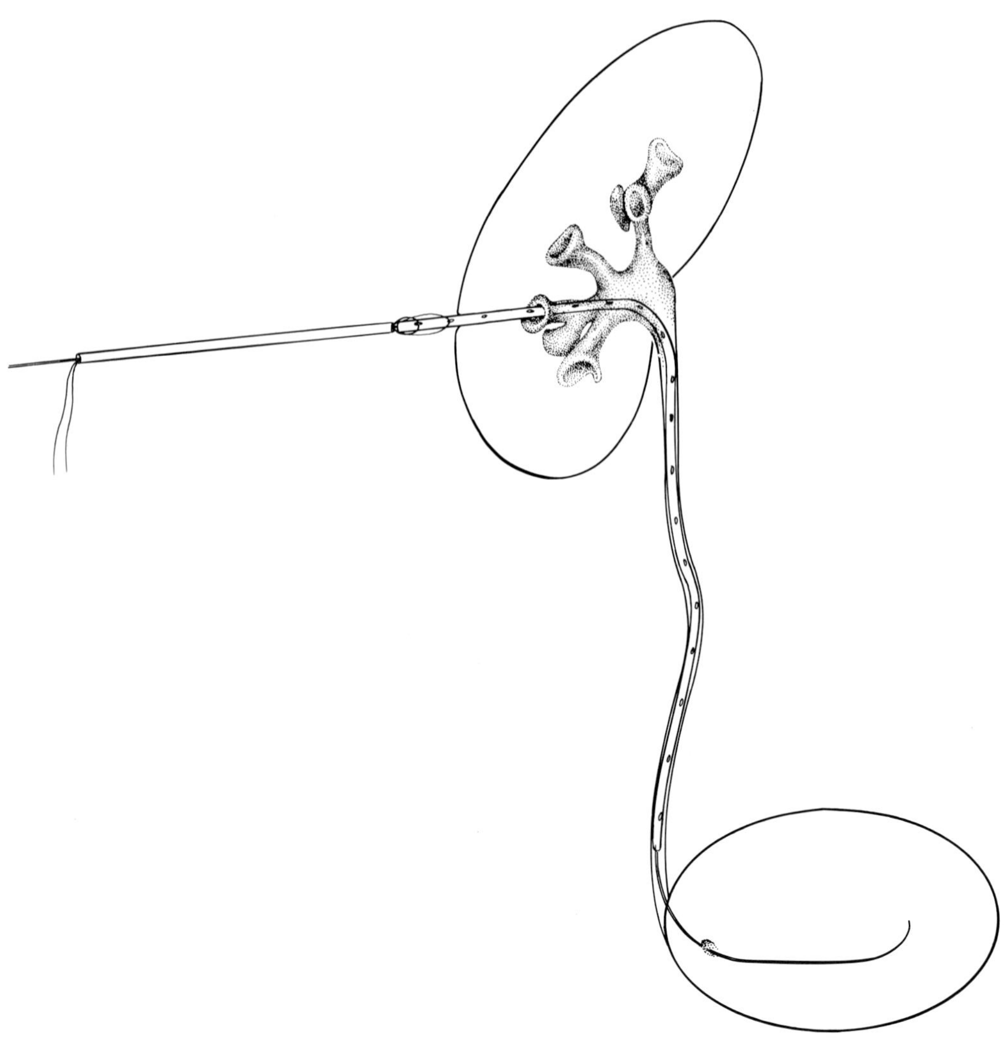

Figure 13.20. The torque wire is guided across the obstruction, stricture, or leak and is advanced into the bladder. The double-J ureteral stent is passed over the wire and pushed into position within the collecting system with the pusher catheter. If the stent has been advanced too far, it can be pulled back with the monofilament.

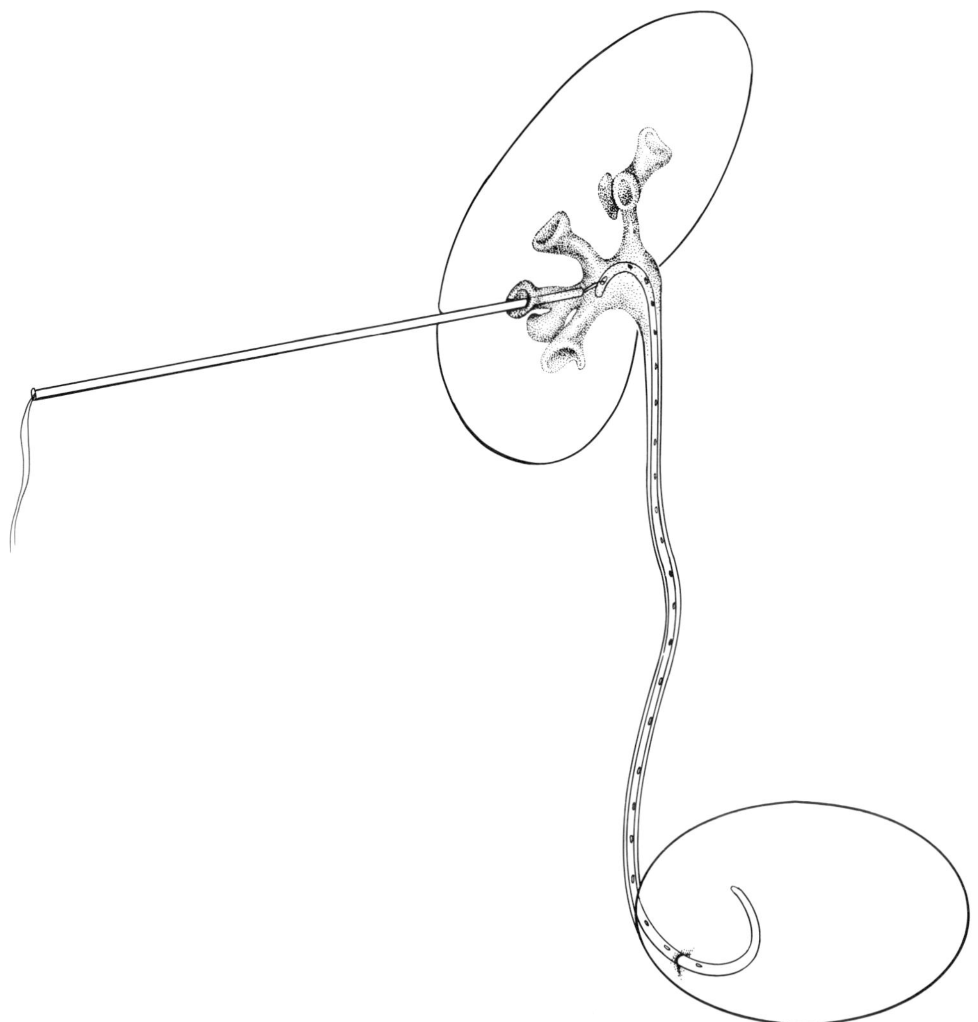

Figure 13.21. Once the stent is in position, the wire is withdrawn and the monofilament is removed while the pusher catheter is still in position in the nephrostomy tract. The pusher catheter can then either be removed immediately or, if desired, replaced with a temporary nephrostomy catheter that will stay in place for 24 hours until good function of the double-J ureteral stent has been confirmed.

When the area of ureteral obstruction is very tight, it is often advisable to place initially a no. 6 French Teflon pyeloureteral catheter across the obstruction for 24–48 hr. This greatly facilitates passage of the relatively soft double-J ureteral stents, which have a tendency to buckle on themselves when tight obstructions are encountered. This is especially true of the popular silicone double-J stents.

COMPLICATIONS

Percutaneous nephrostomies and the other percutaneous procedures described in this chapter, when performed properly, have a relatively low risk of complication, generally estimated at less than 5%. Bleeding and sepsis account for most of the major complications.

Although CT examinations performed after percutaneous nephrostomy reveal a 13% rate of subcapsular or extrarenal hematoma, the hematoma usually is self-limited and of no clinical consequence. Most patients will have macroscopic hematuria for the first day or two after nephrostomy catheter placement. In the vast majority of cases, the hematuria will resolve spontaneously, provided no underlying coagulopathy exists. On the other hand, if a renal arterial branch is inadvertently traversed or lacerated during catheter introduction, significant bleeding into the retroperitoneum or into the collecting system can occur. Other possible sequelae of renal arterial injury are arteriovenous fistulae and pseudoaneurysms. Fortunately, these types of complications often can be managed by angiographic catheter embolization, although occasionally, surgical intervention becomes necessary.

Sepsis is a known complication of percutaneous nephrostomy, especially in the setting of concomitant urinary tract infection or pyohydronephrosis. The risk of sepsis can be reduced, although not eliminated, by adequate antibiotic coverage and by taking care not to overdistend the collecting system at the time of tube insertion.

Occasionally during a percutaneous procedure, a catheter or wire accidentally will pierce through the uroepithelium of the renal pelvis or ureter and protrude into the surrounding soft tissues. Usually these perforations will heal without consequence as long as good external decompression of the collecting system is maintained. In cases of ureteral injury, the operator may wish to leave a ureteral stent in place.

Most late sequelae of percutaneous nephrostomies involve dislodgment or plugging of the nephrostomy catheter. The incidence of catheter dislodgment can be reduced by making the catheter as secure as possible, usually through the use of a Cope loop, Malecot, or Foley catheter. Plugging of a nephrostomy catheter will quickly result in the development of an upper urinary tract infection. A plugged catheter, therefore, should be irrigated or changed promptly. If an upper urinary tract infection has already developed, irrigation is probably not advisable and the catheter should be exchanged for a new one as quickly as possible. The risk of catheter plugging can be reduced by prophylactically changing the catheter every 8–10 weeks.

Suggested Readings

Banner MP, Pollack HM, Ring EJ, Wein AJ: Catheter dilatation of benign ureteral strictures. *Radiology* 147:427, 1983.

Cardella JF, Castaneda-Zuniga WR, Hunter DW, Hulbert JC, Amplatz K: Urine-compatible polymer for long-term ureteral stenting. *Radiology* 161:313, 1986.

Coleman CC, Castaneda-Zuniga W, Miller R, et al: A logical approach to renal stone removal. *AJR* 143:609, 1984.

Cronin JJ, Dorfman GS, Amis ES, Denny DJ Jr: Retroperitoneal hemorrhage after percutaneous nephrostomy. *AJR* 144:801, 1985.

Druy EM, Gharib M, Finder CA: Percutaneous nephroureteral drainage and stenting for postsurgical ureteral leaks. *AJR* 141:389, 1983.

Johnson CD, Oke EJ, Dunnick NR, et al: Percutaneous balloon dilatation of ureteral strictures. *AJR* 148:181, 1987.

Lang EK, Price ET: Redefinitions of indications for percutaneous nephrostomy. *Radiology* 147:419, 1983.

LeRoy AJ, May GR, Bender CE, et al: Percutaneous nephrostomy for stone removal. *Radiology* 151:607, 1984.

LeRoy AJ, Williams HJ Jr, Bender CE, May GR, Segura JW, Patterson DE: Percutaneous removal of small ureteral calculi. *AJR* 145:109, 1985.

Mercado S, Hunter DW, Castanedo-Zuniga WR, et al: The double puncture: An effective percutaneous technique for removing complex, multiple renal calculi. *Radiology* 158:207, 1986.

Picus D, Weyman PJ, Clayman RV, McClennan BL: Intercostal-space nephrostomy for percutaneous stone removal. *AJR* 147:393, 1986.

CHAPTER 14

Percutaneous Extraction of Renal Calculi

STEVAN B. STREEM, MARGARET G. ZELCH,
BARBARA RISIUS, MICHAEL A. GEISINGER

Percutaneous removal of an obstructing renal calculus via an operatively established nephrostomy tract was first described by Rupel and Brown in 1941. Subsequent to that, there were sporadic reports of similar procedures performed successfully, utilizing endoscopic, fluoroscopic, electrohydraulic, and ultrasonic adjunctive measures. While the technique of percutaneous nephrostomy drainage was first reported by Goodwin and associates in 1955, percutaneous removal of calculi via a tract established specifically for that purpose was not described until Fernstrom and Johansson's work was reported 20 years later. Presently, extensive experience has been gained with such procedures at centers throughout the United States and Europe.

INDICATIONS AND CONTRAINDICATIONS

The indications for percutaneous stone extraction are still being defined. In the early 1980s, any patient who would have otherwise required open lithotomy was a potential candidate for percutaneous extraction. Thus, the indications for this procedure included obstruction, pain, infection or significant hematuria resulting from the stone, or active stone growth despite appropriate medical management. However, the recent introduction of extracorporeal shock-wave lithotripsy (ESWL) has had a significant impact on these primary indications. Currently, over 90% of patients who might otherwise have been treated with a percutaneous approach are now managed by ESWL alone or in combination with percutaneous procedures.

At our institution, where ESWL became available in late 1985, the indications for a primary percutaneous approach have narrowed considerably but include patients with extensive "staghorn" calculi, morbidly obese patients, patients with large cystine stones, and patients with distal obstruction.

For those with extensive staghorn calculi, a percutaneous approach is generally performed for "debulking" prior to ESWL. In such cases, the initial percutaneous treatment reduces the stone load for the subsequent ESWL treatment. Furthermore, in these patients who generally have struvite stones, the placement of a large caliber nephrostomy tube at the end of the percutaneous procedure prevents subsequent obstruction in the face of infection and allows passage of much of the stone debris through the nephrostomy tube, reducing the risk of significant "steinstrasse." Finally, the percutaneous nephrostomy provides safe access for chemodissolution, which will at times be required. In our experience with these patients, a well-planned combination of percutaneous debulking followed by ESWL is preferable to ESWL initially, followed by the potential need for emergency intervention in an obstructed, septic patient.

At times, body habitus precludes successful ESWL and, as such, morbid obesity alone is often an indication for percutaneous procedure. Generally, patients weighing more than 300 pounds cannot be adequately positioned to get their stone either at the focal point or within the "power path" for ESWL.

Another indication for a primary percutaneous approach includes those patients with large cystine calculi. It has become evident that these stones do not fragment well with ESWL. Fortunately, however, they are very amenable to ultrasonic fragmentation, and we continue to utilize percutaneous ultrasonic pyelolithotomy for these cases.

Finally, as successful ESWL requires spontaneous passage of stone fragments, obstruction distal to the stone precludes ESWL as primary therapy. In most cases, the obstruction will relate to the ureter or ureteropelvic junction. However, the same may apply to stones in calyceal diverticula or in calyces associated with significant infundibular stenosis. In these cases, we prefer percutaneous stone removal followed by antegrade balloon dilatation or incision of the area in question.

Relative contraindications to a percutaneous approach take into consideration size, composition, configuration, and location of the calculus, though perhaps the most important consideration here is personal experience of the surgeon. There is currently no absolute limit to the size of a calculus that can be removed percutaneously; however, calcium oxalate and/or calcium phosphate calculi present an inconsistent response to ultrasonic disintegration, and those larger than 3 cm should be approached with caution or in conjunction with ESWL. In general, those that have a stippled or a "sunburst" appearance on plain x-ray generally fragment more readily than those that appear shiny or homogenous. Fortunately, struvite and cystine calculi, which tend to be larger on presentation, fragment readily with ultrasound. Furthermore, in such cases, retained fragments may be managed with chemodissolution or ESWL. Large uric acid calculi are often difficult to fragment and in these cases consideration should again be given to combinations of percutaneous extraction, ESWL, and chemodissolution.

As mentioned above, branched or staghorn calculi with multiple "dumbbell"-shaped extensions associated with areas of infundibular stenosis are generally better managed with percutaneous debulking followed by ESWL and chemodissolution where necessary. Occasionally, some smaller calculi may be deemed inaccessible to a percutaneous approach, especially when they are located in upper, lateral calyces that would require access above the 12th rib. Such cases are clearly better managed by ESWL primarily.

The only absolute contraindication to a percutaneous approach is an irreversible coagulopathy.

PATIENT PREPARATION

Of utmost importance, the patient must be apprised of the potential risks and benefits of percutaneous lithotomy versus ESWL or open surgery. It is explained that in some cases percutaneous extraction may require more than one trip to the radiologic or surgical suite and even then, the procedure may be unsuccessful, with open operative intervention ultimately, though rarely, required. However, the vast majority of patients will eventually benefit from a successful percutaneous extraction with a relatively short hospital stay and greatly decreased period of convalescence compared to an open procedure.

Standard preoperative preparation includes "nothing by mouth after midnight" and adequate overnight intravenous hydration. The availability of blood for possible transfusion must also be ensured. At times, the procedure may be performed under local anesthesia and appropriate intramuscular sedation is given on call. Those patients with urinary tract infection require vigorous antibiotic treatment for at least 24 hr prior to any instrumentation other than simple placement of a percutaneous nephrostomy tube. The need for prophylactic antibiotics in the face of sterile urine is unproven; however, we routinely utilize a "short course" antibiotic protocol in this setting. Generally, a first generation cephalosporin is administered intravenously just prior to establishing the percutaneous tract and continued for 48 hr following removal of the calculus.

TECHNIQUE

The exact technique of percutaneous stone extraction varies with the size and position of the calculus. However, the procedure is always performed with the same sequential steps that include establishment of the percutaneous nephrostomy tract, dilatation of the tract, stone manipulation, and postmanipulation drainage and tamponade of the tract. In our clinic, these steps are generally all accomplished on a single day with our access obtained in the radiologic suite and the remainder of the procedure performed in the surgical theater.

Establishment of the Percutaneous Tract

Percutaneous access is established as described in chapter 13 so that a no. 6.5 French "pyeloureteral" catheter is now in place.

Dilatation of the Tract

The patient is brought to a fluoroscopically equipped operating suite where general endotracheal anesthesia is administered. A urethral catheter is placed to accommodate the large amount of irrigating fluid that will flow down the ureter and the patient is placed in the prone position with chest roll protection. The collecting system may now be opacified by injection of contrast through the previously placed percutaneous pyeloureteral catheter.

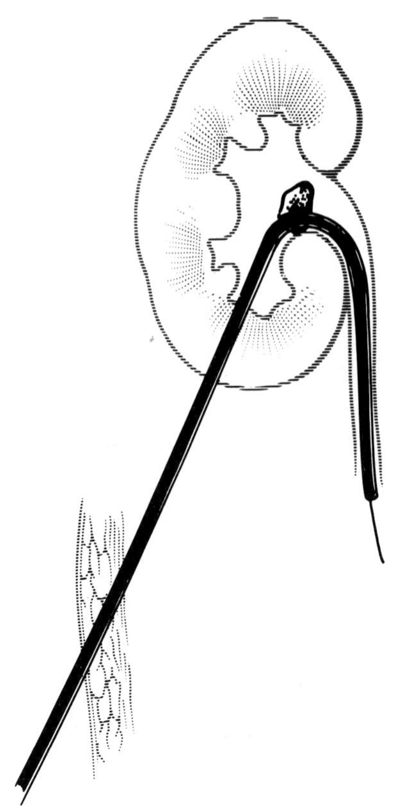

Figure 14.1. Utilizing fluoroscopic control, a 0.038-inch Lunderquist guidewire is placed through the pyeloureteral catheter to the distal ureter or advanced into the bladder. (From Streem SB, Zelch MG, Risius B, Geisinger MA: Percutaneous extraction of renal calculi. *Urol Clin North Am* 12:381, 1985.)

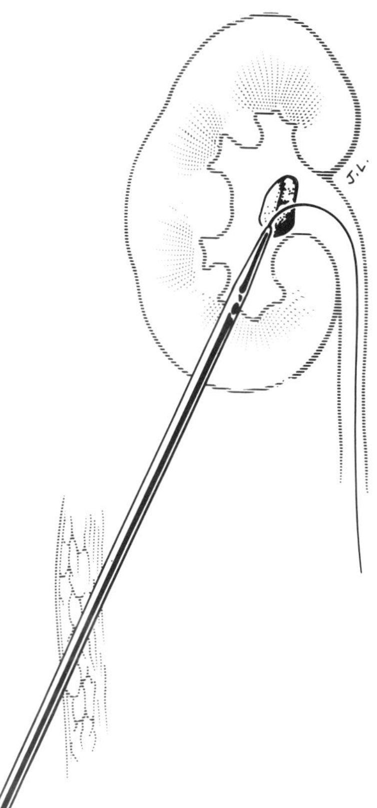

Figure 14.2. The pyeloureteral catheter is removed and the dilatation is accomplished utilizing a sequential polyethylene fascial dilating set, beginning with the no. 8 French dilator. These dilators are passed just to the renal pelvis, taking care not to perforate the medial pelvic wall. (From Streem SB, Zelch MG, Risius B, Geisinger MA: Percutaneous extraction of renal calculi. *Urol Clin North Am* 12:381, 1985.)

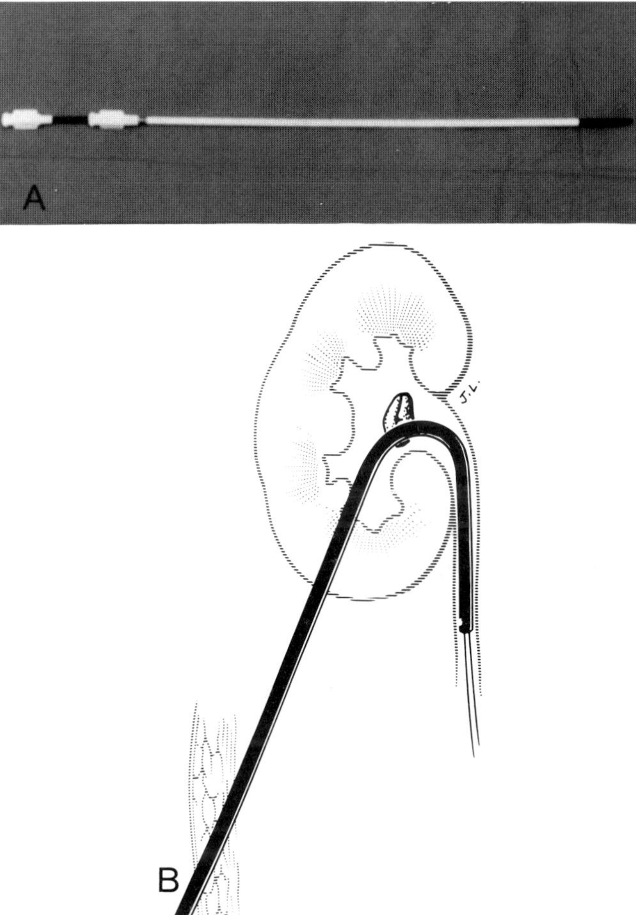

Figure 14.3. During the course of the dilatation, a second guidewire is passed to the distal ureter. This is most easily accomplished utilizing a flexible no. 9 French introducer set that accommodates two guidewires within its lumen as follows. Following dilatation to a no. 16 French catheter with the fascial dilators, the no. 9 French introducer set is passed over the initial guidewire and down the ureter, at which time the inner cannula is removed. A second ''safety wire'' is then placed through the outer sheath of the introducer set and the sheath is withdrawn. The safety wire allows rapid reaccess to the collecting system in case of inadvertent loss of the tract during subsequent dilatation or stone manipulation. (From Streem SB, Zelch MG, Risius B, Geisinger MA: Percutaneous extraction of renal calculi. *Urol Clin North Am* 12:381, 1985.)

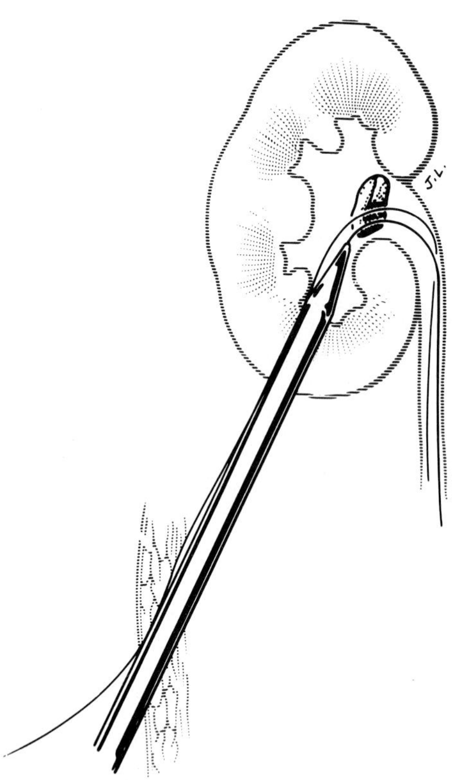

Figure 14.4. Dilatation of the tract is then continued over the Lunderquist wire to an appropriate size. In selected cases, a commercially available ''working sheath'' may be passed over the last dilator and left in place for subsequent stone manipulation, though we generally have not used that system. (From Streem SB, Zelch MG, Risius B, Geisinger MA: Percutaneous extraction of renal calculi. *Urol Clin North Am* 12:381, 1985.)

Stone Extraction—Primary Techniques

Actual stone retrieval may be accomplished with a number of techniques, utilizing either direct vision through a nephroscope, fluoroscopic guidance, or both. At our institution, over 90% of renal stone extractions are accomplished utilizing ultrasonic lithotripsy under direct vision through a rigid nephroscope. This approach was described by Alken and associates in Mainz, West Germany and later popularized in the United States by Segura and his associates at the Mayo Clinic.

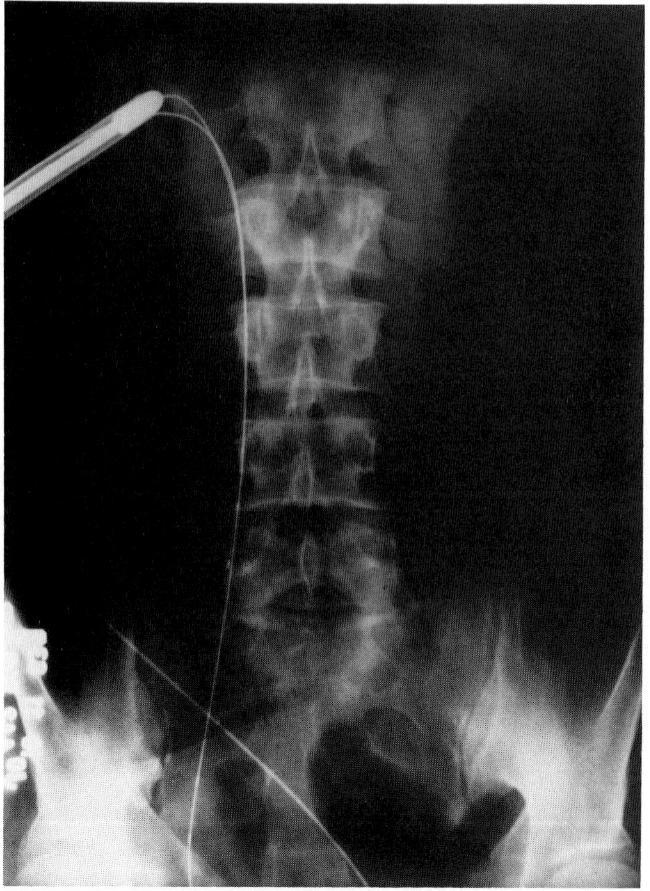

Figure 14.5. Following dilatation of the tract to a no. 24 French catheter, the last dilator is replaced with the rigid no. 24.5 French nephroscope sheath and obturator, which is passed over the Lunderquist guidewire into the pelviocalyceal system. (From Streem SB, Zelch MG, Risius B, Geisinger MA: Percutaneous extraction of renal calculi. *Urol Clin North Am* 12:381, 1985.)

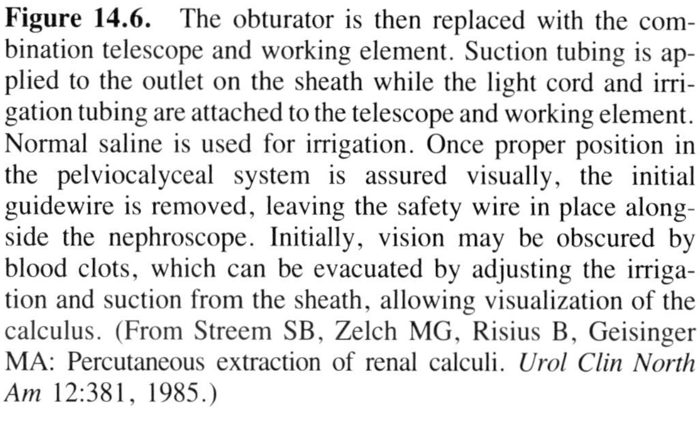

Figure 14.6. The obturator is then replaced with the combination telescope and working element. Suction tubing is applied to the outlet on the sheath while the light cord and irrigation tubing are attached to the telescope and working element. Normal saline is used for irrigation. Once proper position in the pelviocalyceal system is assured visually, the initial guidewire is removed, leaving the safety wire in place alongside the nephroscope. Initially, vision may be obscured by blood clots, which can be evacuated by adjusting the irrigation and suction from the sheath, allowing visualization of the calculus. (From Streem SB, Zelch MG, Risius B, Geisinger MA: Percutaneous extraction of renal calculi. *Urol Clin North Am* 12:381, 1985.)

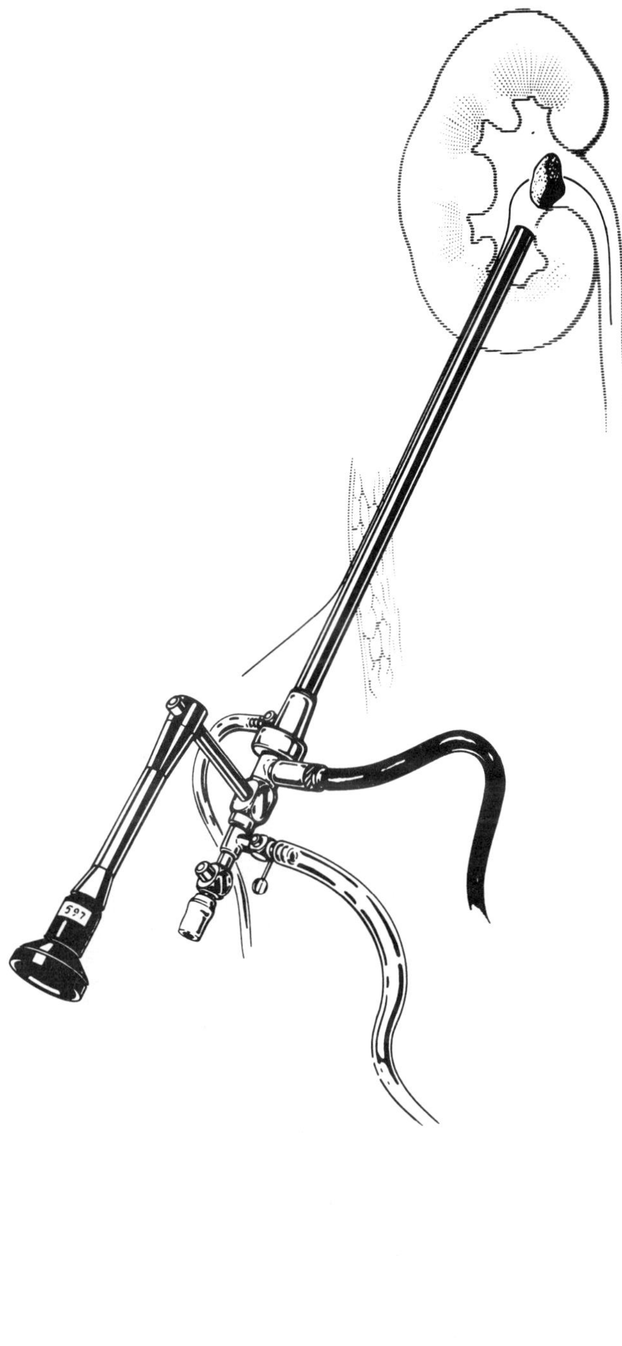

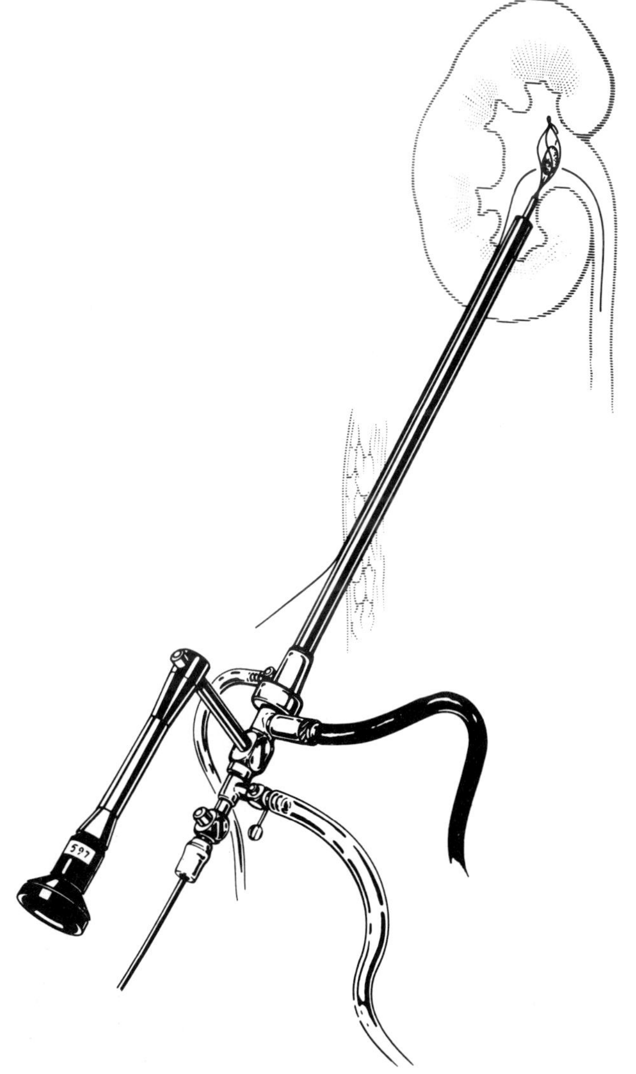

Figure 14.7. Stones less than 7 mm in diameter are small enough to pass through the nephroscope sheath and are grasped under direct vision utilizing a rigid endoscopic forceps or basket passed through the working port. The stone is then extracted by withdrawing the entire working element from the sheath. (From Streem SB, Zelch MG, Risius B, Geisinger MA: Percutaneous extraction of renal calculi. *Urol Clin North Am* 12:381, 1985.)

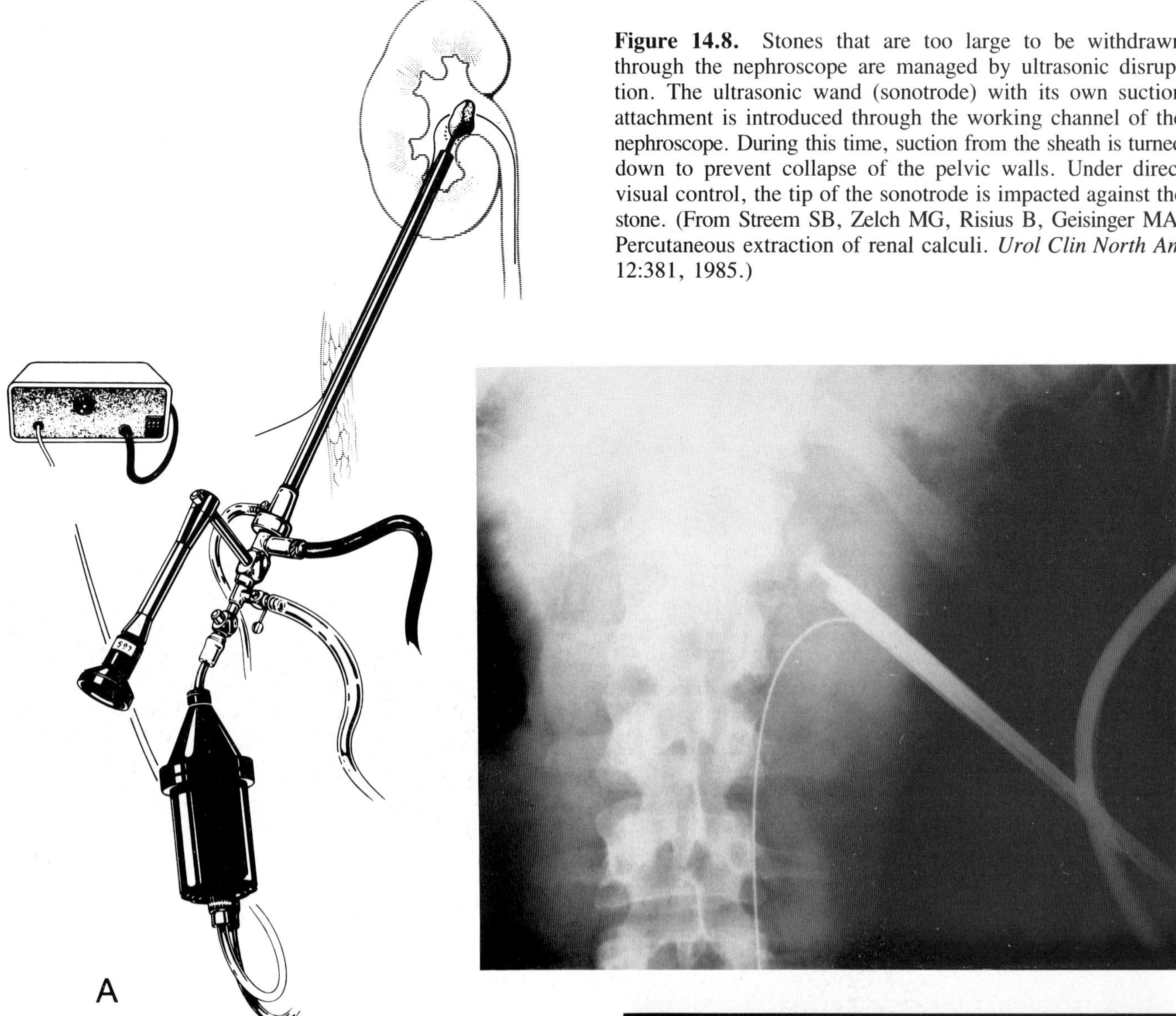

Figure 14.8. Stones that are too large to be withdrawn through the nephroscope are managed by ultrasonic disruption. The ultrasonic wand (sonotrode) with its own suction attachment is introduced through the working channel of the nephroscope. During this time, suction from the sheath is turned down to prevent collapse of the pelvic walls. Under direct visual control, the tip of the sonotrode is impacted against the stone. (From Streem SB, Zelch MG, Risius B, Geisinger MA: Percutaneous extraction of renal calculi. *Urol Clin North Am* 12:381, 1985.)

Figure 14.9. Suction applied through this hollow sonotrode holds the stone in place while stone dust and fragments are evacuated. Remaining fragments that are too large to pass through the sonotrode channel then may be extracted utilizing the previously mentioned grasping techniques or by continuing the ultrasonic fragmentation. Intermittent fluoroscopic monitoring during this procedure and a plain radiograph taken at its termination will help ensure removal of all stone fragments. (From Streem SB, Zelch MG, Risius B, Geisinger MA: Percutaneous extraction of renal calculi. *Urol Clin North Am* 12:381, 1985.)

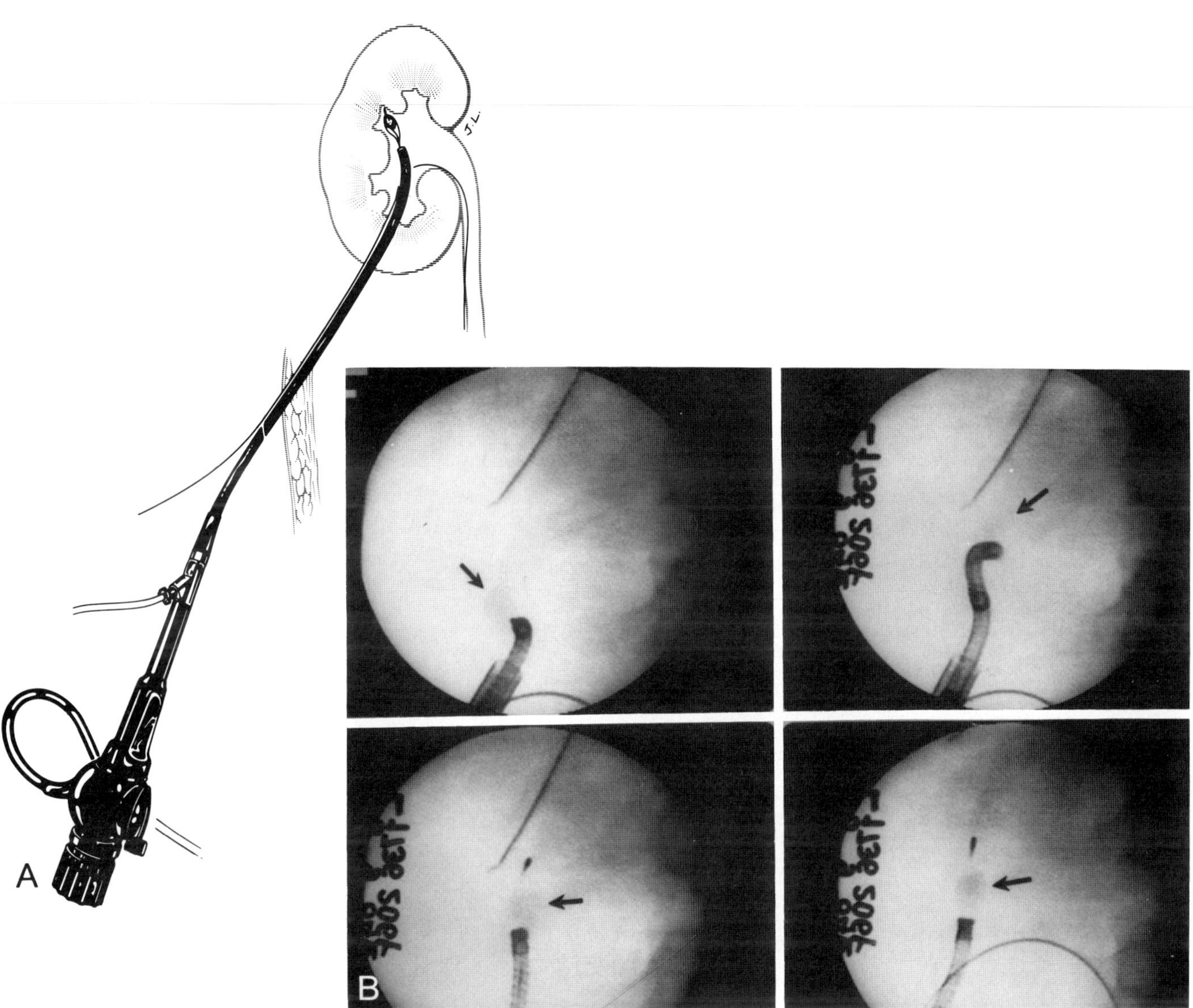

Figure 14.10. Visualization, engagement, and extraction of calyceal or other calculi lying at acute angles to the percutaneous tract may require the use of flexible nephroscopy. Occasionally, the flexible nephroscope may be utilized during the initial attempt at stone manipulation, passing it directly through the sheath of the rigid nephroscope. However, flexible nephroscopy is severely limited by even a small amount of bleeding, which will obscure visualization. Therefore, a nephrostomy tract that has been dilated and left to mature for several days is often a prerequisite for its successful use. Through the mature tract, the flexible nephroscope is passed over one of the guidewires placed through its working channel. The guidewire is removed, at which time thorough inspection of the pelviocalyceal system is accomplished. When the stone is visualized, a grasping forceps, prongs, or basket is passed through the working channel of the nephroscope and the stone is engaged. Extraction is accomplished by withdrawing the entire nephroscope assembly. As a second guidewire had already been placed, the procedure may be easily repeated as often as necessary. Alternatively, the procedure may be performed utilizing a working sheath which will assure patency of the tract for multiple passes. (From Streem SB, Zelch MG, Risius B, Geisinger MA: Percutaneous extraction of renal calculi. *Urol Clin North Am* 12:381, 1985.)

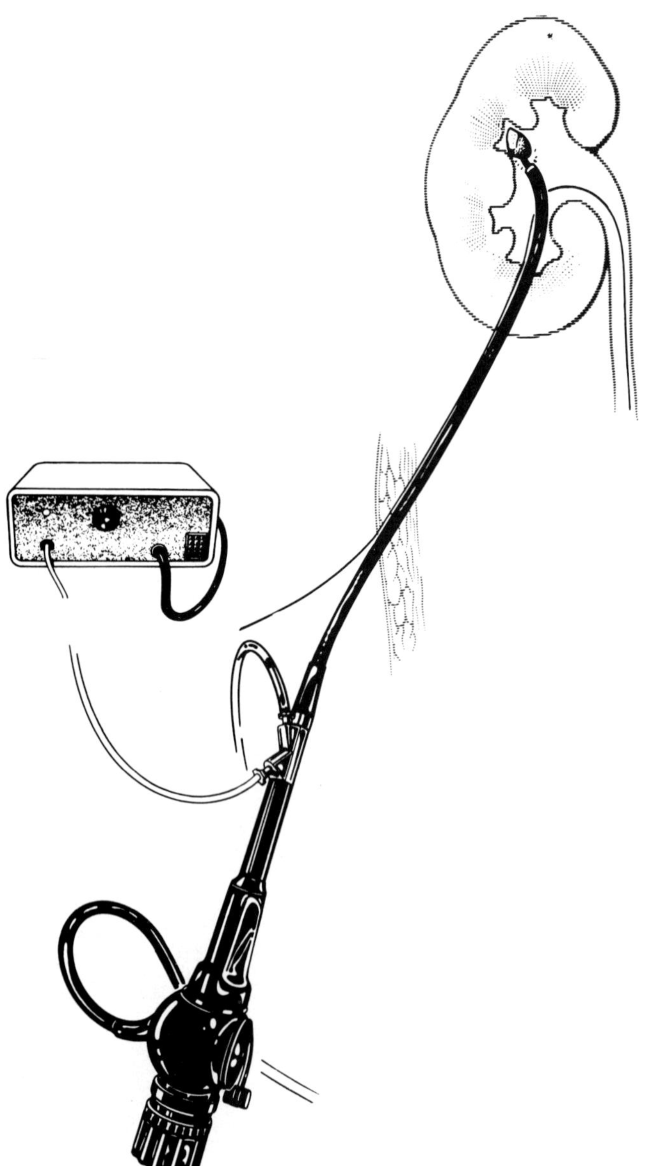

Figure 14.11. Currently, instrumentation is not available to perform ultrasonic lithotripsy in conjunction with flexible nephroscopy. An alternative however, is electrohydraulic lithotripsy, which utilizes a flexible probe. This allows fragmentation of stones which are initially too large to be extracted. Distilled water or one-sixth normal saline must be used as the irrigant in conjunction with this modality. The flexible probe is passed through the working channel or taped to the outside of the flexible nephroscope. Under direct vision, the tip of the probe is placed approximately 1 mm from a rough edge of the calculus. The probe is discharged and the stone fragmented. Electrohydraulic lithotripsy may also be a valuable adjunct for use with rigid nephroscopy when the stone is too large or too hard to be managed by ultrasonic lithotripsy. (From Streem SB, Zelch MG, Risius B, Geisinger MA: Percutaneous extraction of renal calculi. *Urol Clin North Am* 12:381, 1985.)

Stone Extraction—Ancillary Techniques

The following techniques were among those first described for the percutaneous removal of renal calculi in the pioneering work from the University of Minnesota. While occasionally still useful, these modalities have largely been replaced by direct nephroscopic manipulation.

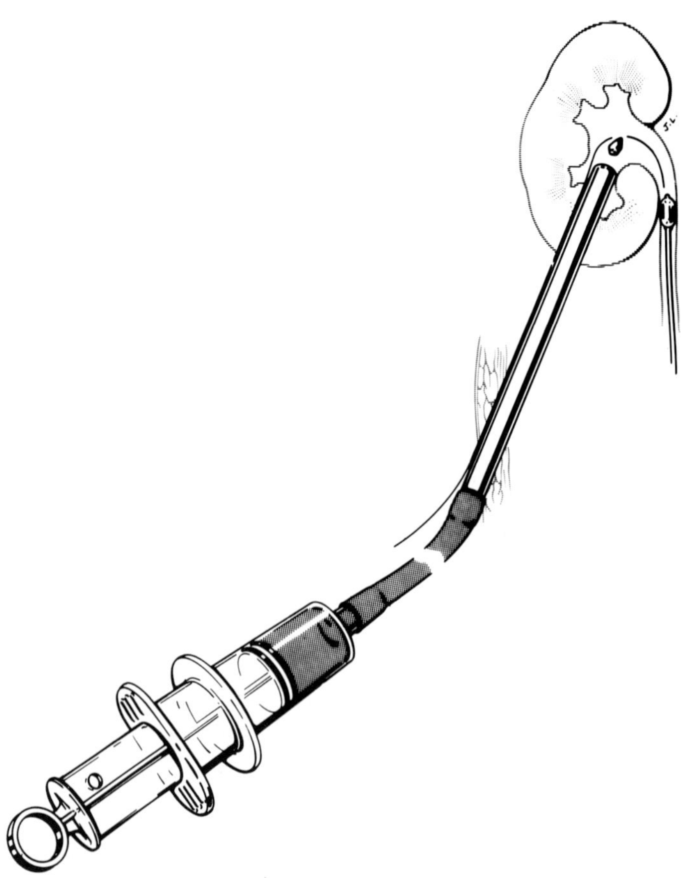

Figure 14.12. Flushing of renal calculi is an alternative technique now used only rarely that may be suitable for smaller calculi that are free-floating within relatively large renal pelves. This technique is performed with fluoroscopic control. The percutaneous tract is dilated to a size that allows placement of a working sheath with an internal diameter larger than the calculus. A piston-type syringe is then adapted to the working sheath utilizing a large bore, stiff plastic tubing. Monitoring with fluoroscopic control to prevent overdistention, dilute contrast is instilled into the renal pelvis in an antegrade or retrograde fashion utilizing either the working sheath assembly or a ureteral catheter placed cystoscopically. Aspiration of the fluid may then yield the calculus, though several attempts will often be required. (From Streem SB, Zelch MG, Risius B, Geisinger MA: Percutaneous extraction of renal calculi. *Urol Clin North Am* 12:381, 1985.)

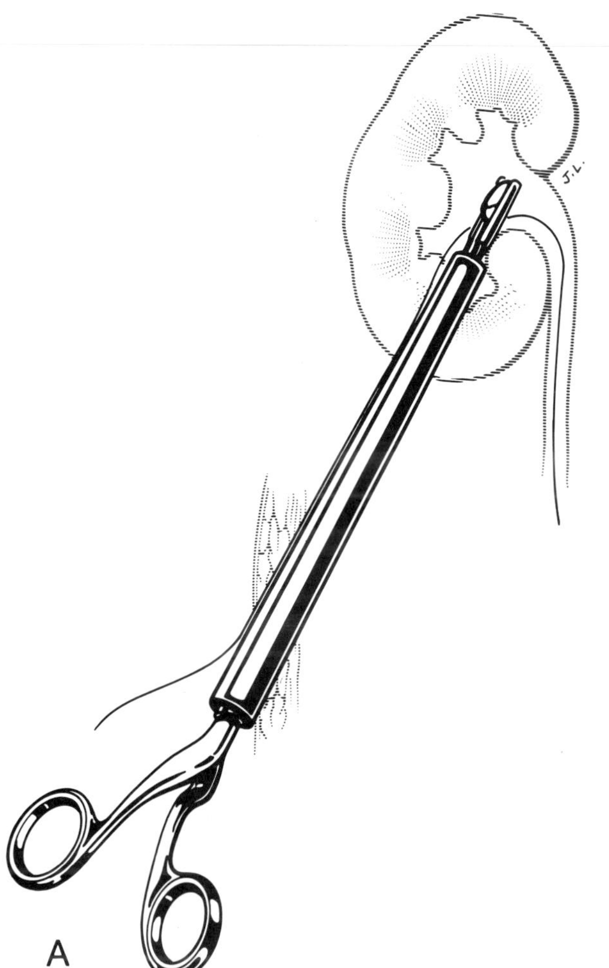

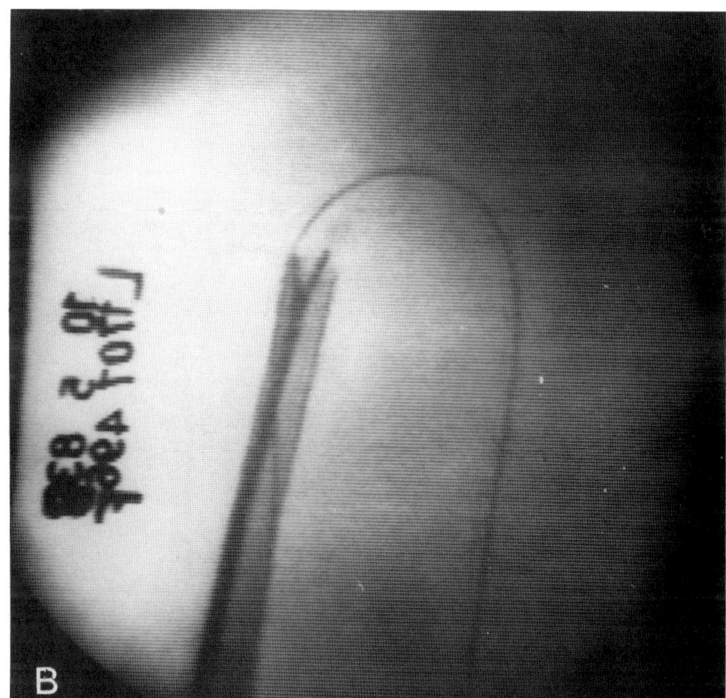

Figure 14.13. Grasping or basketing of calculi may also be performed under fluoroscopic guidance rather than under direct vision and several instruments are available. Again, the tract is dilated to allow placement of a working sheath with a lumen of suitable internal diameter. Whenever possible, the distal end of the sheath is placed just proximal to the calculus so that the grasping forceps or stone basket is easily guided to the stone. Standard Randall stone forceps are difficult to use, as the working sheath limits the opening of the shank portion of the forceps. Excellent alternative instruments include the Mazzariello-Caprini forceps, which open by a rotational rather than scissoring movement, or standard endoscopic alligator forceps. The use of standard filiform stone baskets is somewhat limited for renal calculi, as the basket must generally be passed distal to the calculus before it is opened and withdrawn. This problem may be circumvented by using a modified basket without an end-wire. Stones lying at angles to the working sheath or in the calyces may be extracted utilizing a commercially available ''steerable'' catheter, through which either a grasping forceps or basket may be manuevered. (From Streem SB, Zelch MG, Risius B, Geisinger MA: Percutaneous extraction of renal calculi. *Urol Clin North Am* 12:381, 1985.)

Post Extraction Nephrostomy Drainage and Tract Tamponade

Following extraction of calculi with any percutaneous technique, a plain radiograph of the kidney, ureter, and bladder is taken to ensure complete stone removal.

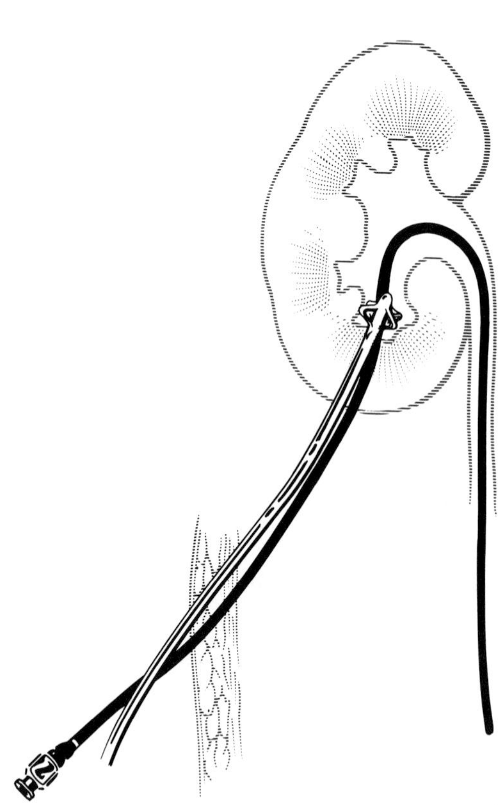

Figure 14.14. One guidewire should still be in place. Utilizing the previously mentioned no. 9 French introducer set, a second guidewire is again passed to the distal ureter and replaced with a no. 6 French, 65-cm long Teflon angiographic catheter as a pyeloureteral catheter. This again allows later access across the ureteropelvic junction if necessary. A no. 24 French Malecot catheter is placed into the pelviocalyceal system over the second guidewire utilizing fluoroscopic control to monitor its position. An ideal catheter for this use is now available commercially in a set that includes a stylet for stiffening the Malecot during insertion. The pyeloureteral catheter and the nephrostomy tube are then secured at the skin level with 0 silk suture, and a protective dressing is placed. The nephrostomy is placed to dependent drainage.

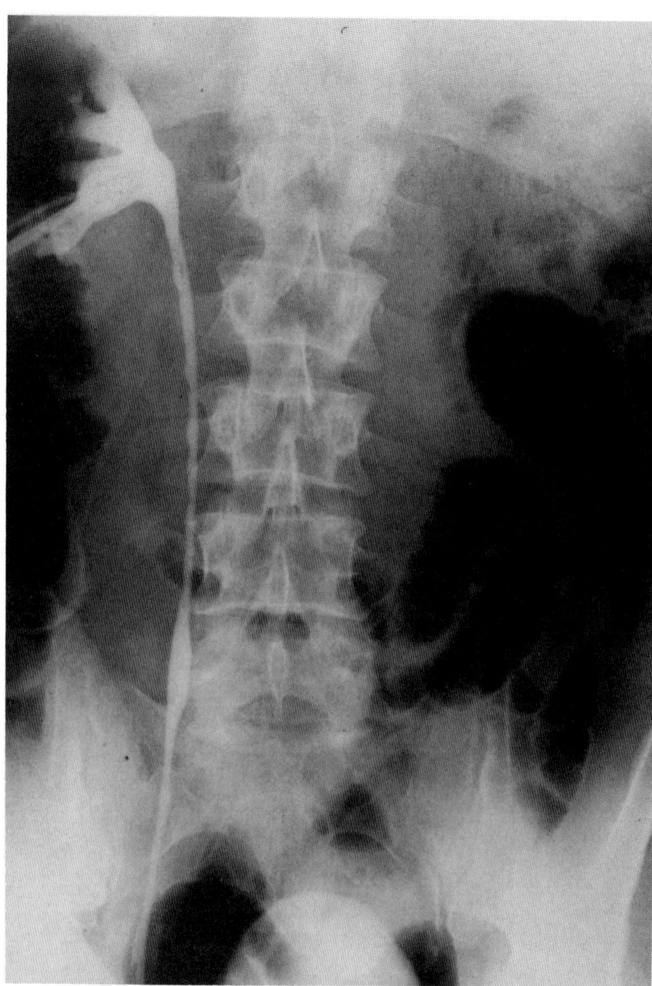

Figure 14.15. A nephrostogram is performed 48 hr following stone removal. Any residual fragments seen on this study may be managed by repeat nephroscopy, which generally requires no anesthetic, or ESWL, depending on the fragment size and location. In those cases where extravasation or obstruction is noted, the nephrostomy tube is left to drain and serial studies are obtained until the problem resolves. Ureteral obstruction noted at this time is usually the result of blood clots, which will lyse, or edema, which will subside spontaneously. Rarely, obstruction may result from small stone fragments in the ureter. Although these generally pass spontaneously, manipulation may occasionally be necessary, and this is more easily accomplished at this time utilizing a stone basket passed antegrade through the pyeloureteral catheter.

Postoperative Care

An accurate determination of irrigation and output is imperative during and following the procedure. Generally, furosemide, 20 mg, is given intravenously when the procedure is near completion. Vital signs are monitored closely and serial blood counts are obtained. Intravenous fluids are administered at a rate that ensures a sustained diuresis. In those patients with documented urinary tract infection associated with the calculus disease, specific antibiotic therapy is continued for a 2-week course, at which time long-term suppressive antimicrobial therapy is considered. In those patients with sterile urine initially, prophylactic antibiotic coverage is generally discontinued within 48 hr of an uncomplicated stone extraction.

When no obstruction or extravasation is noted, the pyeloureteral catheter is removed. The nephrostomy tube is then clamped for 12 hr and removed if there has been no flank pain or fever. The patient is then discharged with a light sterile dressing over the nephrostomy tract site, which will often drain urine for the next 12–48 hr. All patients are allowed to return to full prehospitalization activity and employment 1 week following hospital discharge. We routinely perform a follow-up excretory urogram 1 month later, at the time of the first postoperative visit. (From Streem SB, Zelch MG, Risius B, Geisinger MA: Percutaneous extraction of renal calculi. *Urol Clin North Am* 12:381, 1985.)

Suggested Readings

Alken P, Hutschenreiter G, Gunther R, Marberger M: Percutaneous stone manipulation. *J Urol* 125:463, 1981.

Banner MP, Pollack HM: Percutaneous extraction of renal and ureteral calculi. *Radiology* 144:753, 1982.

Bissada NK, Meacham KR, Redman JF: Nephrostoscopy with removal of renal pelvic calculi. *J Urol* 112: 414, 1974.

Brantley RG, Shirley SW: U-tube nephrostomy: An aid in the postoperative removal of retained renal stones. *J Urol* 111:7, 1974.

Clayman RV, Surya V, Miller RP, et al: Percutaneous nephrolithotomy: Extraction of renal and ureteral calculi from 100 patients. *J Urol* 131:686, 1984.

Fernstrom I, Johansson B: Percutaneous pyelolithotomy. *Scand J Urol Nephrol* 10:257, 1976.

Goodwin WE, Casey WC, Woolf W: Percutaneous trocar (needle) nephrostomy in hydronephrosis. *JAMA* 157:891, 1955.

Harris RD, McLaughlin AP, Harrel JH: Percutaneous nephroscopy using fiberoptic bronchoscope. *Urology* 6:367, 1975.

Karamcheti A, O'Donnell WF: Percutaneous nephrolithotomy: An innovative extraction technique. *J Urol* 118:671, 1977.

Kaye KW: Renal anatomy for endourologic stone removal. *J Urol* 130:647, 1983.

Kurth KH, Hohenfellner R, Altwein JE: Ultrasound litholapaxy of a staghorn calculus. *J Urol* 117:242, 1977.

Marberger M, Stackl W, Hruby W: Percutaneous litholapaxy of renal calculi with ultrasound. *Eur Urol* 8:236, 1982.

Palestrant AM, Sacks BA, Klein LA: Postoperative percutaneous kidney stone extraction. *Radiology* 134:778, 1980.

Raney AM, Handler J: Electrohydraulic nephrolithotripsy. *Urology* 6:439, 1975.

Rupel E, Brown R: Nephroscopy with removal of stone following nephrostomy for obstructive calculus anuria. *J Urol* 46:177, 1941.

Segura JW, Patterson DE, LeRoy AJ, et al: Percutaneous lithotripsy. *J Urol* 130:105, 1983.

Segura JW, Patterson DE, LeRoy AJ: Percutaneous removal of kidney stones: Review of 1,000 cases. *J Urol* 134:1077, 1985.

Streem SB, Zelch M, Risius B, Geisinger M: Single-stage percutaneous extraction of renal calculi. *Cleve Clin Q* 52:15, 1985.

Streem SB, Zelch MG, Risius B, Geisinger MA: Percutaneous extraction of renal calculi. *Urol Clin North Am* 12:381, 1985.

White EC, Smith AD: Percutaneous stone extraction from 200 patients. *J Urol* 132:437, 1984.

Wickham JEA, Kellett MJ, Miller RA: Elective percutaneous nephrolithotomy in 50 patients. An analysis of the technique, results and complications. *J Urol* 129:904, 1983.

CHAPTER 15

Extracorporeal Shock Wave Lithotripsy

STEVAN B. STREEM

"A thousand grains of sand pass through the eye of a needle before a single pebble." W. Spencer

SHOCK WAVE PHYSICS

In order to understand better the clinical aspects of extracorporeal shock wave lithotripsy (ESWL), some basic aspects of shock wave physics need to be reviewed. These include the physical properties of shock waves, the principles of shock wave generation with an underwater spark gap, and the focusing of shock waves. This chapter will be devoted to reviewing the principles and practice of ESWL as applied for use with the Dornier HM-3 lithotriptor. Although this rapidly developing field will no doubt see the introduction of newer generation lithotriptors by the end of this decade, the basic principles of shock wave physics do not change.

Physical Properties of Shock Waves

1. Shock waves are high amplitude/low frequency pressure waves of steep onset and gradual relaxation. This may be contrasted to ultrasonic waves that are of high frequency with a "sinusoidal" curve.
2. Shock waves may be generated in a gas or liquid medium. For practical purposes, the shock waves generated for ESWL are generated in water.
3. Low frequency waves show less damping effect than those of high frequency. Therefore, shock waves (low frequency) have a greater depth of penetration than ultrasonic waves (high frequency).
4. The transmission of shock waves is unimpeded until an acoustic interface is met. Because the density of normal body tissue is essentially the same as the density of water, shock waves that are generated in water will be transmitted through normal body tissue without change. The shock wave will then be reflected at a significant acoustic interface such as is met at a calculus.
5. Shock waves exert a compressive force when they do meet an acoustic interface at a second focal point (F2). At the interface, they are reflected as a tensile force. Both compressive and tensile forces can effect a change at an acoustic interface.

Shock Wave Generation: Underwater Spark Gap

In the Dornier HM-3 system (Dornier Systems Ltd., Friedrichshafen, FRG), the shock wave is generated by a rapid fire, high voltage spark plug that is discharged in water. This underwater spark discharge leads to vaporization of the surrounding fluid, resulting in the local generation of the high amplitude/low frequency shock wave. Obviously, the pressure generated by this system needs to be modulated easily and kept within a range that will both fragment a stone and at the same time be safe to the surrounding tissue. In practical terms, there are three ways to modulate the pressure amplitude:

1. Variation in the electrode separation of the spark gap will change the pressure that is generated. With increasing distance between the electrodes, an increased amplitude of the pressure will be generated when all other variables are kept constant.
2. A change in the discharge voltage of the spark gap condenser will also lead to a change in the pressure amplitude. Again, with all other variables kept constant, increased voltage is associated with an increased pressure that is generated.
3. A change in the rate at which the spark is generated will change the pressure. That is, a discharge of the spark gap over a shorter period of time will lead to an increased pressure amplitude of the shock wave.

Shock Wave Focusing: Semiellipsoid

For practical purposes, safe destruction of a calculus in vivo requires the ability to focus the shock wave within narrow limits so that the targeted calculus receives maximum pressure while the surrounding, normal tissue is left intact. In the Dornier system, this is accomplished by focusing the shock wave through the use of a brass, symmetrical semiellipsoid reflector. The maximum semiaxis of this semiellipsoid is 11 cm whereas the minimum axis is 6.5 cm.

The spark gap generator is positioned at the F1 focal point

of the semiellipsoid. The generated shock waves will then be focused at a distance from this F1 focal point known as the F2 focal point. It is here at the F2 focal point where the pressure amplitude of the shock wave will be greatest. Theoretically then, the calculus needs to be positioned at the F2 focal point to receive the maximum shock wave pressure. (In the Dornier system, the F2 focal point is fixed. Thus, the calculus is brought to the focal point. In some other systems, the focal point may be moved to the stone.)

Shock Wave Generation and Focusing: Damping Effect

As mentioned above, these low frequency shock waves show relatively little damping effect. However, accurate pressure generation and focal point localization must take into account the potential damping effect of normal body tissue. In fact, the interposition of normal tissues such as fat or muscle will result in a relatively small but clearly detectable change in the maximum pressure amplitude generated at the focal point. However, the interposition of the same amount of fat or muscle will not change the location of the F2 focal point.

EXTRACORPOREAL SHOCK WAVE LITHOTRIPSY: ANIMAL EXPERIENCE

During the initial development of ESWL, an excellent dog model was developed by the Dornier company in conjunction with the Urology Department at the University of Munich. Initially, shock waves were generated and focused onto normal organs. Blood studies were then obtained and the animals were sacrificed for histologic and pathologic study. When biologically tolerable amplitudes of the shock waves were known, a more practical system was developed to test the feasibility of fragmenting stones in vivo. In those studies, hydronephrosis was unilaterally induced by placing a ligature around the distal ureter of a dog. One week later, after dilatation of the collecting system developed, a pyelotomy was performed at which time human urinary stones were implanted. At the same time ureteroneocystostomy was performed to relieve the distal obstruction. Shock waves were then induced utilizing ultrasonic localization of the stone or of the kidney itself.

Through those studies, it became evident that clinically useful fragmentation could be accomplished utilizing relatively lower pressures with greater number of shocks. At higher pressures, fragmentation was obtained. However, the fragmentation in those cases resulted in large pieces of stone rather than small, easily passible particles. It was through those studies that the currently applicable pressure ranges were developed.

Target Localization

Although ultrasonography provided a reasonable means of localizing stones in the experimental model, the resolution in the initial studies that was provided by ultrasonography was not great enough to predict accurate stone fragmentation. Thus, a high resolution fluoroscopic system suitable for use under water was developed. Utilizing image intensification, two fluroscopes placed at nearly 90° angles were utilized to place the calculus accurately at the F2 focal point. Although technical advances will soon allow the use of high resolution ultrasonography to monitor the progress of fragmentation, the only practical systems currently available in the United States utilize such fluoroscopic control.

EXTRACORPOREAL SHOCK WAVE LITHOTRIPSY: CLINICAL ASPECTS

It became apparent in the early 1980s at the University of Munich (and later at other centers in West Germany) that ESWL provided an excellent, noninvasive means to manage renal and some upper ureteral calculi in the majority of patients. Initially, the treatment was limited to relatively small, opaque stones in otherwise healthy patients. With experience though, these treatments were extended to patients with large or otherwise complex stones as well as those patients with multiple medical problems. In 1984, a multicenter trial involving six institutions was begun in the United States. In less than 1 year, Food and Drug Administration (FDA) approval was given for ESWL as an effective and safe modality for the treatment of renal and some ureteral calculi in the United States.

Patient Selection

The indications for intervention have not changed. Thus, patients in whom the stones are increasing in size despite appropriate medical management or patients in whom the stones are associated with obstruction, refractory pain, urinary tract infection, or significant bleeding may all be initially considered as candidates for ESWL. In fact, ESWL is the primary treatment of choice for almost all such patients and, therefore, it is perhaps more pertinent to note contraindications to this treatment modality. Currently, absolute contraindications include an irreversible coagulopathy, pregnancy, or vascular calcification in close proximity to the stone. Obstruction distal to the stone is a contraindication to ESWL as sole therapy. However, even in those patients, ESWL, at times, may be combined with percutaneous techniques for optimal management.

Relative contraindications include body habitus considerations. In the Dornier HM-3 system, the support apparatus was designed for height between 4 feet and 6 feet, 6 inches. However, minor modifications have allowed successful treatment for patients outside those parameters at most centers. Weight greater than 135 kg may also preclude successful treatment due to inability to place the calculus at the F2 focal point and because of weight restriction on the support mechanism. However, treatment in the "power path" of the shock wave may allow success even in this setting. Patients with calculi in congenital pelvic or transplanted kidneys have also been considered poor candidates for ESWL. Again though, some centers have reported modifications in patient positioning such as placement in the prone position to allow successful fragmentation. Similarly, lower ureteral calculi, at times, may be treated successfully when patient position is modified. Although patients with cardiac pacemakers do not have FDA approval for ESWL, many such patients, in fact, may be treated successfully though each must be individualized and monitored closely during treatment.

Urinary tract infection is not itself a contraindication to

ESWL. However, all attempts should be made to sterilize the urine before ESWL, and the shock wave treatment should not be performed in the face of acute pyelonephritis or urinary sepsis. Patients with chronic infection associated with their stones should be treated with 24–48 hours of intravenous antibiotics before ESWL. Currently, a role for "prophylactic" antibiotics in patients with sterile urine is unproven.

There is no absolute size of a stone that would preclude successful ESWL treatment. However, patients with larger stones generally require adjunctive techniques to prevent significant sequelae from the large burden of stone fragments. In our experience, significant morbidity and the need for emergent secondary and more invasive intervention can be reduced by the judicious use of indwelling stents, percutaneous nephrostomy drainage, and percutaneous ultrasonic debulking before planned ESWL. The optimal use of such ancillary techniques takes into consideration the following factors:

1. Stone size
2. Stone composition
3. Intrarenal anatomy
4. Urinary diversions
5. Solitary kidneys

In general, indwelling stents should be placed for stones greater than 1.5–2.0 cm. These internal stents will generally allow fragments to pass more uneventfully. Furthermore, they will prevent large pieces from migrating down the ureter before a secondary treatment can be performed where indicated. For stones larger than 3 cm, consideration should be given to percutaneous removal or at least "debulking" before ESWL. This is especially true for patients with struvite stones. Not only are these stones generally larger to begin with, but because they are associated with infection, post-ESWL obstruction can be associated with pyelonephritis and/or sepsis. A nephrostomy tube placed pre-ESWL not only prevents obstruction in the face of infection, but allows access for antegrade manipulation or chemolysis where necessary post-ESWL. Our general approach is that if a nephrostomy tube is to be placed before the shock wave treatment, the tract is utilized to debulk the stone.

Patients with urinary diversions present special problems as retrograde access to the upper tract is generally impossible pre- or post-ESWL. Furthermore, the stones in these patients are often struvite and again, there is a greater risk of obstruction associated with infection post-ESWL. Therefore, nephrostomy drainage with or without "debulking" before ESWL is recommended in all but the most uncomplicated stones in those patients with urinary diversion.

Obstruction post-ESWL is potentially most devastating in those patients with solitary kidneys or otherwise compromised renal function. Thus, internal stents and pre-ESWL percutaneous procedures have been utilized even more liberally in this group of patients.

Cystine stones respond poorly to ESWL. Therefore, cystine stones are managed primarily with alkalinization, fluids, and D-penicillamine as necessary. Failures of such medical regimens are generally managed with percutaneous and ureteroscopic techniques with or without percutaneous chemodissolution.

Finally, uric acid stones are relatively radiolucent and, therefore, difficult to visualize fluoroscopically. Fortunately, almost all pure uric acid stones may be managed successfully with oral or percutaneous dissolution. When such stones are treated with ESWL, they are visualized as filling defects after contrast-injected retrograde or antegrade.

TECHNIQUE

The procedure is generally performed with general endotracheal or regional (epidural) anesthesia. Our preference is for general endotracheal anesthesia as this allows control over the otherwise significant respiratory excursions associated with epidural anesthesia. In selected patients, simple intravenous sedation with local anesthetic skin infiltration can be utilized effectively.

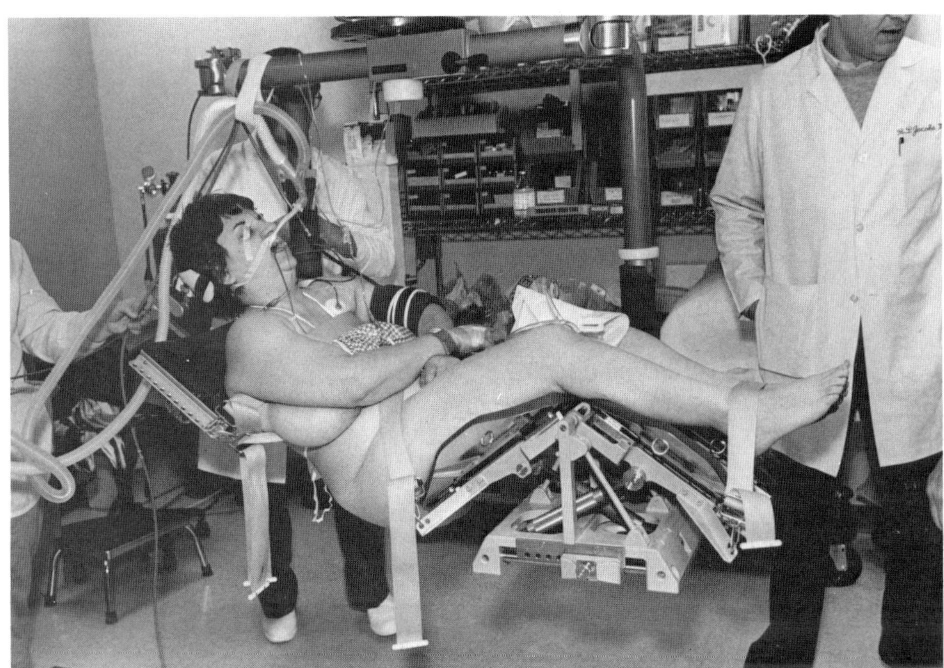

Figure 15.1. The patient is positioned in the hydraulically controlled gantry and strapped into place to prevent subsequent flotation out of proper position once they are in the water bath.

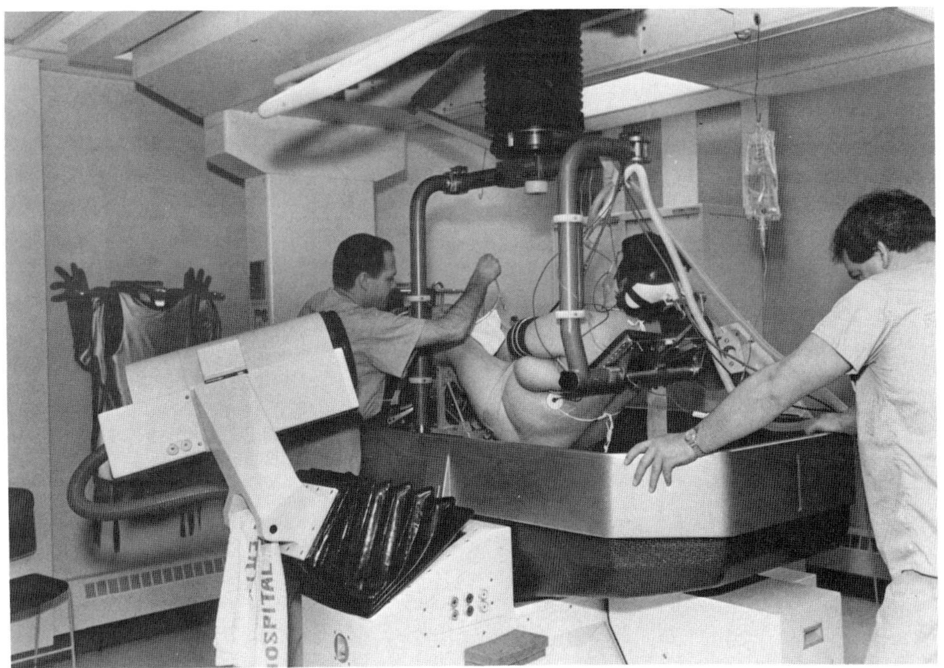

Figure 15.2. The gantry is swung into position and the patient lowered into the tub.

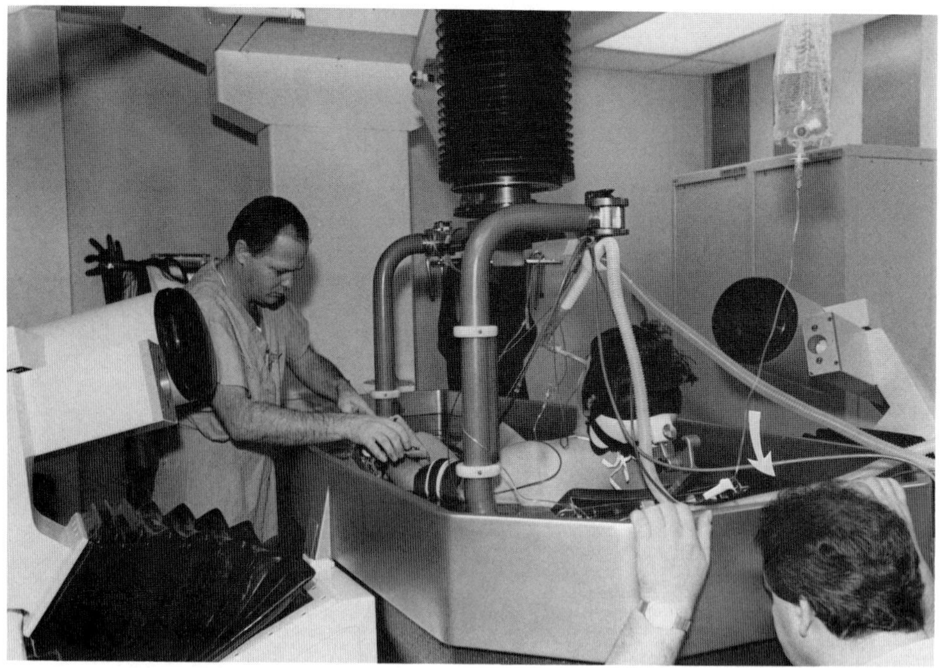

Figure 15.3. Gross visual positioning of the patient is performed by the technician *(arrow)* to place the stone as close to the F2 focal point as possible. This will help reduce the subsequent fluoroscopic imaging time.

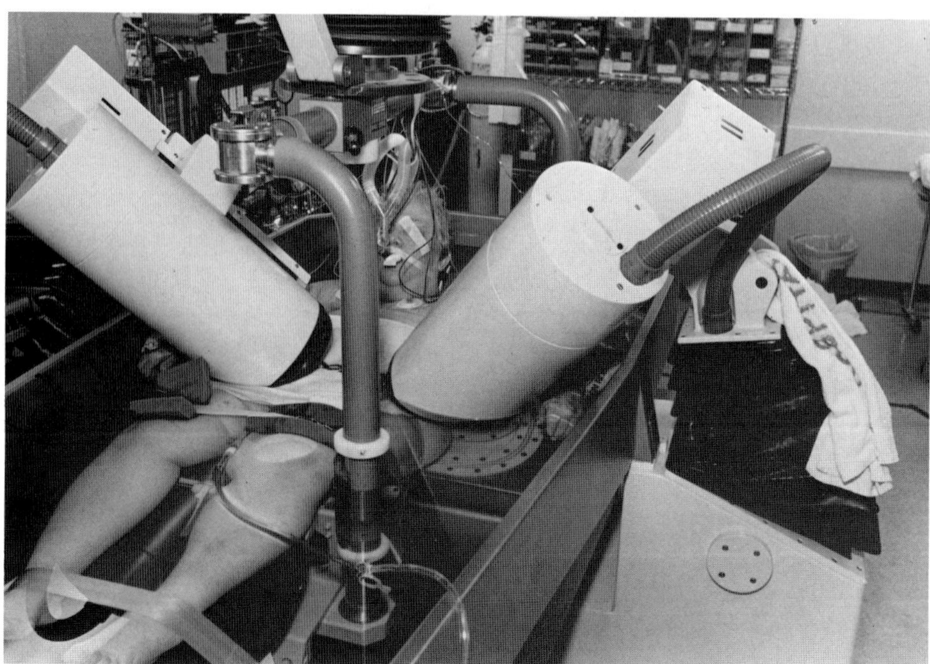

Figure 15.4. The fluoroscopes are lowered into position.

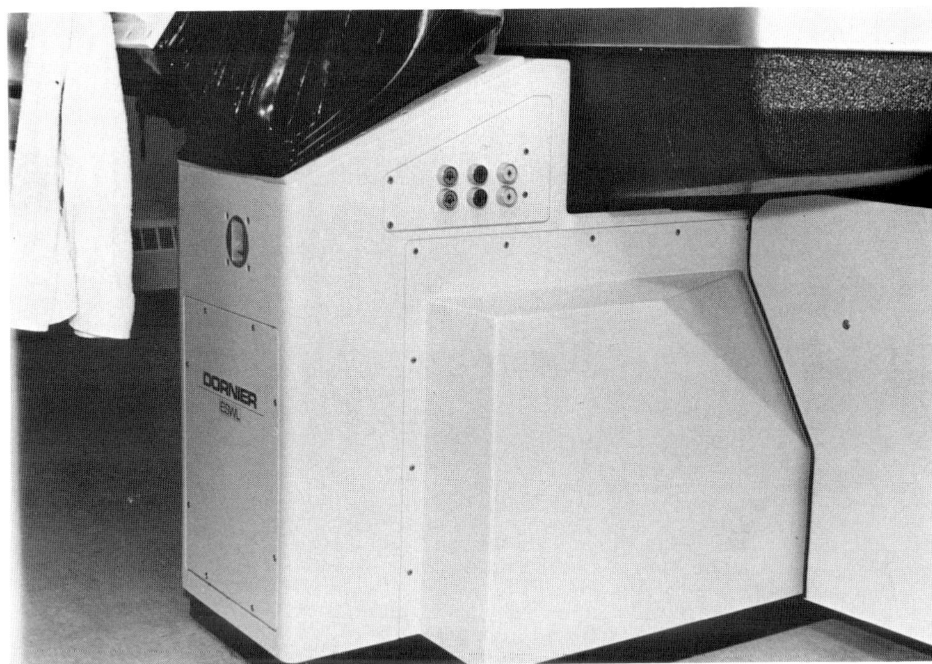

Figure 15.5. The water displacing balloons in the bottom of the tub are inflated using the controls on the side of the tub. Inflation of these balloons will improve the subsequent fluoroscopic image.

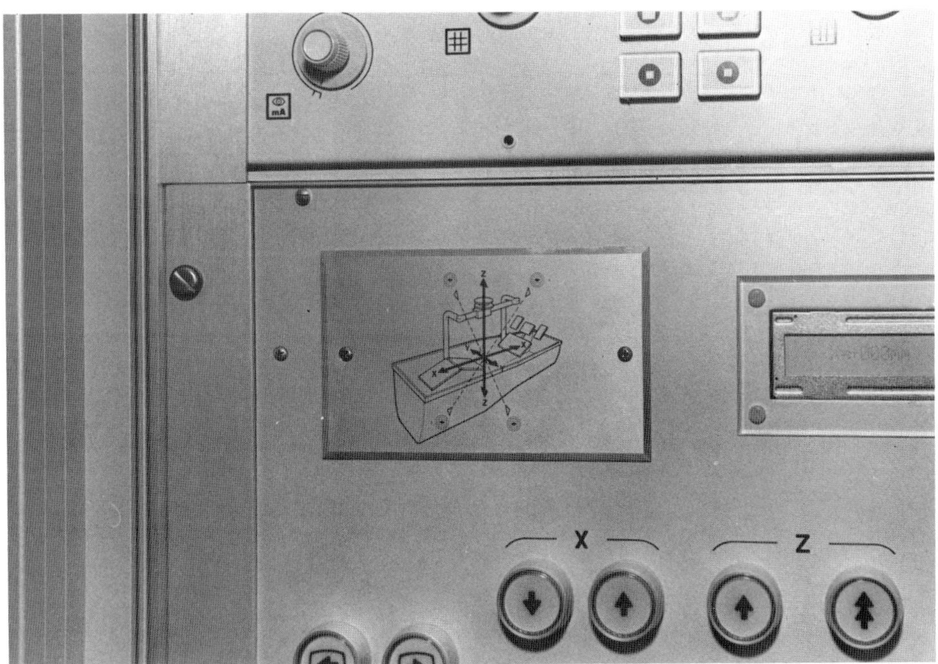

Figure 15.6. Final positioning of the stone at the F2 focal point will be accomplished in the x, y, and z axes. In most instances, changes in the x and "integrated" planes are all that are required.

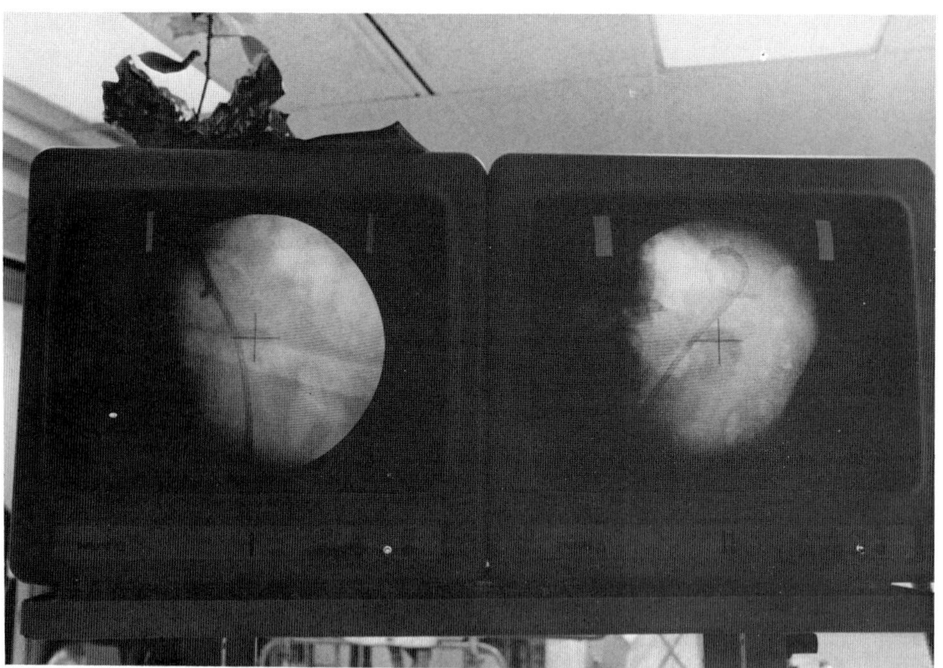

Figure 15.7. Fluoroscopic monitoring is utilized during this time to localize the stone to the F2 focal point. "Coned down" images are used in all cases so that radiation exposure is minimized. "Quick pics" are obtained only when the stone cannot otherwise be visualized or for a final determination as to whether fragmentation has been completed. In many cases, a whistle tip catheter is placed cytoscopically at the outset of the procedure for better stone localization. Internal stents are utilized selectively as discussed above.

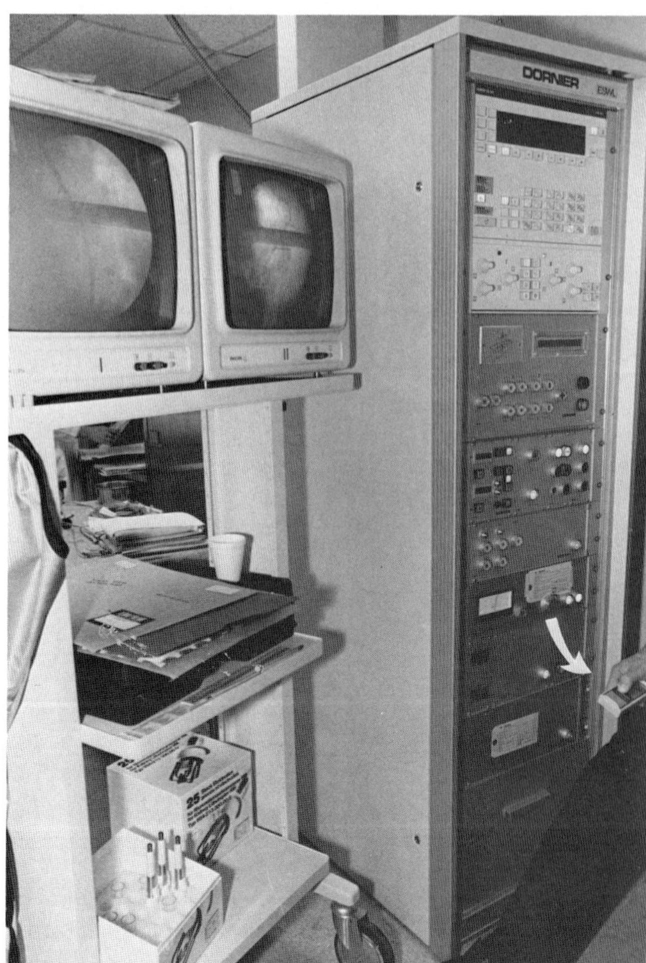

Figure 15.8. The voltage is set at 18–20 kv. The balloons are deflated and treatment is begun. We prefer the standard technique utilizing the right thumb to generate a downward force on the hand-held red button *(arrow)*. Similar results have been obtained at other centers utilizing the left thumb or other body parts. The shock waves are coordinated to the R wave of the patient's cardiographic tracing to prevent arrhythmias.

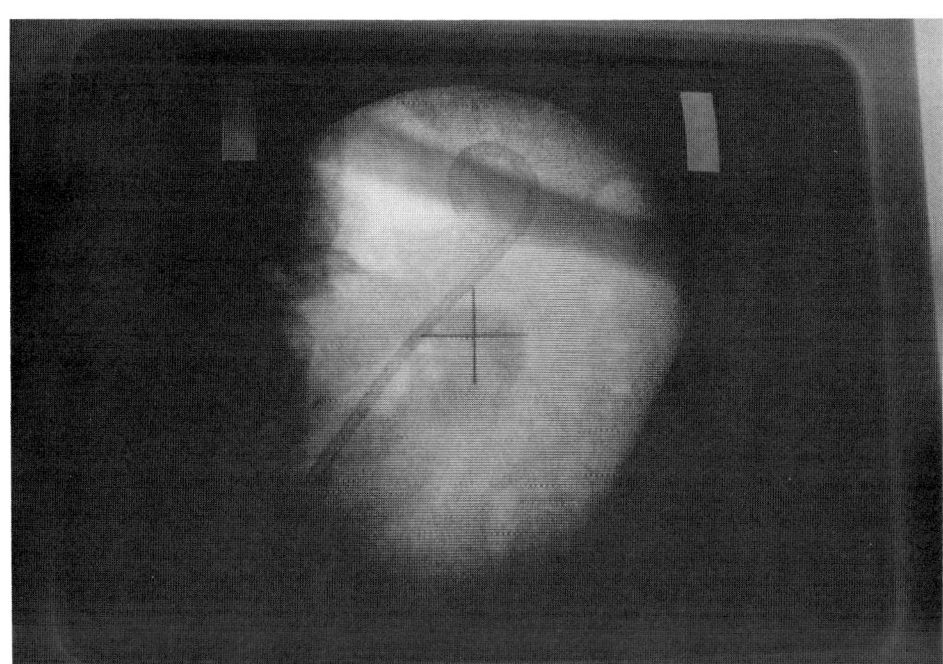

Figure 15.9. The procedure is monitored fluoroscopically every 200–300 shocks. Minor positional adjustments are made as necessary during this time and progress of the fragmentation is noted. The FDA has given approval to a maximum of 2000 shocks per treatment to each renal unit. However, we occasionally give more if we believe a secondary treatment will be obviated.

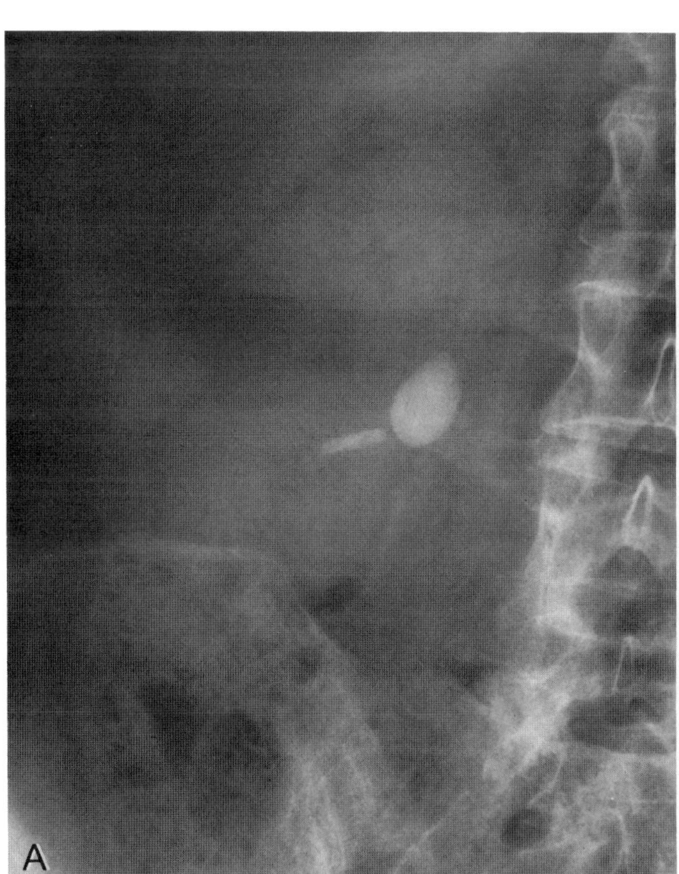

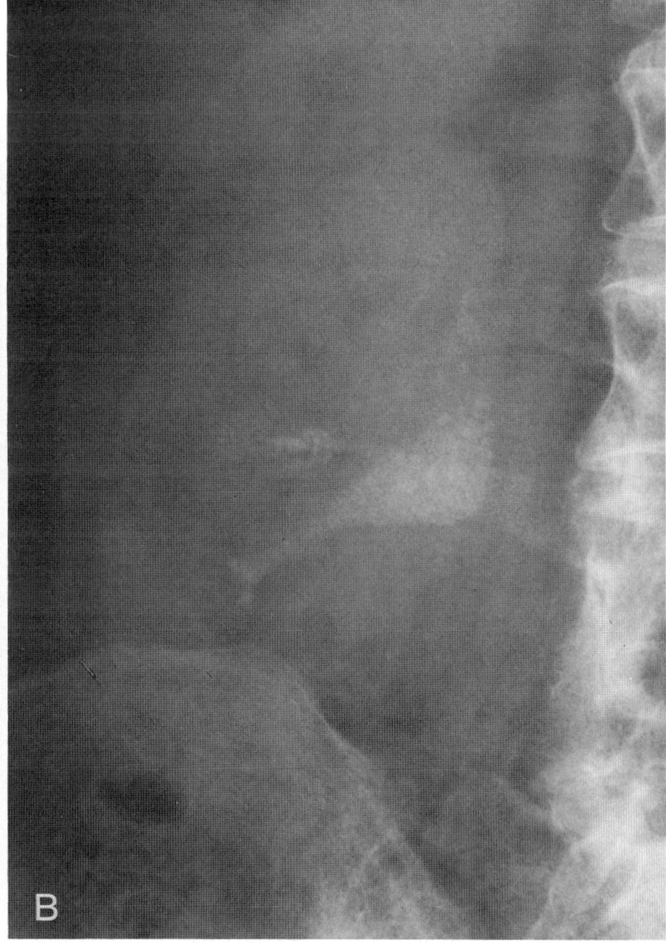

Figure 15.10. At the end of a successful treatment, stone fragmentation is generally obvious. With larger calculi, a ''powder pyelogram'' may be evident as particles of the stone spread out to fill the collecting system.

Ureteral Calculi

Patients requiring intervention for upper and midureteral calculi are generally best managed by ESWL. As stones in the ureter do not fragment as well as renal calculi, the initial procedure should be an attempt at retrograde flushing of the stone to the kidney, with placement of a ureteral catheter or internal ureteral stent until ESWL can be performed. Stones that can not be flushed to the kidney may be treated in situ. However, better results will be attained in those cases if a ureteral catheter or internal stent can be passed beyond the stone. A stone that cannot be manipulated or at least bypassed with a catheter or stent utilizing standard techniques may be managed with ureteroscopic techniques as described in Chapter 39. The ureteroscopic techniques may be utilized either for stone manipulation or to manage the stone definitively.

Ureteral calculi are better visualized during ESWL if the patient is placed in the tub with the affected side obliqued downward to throw the stone off the spine. The kv is set higher than for renal calculi and therapy is routinely begun at 20 kv and increased to 24 kv as necessary.

At our center, distal ureteral calculi are generally managed primarily with endoscopic techniques. Occasionally, however, a failure of such therapy may be salvaged with ESWL.

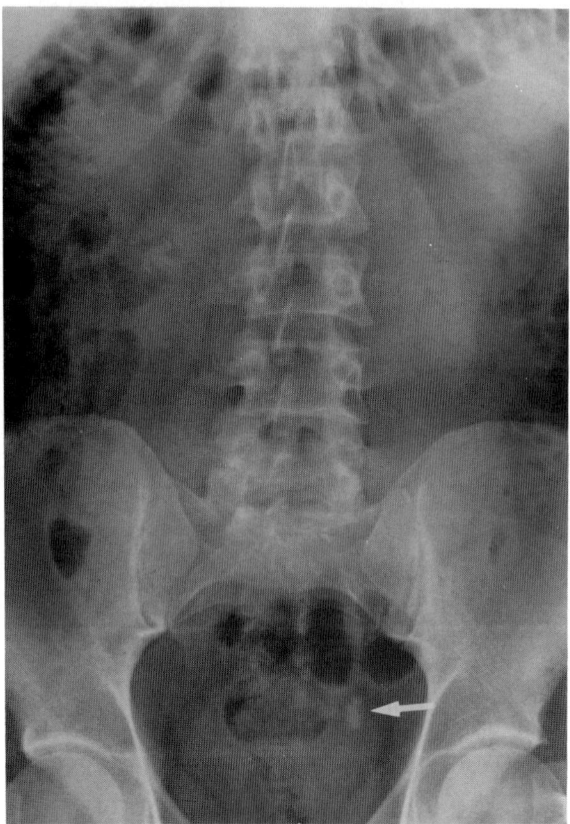
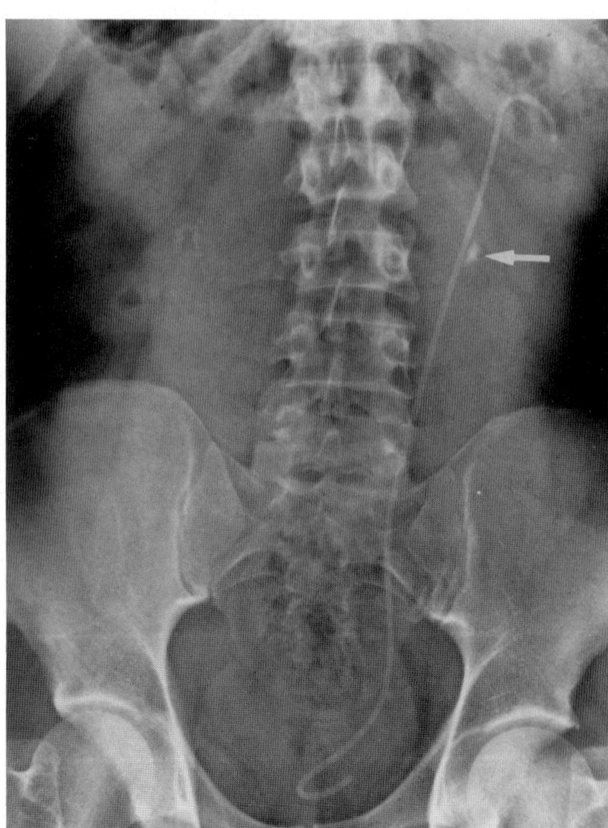

Figure 15.11. In some cases, distal ureteral calculi are managed by retrograde manipulation to the kidney or to a higher point in the ureter, at least above the sacroiliac bone.

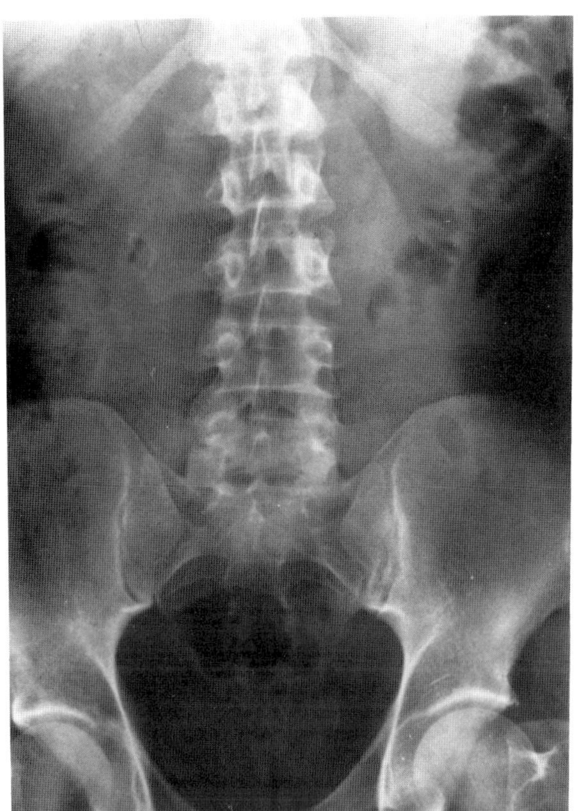

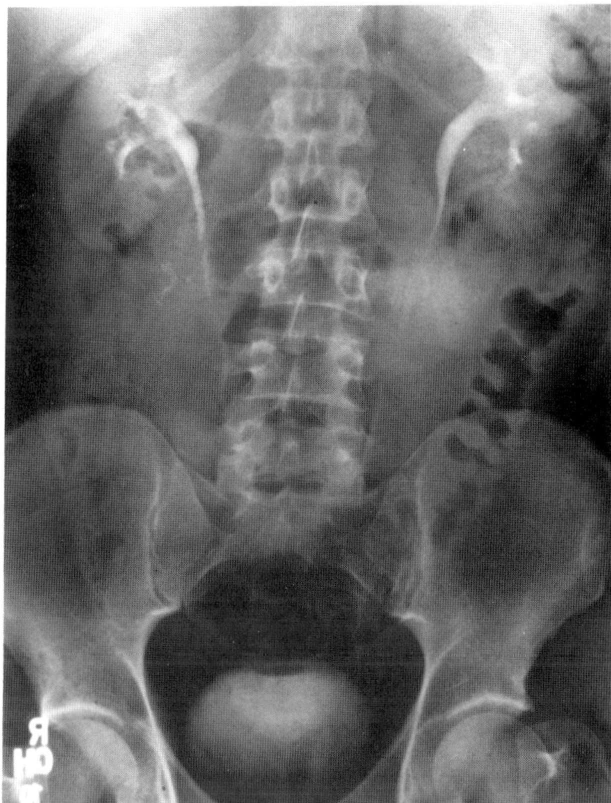

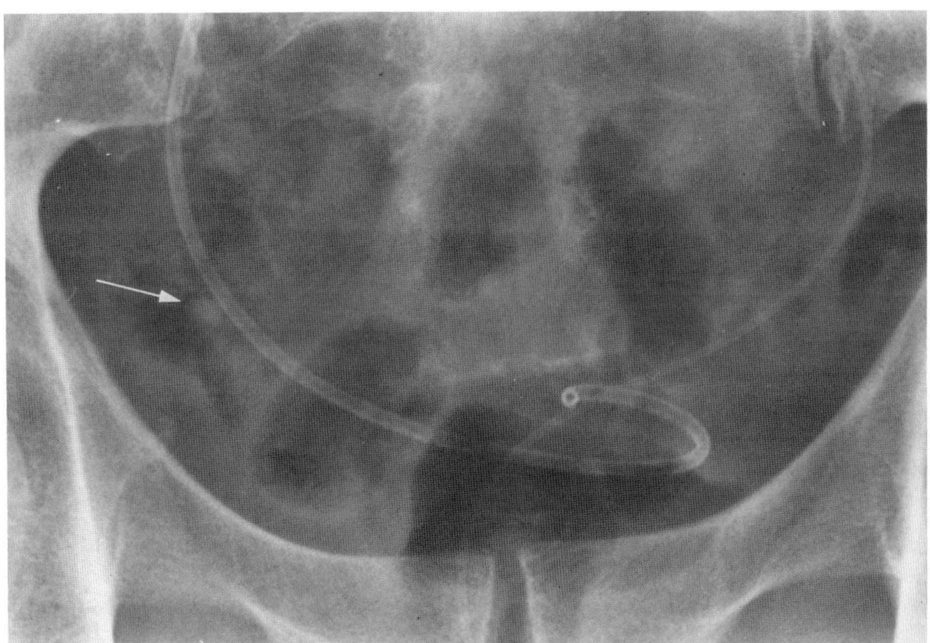

Figure 15.13. In some cases, ESWL may be used successfully to treat distal ureteral calculi in situ. Again, treatment is more likely to be successful if a catheter can be passed beyond the stone. This allows better visualization fluoroscopically and also provides room within the ureteral lumen for the stone to fragment. ESWL for distal ureteral calculi requires placement of the patient in a exaggerated cephalad position in the gantry.

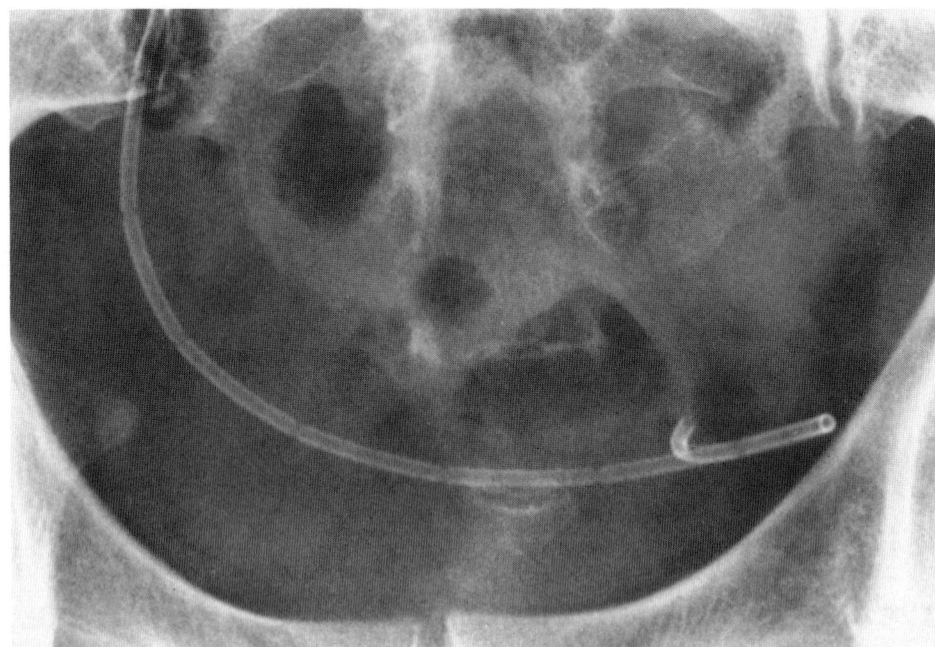

Figure 15.14. Plain film immediately after ESWL reveals excellent fragmentation of this distal stone.

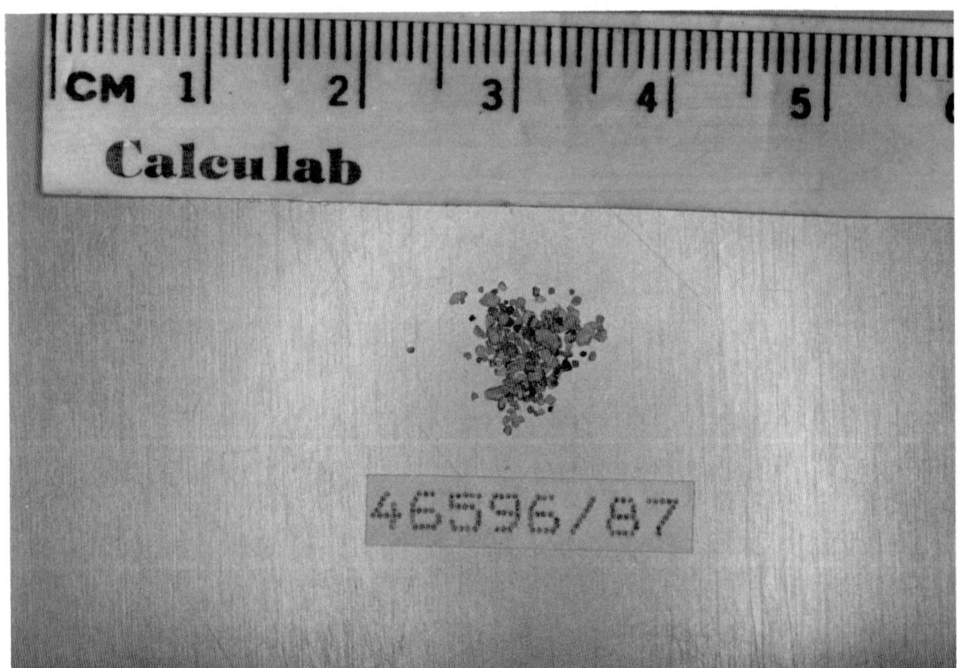

Figure 15.15. Fragments passed after ESWL of this distal stone.

Large Volume Calculi

To lessen the risk of "steinstrasse" after ESWL of larger volume stones, ancillary procedures are generally performed. We often utilize internal stents for stones 1.5–2.0 cm and use them routinely for stones measuring 2–3 cm. For stones larger than 3 cm, percutaneous procedures or combinations of percutaneous techniques and ESWL may be required.

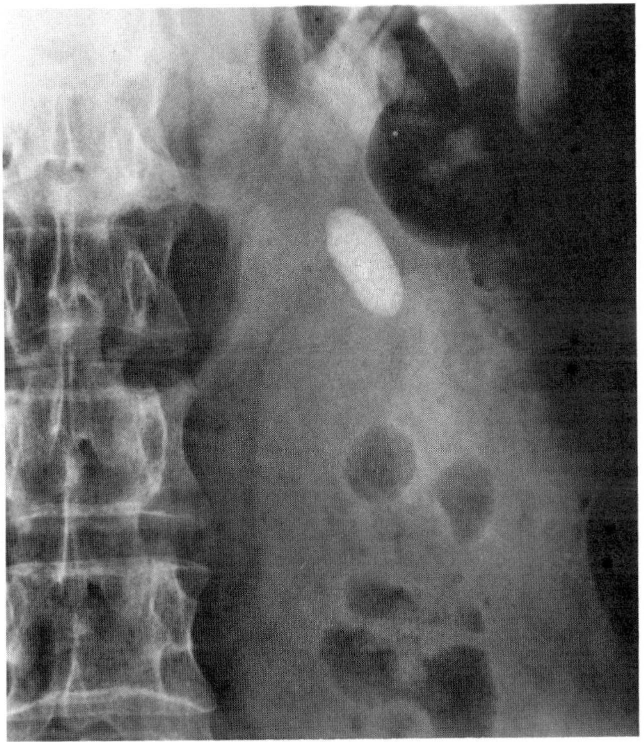

Figure 15.16. Plain film reveals 3.0 × 1.5 cm pelvic stone. An internal stent was placed at the time of ESWL.

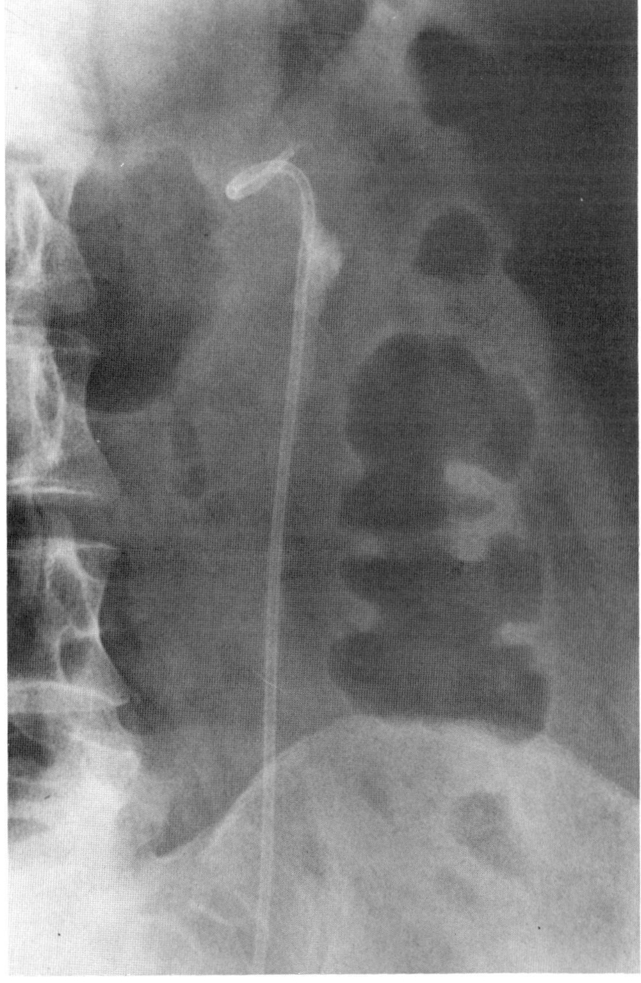

Figure 15.17. Plain film 24 hr after single ESWL treatment reveals excellent fragmentation. The stone fragments are migrating down the ureter along the stent.

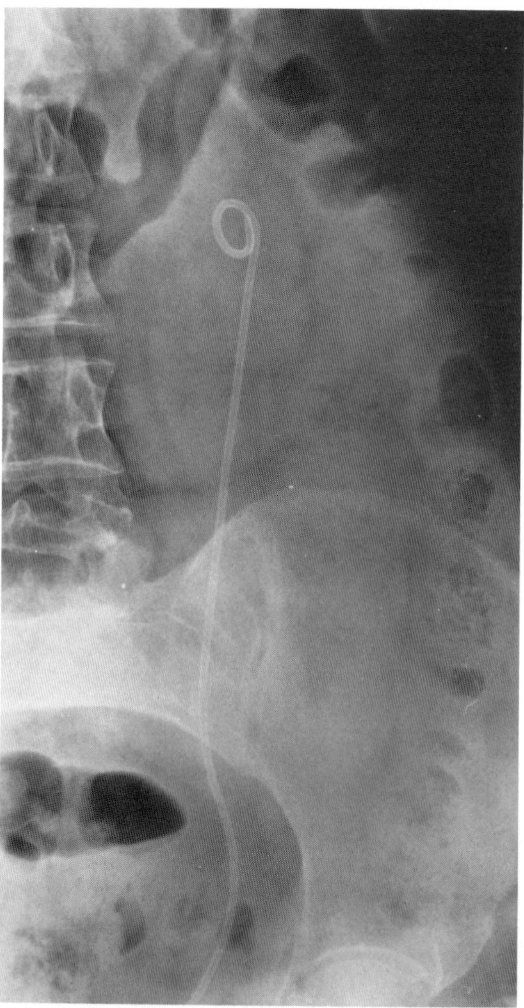

Figure 15.18. In these cases, the patient is seen 3–4 weeks after ESWL and a plain film is attained. If no significant residual fragments remain, the stent is removed. If there are significant residual fragments remaining, a second shock wave procedure is performed at this time. The stent is removed at the end of the second shock wave treatment.

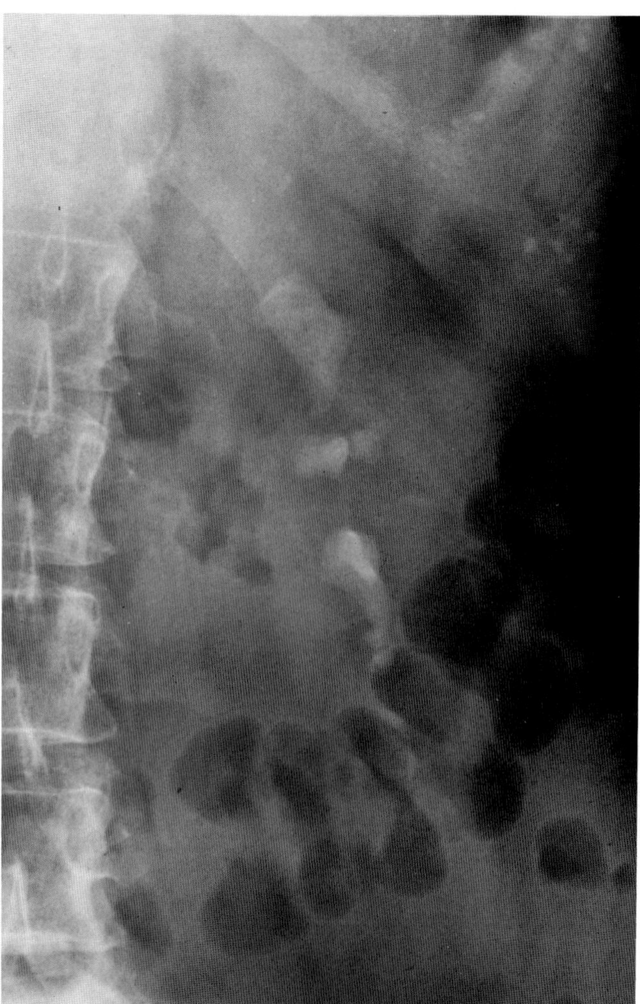

Figure 15.19. Some partial staghorn calculi may be treated with ESWL and internal stenting. This plain film reveals such a calculus involving parts of the upper, mid- and lower infundibulocalyceal systems. Again, an internal stent is placed at the outset of the primary ESWL procedure.

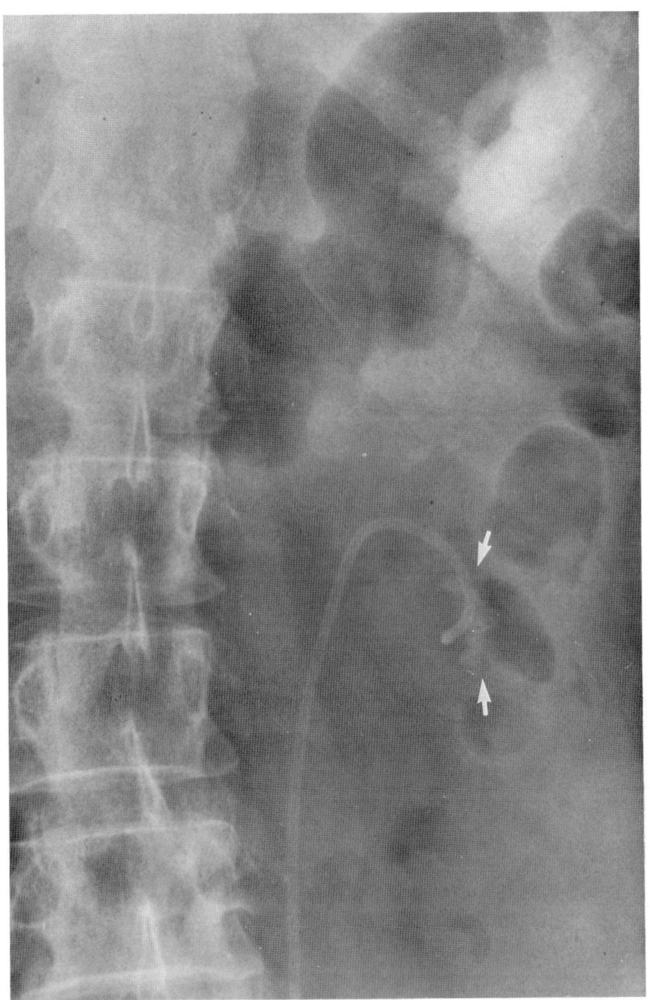

Figure 15.20. A plain film 4 weeks later reveals residual lower calyceal stone. That area was not treated at the first ESWL procedure. Secondary ESWL and stent removal are performed at this time.

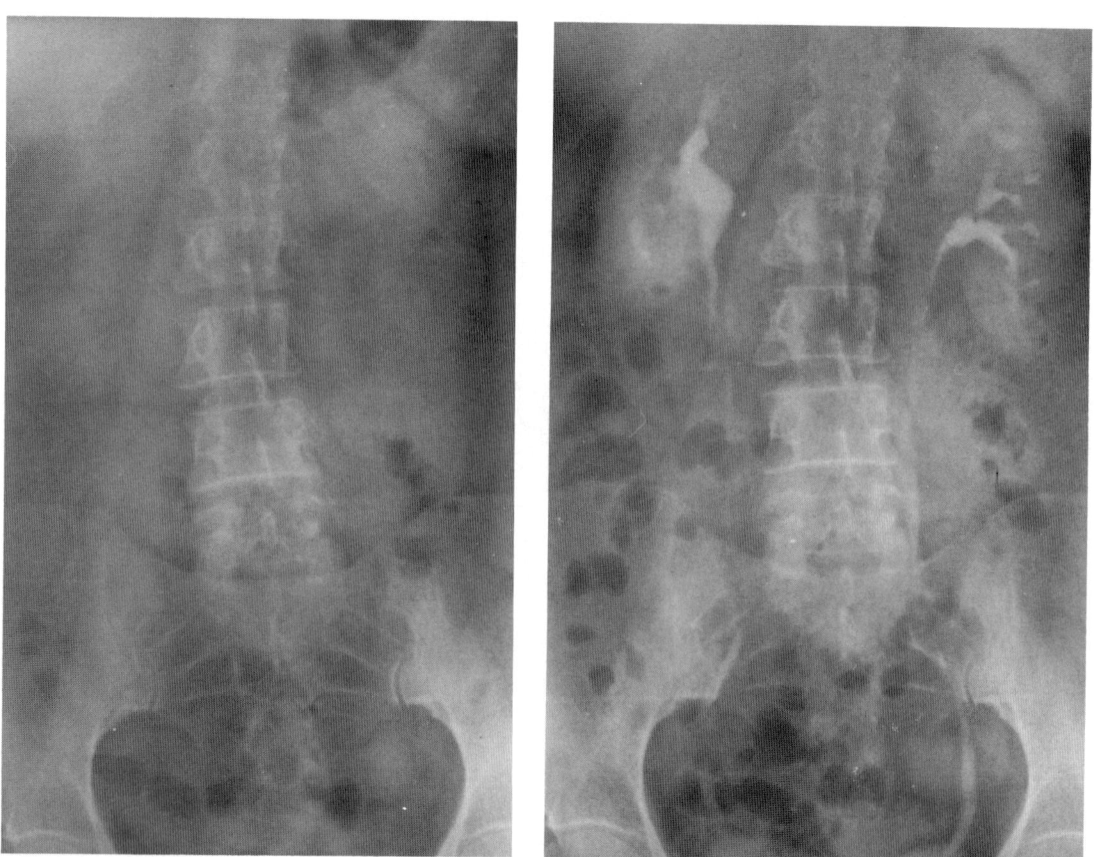

Figure 15.21. Intravenous urography 1 month later reveals freedom from residual stones or obstruction.

Extensive Staghorn Calculi

Patients with extensive staghorn calculi are managed with a combination of percutaneous "debulking" and ESWL. Primary debulking will decrease the total amount of shock waves ultimately required. Furthermore, the presence of a large caliber nephrostomy tube that is placed at the termination of the percutaneous procedure gives protection from obstruction after ESWL. It also allows an additional route of egress for the fragments. Finally, it provides a route for chemolysis that is often necessary in these patients.

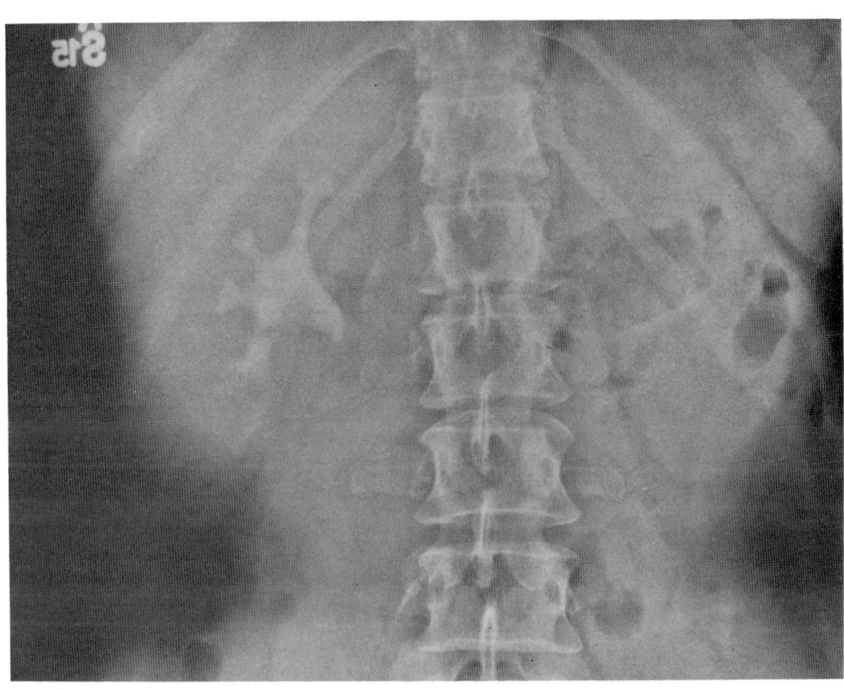

Figure 15.22. Plain film reveals extensive right staghorn calculus.

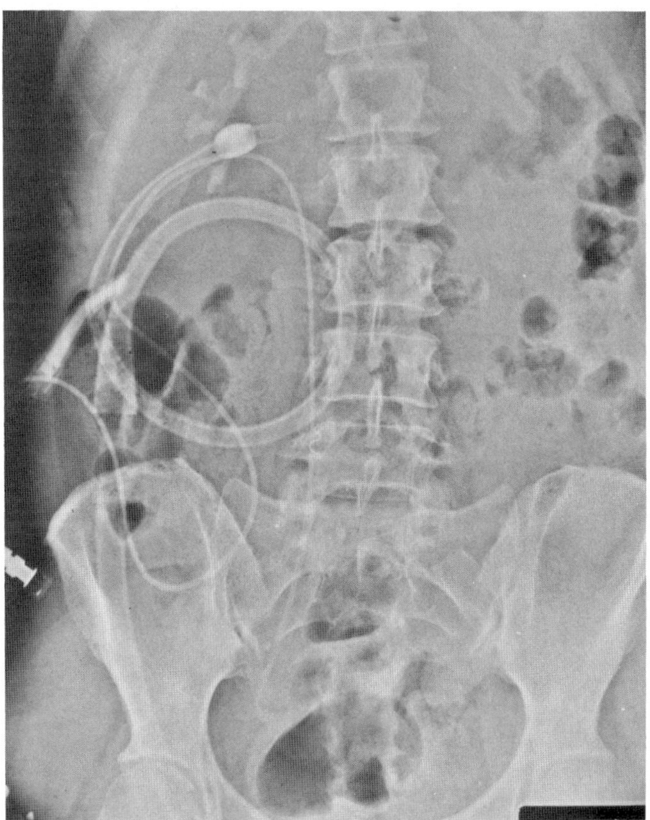

Figure 15.23. The access for percutaneous debulking is attained through the mid- or lower infundibulocalyceal system that allows ultrasonic lithotripsy of the greatest stone bulk. Ultrasonic lithotripsy is performed as described in the previous chapter.

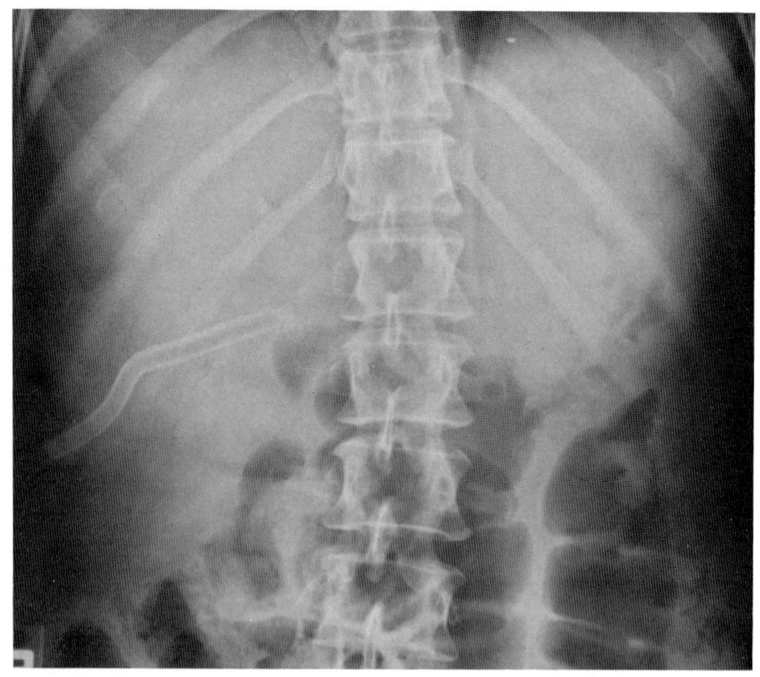

Figure 15.24. The infundibulocalyceal extensions of the stone that remain after primary percutaneous ultrasonic debulking are treated 4 days later with ESWL. After ESWL to the residual fragments, only "dust" remains as seen here. After ESWL, there may still be residual fragments that can be treated with percutaneous irrigation, secondary percutaneous procedures (often performed through the mature tract) or secondary ESWL as necessary.

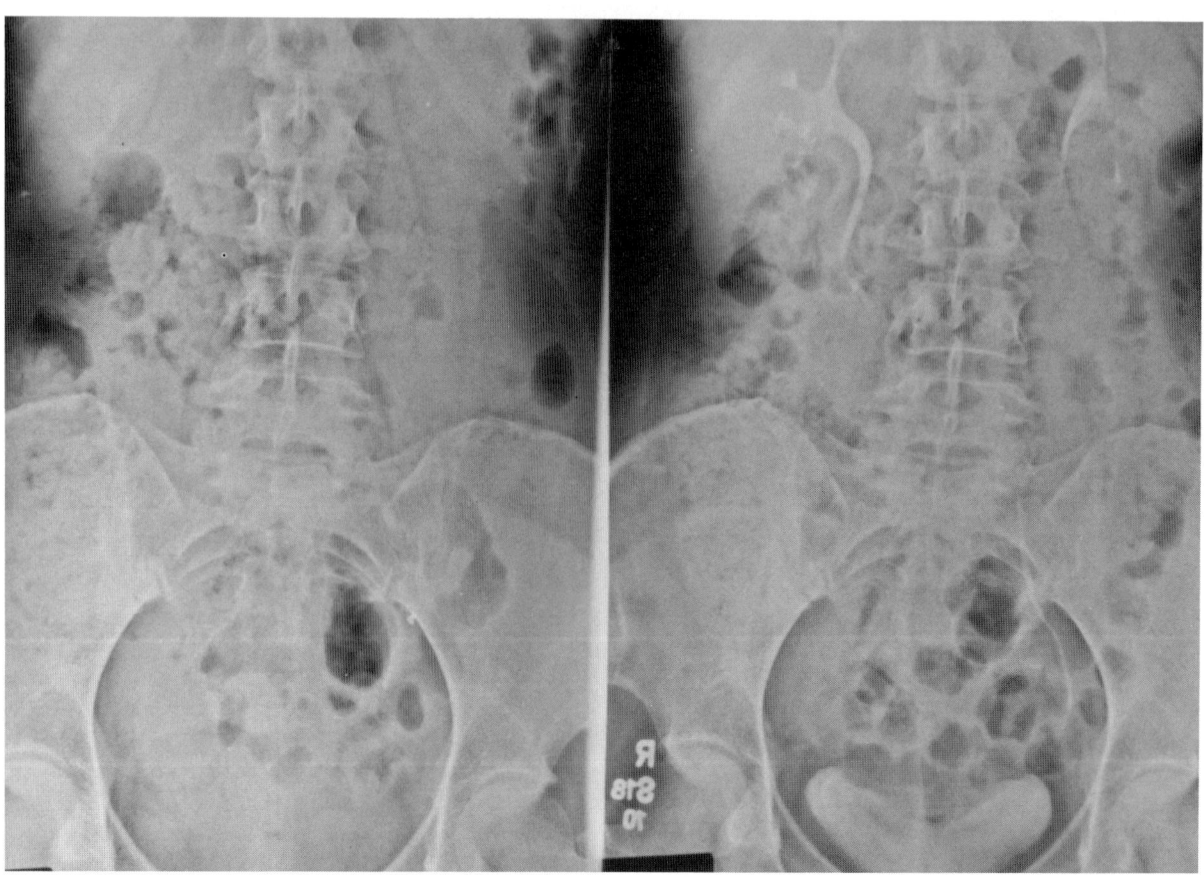

Pediatric Patients

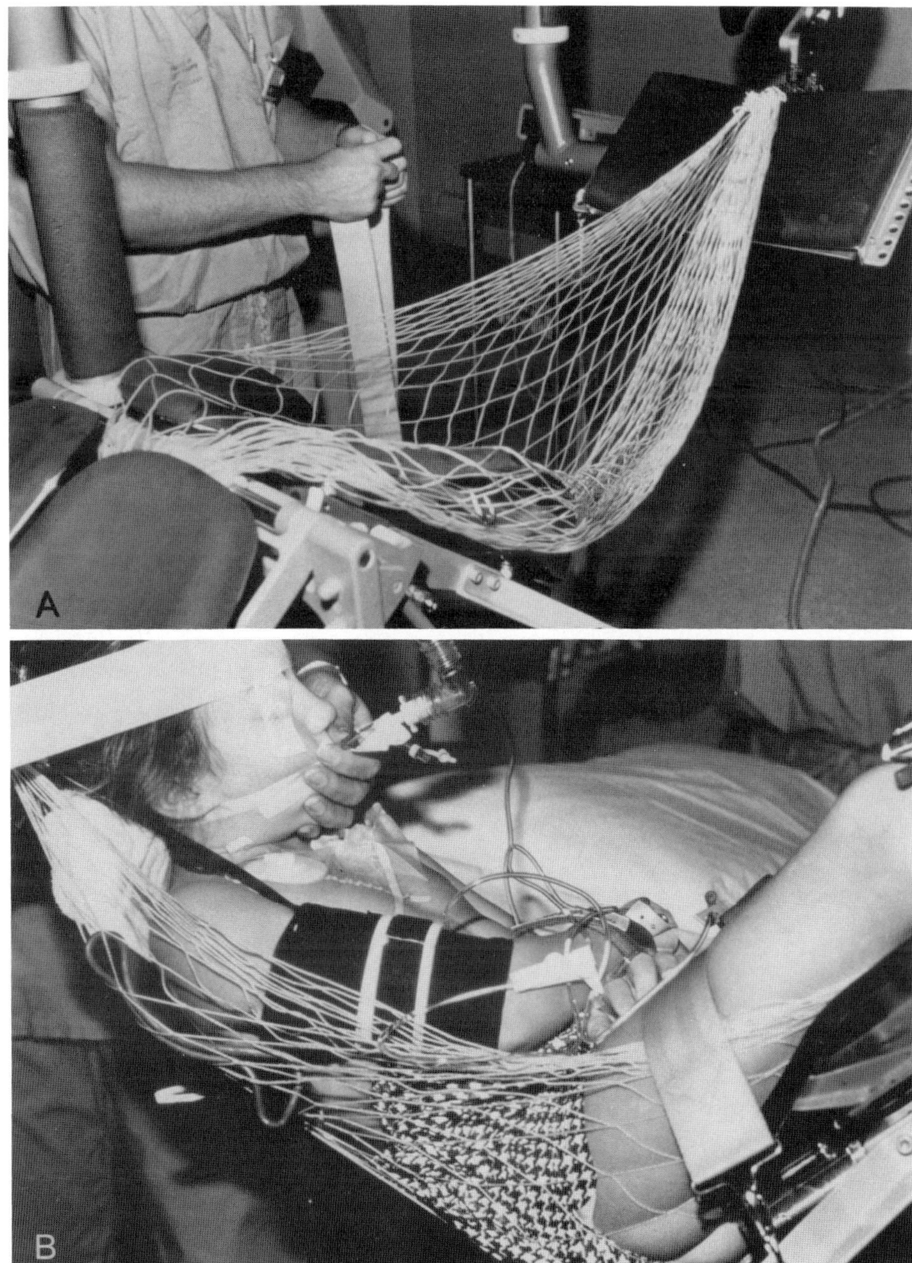

Figure 15.26. Patients less than 4 feet tall may be treated with ESWL. However, the gantry must be modified to accommodate them. We utilize a hammock that is simply tied to each end of the gantry to support the patient. In these cases, the lungs must be protected from the shock waves to prevent a possible pulmonary contusion at the water/air interface. At our center, we place a lead lined glove under the patient's back. Its position can then be monitored fluoroscopically during ESWL to make sure the lung but not the stone is adequately protected from the shock waves.

Management of Steinstrasse

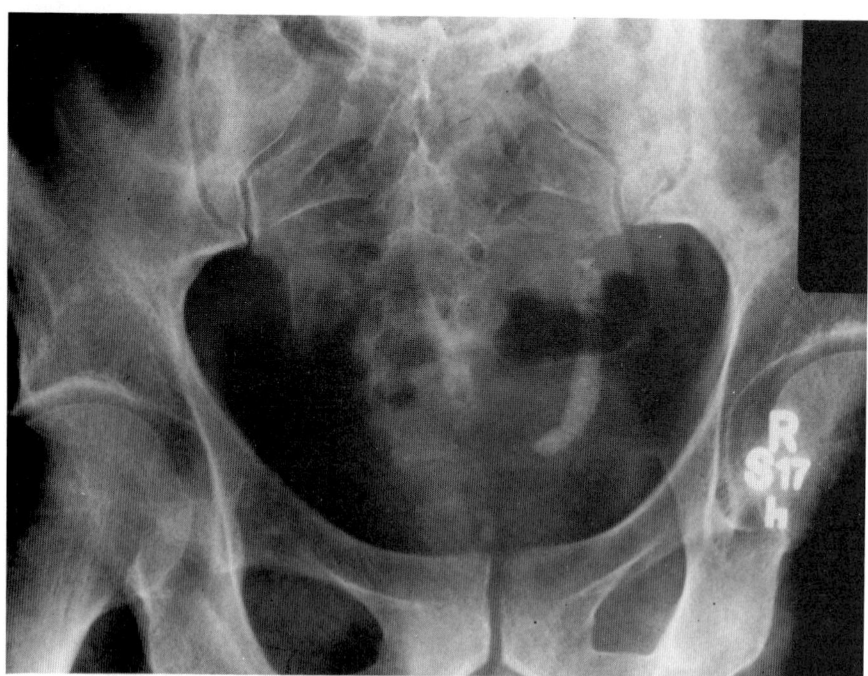

Figure 15.27. Ureteral obstruction from stone fragments is the most common complication of ESWL. In general, the potential for this complication increases with increasing size of the stone that was treated. However, this complication has been seen with much less frequency with the more liberalized use of internal stents and percutaneous debulking before ESWL.

In most cases, this problem can be managed conservatively with analgesia, hydration, and reassurance. However, infection associated with the obstruction, progressive hydronephrosis, or persistent pain require intervention.

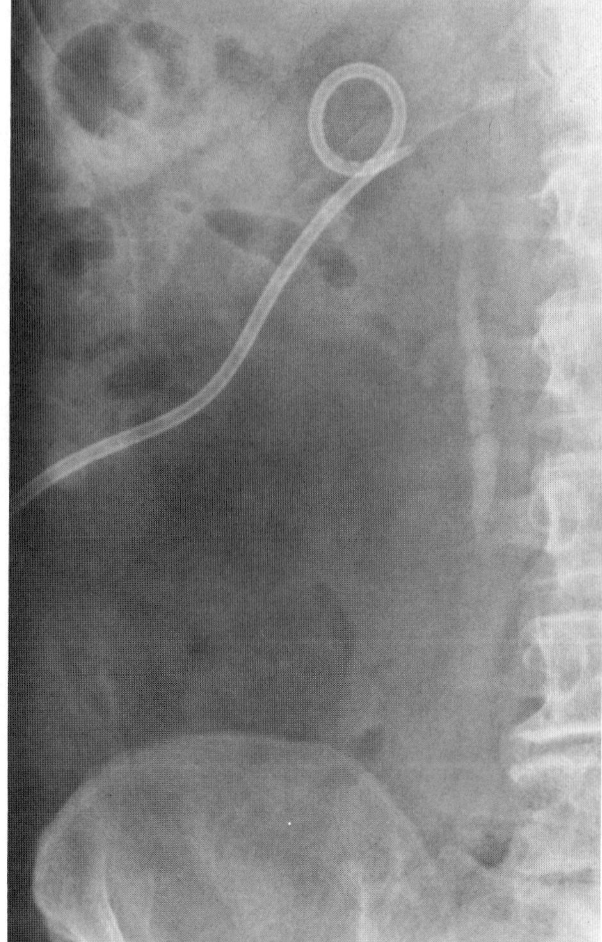

Figure 15.28. For those patients with infection and obstruction or extensive steinstrasse, percutaneous nephrostomy is the procedure of choice. The ureteral fragments may then pass spontaneously over the next few days or weeks. If the obstruction results from a few discreet fragments or if there is a large "lead" fragment to the steinstrasse, ureteroscopic or other retrograde manipulation with or without repeat ESWL may be appropriate.

Postoperative Care

After ESWL, intravenous hydration is continued until adequate oral alimentation is established. Parenteral pain and antimetic medication may be required in first few hours after treatment, although most patients can be discharged the evening of the procedure or the next morning. A plain x-ray is obtained routinely at the time of discharge. Other radiographic evaluation in the early post-ESWL period is reserved for those patients with continued symptoms of flank pain or fever. In those cases, ultrasonography is attained to exclude a perinephric hematoma or ongoing obstruction. Further evaluation and treatment is then performed as necessary.

After hospital discharge, patients are instructed to drink at least 2 quarts of water daily and to strain the urine for gravel that will subsequently be sent for analysis. The patient is seen in follow-up 3–4 weeks later. At that time, either a plain film and ultrasonography or intravenous urography is performed. The urine is examined for possible infection, the gravel is sent for analysis, and further recommendations regarding preventive therapy are then offered.

Suggested Readings

Bush WH, Jones D, Gibbons RP: Radiation dose to patient and personnel during extracorporeal shock wave lithotripsy. *J Urol* 138:716, 1987.

Chaussy CH: *Extracorporeal Shock Wave Lithotripsy*. Basil, Karger, 1982.

Chaussy C, Schmiedt E, Jocham D, Brendel W, Forssman B, Walther V: First clinical experience with extracorporeally induced destruction of kidney stones by shock waves. *J Urol* 127:417, 1982.

Coptcoat MJ, Webb DR, Kellett MJ, Fletcher MS, McNicholas TA, Dickinson IK, Wickham JEA: The complications of extracorporeal shock wave lithotripsy: Management and prevention. *Br J Urol* 58:578, 1986.

Drach GW, Dretler S, Fair W, et al: Report of the United States cooperative study of ESWL. *J Urol* 135:1127, 1986.

Hunter PT, Finlaysan, Hirko RJ, et al: Measurement of shock wave pressures used for lithotripsy. *J Urol* 136:733, 1986.

Kaude JV, Williams CM, Milner MR, Scott KN, Finlayson B: Renal morphology and function immediately after extracorporeal shock wave lithotripsy. *AJR* 145:305, 1985.

Lingeman JE, Newman D, Mertz JHO, et al: Extracorporeal shock wave lithotripsy: The Methodist Hospital of Indiana Experience. *J Urol* 135:1134, 1986.

Lingeman JE, Shirrell WL, Newman DM, Mosbaugh PG, Steele RE, Woods JR: Management of upper ureteral calculi with extracorporeal shock wave lithotripsy. *J Urol* 138:720, 1987.

Miller K, Fuchs G, Rassweiler J, Eisenberger F: Treatment of ureteral stone disease: The role of ESWL and endourology. *World J Urol* 3:53, 1985.

Riehle RA, Fair WR, Vaughan ED Jr: ESWL for upper urinary tract calculi: One year's experience at a single center. *JAMA* 255:2043, 1986.

Rubin JI, Arger PH, Pollack HM, Banner MP, Coleman BG, Mintz MC, VanArsdalen KN: Kidney changes after extracorporeal shock wave lithotripsy: CT evaluation. *Radiology* 162:21, 1987.

Schmiedt E, Chaussy C: Extracorporeal shock wave lithotripsy (ESWL) of kidney and ureteric stones. *Internat Urol Nephrol* 16:273, 1984.

Schulze H, Hertle L, Graff J, et al: Combined treatment of branched calculi by percutaneous nephrolithotomy and ESWL. *J Urol* 135:1138, 1986.

Sigman N, Laudone VP, Jenkins AD, Howards SS, Riehle R Jr, Keating MA, Walker RD: Initial experience with extracorporeal shock wave lithotripsy in children. *J Urol* 138:839, 1987.

Streem SB, Geisinger MA, Risius B, Zelch MG, Siegel SW: Endourologic "Sandwich" therapy for extensive staghorn calculi. *J Endourol* (in press), 1988.

CHAPTER 16

Pyelolithotomy

J. PATRICK SPIRNAK
MARTIN I. RESNICK

The operative removal of renal calculi, as documented in both the Greek and Roman literature, usually occurred incidental to the drainage of a renal or perirenal abscess. Although Celsus and Galen mentioned kidney stones in their writings, neither believed surgical removal to be safe or feasible. In the 1500s Cardan of Milan reportedly extracted 18 renal stones while draining a renal abscess (1). Other isolated accounts of renal stone removal appeared during the 16th and 17th centuries. Hevan in 1775 believed that renal operations for the removal of stones be limited solely to infected pyonephrotic kidneys (2). If the stones were not identified at the time of the drainage procedure, they often would pass spontaneously through a fistulous tract.

Dr. William Ingalls in 1872 performed what is believed to be the first planned nephrotomy on a patient who earlier had a perirenal abscess drained (3). In 1880, an English surgeon, Sir Henry Morris performed the first nephrolithotomy on a kidney free of abscess (4). In the same year, Vincenz Czerny is credited with performing the first pyelolithotomy (5). Controversy raged over which method of stone removal was preferable. Prior to the discovery of the roentgen ray in 1895, and the development of clinically useful radiography, nephrolithotomy afforded the stone surgeon a direct view of the intrarenal collecting system and was thus the surgical technique of choice. In 1898 Sir Henry Morris published the results of 34 nephrolithotomies and reported only one death. His successful results helped disprove the dangers of nephrolithotomy and promoted stone removal before the kidney was converted into an abscess sac. Progress in the field of renal stone surgery continued into the 20th century with emphasis being placed on identifying the most atraumatic route to the intrarenal collecting system. The development of intravenous and retrograde pyelography made it possible for the stone surgeon to preoperatively identify and precisely locate the site of the stone in the collecting system. With this new capability came a renewed interest in pyelolithotomy. Lower in 1913 advocated pyelolithotomy as the procedure of choice for the removal of all pelvic stones (6). Pyelolithotomy via a vertical incision in the renal pelvis thus replaced nephrolithotomy as the procedure of choice for the removal of uncomplicated renal pelvic stones.

In the 1960s, Gil-Vernet studied the functional anatomy of the renal pelvic musculature and described the presence of spiral muscle fibers arranged in circular fashion (7). He concluded that a transverse pyelotomy incision was less likely to disrupt ureteropelvic peristalsis when compared to the standard vertical incision. Based on his anatomical studies, the vertical pyelotomy with all of its potential drawbacks, including pelvic hypotonia and inadvertent tearing of the ureteropelvic junction, was abandoned by many in favor of the transverse incision. It was also at this time that Gil-Vernet described an atraumatic approach to the intrarenal collecting system (extended pyelolithotomy) that allowed the removal of large branched calculi without incising the renal parenchyma or compromising the renal blood supply. With the development of percutaneous techniques and extracorporeal shock wave lithotripsy, the majority of renal stones are currently managed without a surgical incision. We expect that, in the future, open stone removal will be reserved for patients with complex stones associated with anatomic abnormalities or when other less invasive techniques have failed.

The indications for surgical stone removal include intractable urinary infection, obstruction, progressive renal damage, pain, or gross hematuria. The objectives of stone surgery include: removal of all calculi, repair of associated anatomic abnormalities, eradication of associated urinary tract infection, preservation of renal function, and prevention of recurrent stone formation. Selection of the appropriate surgical approach is based on achieving these objectives.

STANDARD PYELOLITHOTOMY

The surgical approach to the kidney depends on multiple factors including the anatomic position of the kidney, the patient's body habitus, a prior history of renal surgery, and perhaps most important of all, the training and personal preference of the surgeon. The standard approach is through a flank incision; however, in some centers the posterior lumbotomy incision has replaced the flank incision for the removal of uncomplicated pelvic stones.

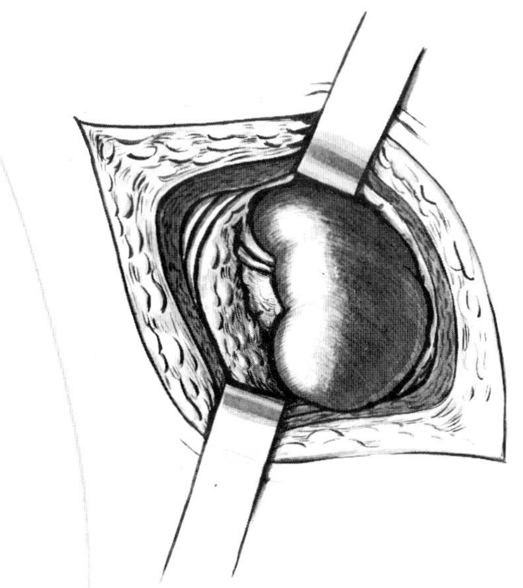

Figure 16.1. A posterior longitudinal incision is made in Gerota's fascia and the kidney is identified. In the presence of a solitary pelvic stone, it is usually not necessary to free the entire kidney. The dissection is limited to identifying the proximal ureter and posterior renal pelvis. Excessive mobilization of the kidney leads to extensive perirenal scarring and complicates future surgical procedures.

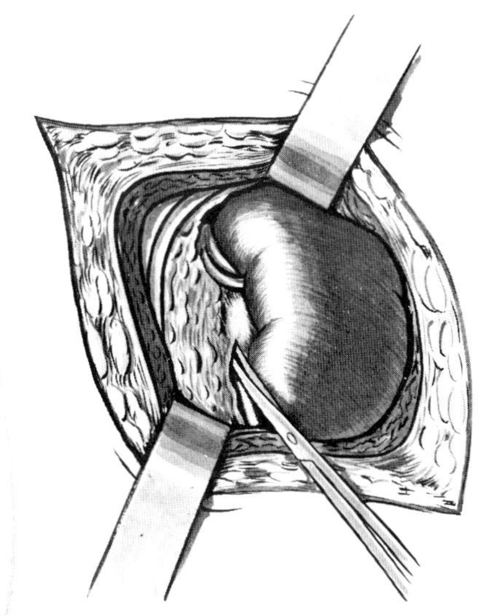

Figure 16.2. The upper ureter is identified as it lies on the psoas muscle and is dissected free of surrounding tissue. A small Penrose drain or vessel loop is placed around it. Tightening the Penrose drain at the time of stone manipulation guards against distal migration of stone fragments and ureteral obstruction. The ureter is followed proximally until the posterior renal pelvis is identified.

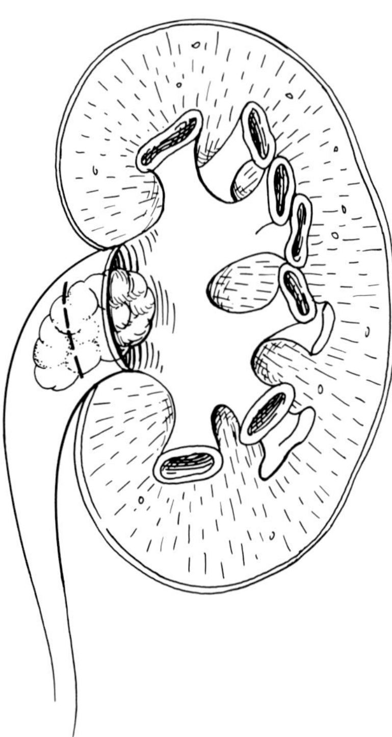

Figure 16.3. A transverse pyelotomy incision is planned well away from the ureteropelvic junction.

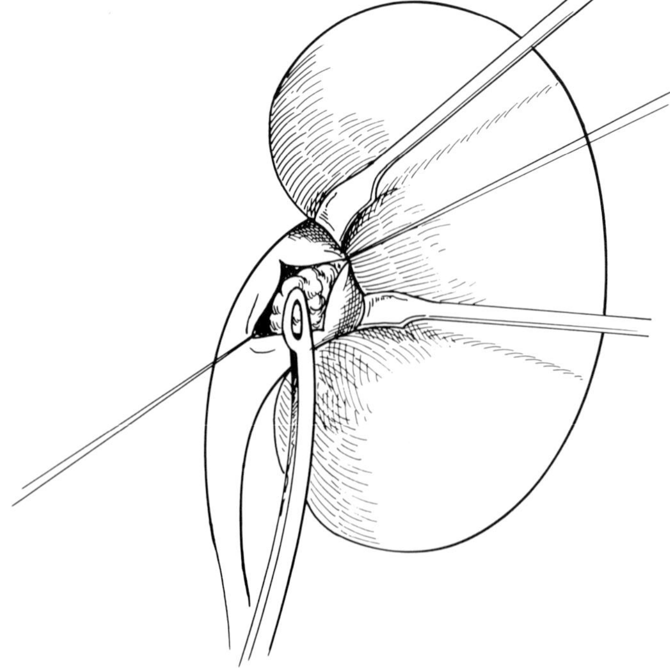

Figure 16.4. In the presence of an intrarenal pelvis, exposure may be improved by gently retracting the posterior lip of renal parenchyma with a small Richardson or vein retractor. The incision is initiated with a curved scalpel blade and may be extended with vascular or Potts' scissors. Mild traction placed on stay sutures of 4–0 chromic catgut located on either side of the incision will facilitate direct visualization of the calculus. The incision is made large enough to allow stone removal without tearing the renal pelvis. When the stone is very large, extending the incision in "visor" fashion onto the anterior pelvic wall will avoid undue trauma to the renal pelvis.

Nerve hooks, spatulae, or vascular forceps are helpful in freeing the stone from the mucosa. The calculus is grasped with Randall stone forceps and removed. A no. 10 French straight catheter is passed into the bladder to demonstrate the patency of the ureteropelvic junction and ureter. With the catheter in place, the pelvis is irrigated with saline. The pyelotomy is closed in watertight fashion with 5–0 absorbable suture. A Penrose or suction-type drain is placed near the pyelotomy incision and brought out dependently through a separate stab incision. Gerota's fascia is reapproximated and the incision closed in standard fashion.

EXTENDED PYELOLITHOTOMY

In 1866, Henle defined the renal sinus as a rectangular space containing the renal pelvis, intrarenal collecting system, renal blood vessels, lymphatics, and nerves. In 1891, Disse showed that fibrous extensions of the renal capsule extended onto the posterior renal pelvis, forming a tissue diaphragm and closing the renal sinus from the retroperitoneal space. Based on the above anatomic observations, Gil-Vernet in 1965 described a modification of the simple transverse pyelotomy incision that allowed complete access to the intrarenal collecting system. This approach offered the stone surgeon an alternative to nephrolithotomy as the treatment of staghorn calculi without the risks associated with parenchymal incisions. Complex stones are frequently associated with chronic urinary infections and extensive perirenal scarring. We therefore avoid the posterior approach and routinely use a flank incision.

The kidney is completely mobilized and the vascular pedicle isolated. In the presence of a complex stone, intraoperative radiographs are routinely obtained to document complete stone removal. Clamping the renal artery and cooling the kidney produces a softening of the renal parenchyma that may facilitate localization of elusive stone fragments.

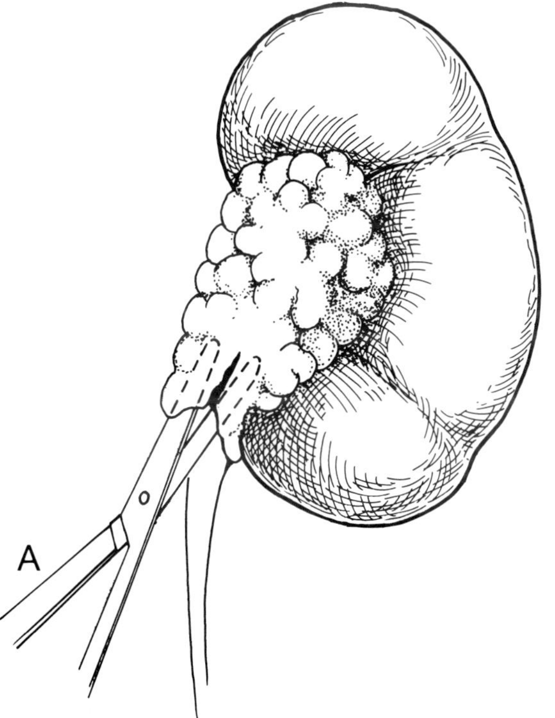

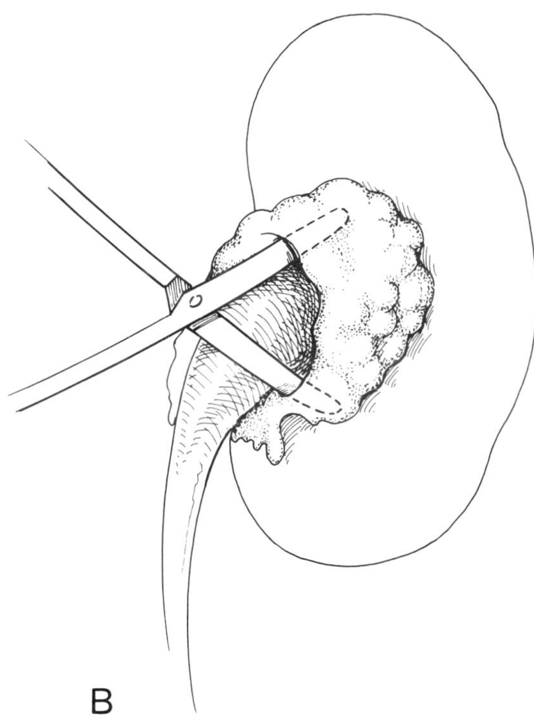

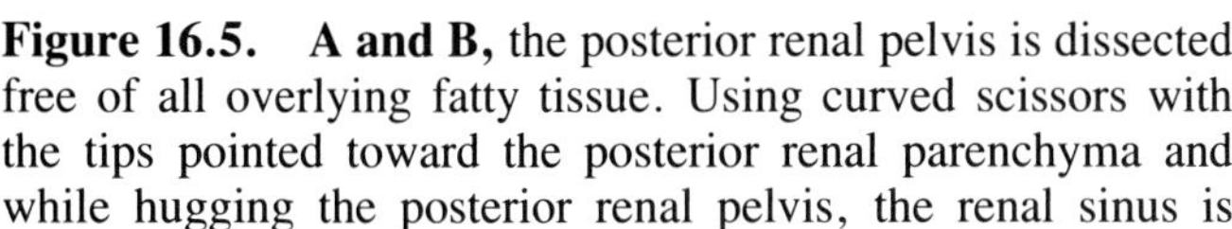

Figure 16.5. A and B, the posterior renal pelvis is dissected free of all overlying fatty tissue. Using curved scissors with the tips pointed toward the posterior renal parenchyma and while hugging the posterior renal pelvis, the renal sinus is entered by incising the fibrous diaphragm. Dissection of the renal sinus is begun by placing a small retractor beneath the posterior lip of renal tissue and by gently retracting this tissue in an anteromedial direction.

Figure 16.6. Bluntly packing the renal sinus with a moist gauze sponge facilitates and completes the exposure of the intrarenal infundibula and calyces. The packing is removed and several small retractors are placed beneath the posterior lip of parenchyma.

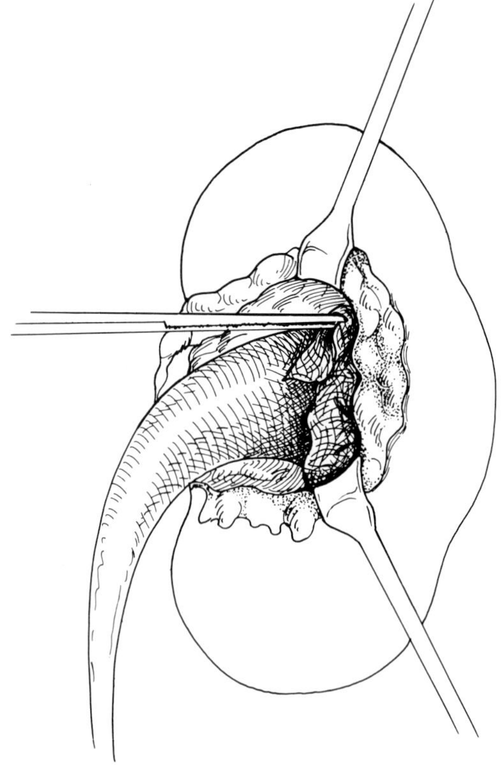

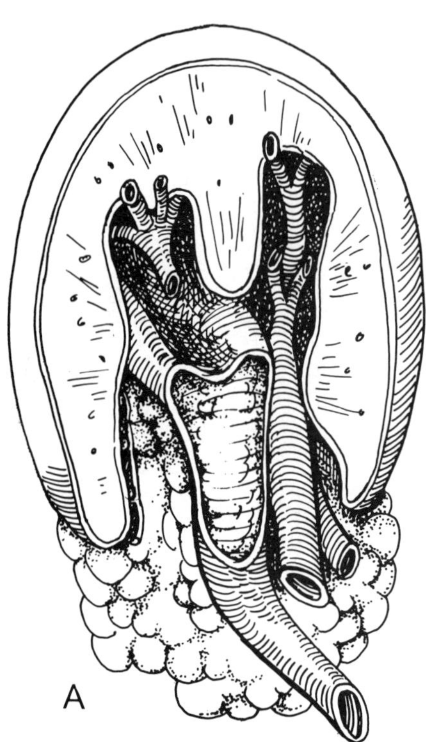

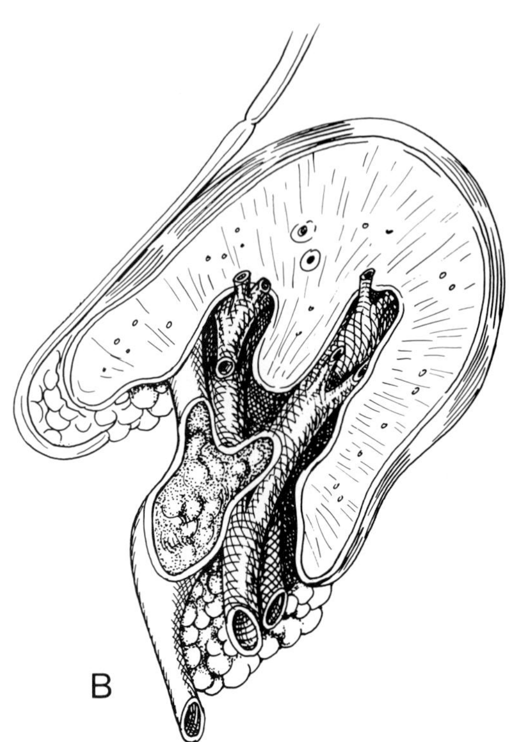

Figure 16.7. A and B, gentle traction now exposes the entire intrarenal collecting system, while avoiding vascular injury.

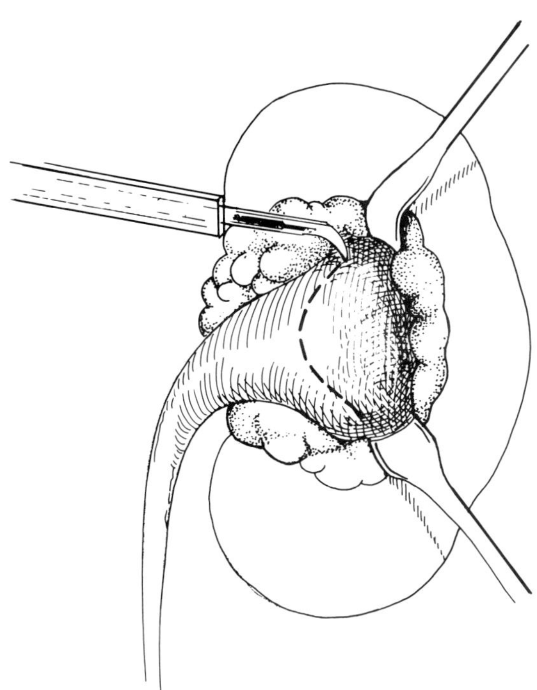

Figure 16.8. A curved transverse pyelotomy incision conforming to the configuration of the intrarenal collecting system is made with a curved scalpel blade. The incision is extended longitudinally onto the upper and lower infundibula. This, in effect, creates a flap of renal pelvis. The entire stone is freed from the pelvic mucosa using a blunt probe or nerve hook and is removed. Dumbbell-shaped calyceal extensions are best removed by radial nephrotomy. A catheter is passed down the ureter and the entire collecting system is irrigated to remove all mucosal calcifications and debris. Intraoperative x-rays are obtained to confirm complete stone removal. The flexible nephroscope or intraoperative ultrasound may help locate residual fragments identified on x-ray.

The pyelotomy incision is closed with 5–0 absorbable suture. It is not necessary to completely close the infundibular incisions, as the renal parenchyma, when returned to its normal position, will cover the incision. The flank is drained with a Penrose or suction-type drain and the incision is closed in routine fashion.

COAGULUM PYELOLITHOTOMY

Coagulum pyelolithotomy was initially described by Dees in 1943 (8). However, the procedure did not gain widespread urologic acceptance until being rediscovered by Patel in 1973 (9). In an effort to simplify the technical aspects of the procedure, decrease the associated morbidity, and improve the surgical results, the coagulum recipe has undergone a number of modifications. We have primarily used the technique described by Burns and Finlayson (10) and have achieved excellent results.

The formation of a coagulum suitable for stone removal is based on the local conversion of fibrinogen to fibrin with

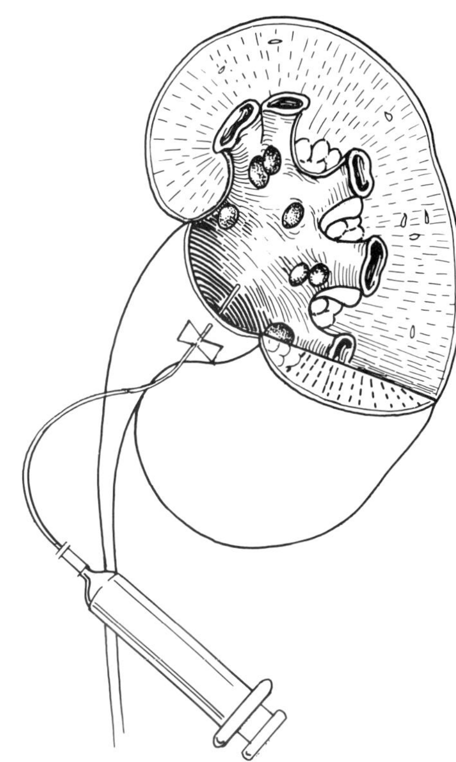

Figure 16.9. The ideal candidate for coagulum pyelolithotomy has a large extrarenal pelvis with multiple small calculi scattered throughout the intrarenal collecting system. Coagulum pyelolithotomy may also be used in conjunction with anatrophic nephrolithotomy or extended pyelolithotomy when there are multiple stones present. It is not helpful in removing calyceal stones associated with infundibular stenosis.

thrombin acting as the catalyst. Cryoprecipitate is used as the source of fibrinogen. Calcium chloride serves to neutralize the anticoagulant (citrate) present in the cryoprecipitate and acts as a cofactor in the conversion of prothrombin to thrombin.

The kidney is exposed in the usual manner and the upper ureter is identified and occluded with a soft vessel loop. One ampule of topical thrombin (5000 units) is reconstituted with 5 ml of normal saline. Ten ml of 10% calcium chloride is placed in a small sterile basin and to it is added 0.25 ml of the thrombin solution. Four units of cryoprecipitate (40–60 ml) are mixed with several drops of methylene blue in a separate sterile container. The addition of methylene blue facilitates removal of the entire coagulum.

A 19-gauge butterfly or angiocatheter is positioned in the renal pelvis. The volume of the renal pelvis is measured by aspirating all of the urine. A similar amount of cryoprecipitate is aspirated in a 50-ml syringe and to this is added 1.0 ml of the thrombin-calcium chloride solution. If the capacity of the renal pelvis is greater than 50 ml, 2.0 ml of the thrombin-calcium chloride solution is used. The measured amount is then injected to completely fill the pelvis. Overdistention results in pyelovenous backflow and is to be avoided. Clotting typically begins in 30–45 sec after mixing the solutions.

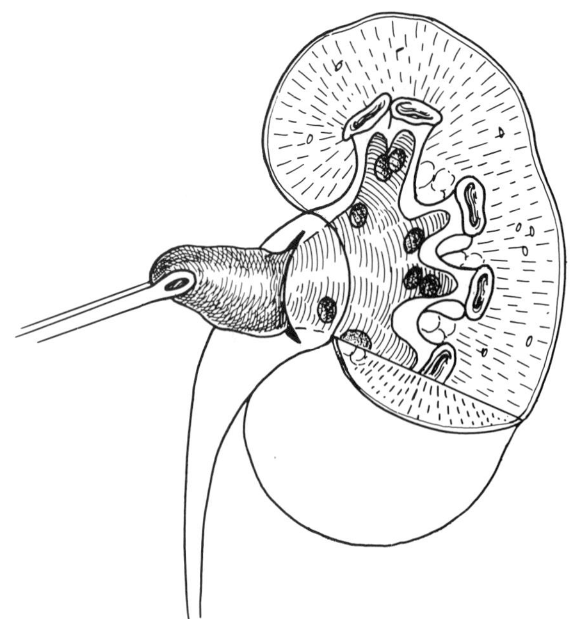

Figure 16.10. After 5 min, the renal pelvis is transversely incised and the coagulum with the entrapped stones is gently removed. X-rays are routinely obtained to confirm complete stone removal.

Kalash and associates in 1982, further simplified the procedure by deleting thrombin from the coagulum recipe (11). They mixed 1 unit (10–15 ml) of cryoprecipitate with 1 ml of 10% calcium chloride and have reported excellent results.

Coagulum pyelolithotomy has generally been considered to be a safe procedure. However, Pence has reported one case of a fatal pulmonary embolism directly related to to the procedure (12). The pulmonary embolism is believed to have occurred as a result of overdistending the renal pelvis with subsequent pyelovenous backflow and dissemination of the thrombogenic material into the systemic circulation. Studies on dogs have confirmed this theory. To avoid this potentially lethal complication, one must carefully measure the pelvic capacity and avoid overdistention of the renal pelvis. Deleting thrombin from the coagulum recipe might further enhance the safety of this procedure. Retained clots pose little threat to the patient and will usually be dissolved within 24–48 hr.

POSTOPERATIVE CARE

Postoperative management of the stone patient is similar to that of any patient following a major operation. Intravenous fluids are maintained until the patient has fully recovered from the effects of anesthesia and is able to tolerate a clear liquid diet. It is desirable to maintain a urine output of at least 50 ml hr to help clear any debris or small clots from the collecting system. Intravenous antibiotics are selected on the basis of preoperative urine culture and sensitivity results and, in the presence of infection or struvite stones, are maintained for at least 3–5 days. Appropriate oral antibiotics are then selected based on repeated urine culture results. Patients with infectious stones are discharged receiving prophylactic antibiotic therapy and require close urologic follow-up.

Intraoperatively placed drains are removed when all drainage has stopped, usually by the 5th postoperative day. Routine 24-hr urine collection for calcium, phosphorus, creatinine, and uric acid is obtained at least 6 weeks from the time of surgery and after the patient has resumed his or her normal life-style. If metabolic abnormalities are detected, appropriate therapy is then instituted.

References

1. Murphy JT: *The History of Urology*. Springfield, IL, Charles C Thomas, 1972, p. 77.
2. Hevan P: Recherches historiques et critiques sur la nephrotomie ou taille du rein. *Mem Acad R Chir* 3:238, 1778.
3. Bundy FE, Ingalls W: Nephrolithotomy. *Boston Med Surg J* 106:483, 1882.
4. Morris H: A case of nephro-lithotomy in the extraction of a calculus from an undilated kidney. *Trans Clin Soc Lond* 14:31, 1881.
5. Gil-Vernet JM: Pyelolithotomy. In Roth RA, Finlayson F (eds): *Stones: Clinical Management of Urolithiasis*. Baltimore, Williams & Wilkins, 1983, pp. 297–331.
6. Lower WE: Conservative surgical methods in operating for stone in the kidney. *Cleve Med* J 12:260, 1913.
7. Gil-Vernet JM: New surgical concepts in removing renal calculi. *Urol Int* 20:255, 1965.
8. Dees JE: The use of intrapelvic coagulum in pyelolithotomy. *South Med J* 36:167, 1943.
9. Patel VJ: Coagulum pyelolithotomy. *Br J Surg* 60:230, 1973.
10. Burns JR, Finlayson B: Coagulum pyelolithotomy. In Resnick MI (ed): *Current Trends in Urology*, Vol. 2. Baltimore, Williams & Wilkins, 1982, pp. 31–44.
11. Kalash SS, Young JD, Harne G: Modification of cryoprecipitate coagulum pyelolithotomy technique. *Urology* 19:467, 1982.
12. Pence JR, Airhart RA, Novicki DE, Williams JL, Ehler WJ: Pulmonary emboli associated with coagulum pyelolithotomy. *J Urol* 127:572, 1982.

CHAPTER 17

Anatrophic Nephrolithotomy

RALPH A. STRAFFON

Staghorn calculi present a difficult problem in management to the urologist for several reasons: *(a)* they are surgically difficult to remove completely; *(b)* they are usually associated with infection and/or obstruction; and *(c)* they tend to recur. These calculi are usually composed of magnesium ammonium phosphate alone or combined with hydroxyapatite.

In each patient with staghorn calculi, a decision must be made as to the need for surgical removal of the calculus. Factors that influence this decision are the age and general condition of the patient, the status of the renal function, and the presence of infection and/or obstruction. In a young, good risk patient, it is well worth the surgical effort to remove the calculi, for only after removing all the foreign bodies can one effectively treat the coexisting urinary infection. In an older, poor risk patient, it may be better to treat the patient conservatively, particularly if he has had a number of stones removed in the past. In these cases, surgical intervention is necessary only if the patient continues to lose renal function, becomes septic, or has persistent pain.

Longitudinal Nephrotomy of Boyce

This is the surgical procedure of choice for removing staghorn calculi in a kidney with an intrarenal pelvis or in a patient who has had one or more operations for stones removed from the renal pelvis, which may make it difficult to dissect this area free from surrounding tissue. The patient is placed in the lateral position used in the classic flank incision. The 12th rib may be removed if it overlies the kidney. It is important to extend the incision medially to the edge of the rectus muscle. This will allow the kidney, when dissected free from the perirenal tissue, to be pushed forward, giving good exposure to its posterior surface. The right kidney will be demonstrated in the following illustration.

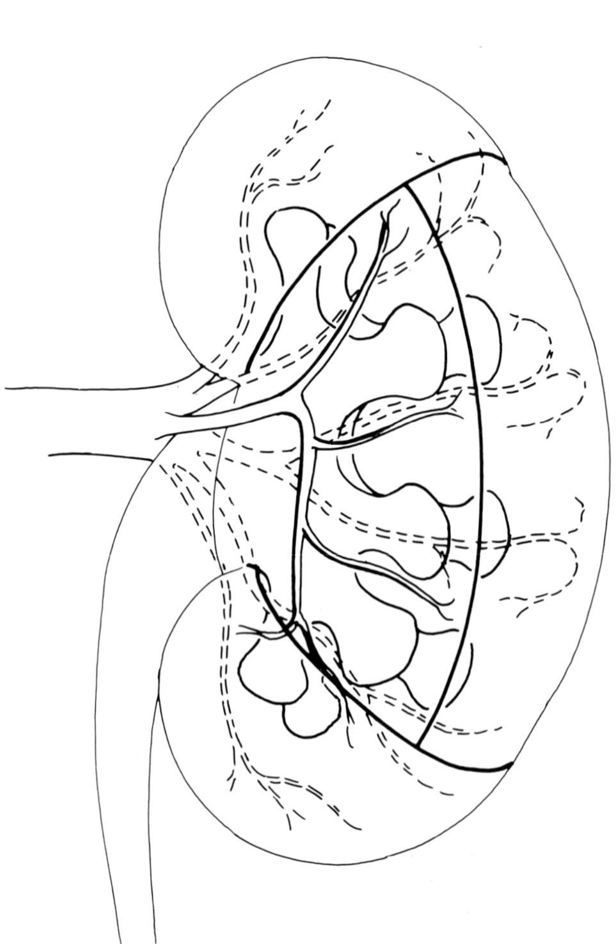

Figure 17.1. It is wise to review some of the surgical anatomy of the kidney as it relates to the surgery of staghorn calculi. There are four surgical segments of the kidney: apical, basilar, anterior (superior and inferior), and posterior. There are two major divisions of the renal artery, anterior and posterior, with the anterior divisions supplying the apical, anterior, and basilar segments of the kidney, and the posterior division supplying only the posterior segment. The posterior surface of the right kidney is shown here. It is important to note the junction of the anterior and posterior division blood supply, which is on the posterior surface of the kidney, and is about two-thirds of the distance from the hilar margin to the lateral surface of the kidney. Each segmental vessel next divides into interlobar branches, which originate in pairs at the base of each major calyx, and course toward the papillae to become transmedullary arteries. These arteries pass through the medulla and end as arcuate arteries at the cortical-medullary junction.

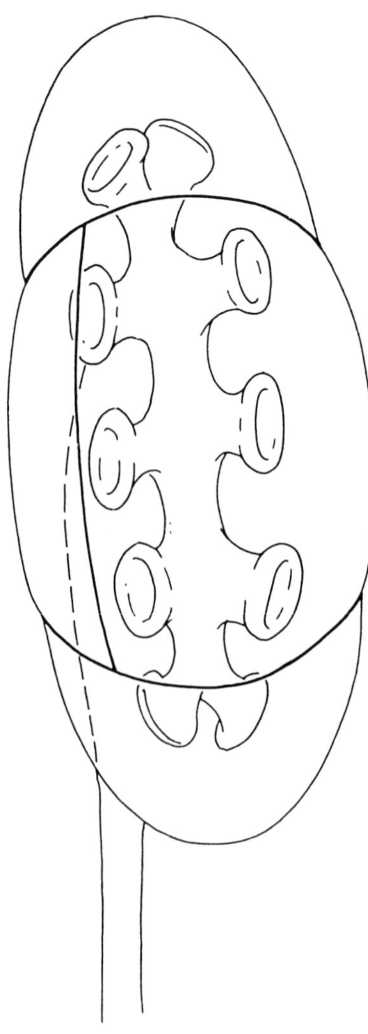

Figure 17.2. There are 8–10 major calyces that open into the renal pelvis. The apical segment has one major calyx that lies in the midfrontal plane and receives two minor calyces (lateral and medial). The basilar segment has a single major calyx in the median plane and receives two minor calyces (anterior and posterior). There are three major calyces in the anterior segment that enter the renal pelvis at a 20° angle to the midfrontal plane and three major calyces in the posterior segment that enter the renal pelvis at a 75° angle to the midfrontal plane. Although the anatomy of the kidney is fairly constant, each case should be studied with pyelography to identify the calyceal system and renal angiography to visualize the arterial blood supply. With this information in hand, the surgeon then can plan the best surgical approach for the removal of the staghorn calculus.

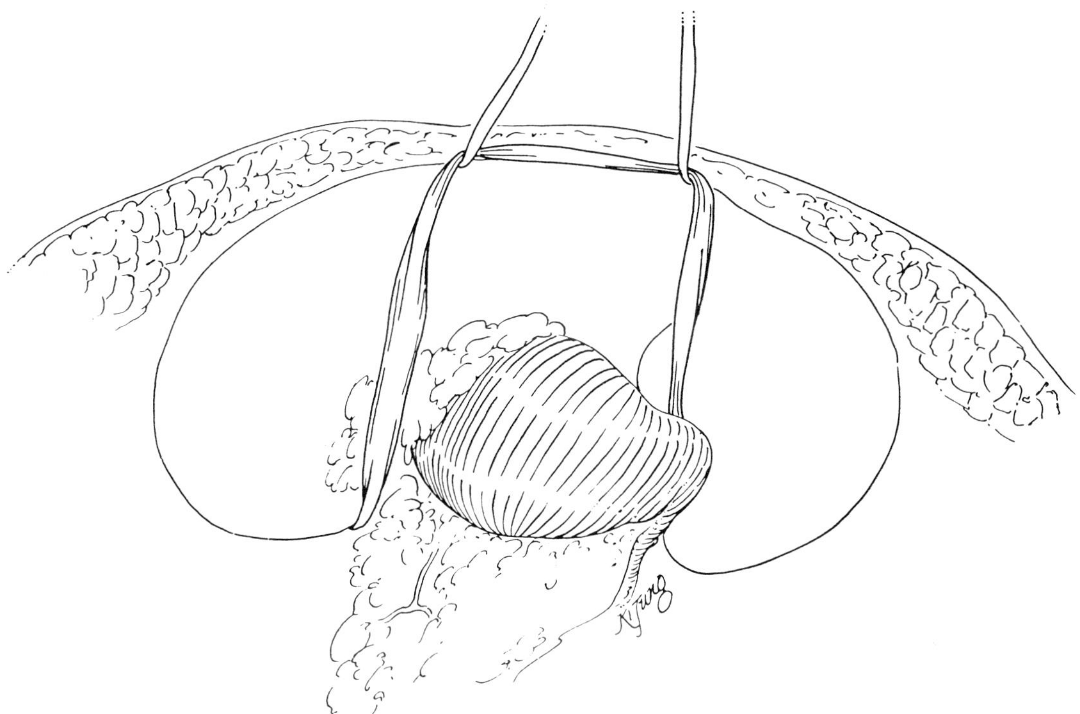

Figure 17.3. The ureter is identified and dissected upward toward the renal pelvis. The entire kidney is then mobilized by sharp and blunt dissection around its periphery. Once the kidney has been completely mobilized, leaving only the renal pedicle, a surgical tape can be placed around each pole and used as a sling to facilitate handling of the kidney.

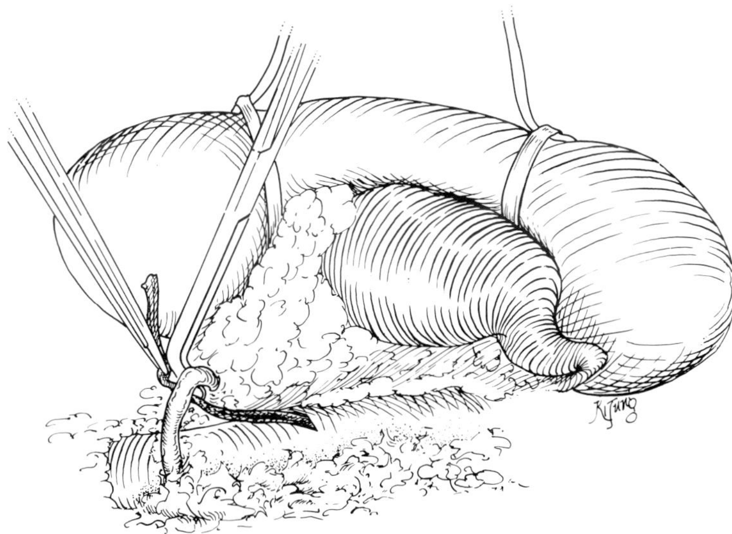

Figure 17.4. The kidney then is pushed medially and the renal artery can be identified by palpation in the renal pedicle. The artery is dissected free from surrounding tissue and, using the preoperative selective renal angiogram as a roadmap, the posterior division can be easily identified. A segment of polyethylene tubing is then placed around the artery to aid in handling the vessel. In many cases, it is more convenient and effective to occlude the entire main renal artery, as is shown here.

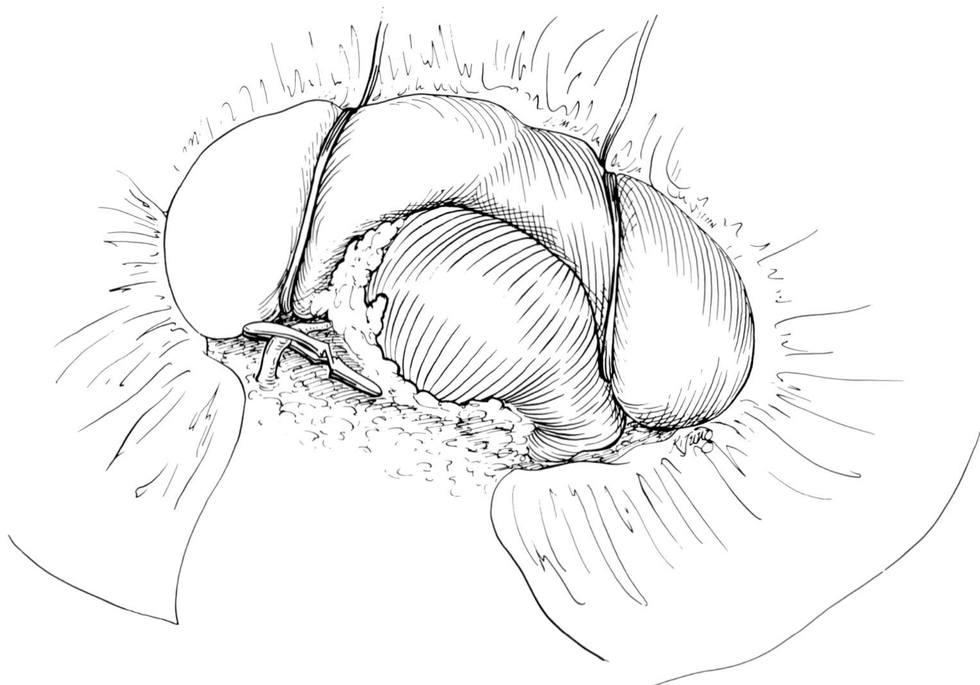

Figure 17.5. Renal hypothermia is a valuable adjunct to this surgical procedure. With the kidney suspended by a surgical tape, a plastic dam is wrapped around the renal pedicle, to furnish a container for the kidney into which the cooling solution can be poured. Renal core temperatures of 12–18°C can be obtained easily with simple surface cooling, once the renal artery is occluded. Iced saline slush is used to cool the kidney after a bulldog clamp has been placed on the renal artery.

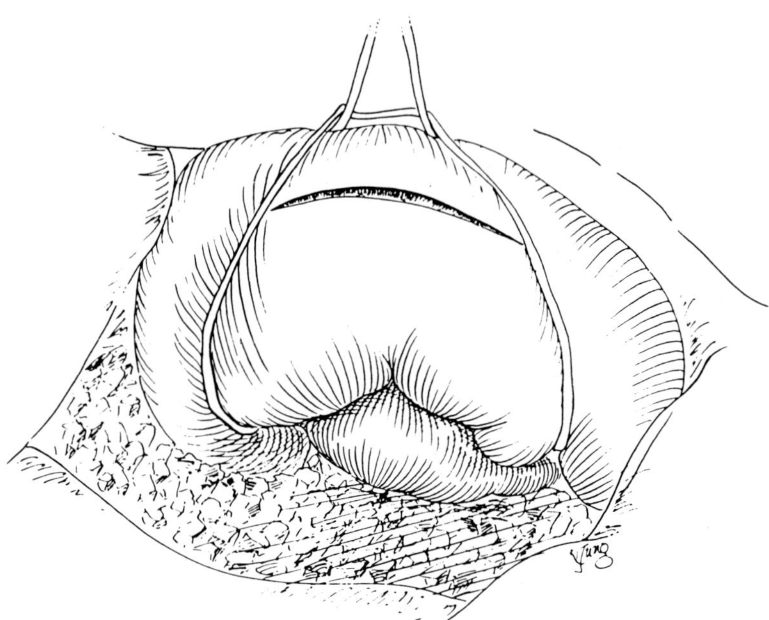

Figure 17.6. An incision is made in the capsule of the kidney on its posterior surface, at the junction of the anterior and posterior segments. This may extend up but not into the apical segment, and down but not into the basilar segment. To aid in identifying the position of this incision, the posterior division of the renal artery may be injected with 2 ml of indigo carmine, which will clearly outline the posterior segment and help in placement of the capsular incision.

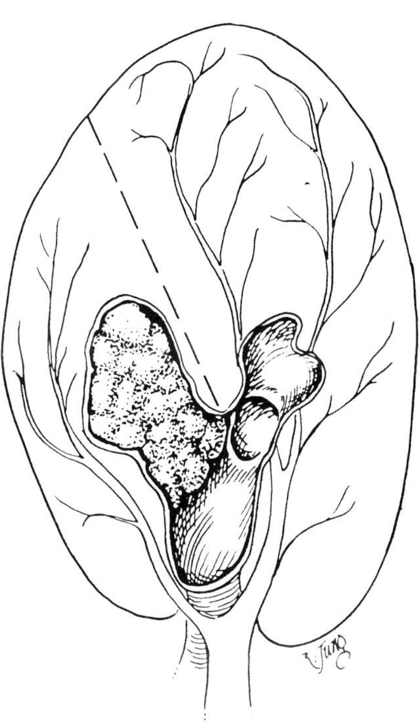

Figure 17.7. Once the capsule has been incised, the blunt end of the knife can be used to divide the renal parenchyma. It is important to enter the proper plane, shown here. If the dissection is too far forward, which is the natural tendency of the surgeon, one encounters the large peripelvic venous plexus, and much bleeding will occur. If the dissection is too far posterior, the blood supply to the posterior segment will be damaged. The correct plane is nearly avascular and should lead to the anterior surface of the major calyces of the posterior segment.

Boyce (1977) has developed two approaches to the collecting system. The *posterior segment* approach is preferred for staghorn calculi that extend into the posterior calyces. It may also be used if only the posterior calyces contain calculi. The posterior calyces are approached on their anterior surface and opened through a transverse incision in the midportion of the calyx. An incision may be made in each of the posterior calyces containing a calculus and these may then be joined by extending the incisions into the renal pelvis. Care is taken to stay away from the renal papillae so as to avoid damage in this area.

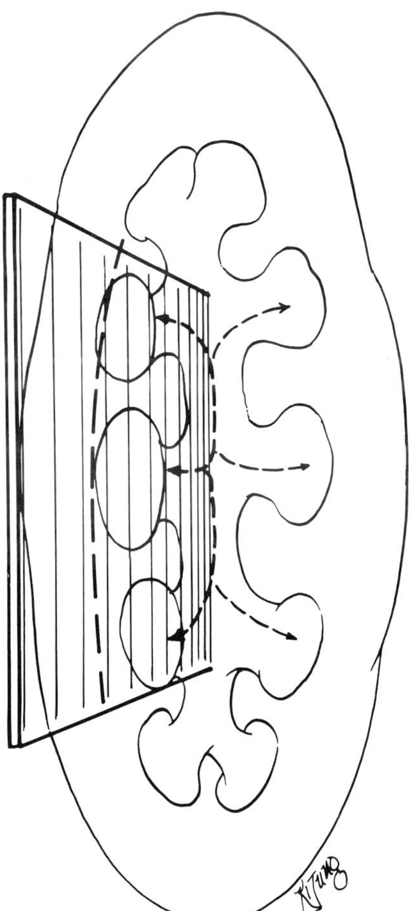

Figure 17.8. The *intersegmental approach* is the route we prefer and use in most patients. In this procedure, the incision in the renal parenchyma is made just in front of the posterior calyces, entering the posteriolateral aspect of the renal pelvis. The presence of a large staghorn calculus in the renal pelvis extending into the major calyces is very helpful in identifying the landmarks as one approaches the pelvis. Once the pelvis has been entered, the incision then can be enlarged in both the cephalad and caudad directions. It may also be extended into the posterior calyces by a transverse incision on the anterior surface and into the anterior segment calyces by a transverse incision on the posterior surface. The apical and basilar segments may be opened on their lateral margins in the midfrontal plane if necessary, for removal of staghorn calculi extending into these calyces.

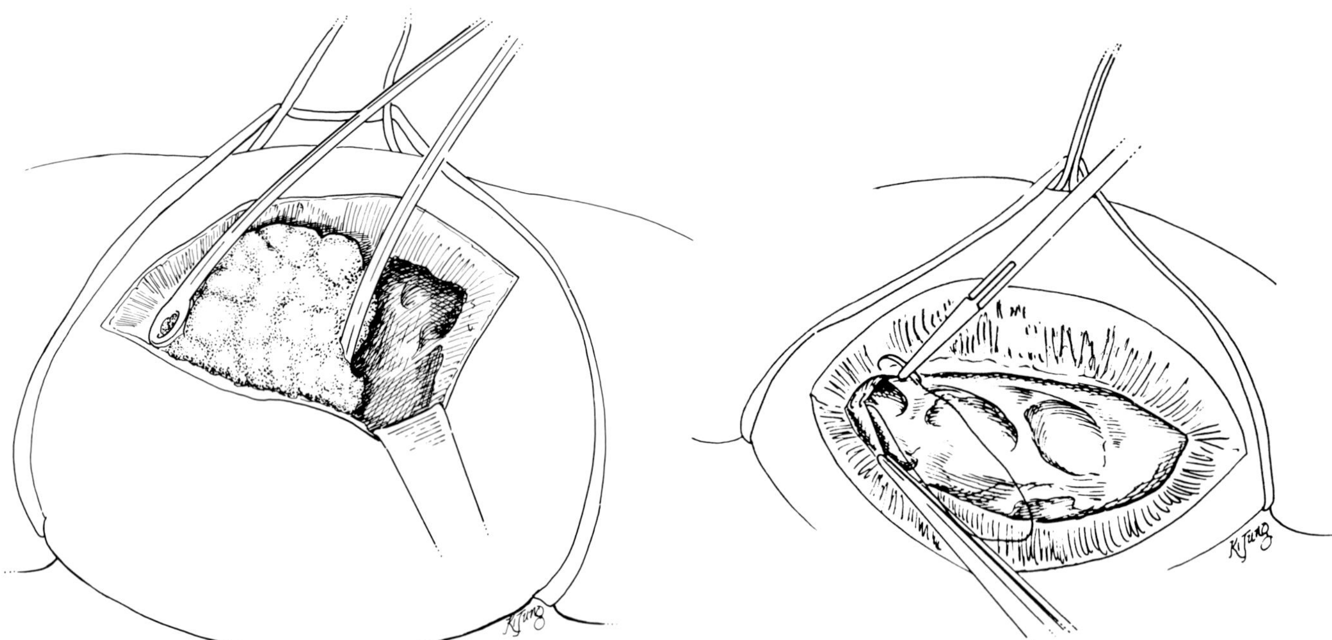

Figure 17.9. Once the collecting system is opened adequately, the staghorn calculus usually can be removed with a Randall stone forceps. During this manipulation, it is wise to occlude the ureteropelvic junction to prevent any fragments of stone from passing down the ureter. In some cases, an extension of a calculus into a major calyx will break off and this will have to be removed separately. It is imperative to inspect each major calyx carefully to be sure that all the stones are removed. The entire area is then thoroughly lavaged with saline.

Figure 17.10. Once all the calculi are removed, a small red rubber catheter (no. 6 or 8 French) is passed down the ureter to the bladder to be sure the ureter is patent. The bulldog clamp is then removed from the renal artery and all bleeding vessels are suture ligated with 4–0 chromic ligatures to ensure good hemostasis. If the incision in the parenchyma has been placed in the proper anatomic position, bleeding encountered after removing the bulldog clamp is minimal. At this time, an intraoperative roentgenogram is obtained of the isolated kidney using a small film. This is done in each case to be sure every stone fragment has been removed. The collecting system is then closed with both running and interrupted 4–0 chromic sutures.

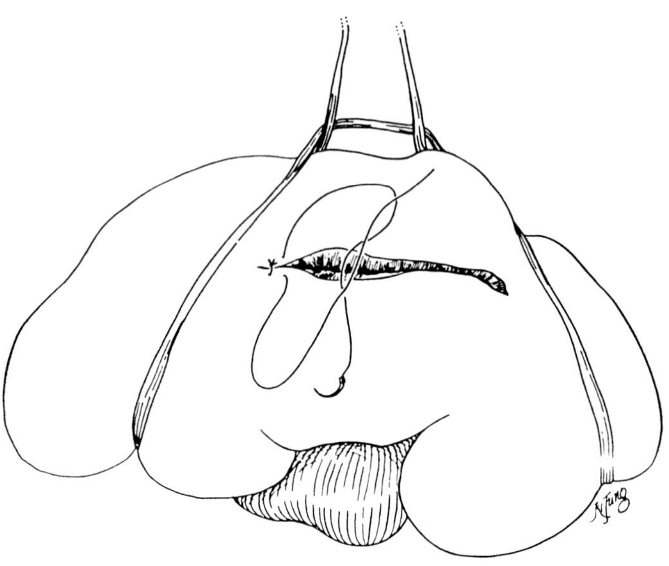

Figure 17.11. When the collecting system has been closed and good hemostasis has been obtained, it is not necessary to place any sutures in the renal parenchyma. The capsule is simply approximated with interrupted 3–0 or 4–0 chromic sutures. A nephrostomy tube is not used routinely but may be used in selected cases. A stent is not placed down the ureter.

The flank incision is then closed in layers, after a Penrose drain is placed in the retroperitoneal space behind the kidney, and brought out through a stab wound below the incision. When the nephrotomy is well closed, there is usually little or no urinary leakage in the postoperative period.

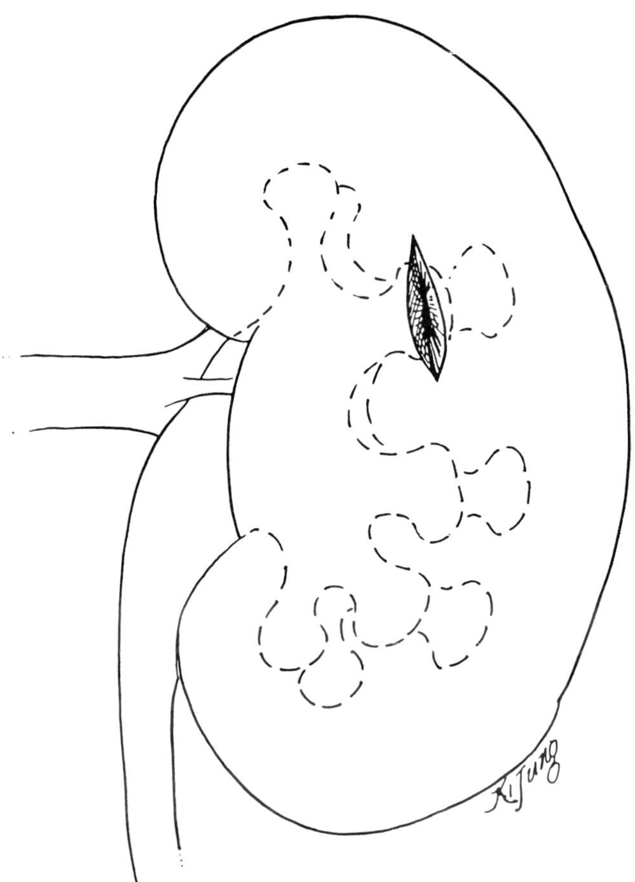

Figure 17.12. In selected patients, it may be impossible to remove some calculi in major or minor calyces through the incision in the renal pelvis. In these cases, isolated nephrotomies are used for removal of these stones. There are certain rules that should be kept in mind when placing a nephrotomy in the renal parenchyma: *(a)* the incision should be limited to one segment of the kidney; *(b)* the incision should be in a straight line; *(c)* the incision should be placed so it does as little damage as possible to the blood supply of the segment; and *(d)* the renal artery should be clamped and the kidney cooled before making an incision.

The placement of the nephrotomy incision in the kidney should be planned carefully. Exceptions to these principles are in cases where the renal cortex is so thin over the calyx that it makes little difference how the incision is placed, as there is very little functioning parenchyma that will be damaged.

In the posterior segment, all nephrotomies should be placed along the longitudinal nephrotomy described by Boyce and Smith. In the anterior segment, the incision should be transverse so it parallels the interlobar arteries. Nephrotomies in the apical segment should be made in the midfrontal plane, starting at the apex and extending along the lateral margin of the kidney. The pyelotomy incision can be extended posteriorly into the basilar segment at the junction of the posterior and basilar segments.

In making a nephrotomy, the capsule is incised and the parenchyma separated with blunt dissection to the major and minor calyx containing the stone. The calyx is opened on its anterior or posterior surface, taking card to avoid injury to the renal papillae. The stone is removed, the area is irrigated, and an intraoperative x-ray is obtained to be sure the stone removal is complete. Hemostasis is secured after removing the vascular clamp from the renal artery; the collecting system and capsules are then closed.

Partial Nephrectomy

It is easy to combine a lower pole partial nephrectomy with pyelocalycotomy to remove a staghorn calculus. This technique is used more frequently in Europe than it is in the United States; its proponents believe that removing a scarred lower pole of the kidney with its dependent collecting system will decrease the chance that recurrent calculi will form. The disadvantage, of course, is that one removes some viable renal tissue in this procedure.

Nephrectomy

In selected patients, in whom a staghorn calculus associated with infection and obstruction has virtually destroyed the kidney, nephrectomy is the surgical treatment of choice. An effort should always be made to conserve renal tissue, but sometimes this is simply not feasible.

POSTOPERATIVE MANAGEMENT

After removing the calculi, the coexisting urinary tract infection should be treated vigorously with the antibiotic of choice followed by long-term chemotherapy. The patient is instructed to eliminate milk and milk products from his or her diet and to force fluids. If the infection can be cleared, then there is hope that recurrent calculi may be prevented. Continued follow-up care is imperative, with periodic renal function studies, intravenous pyelography, and urine cultures performed at appropriate intervals.

Suggested Readings

Boyce WH: The localization of intrarenal calculi during surgery. *J Urol* 118:152, 1977.

Boyce WH, Smith MBJ: Anatrophic nephrotomy in plastic calyorrhaphy. *Trans Am Assoc Genitourin Surg* 59:18, 1967.

Braasch WF, Carman RD: Renal fluoroscopy at the operating table. *JAMA*, ixxiii: 1751, 1919; *Radiology* 222, 1924.

Brödel M: The intrinsic blood vessels of the kidney and their significance in nephrotomy. *Bull Johns Hopkins Hosp* 12:10, 1901.

Graves FJ: The anatomy of the intrarenal arteries in health and disease. Br J Surg 43:605, 1956.

Harrison LH, Nordan JM: Anatrophic nephrolithotomy for removal of renal calculi. *Urol Clin North Am* 1:333, 1974.

CHAPTER 18

Operative Nephroscopy

DONALD E. NOVICKI

Since the time that urology emerged as a surgical subspecialty, practitioners have taken pride in their ability to define intrarenal pathology by palpation and to extract intrarenal calculi bluntly. Many erroneous diagnoses and kidneys with retained stones resulted. Early attempts to visualize the intrarenal collecting system with standard cytoscopic instruments were frustrated by the poor maneuverability of these instruments in a closed space. In 1949, Leadbetter developed a right-angled nephroscope that allowed good visibility and improved maneuverability in the kidney (1). Various devices could be passed beside the instrument to manipulate visualized lesions. Refinements of this instrument provided a suitable operative tool somewhat limited by its rigidity that allowed less than ideal access to portions of the collecting system. Subsequent development of the flexible nephroscope incorporated the desirable features of previous instruments with maneuverability and excellent optics allowing one to visualize all of the intrarenal collecting system with minimal trauma (2). Spectacular technologic advances in the last decade have provided the urologist with a variety of reasonable options to visualize and manipulate intrarenal collecting system lesions. Reliable and durable ureteroscopes, excellent techniques, and instruments for percutaneous renal surgery and extracorporeal shock wave lithotripsy (ESWL) have relegated operative nephroscopy to a secondary position (3–5). The busy practitioner will still encounter circumstances when this procedure is indicated and should attempt to master the technique.

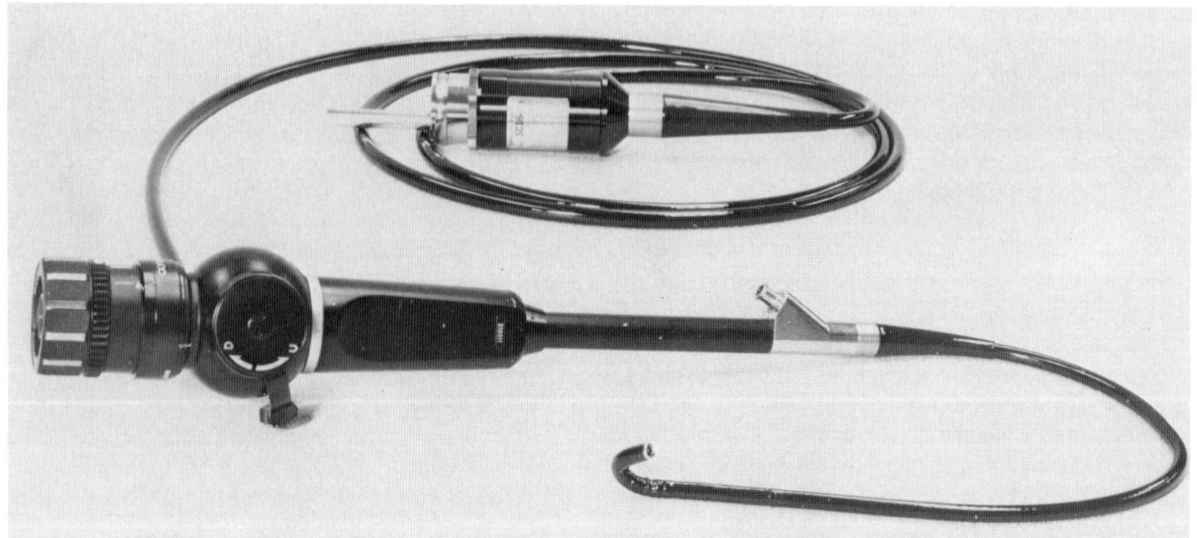

Figure 18.1. Flexible nephroscopes contain a distal working element controlled by a thumb-operated lever or rotator that provides flexion in one plane. The length of the working element and degree of flexion varies with different instruments. In general, shorter instruments are more useful for intraoperative nephroscopy, whereas longer instruments are more suitable for percutaneous techniques.

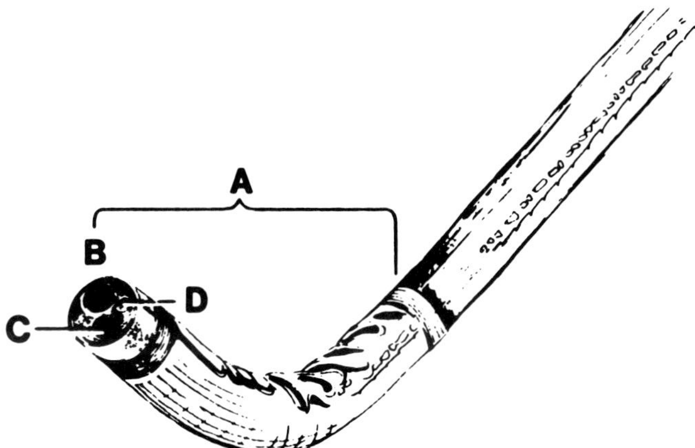

Figure 18.2. The working element of the flexible nephroscope contains: **A,** a flexible shaft; **B,** an irrigation/working channel; **C,** an objective lens; and **D,** a light carrier. A variety of forceps, baskets, and brushes can be passed through the working channel. An eyepiece, inlet port, and light cable plug complete the instrument.

Efficient nephroscopy requires familiarity with the instrument and its accessories. Habit patterns acquired during standard cystoscopic procedures must be disregarded when performing nephroscopy. Practice is necessary to visualize systemically all of the collecting system; several practice sessions using animal or cadaver kidneys should be performed before clinical use. During these periods, one should become familiar with the typical appearance of the major infundibula, calyces, and papillae, and should develop a systematic method to inspect the entire kidney. Forceps and brushes should be used to familiarize the surgeon with their appearance and maneuverability through the nephroscope. Confidence may be gained by having an assistant place small foreign objects in unknown portions of the practice kidney for detection and retrieval. Procedures should be performed with various irrigation fluid flow rates. Once these techniques are mastered, clinical application is easier and more rewarding.

CALCULI

Despite newer approaches to renal stone disease, circumstances requiring surgical removal of calculi still exist. Calculi in kidneys with reparable anatomic abnormalities, large stone burdens, and obesity or skeletal abnormalities contraindicating percutaneous stone removal or ESWL represent a few situations where open surgery is appropriate. Operative nephroscopy may be a useful adjunct in these cases.

Preoperative localization of calculi should be accomplished with the usual imaging techniques. The kidney is exposed in any standard fashion. The renal pelvis and upper ureter are freed and the kidney is mobilized sufficiently to obtain easy access for a posterior pyelotomy. If concurrent pyeloplasty is anticipated, the pyelotomy is performed after planning the pyeloplasty incisions. An intraoperative x-ray is taken before opening the collecting system for comparison to subsequent organ films. The nephroscope and ancillary equipment are inspected to ensure proper function. A generous pyelotomy, adequate to allow easy insertion of the nephroscope and free egress of irrigating fluid is performed. Any stones visible in the pelvis are gently removed. Trauma to the collecting system must be avoided as minimal bleeding will easily impair one's vision. Irrigation flow is initiated through the instrument and the flexible end of the nephroscope is inserted into the pelvis under direct vision. The collecting system is inspected completely.

TUMORS

Most epithelial tumors of the upper collecting system should be managed by standard surgical techniques. When the nature of intrarenal filling defects remains unclear despite preoperative evaluation or when nephron-sparing procedures are indicated, nephroscopy may be useful.

The approach described for calculi is employed, but additionally, complete renal mobilization is accomplished to allow isolation of the kidney with surgical sponges or a rubber dam. Multiple suction devices should be available to limit contamination of surrounding tissue with irrigation fluid containing tumor cells. Systematic visualization of the collecting system allows assessment of the nature and extent of the lesion, which is often underestimated properatively. Direct-vision biopsy or brushing biopsy of suspicious areas with immediate pathologic examination of the specimen may also aid in deciding treatment. When conservative management is chosen, lesions can be fulgurated using a catheter electrode placed through or next to the working element. When partial or total nephrectomy is indicated, the pyelotomy is closed and surgery proceeds in the usual fashion.

RENAL HEMORRHAGE

Unilateral renal hemorrhage, undefined by the usual evaluation, may be directly investigated with the nephroscope (6). A surgical approach similar to that used in dealing with known

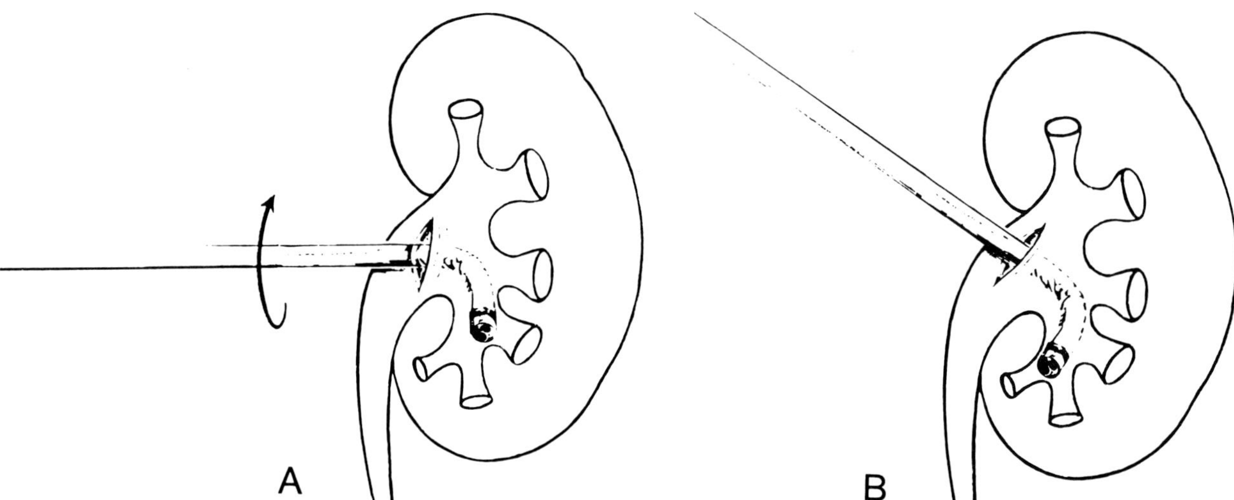

Figure 18.3. The nephroscope flexes in one plane only and will not negotiate complex angles. When attempting to enter polar infundibula, it may be necessary to rotate or tip the instrument to gain access depending on the flexibility of the instrument. **A,** most inferomedial infundibula and calyces cannot be visualized or entered despite maximum deflection of shaft. Visualized stones may be removed by several methods. Direct extraction using grasping forceps or a stone basket placed through the working channel is most suitable for small stones up to about 5 mm in diameter. **B,** the nephroscope is rotated cephalad, allowing access to previously obscured collecting system. Because the forceps are quite stiff, they should not be forced through the flexed instrument or damage to the light bundles may occur. When the stone is too large to grasp or the forceps cannot negotiate the instrument, thin forceps or a stone basket are passed next to the instrument to grasp the stone. If the stone is too large to remove throughout the infundibulum, nephrotomy and extraction with adherence to anatrophic techniques are recommended. When multiple small stone fragments are present, irrigation through the water inlet will often wash the stones free. A commercial pulsatile irrigating device or hand-held 60-ml syringe may be attached to the water inlet port to accomplish irrigation. The upper ureter should be occluded temporarily when washing out fragments to preclude distal migration of small stones.

Nephroscopy can be used in conjunction with coagulum pyelolithotomy or anatrophic nephrolithotomy. When the former procedure is performed, the nephroscope is inserted after coagulum extraction. Residual fragments of coagulum may be removed and stone fragments that were not extracted may then be managed as previously described. The instrument is inserted easily through an anatrophic nephrolithotomy incision and will visualize portions of the collecting system not seen directly through the incision.

After inspection of the entire collecting system, a final organ x-ray is obtained to ensure that the kidney is stone-free. Any residual stone fragments are localized radiographically and the collecting system is reinspected using the nephroscope. Renal closure and drainage are accomplished in the standard fashion.

or suspected malignancies is employed. Gentle tissue techniques are necessary to preclude confusion from operation-induced hemorrhage. When indicated, biopsy or fulguration of bleeding areas is accomplished. Partial nephrectomy may be used for larger benign lesions not amenable to simple fulguration.

LIMITATIONS OF NEPHROSCOPY

Nephroscopic procedures are limited by unfavorable anatomy, the skill and experience of the surgeon, and the inherent limitations of the instrument. Scarred kidneys that cannot be mobilized, small intrarenal pelves, collecting system anomalies, and narrow infundibula limit intrarenal mobility of the instrument. At times, narrowed infundibula can be dilated gently under direct vision with forceps or balloon catheters to allow insertion of the instrument. Acute renal infection or an inflamed, easily traumatized collecting system contraindicates nephroscopy.

Total familiarity with the mechanics, care and handling, and accessory equipment is mandatory before using the nephroscope. Gentle manipulation of the instrument, atraumatic techniques when dealing with tissue, and persistence, tempered with patience on the part of the nephroscopist are essential for a successful examination. As technologic advances are made and miniaturization of equipment improves, the application and utility of nephroscopy will likely advance further.

References

1. Leadbetter WF: Instrumental visualization of the renal pelvis at operation as an aid to diagnosis. Presentation of a new instrument. *J Urol* 63:1006, 1950.
2. Wilbur HJ: The flexible choledochoscope: A welcome addition to the urologic armamentarium. *J Urol* 126:380, 1981
3. Lyon ES, Huffman JL, Bagley DH: Ureteroscopy and ureteropyeloscopy. *Urology* 23 (Suppl 5):29, 1984.
4. Segura JW, Patterson DE, Leroy AJ, May GR, Smith LH: Percutaneous lithotripsy. *J Urol* 130:1051, 1983.
5. Chaussy C, Schmiedt E, Jocham J, Brendel W, Forssmann B, Walther V: First clinical experience with extracorporeally induced destruction of kidney stones by shock waves. *J Urol* 127:417, 1982.
6. Gittes RF, Varady S: Nephroscopy in chronic unilateral hematuria. *J Urol* 126:297, 1981.

SECTION 5

Surgery for Other Benign Renal Disorders

CHAPTER 19

Simple Nephrectomy

DROGO K. MONTAGUE

Renal surgery has its origin some 400 years before Christ, with the drainage of abscesses and with the removal of calculi from renal fistulae. In the early 19th century, kidneys were sometimes removed inadvertently during attempted ovarian surgery, with the observation that the remaining kidney continued to produce normal amounts of urine. It was not until 1869, however, that Gustave Simon performed the first planned nephrectomy. There was great controversy among early surgeons regarding the relative merits of retroperitoneal versus transperitoneal exposure of the kidney. However, because of the potentially serious postoperative complications of peritonitis and intestinal obstruction, most urologists adopted a retroperitoneal flank approach to the kidney during the first half of this century. Then, with the advent of antibiotic therapy and the development of vascular surgery, Poutasse and others again popularized various anterior approaches to the kidney.

Simple nephrectomy is indicated when the function of a kidney has been irreparably damaged due to long-standing infection, calculus disease, or obstruction. Occasionally, a kidney may be removed because of a persistent urinary fistula. Nephrectomy may also be indicated in cases of uncontrollable renovascular hypertension, when the patient's general condition is too poor to permit revascularization or when ischemic atrophy is so severe as to preclude functional recovery.

The procedure can be performed through a variety of incisions. A flank approach is usually preferable when the kidney is chronically infected, when the patient is extremely obese, or when multiple abdominal operations have previously been performed. In cases where severe inflammatory reaction or adhesions obscure anatomic relationships between kidney and surrounding structures, subcapsular nephrectomy is the procedure of choice. In slender patients, simple nephrectomy can be performed easily through an anterior extraperitoneal approach and this is especially appropriate when there has been previous surgery through the flank. Bilateral nephrectomy is often performed in patients being prepared for renal transplantation. This is usually done through a midline transperitoneal incision, which decreases operating time and minimizes blood loss.

Simple unilateral nephrectomy in the patient who does not have end-stage renal disease should, of course, never be performed without the knowledge of the presence and functional status of the contralateral kidney. This is particularly important in emergency situations. Diseased or ectopic kidneys have, on occasion, been removed, only to find later the ''kidney'' that was palpated on the opposite side did not exist. Under such conditions, appropriate urographic studies must always be performed before the final decision is made to proceed with nephrectomy.

STANDARD TECHNIQUE

The principles employed in simple nephrectomy are the same, regardless of the approach or of the side on which the operation is done. Gerota's fascia is opened initially and the kidney mobilized by blunt and sharp dissection. Care should be taken to protect adjacent bowel structures and the renal pedicle should be sufficiently well developed to ensure satisfactory hemostasis. The ureter may be transected first and used as a handle to help develop the pedicle in cases where extensive perinephric adhesions are present.

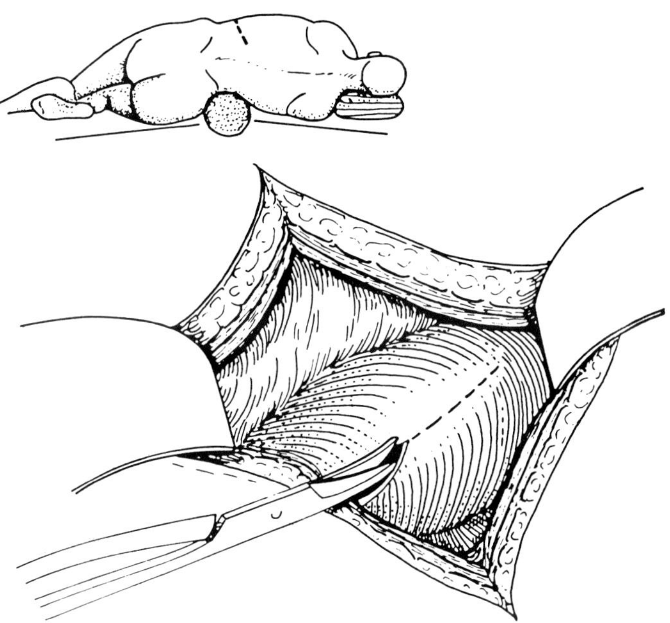

Flank Approach

Figure 19.1. With the patient in the left flank position, Gerota's fascia is opened posteriorly, so that the peritoneal cavity is not entered.

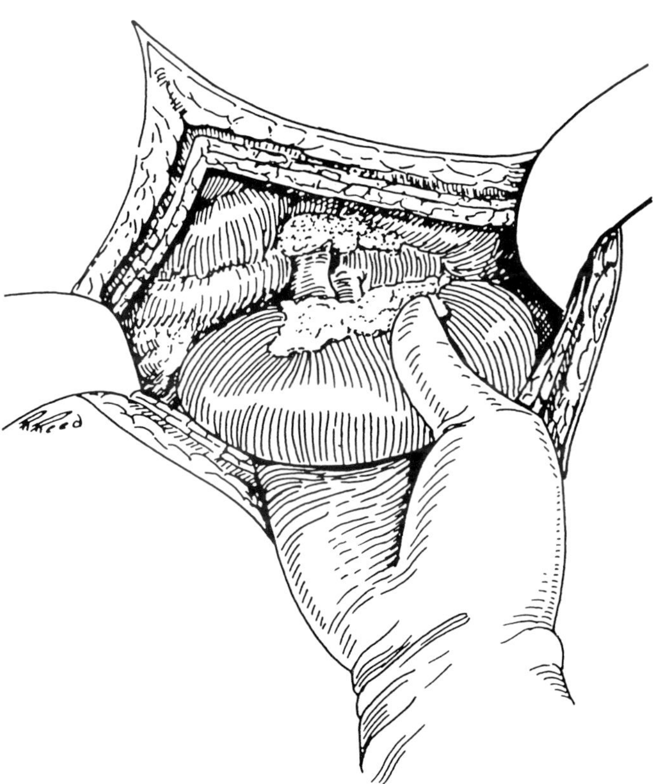

Figure 19.2. The kidney is mobilized by blunt dissection and the pancreas and duodenum are carefully reflected medially along with the peritoneum to avoid injury to these structures. Small vessels and fascial bands can be secured by electrocautery or silver clips as they are encountered, thus ensuring hemostasis.

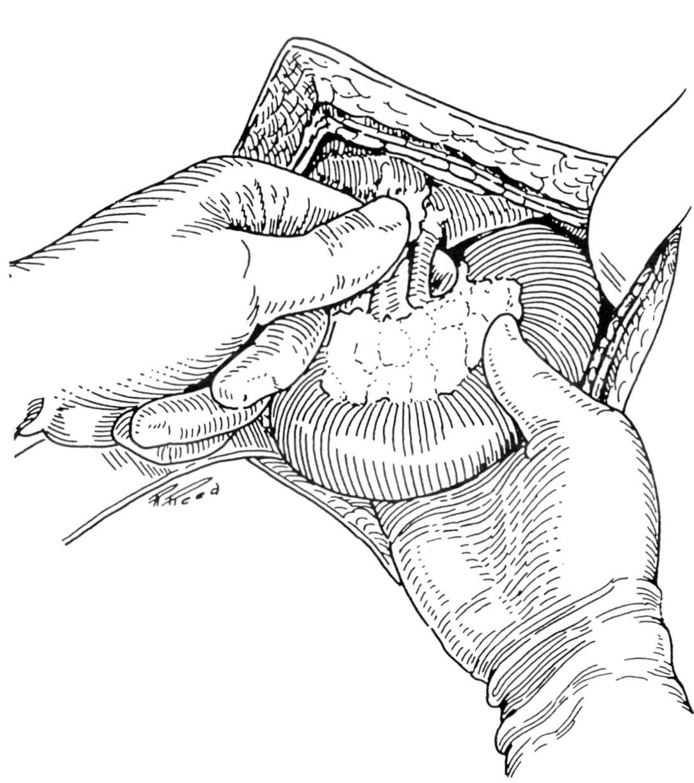

Figure 19.3. The renal artery and vein are separated from surrounding fatty and lymphatic tissues by blunt dissection with the thumb and forefinger.

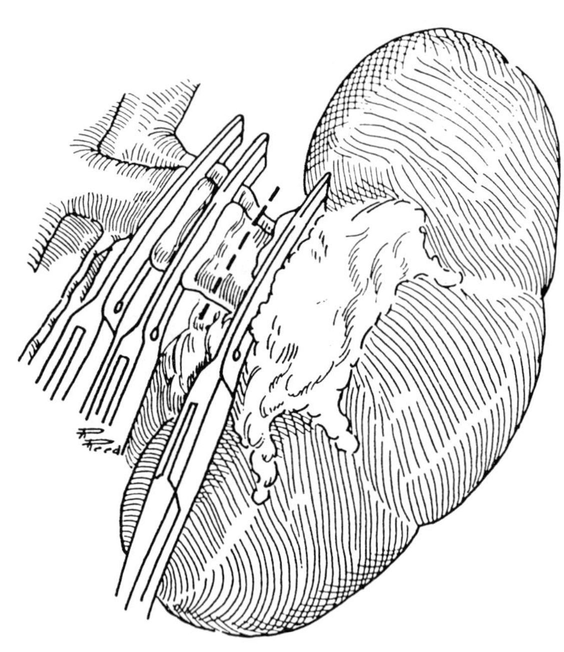

Figure 19.4. With the kidney retracted laterally and the peritoneum and duodenum medially, a generous length of the renal pedicle is isolated. If length permits, two pedicle clamps are placed proximally and one clamp is placed distally at the hilus of the kidney. The pedicle is transected between the second and third clamps. If the pedicle is particularly short or exposure is difficult, then a single pedicle clamp will suffice, transecting the pedicle distal to this clamp, as close to the hilus of the kidney as possible. Care should be taken not to include portions of the renal pelvis in the pedicle, as this can serve as a focus of infection after operation.

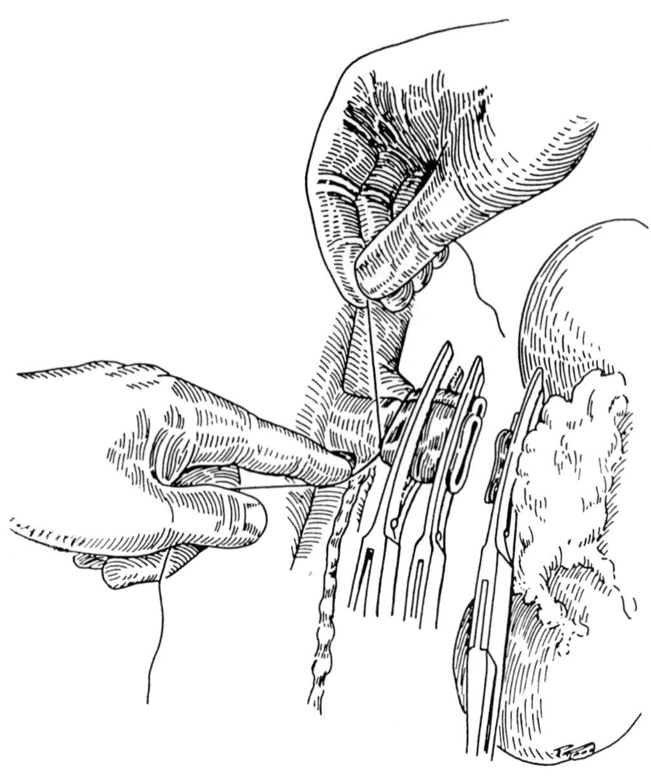

Figure 19.5. The pedicle is secured with two separate heavy silk or catgut ligatures, the first being placed proximal to the medial clamp. As recommended by Nesbit, the knot must be laid down along the inferior margin of the clamp, thus, avoiding injury to the proximal pedicle or slippage as the clamp is removed. Suture ligature of the pedicle proximal to the first clamp should be avoided, as arteriovenous fistulae secondary to this technique have been reported. A second ligature is placed proximal to the second clamp and similarly secured. When possible, the gonadal and adrenal veins are left undisturbed, lying proximal to the level where the pedicle is ligated.

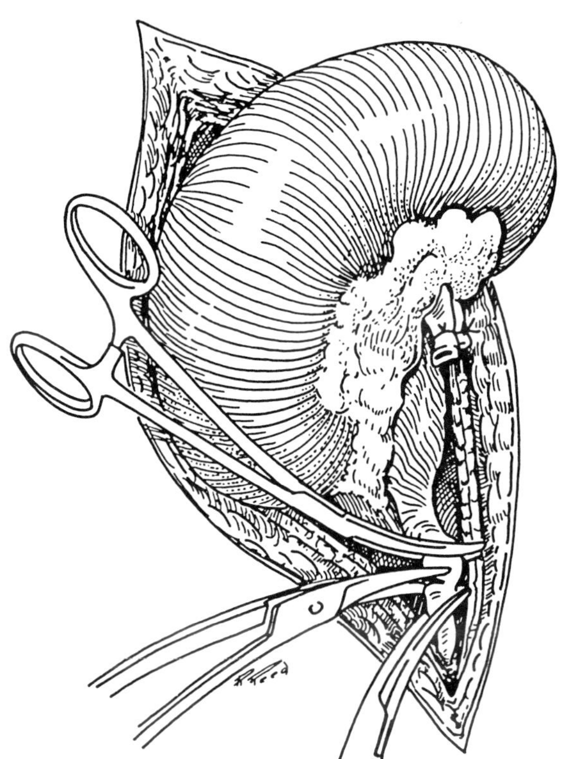

Figure 19.6. The kidney is then mobilized into the incision and the ureter is secured between hemostats, divided, and distally ligated with a 2–0 or 3–0 chromic catgut suture. If extensive adhesions are present and the pedicle is particularly short, the ureter may be transected first and used as a handle to help develop the renal pedicle in a more satisfactory fashion.

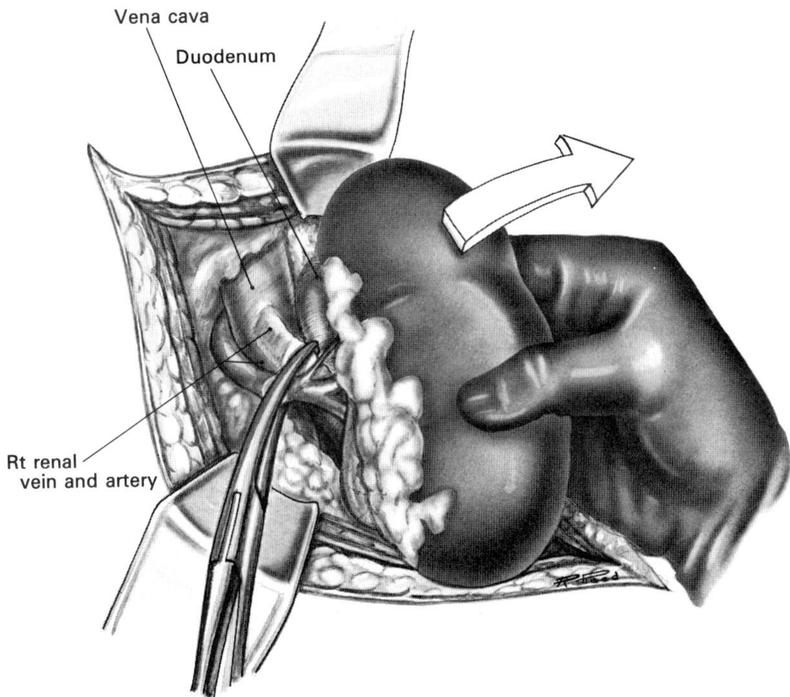

Figure 19.7. Simple nephrectomy on the right side is performed through the flank with the same technique and for the same reasons as described for the left. Care must be taken to reflect the peritoneum and second portion of the duodenum medially to avoid injury to these structures and to gain maximum exposure of the pedicle before it is transected. It is absolutely imperative to avoid including the duodenum or colon in the proximal clamp, which should be carefully placed under direct vision.

Transperitoneal Approach

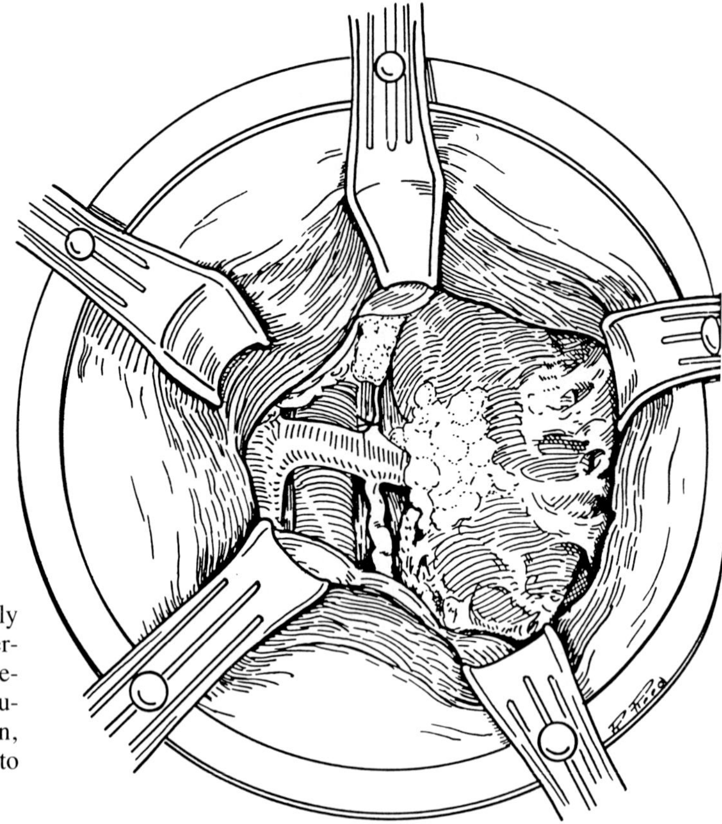

Figure 19.8. The transperitoneal approach is particularly useful in cases where multiple operations have been performed previously through the flank and there are dense adhesions or inflammatory reaction about the kidney. In this situation, the peritoneal cavity is entered, and the left colon, pancreas, and spleen are reflected upward and medially to expose the left renal vein.

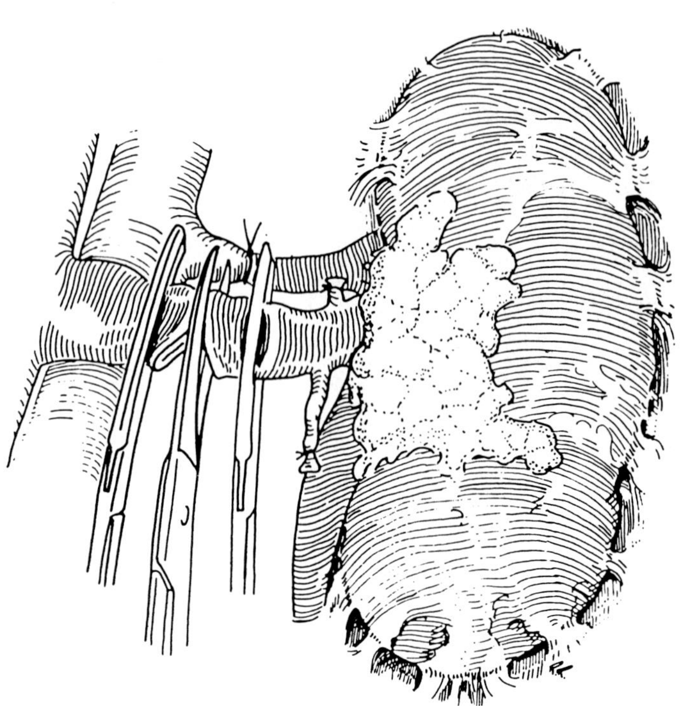

Figure 19.9. The left adrenal vein and gonadal vein are transected between hemostats and doubly ligated with 2–0 silk sutures. The left renal vein and artery can then be mobilized individually or together, depending upon the ease of dissection and the preference of the operating surgeon. The pedicle is then secured either by mass ligature or by individual exposure and ligation of the artery and vein. Should the artery and vein be ligated separately, it is best to occlude the artery first to avoid excessive blood loss into the kidney itself.

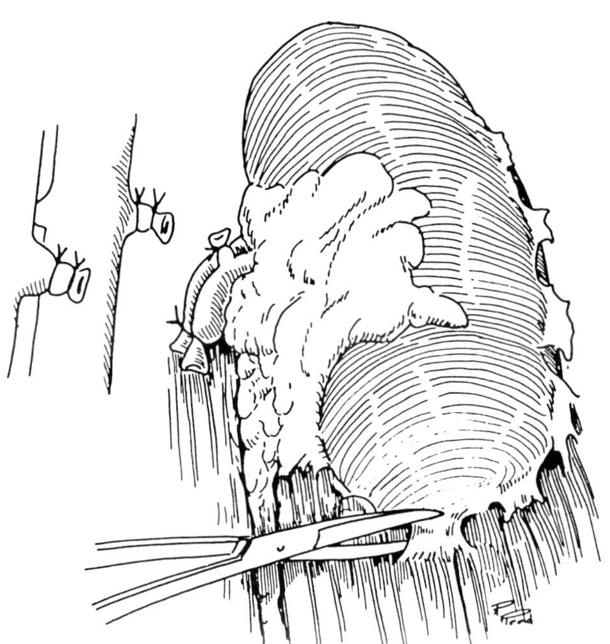

Figure 19.10. After double ligature of the renal artery and vein proximally with heavy silk or catgut sutures, the distal vessels may be ligated en masse or individually. A heavy suture should be used and left long to aid the pathologist in identification. The kidney is then mobilized laterally, superiorly, and inferiorly by sharp and blunt dissection. It is wise to begin the dissection laterally in most cases, in order to gain maximum mobilization before reaching the area of friable lumbar veins that occur just behind and medial to the hilus of the kidney. In many cases, the inflammatory response is severe and adhesions to the psoas fascia necessitate removal of some of these tissues along with the kidney itself.

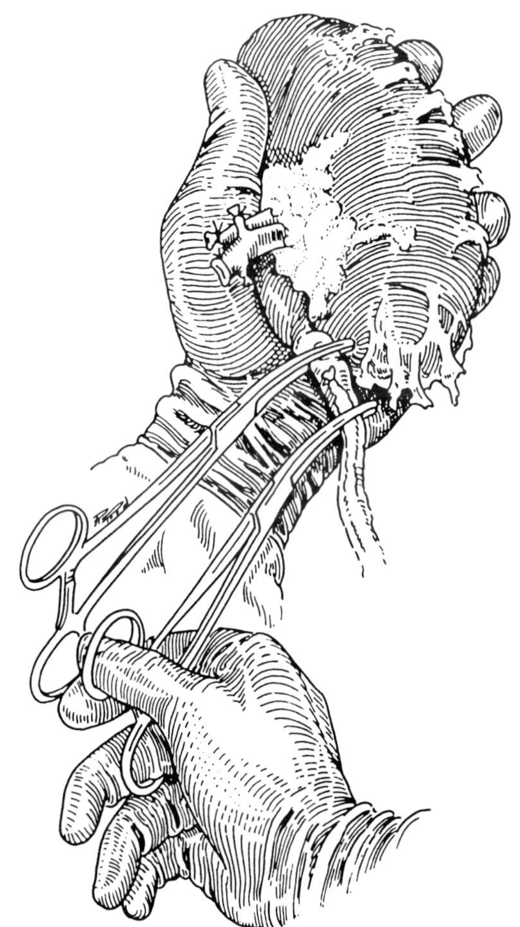

Figure 19.11. After complete mobilization of the kidney, the ureter and renal pelvis can be identified easily and the ureter can be transected between hemostats. A Penrose drain is placed in the renal fossa and brought out laterally through a separate stab incision whenever the kidney is removed for inflammatory disease or where oozing persists in the renal fossa. The colon is then replaced and, whenever possible, the lateral peritoneum is closed with running 2–0 or 3–0 silk sutures. The main incision is then closed in layers in the usual fashion.

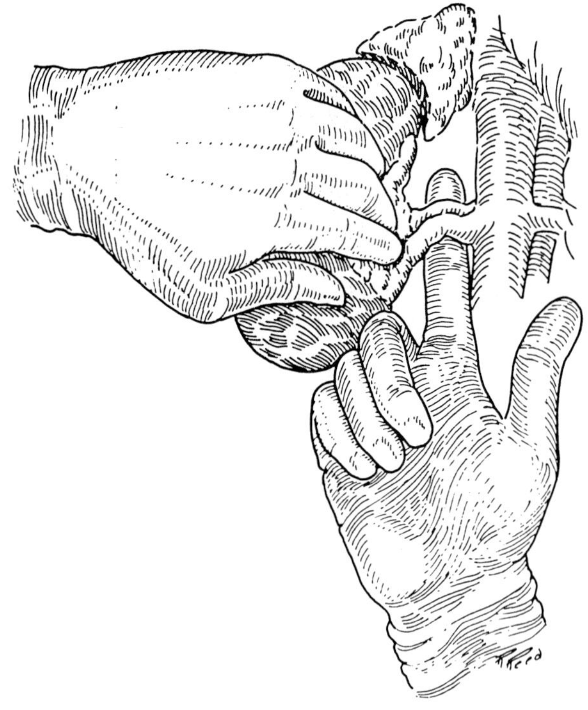

Figure 19.12. When the transperitoneal approach is employed on the right side, the colon should be reflected medially and the right renal artery and vein first dissected free from surrounding structures. With the kidney retracted laterally, it is possible to isolate the right renal vein without disturbing the adrenal gland or the right internal spermatic or ovarian veins. Care should be taken not to traumatize large lumbar veins that may enter the vena cava at the entrance of the renal vein. Both the artery and the vein can frequently be mobilized and the mass can be ligated as a single pedicle with two heavy silk or catgut ligatures.

SUBCAPSULAR TECHNIQUE

Subcapsular nephrectomy is indicated when severe inflammatory reaction about the kidney precludes satisfactory dissection between the renal pedicle and surrounding structures. Often this procedure is done as a second stage after incision and drainage of perinephric or renal abscesses. The procedure was apparently accompanied by technical difficulties in the early days, with more than one surgeon describing "furious hemorrhage" after piecemeal removal of renal parenchyma from within the capsule. However, with modern surgical exposure and careful preservation of the vessels as they enter the hilus of the kidney, these complications by and large can be avoided.

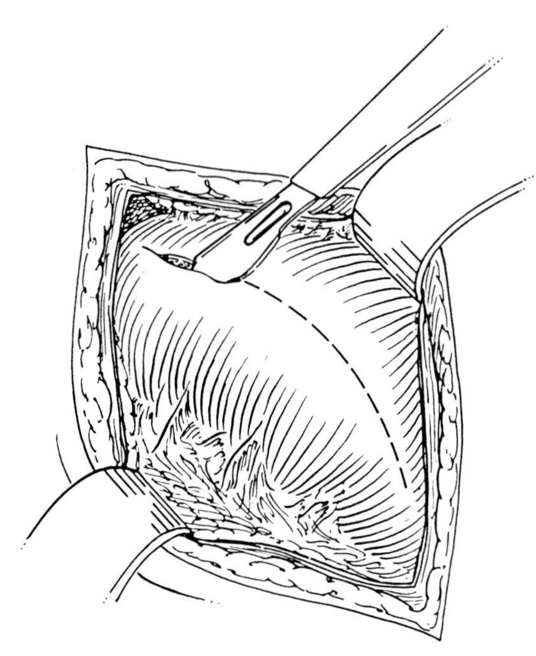

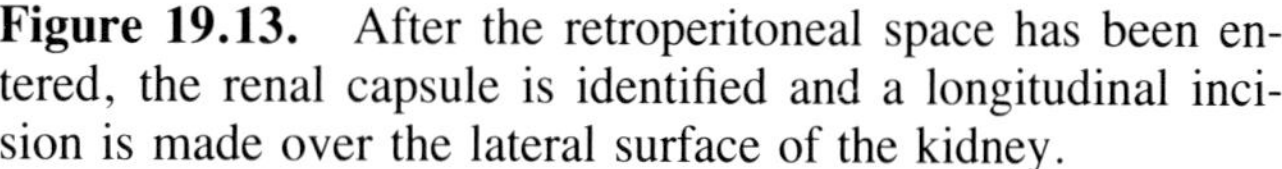

Figure 19.13. After the retroperitoneal space has been entered, the renal capsule is identified and a longitudinal incision is made over the lateral surface of the kidney.

Figure 19.14. Once the capsule has been entered, a plane is developed very easily between renal parenchyma and capsule over the entire surface of the kidney down to the level of the hilus.

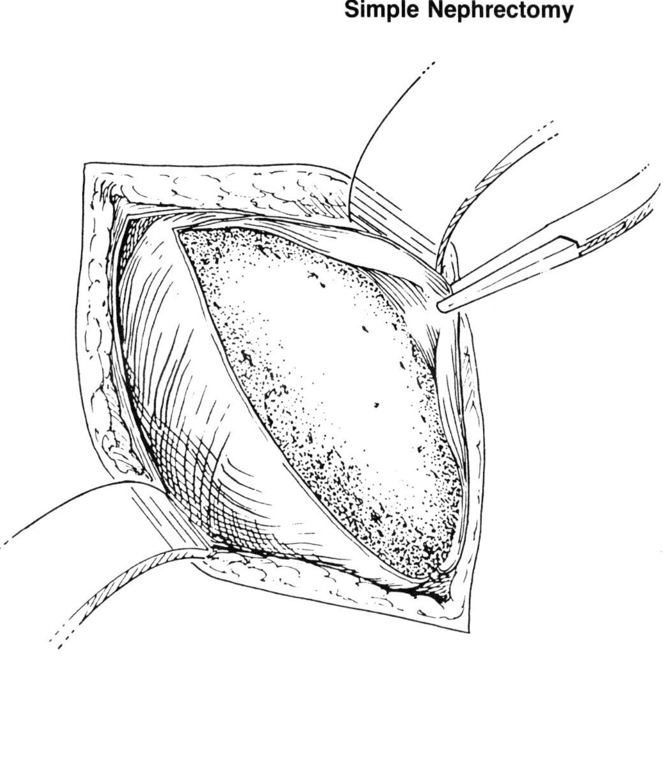

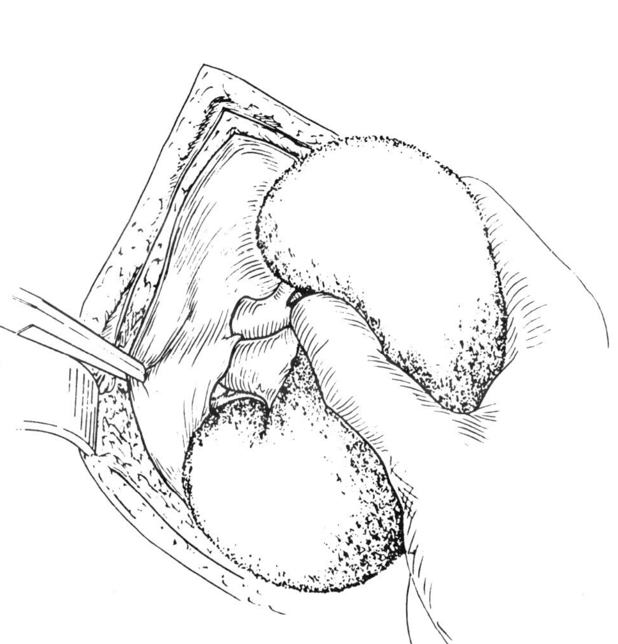

Figure 19.15. The renal parenchyma is then retracted laterally to expose the hilar vessels as they enter the hilus of the kidney.

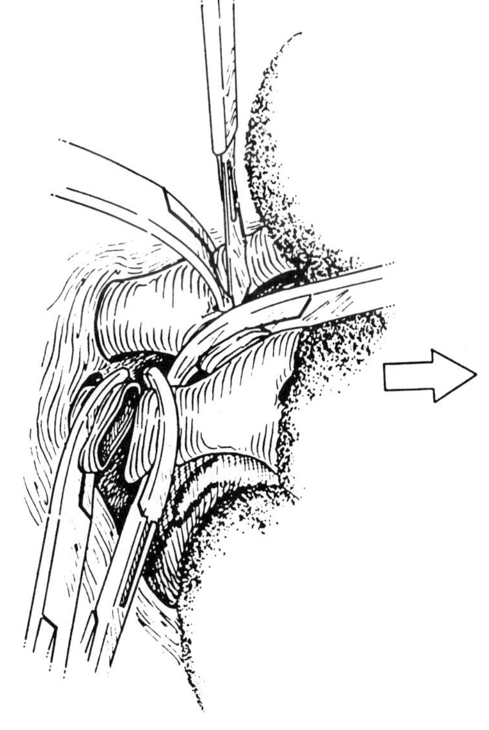

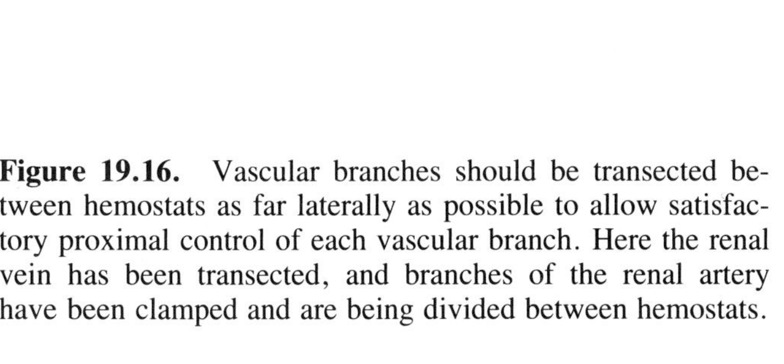

Figure 19.16. Vascular branches should be transected between hemostats as far laterally as possible to allow satisfactory proximal control of each vascular branch. Here the renal vein has been transected, and branches of the renal artery have been clamped and are being divided between hemostats.

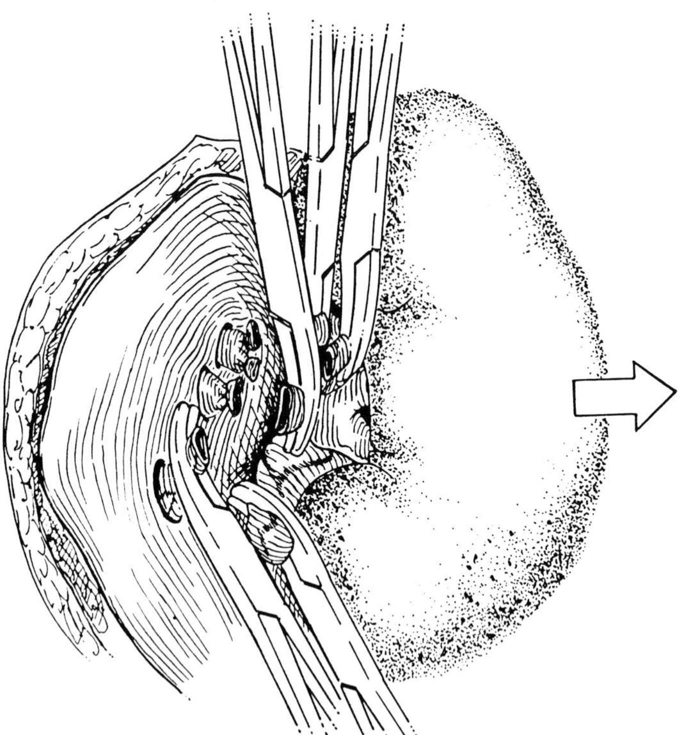

Figure 19.17. The proximal vascular segments are ligated, allowing further lateral retraction of the kidney. The renal pelvis and upper ureter are then brought into view and are divided between hemostats. After transection of the upper ureter and removal of the kidney, the ureteral stump is ligated with a heavy catgut suture. Hemostasis is completed with electrocautery and a Penrose drain is placed down into the confines of the capsule and brought out through a separate stab incision. After copious irrigation with appropriate antibacterial solutions, the incision is closed in layers in the usual fashion.

BILATERAL NEPHRECTOMY

Bilateral simple nephrectomies before renal transplantation are no longer performed routinely. When indicated, however, both kidneys can be removed through a variety of incisions. Large, polycystic kidneys are best removed via a xiphoid to pubis midline abdominal incision (chapter 2). Small end-stage kidneys may be removed through separate posterior incisions by two teams operating simultaneously. Of course, each kidney may be removed separately though a flank incision; but because this requires repositioning, prepping, and draping the patient, this approach is not often used.

POSTOPERATIVE CARE

Postoperative care should be essentially the same for any major abdominal or retroperitoneal procedure. After simple nephrectomy, the incision is closed in layers without drainage in cases where incision and urinary drainage have not occurred. In most patients, however, the kidney was removed because of conditions that result in chronic infection and the retroperitoneal space should be adequately drained for a period of at least 7–10 days. In such cases, spillage of urine during the operation should be avoided, if possible, and the ureteral stump should be lightly cauterized and the wound copiously irrigated with antibacterial solution throughout the operation. A delayed primary closure should be considered in patients where gross contamination occurred while the kidney was mobilized and removed.

Reflex ileus, which can be quite variable in its severity and duration, occurs in most patients after dissection in the retroperitoneal space. Although nasogastric suction is rarely necessary, postoperative intravenous fluids should be maintained until satisfactory gastrointestinal function has resumed. Systemic antibiotic therapy with the drug of choice should be maintained for at least 1 week after operation in patients with urinary infection. Long-term therapy may be necessary in patients who have developed chronic inflammatory changes in the contralateral kidney, ureters, or bladder.

Suggested Readings

Alcock NG: Two step nephrectomies. *J Urol* 14:239, 1925.
Anson BJ, Daesler EH: Common variations in renal anatomy affecting blood supply, form and topograhy. *Surg Gynecol Obstet* 112:439, 1961.
Ballenger EG, Frontz WA, Hamer HG, Lewis B: *History of Urology*. Prepared under the Auspices of the American Urological Association. Baltimore, Williams & Wilkins, 1933.
Culp OS: Anterior nephroureterectomy—advantages and limitations of a single incision. *J Urol* 85:193, 1961.
Chute AL: Secondary nephrectomy. *NY Med J* 3:931, 1920.
Derrick FC, Hughes JC, and Lynch HM Jr: Combined abdomino-lumbar subcapsular nephrectomy. *J Urol* 96:635, 1966.
Grayhack JT, Graham JB: Surgery of the kidney. In Glenn JF, Boyce WH (eds): *Urologic Surgery*. New York, Harper & Row, 1969, pp. 37–71.
Hellstrom J, Franksson C: Operations of the kidneys. In Alksen CE, Dix VW, Weyrauch HM, Wildbolz E (eds): *Encyclopedia of Urology*, Vol. 13, Chap. 7. Berlin, Springer, 1961.
Kimbrough JC, Morse WH: Subcapsular nephrectomy. *Surg Gynecol Obstet* 96:235, 1953.
Kittredge WE, and Fridge JC: Subcapsular nephrectomy. *JAMA* 168:758, 1958.
Lyon R: An anterior extraperitoneal incision for kidney surgery. *J Urol* 79:383, 1958.
Marchioro TL, Brittain RS, Hermann G, Holmes J, Waddell WR, Starzl TE: Use of living donors for renal hemotransplantation. *Arch Surg* 88:711, 1964.
Marshall M Jr, Johnson SH: A simple direct approach to renal pedicle. *J Urol* 84:24, 1960.
Mathé CP: Two-stage nephrectomy. *J Urol* 39:469, 1938.
Morris H: *On the Origin and Progress of Renal Surgery*. The Hunterian Lectures for 1898. Caswell, London, 1898.
Nesbit RM: Personal communication, 1961.
O'Conor VJ Jr, Logan DJ: Nephroureterectomy. *Surg Gynecol Obstet* 122:601, 1966.
Poutasse EF: Anterior approach to the upper urinary tract. *J Urol* 85:199, 1961.
Scott HW, Cantrell JR, Bunce PL: The principle of aortic compression in the management of massive hemorrhage from the renal pedicle after nephrectomy. *J Urol* 69:26, 1953.
Scott RF Jr, Selzman HM: Complications of nephrectomy: review of 450 patients and description of modification of transperitoneal approach. *J Urol* 95:307, 1966.
Smith DP: An anchored mechanical retractor. *Am J Surg* 83:717–720, 1952.
Thornton JK: *The Surgery of the Kidneys*. The Haverian Lectures. London, Griffen, 1890.
Watson FS: Historical sketch of genito-urinary surgery in America. In Cabot H (ed): *Modern Urology*, Vol I. Philadelphia, Lea & Febiger, 1918.
Yeates WK: Post-nephrectomy arteriovenous fistula. *Proc R Soc Med* 60:112, 1967.
Young HH, and Davis DM: In Young HH (ed): *Practice of Urology*. Philadelphia, WB Saunders, 1926, pp. 250–301.

CHAPTER 20

Partial Nephrectomy for Benign Disease

MARK J. NOBLE

GENERAL TECHNIQUE FOR BENIGN DISEASE

Partial nephrectomy literally means removal of a part of one kidney. Although this technically may include renal biopsy, most now use the term to indicate resection of a major percentage of a renal unit. Because a careful partial nephrectomy requires understanding of segmental, renovascular anatomy and often involves time-consuming repair of the portion of kidney remaining in the patient, it is generally a more difficult procedure than simple nephrectomy.

Partial nephrectomy is hardly new; it was first performed by Czerny in 1887 for removal of an angiosarcoma (1). Others have used partial nephrectomy for conserving undamaged renal tissue after traumatic injury; for removing areas damaged by stones, obstruction, or other inflammatory disorders; for excising clinically symptomatic segments with vascular disease (arteriovenous fistula with bleeding or an ischemic area with hypertension); and for elimination of congenitally abnormal segments that pose immediate or future risk to the patient. Partial nephrectomy is also applicable for malignancy in a solitary kidney; techniques for management of this problem usually differ somewhat (and sometimes greatly) from methods employed for benign conditions and are discussed in chapter 11.

One might question the need for this procedure, especially because actuarial tables demonstrate virtually the same life expectancy for persons with one (normal) kidney as for persons with two kidneys. In fact, it might be safer for an older or higher risk patient to have a complete nephrectomy for localized, benign disease technically curable by partial nephrectomy; a partial nephrectomy is probably not appropriate in such individuals whose opposite kidney is normal. Complications such as persistent urinary leakage, delayed rupture and bleeding, or eventual hypertension are not totally preventable and may require subsequent nephrectomy anyway, with its attendant increase in morbidity and mortality.

In this author's opinion, partial nephrectomy should be reserved for patients of fairly good operative risk and reasonable life expectancy, such that the remaining portion of the renal unit would be adequate to support the patient (off dialysis) should the other kidneys be rendered nonfunctional. Usually this implies that the preserved renal segment should provide 20% or more of the total renal function after surgical recovery is complete. With physiologic renal scanning, such estimates often can be made preoperatively with fair accuracy. Obviously, risks are justified with a solitary kidney or in a patient with significant or progressive disease in the other kidney because chronic dialysis carries significant morbidity also.

Because recent studies (2) have shown in animals (with some correlation in humans) that high dietary protein intake (the common American diet) may be injurious to nephrons over a number of years in persons with reduced renal mass, urologists and other clinicians with an interest in kidney disorders have tried to conserve renal mass whenever possible. This is definitely worth the effort when life expectancy and other considerations listed above provide appropriate justification.

Although there are various techniques for partial nephrectomy, this author prefers the anatomic (vascular) method for most circumstances. This method implies careful exposure, dissection, and control of the renal vessels and major branches with removal of tissue primarily supplied by one or more segmental arteries (venous cross-circulation is much more extensive than is arterial circulation). When there is a duplication anomaly (discussed later in this chapter), the area for separation is often apparent and the abnormal segment clearly demarcated. In the average kidney with localized, benign pathology, however, separation is not always straightforward and the vascular method seems to provide the most consistent results with respect to minimized blood loss, demarcation of tissue to be excised (so as to avoid leaving ischemic remnants), and limitation of injury to normal cortex. Closure of the collecting system, control of bleeding vessels in the raw parenchymal surface, and proper coverage of the defect are other principles critical to a good result.

Although the methods to be described below are fairly applicable to any type of benign, localized disorder, one should employ bench (extracorporeal) surgical techniques for hilar lesions or large central lesions requiring extensive control and repair of branch vasculature (see chapter 12). Traumatic injuries requiring partial nephrectomy and debridement are described in a later chapter as well (chapter 23) and will not be discussed here.

Most often, partial nephrectomy for benign disease is elective and preoperative study is important in planning one's approach. A preoperative renal scan, an angiogram (digital subtraction technique often suffices), and a computerized tomographic study enable proper choice of therapy in most instances. In order to perform best a partial nephrectomy with vascular emphasis, an anterior, transperitoneal approach through a midline or subcostal incision is preferred, although a generous flank incision also can be used with success by a skillful surgeon in many instances. In the illustrations below, exposure is obtained through an anterior transperitoneal approach and the pathologic lesion illustrated is an atrophic lower pole causing hypertension.

Figure 20.1. The right main renal artery and vein plus major branches have been exposed through an anterior, transperitoneal approach with reflection of the colon and duodenum medially. A diseased branch renal artery, responsible for atrophy of the lower pole, is identified, secured with mosquito clamps, divided, and ligated with 3–0 silk suture proximally and distally. This demarcates as a dusky area of parenchyma adjacent to pink cortex in the normal segment. Care is taken not to place undue traction on the kidney or other branches might go into spasm and make demarcation more difficult.

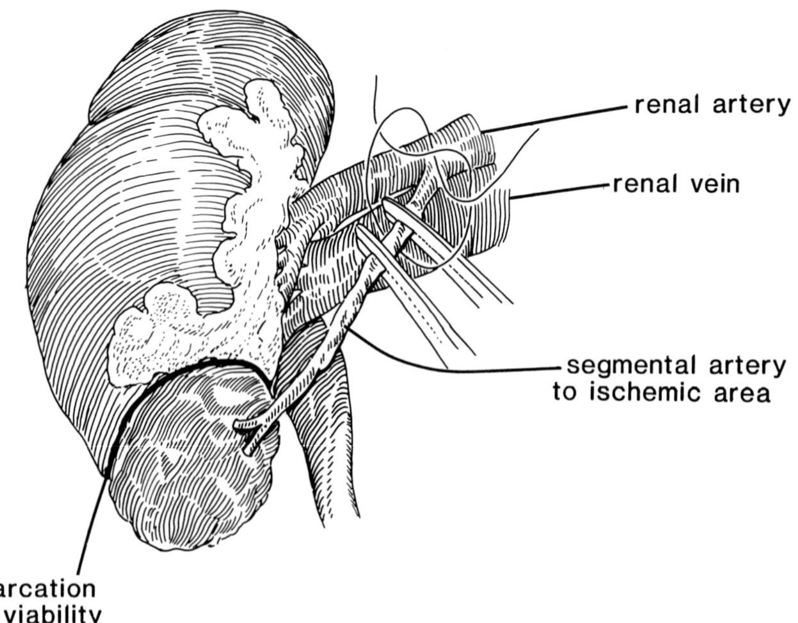

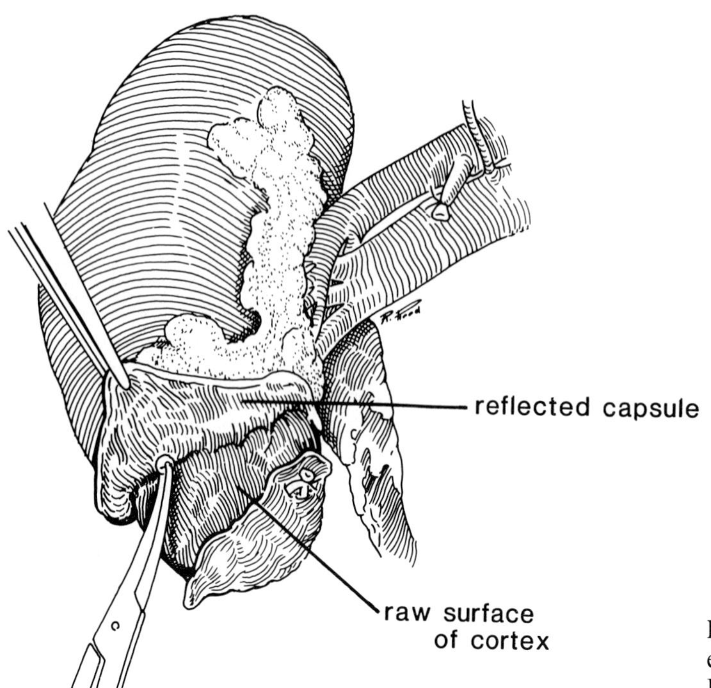

Figure 20.2. Capsule is incised and reflected off the diseased parenchyma so that it will be available for closure later. Blunt dissection usually suffices, but occasional sharp division of small areas adherent to cortex may be necessary.

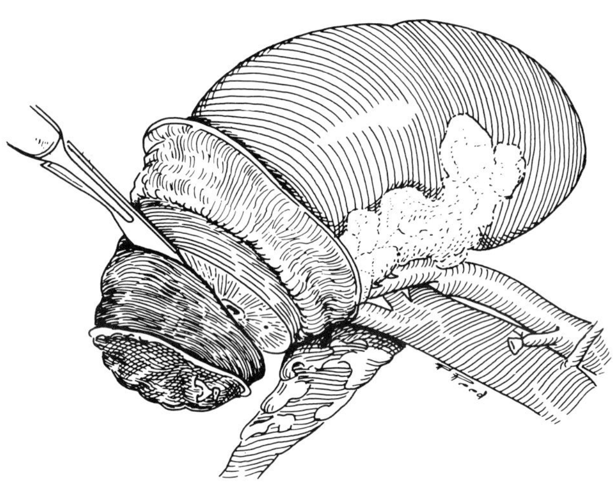

Figure 20.3. The demarcated segment of parenchyma is excised completely; if any cortex looks only partly perfused, it is best to excise this marginal tissue as well so as to avoid leaving ischemic cortex. Major bleeding on the raw cortical surface may be controlled temporarily with pressure (or, rarely, with clamping of the renal artery) until suture ligatures can be placed.

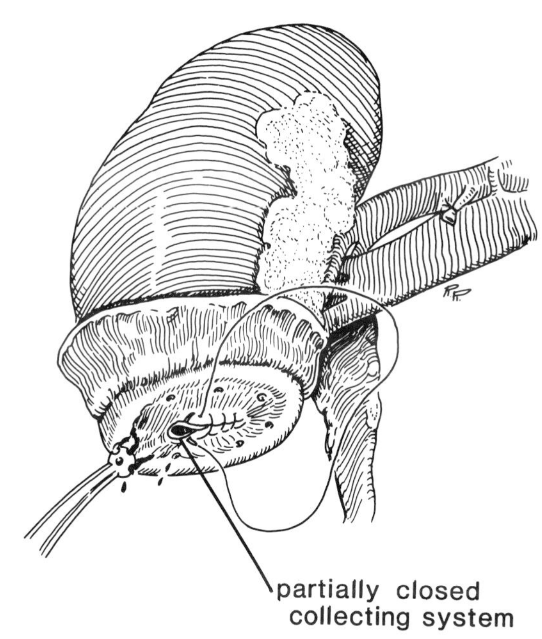

Figure 20.4. The collecting system is closed with 4–0 or 5–0 absorbable suture in a running fashion, and any remaining bleeders sewn with figure-eight 4–0 or 5–0 absorbable sutures. If the partial nephrectomy were for infection stone disease, one might wish to place an open nephrostomy (chapter 24) for hemiacidrin irrigation postoperatively. In most other cases, when the ureter is unobstructed, nephrostomy should not be needed.

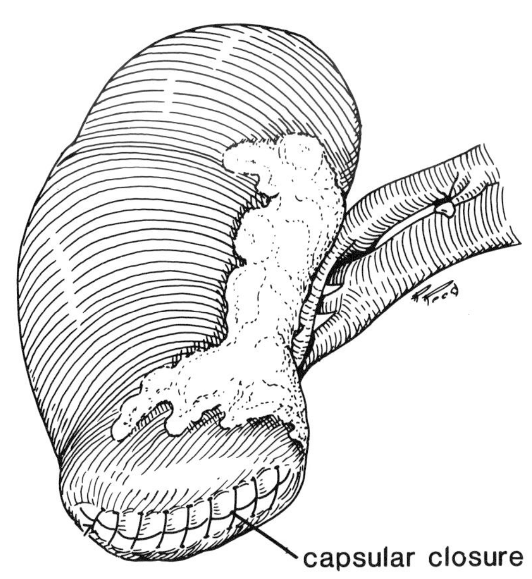

Figure 20.5. After collecting system closure and control of major bleeding vessels, the capsule is closed with running 3–0 absorbable sutures to cover the defect. If capsule is unavailable, omentum may be used (chapter 5) to cover the area. A drain, preferably of the suction type, is placed near the operative site and brought through a stab wound through the flank, if possible. The bowel is repositioned (suturing for reperitonealization is optional) and the incision closed in the usual manner. The drain is usually left for 8–10 days to obviate delayed urinary leak. Follow-up excretory urography or at least a renal scan should be obtained at 1 and 6 months postoperatively; more often, if the clinical situation warrants. Blood pressure should be checked at those occasions as well, after partial nephrectomy for any reason, in case a segment becomes ischemic and the patient requires medication for hypertension.

HEMINEPHROURETERECTOMY

Heminephroureterectomy is appropriate for benign disease confined to one segment of a kidney whose remaining segment has no significant abnormalities (3). The usual situation involves a duplicated kidney where the upper segment has been chronically obstructed, has little function, and is causing pain or recurrent infection. On occasion the ureter from the abnormal segment will insert ectopically; a well-known example is the female with a lifetime of mild incontinence secondary to a "cap" of poorly functioning tissue on one upper renal pole that drains into the genital tract. Because it excretes contrast very poorly, such a segment fails to visualize on excretory urography and imparts a "drooping flower" appearance to the collecting system of the normal renal segment (4). Another instance is the rare Ask-Upmark renal segment, which is severely dysplastic, may have a dilated ureter, and causes hypertension by excess renin production (5). In all such cases, the principles are similar to those discussed earlier and involve control of segmental and larger parenchymal bleeding vessels, careful tissue handling so as to minimize cortical damage or devitalization, and watertight closure of the renal collecting system.

When the ureter is not significantly dilated and does not reflux, one may ligate the ureter of the removed segment at any convenient point below the ureteropelvic junction; there is no need to resect it extensively in such circumstances. The diseased ureter, on the other hand, needs to be removed as completely as possible (without jeopardizing the normal ureter adjacent to it). Care is required to avoid impairing the adventitial blood supply of the ureter remaining behind. This usually can be accomplished by stripping the adventitia from the wall of the ureter being excised; this "close dissection" results in all of the adventitia (and blood supply) remaining with the normal ureter.

The choice of incisions for nephroureterectomy is primarily made after review of the patient's habitus and clinical problem. The entire procedure may be performed through a single midline or paramedian transperitoneal incision if one wishes. More often, an extraperitoneal approach is utilized via flank, anterior subcostal, or even dorsolumbotomy incision for access to the kidney, with the distal ureter resected through a Gibson-type or other separate lower abdominal incision. In the illustrations below, heminephrectomy in a duplicated segment is depicted through a flank approach.

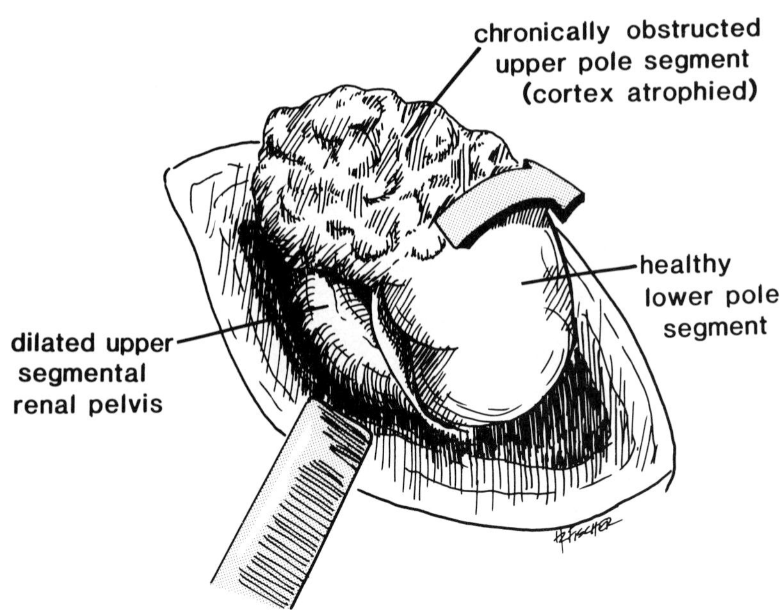

Figure 20.6. The kidney has been exposed and mobilized through an incision appropriate for the patient and convenient for the surgeon (right flank incision illustrated). In this example, the upper segment has thin, atrophic cortex and the upper ureteral segment is chronically dilated. One begins by rotating the kidney medially for exposure of the collecting system. The abnormal renal pelvis and upper segmental ureter are dissected and isolated from the adjacent normal structures. It is best if the normal (lower segmental) pelvis and ureter are minimally disturbed; this helps avoid late fibrosis that might impair peristalsis and better maintains the blood supply to the middle portion of the ureter. If an upper pole branch vessel (not shown) passes posterior to the dilated pelvis, it should also be exposed and isolated at this time.

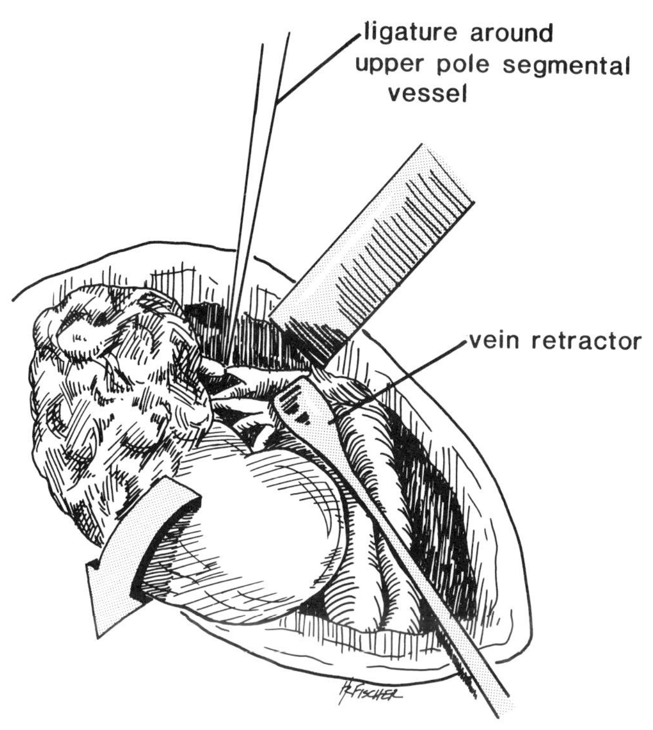

Figure 20.7. The kidney is now externally rotated *(arrow)* in order to bring the hilar vessels into view. The renal vein is usually anterior and can be dissected and retracted inferiorly to expose segmental arterial branches as shown. If required, the vena cava may be mobilized in order to permit better retraction of the renal vein. Usually, the segmental vessels to the diseased segment can be identified, ligated proximally and distally with 3–0 or 4–0 silk, and divided. If there is doubt concerning vascular distribution when a branch enters near the junction of the normal and abnormal segments, gentle compression of an arterial branch permits one to check carefully the parenchyma for ischemic zones in the normal renal segment. (Be sure also to check posteriorly if doing this). Rather than induce a significant ischemic area in normal parenchyma, it is better to leave the branch vessel intact and control bleeding on the raw surface of the preserved lower pole. Creation of large ischemic zones obviously risks emergence of hypertension at a later date.

Figure 20.8. For coverage of the raw cortex of the lower pole, a flap may be created from capsule overlapping the diseased upper segment. Many times, however, this is not feasible due to scarring and fibrous reaction cementing capsule to diseased parenchyma. In these circumstances, sharp division of the diseased from the normal segment becomes necessary. Often, a demarcation line is visible that facilitates this. One simply incises sharply through the capsule and either sharply or bluntly through parenchyma, as depicted. Traction on the diseased segment by an assistant helps maintain exposure, while compression of the normal parenchyma between thumb and forefinger controls bleeding from arcuate vessels. It is important to have the kidney rotated so that one can see the separate collecting systems; this helps in planning the incision and creating a clean separation of segments. Although a theoretical plane of decreased vascularity exists between segments, frequently brisk bleeding is encountered and small parenchymal vessels must be oversewn with 4–0 or 5–0 absorbable figure-eight sutures. When diseased tissue does not dissect free cleanly, sharp trimming is essential to avoid leaving abnormal tissue behind, even though this may mean additional suturing of bleeders.

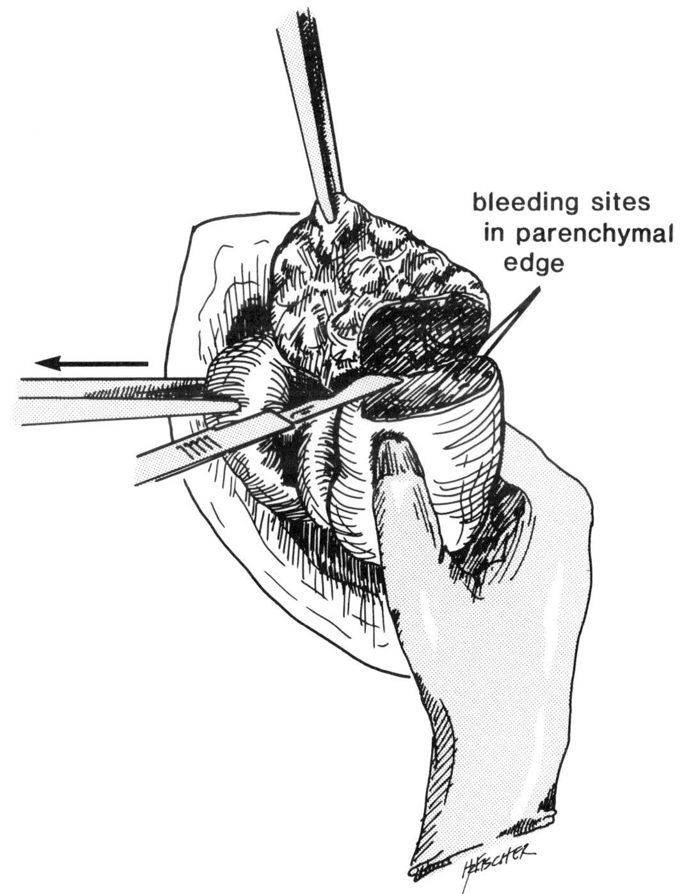

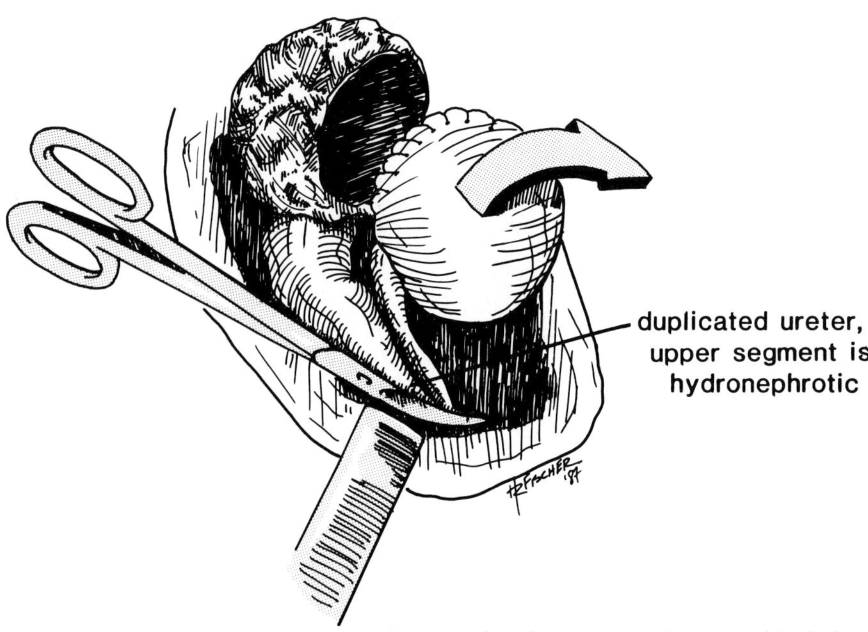

Figure 20.9. With the diseased segment separated, any portion of the normal collecting system that was entered must be closed in a watertight fashion with 4–0 or 5–0 absorbable suture; the raw parenchyma may then be covered with capsule brought together with additional 3–0 or 4–0 absorbable suture, if sufficient capsule is present. Alternately, a flap of perirenal fat (or omentum harvested through a peritoneal window) can be used to cover this surface and is secured to capsule along the perimeter with 3–0 absorbable sutures. Although coverage is not absolutely required, it does seem to speed healing (should small areas of urinary leakage develop) and helps prevent fixation should the remaining segment ever require reoperation or removal. The diseased ureter is dissected from normal ureter as far inferiorly as possible, leaving as much of the adventitia as one can.

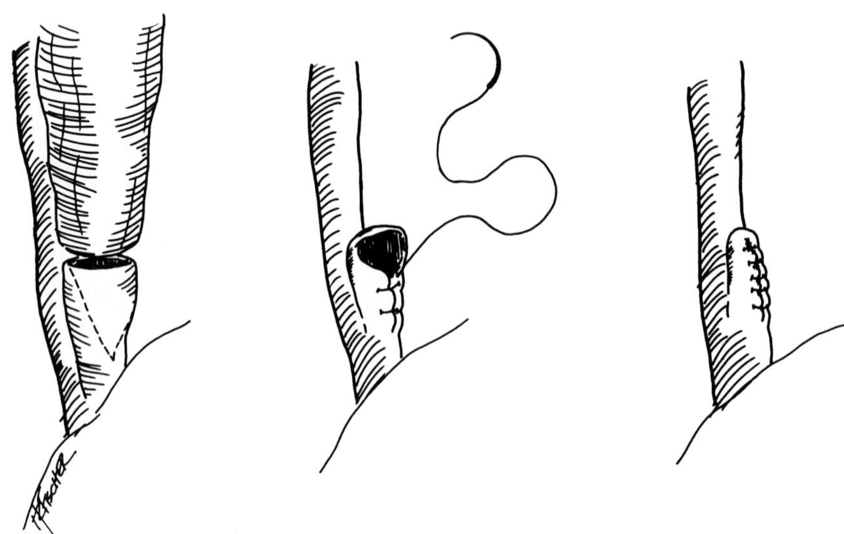

Figure 20.10. In cases of incomplete duplication, the diseased ureter is divided very near its point of fusion with the normal ureter, tailoring the tissue to enable smooth closure without creating a pucker or stricture. A 4–0 or 5–0 absorbable suture is used to close the small stump, obliterating the abnormal lumen as shown. Suction drains (Jackson-Pratt or equivalent) are placed in this area and at the renal level and brought through separate stab wounds; the incision(s) are closed in usual fashion. Drainage is generally maintained 7–10 days or longer to obviate the risk of delayed leakage.

In cases of complete duplication, judgment rarely may dictate resection of the entire diseased ureteral segment. If the intramural ureters are within a common sheath and prove difficult to separate after both intra- and extravesical dissection, it may be best to reimplant the normal ureter using the extramural, well-vascularized portion rather than risk fibrosis of its tip. This decision is obviously one of surgical choice based on the specific clinical circumstance.

EXCISION OF CALYCEAL DIVERTICULUM

A calyceal diverticulum is a small, usually solitary cystic space containing urine and having a slender communication with a calyx (6). It is lined by transitional epithelium and is generally peripheral to the calyces. Most commonly, it has a diameter of 1–3 cm and is picked up as an incidental finding when a patient undergoes intravenous pyelography for unrelated reasons. Occasionally, however, it may be symptomatic and can be a source of infection, pain, or may contain one or more calculi. Because one rarely finds a calyceal diverticulum in the pediatric age group, it is believed that the lesion is probably not congenital (7).

When symptomatic, a calyceal diverticulum may be removed by partial nephrectomy (previous section) or by marsupialization and excision (marsupialization is illustrated). Even with methods such as methylene blue instillation into the renal pelvis (with temporary compression at the ureteropelvic junction), the communication with a deeper calyx is often difficult to demonstrate at surgery; if not found, it will probably seal itself provided the area is drained adequately during the postoperative period. Some, occasionally, have found intraoperative ultrasound useful for localization; if a sizable calculus is present or if the parenchyma is thin over the diverticulum, it should not be hard to find by simple palpation. The technique for excision of a calyceal diverticulum is illustrated below.

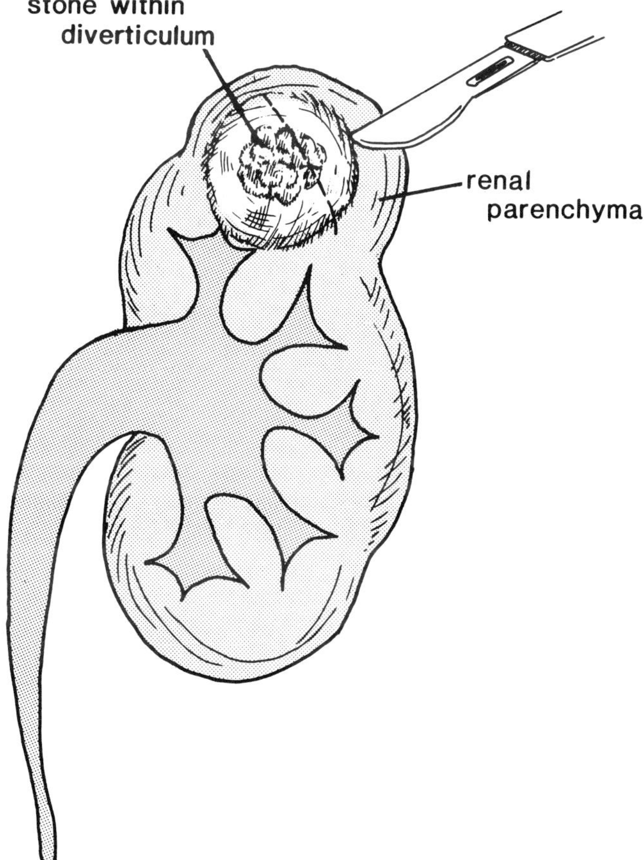

Figure 20.11. The kidney is mobilized through an incision of surgeon's choice, usually flank, and the capsule generously exposed in the region of the diverticulum. A capsular incision is made and then bluntly deepened until a pseudocapsule is encountered. This is usually thickened and has a different feel than ordinary cortex.

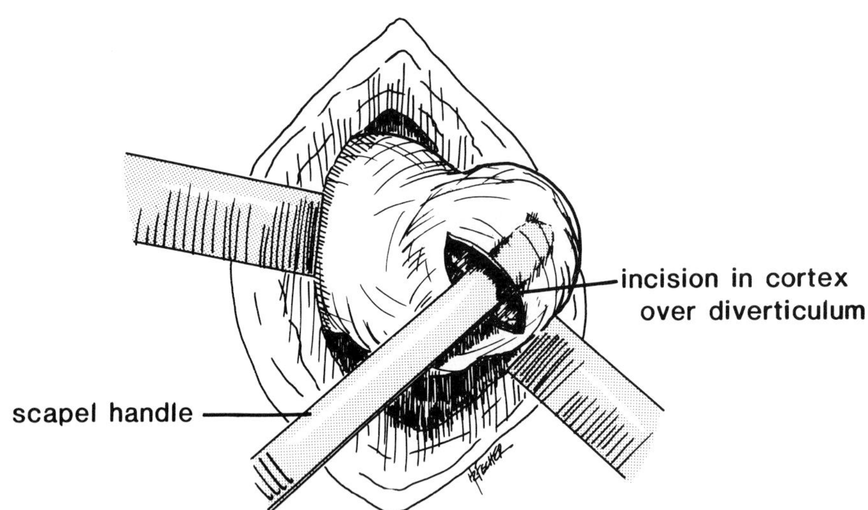

Figure 20.12. As with a sebaceous cyst of the integument, a calyceal diverticulum can be marsupialized and exteriorized by following the natural plane between normal parenchyma and pseudocapsule. It should ''shell out'' fairly easily with blunt dissection, but there may be an occasional adherent spot where inflammatory reaction has been pronounced. If one imagines where the curvature seems to be heading, or if a deeper spot can be dissected and the two ''known'' areas joined, one simply can cut sharply and resume at the next area where the mass dissects easily. There will be times that such does not succeed and normal parenchyma is resected or even torn with subsequent brisk bleeding. If this occurs, it can be controlled with pressure until the cyst is excised; one then can suture and ligate the bleeding vessels with better exposure. If the cyst is entered accidently, a culture is taken and one continues to excise its wall, palpating from inside to help to define it better.

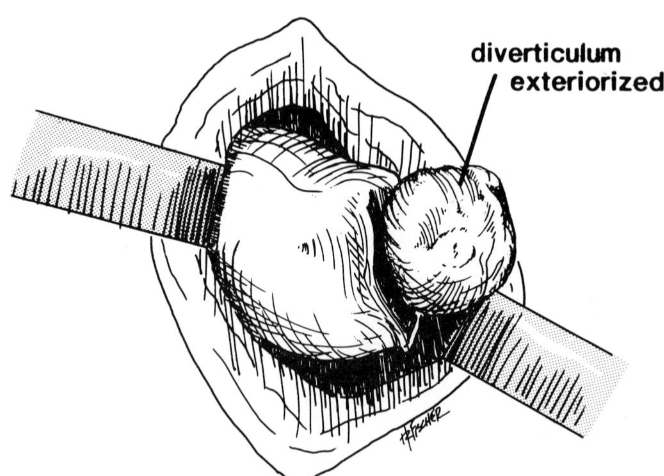

Figure 20.13. When the diverticulum is free from surrounding tissue, it can be exteriorized and a tract may be seen in some instances, presumably leading to the subjacent calyx. This should be closed with a fine absorbable suture if possible. Most often, no tract will be identifiable and the mass is simply delivered and sent for pathologic examination. Any stones from the diverticulum should be analyzed.

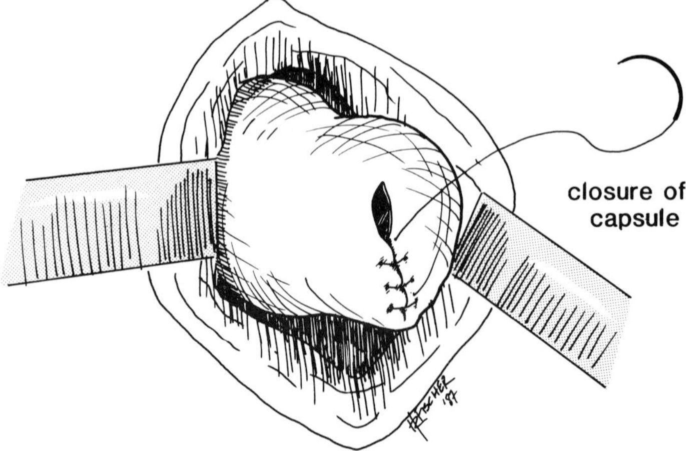

Figure 20.14. Any major bleeding points can now be sutured with figure-eight fine absorbable material (4–0 or 5–0). The parenchyma then usually can be approximated, redundant capsule excised, and the capsule closed with running or interrupted 3–0 absorbable sutures. Alternate methods include leaving the area open with an inlay of perirenal fat, omentum, or even absorbable collagen sponge. A suction drain is placed nearby, brought through a separate stab wound, and the incision closed in the standard manner. If purulent material begins draining during the procedure, then after removal, treatment with copious antibiotic irrigation, followed by drainage (as with a renal carbuncle) is wise. The skin and soft tissues may be left open and packed in such instances.

References

1. Mathe CP: Kidney surgery. In Ballenger EA (ed): *History of Urology*, Vol. 1 Baltimore, Williams & Wilkins, 1933.
2. Smith S, Laprad P, Grantham J: Long-term effect of uninephrectomy on serum creatinine concentration and arterial blood pressure. *Am J Kidney Dis* 6:143, 1985.
3. Culp OS: Heminephroureterectomy: Comparison of one-stage and two-stage operations. *J Urol* 83:369, 1960.
4. Gross RE, Chait A: Renal duplication with hydronephrotic segment. *AJR* 101:728, 1967.
5. Ljungquist A, Lagergran C: The Ask-Upmark kidney. *Acta Pathol Microbiol Scand* 56:277, 1962.
6. Devine CJ, Guzman JA, Devine PC, Poutasse EF: Calyceal diverticulum. *J Urol* 101:8, 1969.
7. Williams G, Blandy JP, Tressider GC: Communicating cysts and diverticula of the renal pelvis. *Br J Urol* 41:163, 1969.

CHAPTER 21

Procedures for Ureteropelvic Junction Obstruction

ROBERT KAY

Ureteropelvic junction obstruction is one of the most common congenital anomalies found in urology. It is the most frequent cause of upper urinary tract obstruction in children. Historically, treatment for the relief of hydronephrosis consisted of loin massage, needle aspiration, ureteric catheterization, nephropexy, nephrotomy with fistula formation, and, commonly, nephrectomy.

Reconstructive surgery was first performed by Trendlenburg in 1886. This operation consisted of an opening into the kidney and, through an extensive nephrotomy, the adjacent ureteric and pelvic wall were divided and reanastomosed. The patient died secondary to postoperative complications. The first successful pyeloplasty was performed in 1891 by Ernest Kuster. This was done by dividing the ureter and reanastomosing it to the pelvis in a forerunner to the more modern dismembered pyeloplasty.

The Heineke-Mickulicz principle was applied to ureteropelvic junction obstructions by Fenzer in 1892. Other developments in surgery of this obstructive lesion included the Y-V pyeloplasty initiated by Schwyzer in 1916 (5) and improved by Foley 1937 (3). In 1943, David M. Davis reported the intubated ureterostomy for a long stricture of the upper ureter. This had been done previously by Fiori in 1905, Albarran in 1909, and Keyes in 1915. In 1949, two English surgeons, Anderson and Hynes (1), described the dismembered pyeloplasty that is the most common reconstructive procedure for ureteropelvic junction obstruction used today. Culp and DeWeerd in 1951 (2) and Scardino and Prince in 1953 (4) returned to using the redundant pelvis as a flap to reconstruct the ureteropelvic junction. This idea was carried further in 1969 when Thompson and associates (6) suggested a capsular flap pyeloplasty for renal pelvic reconstruction when sufficient pelvic tissue was not present for use in repair.

Today, most urologists use a form of a dismembered pyeloplasty, although flap procedures such as the Foley Y-V (3), Culp (2), or Scardino (4) are applicable in selected cases. In any repair of the ureteropelvic junction, one must remember Foley's criteria for a successful pyeloplasty that should apply to any form of repair:

1. Formation of a funnel
2. Dependent drainage
3. Watertight anastomosis
4. No tension

One should have an understanding and the ability to perform many types of pyeloplasty repairs and apply the proper technique to the individual ureteropelvic junction obstruction.

The controversy regarding the use of stenting catheters and nephrostomy tubes continues today as much as in the past. Advantages of stenting catheters and nephrostomy tubes include prevention of pelvic distension and subsequent disruption and leak. Disadvantages include increased hospital stay, possible route of infection, and renal injury in placing the catheter. Although the use of tubes should be individualized, we prefer to use them in small infants, except in the presence of infection, presence of stones, poorly functioning kidneys, or technical problems during surgery. In adults, we prefer the use of an indwelling double J stent, that can be removed in 7–10 days or 3–6 weeks depending on the underlying problem. Its use in children is limited as its removal does necessitate endoscopy. In children, this would require an anesthetic as well as the risk of urethral injury. In adults, the stent may be removed under local anesthesia thereby eliminating any serious problem with its removal.

Exposure

The approach to the ureteropelvic junction may be done through any standard approach to the kidney. Advantages of the anterior approach are that the structures are distorted less and the spatial relationships are better preserved with the patient in the supine position. In slender patients and children, an anterior extraperitoneal approach gives satisfactory exposure. However, in heavily muscled and obese patients, the transperitoneal approach may be necessary. The flank procedure allows an excellent extraperitoneal approach to the ureteropelvic junction and its repair may be performed without difficulty. A major advantage is that the peritoneum has not been entered and, therefore, the risk of intestinal adhesions and subsequent obstruction are nonexistent. Transperitoneal approaches should be avoided in children for this reason. A posterior lumbotomy approach also is excellent in children but caution must be exercised if the pelvis is anterior or if other anatomic aberrations are present.

Anderson-Hynes Dismembered Pyeloplasty

Dismembered pyeloplasty (1) may be used in any form of ureteropelvic junction and is the most widely used repair today.

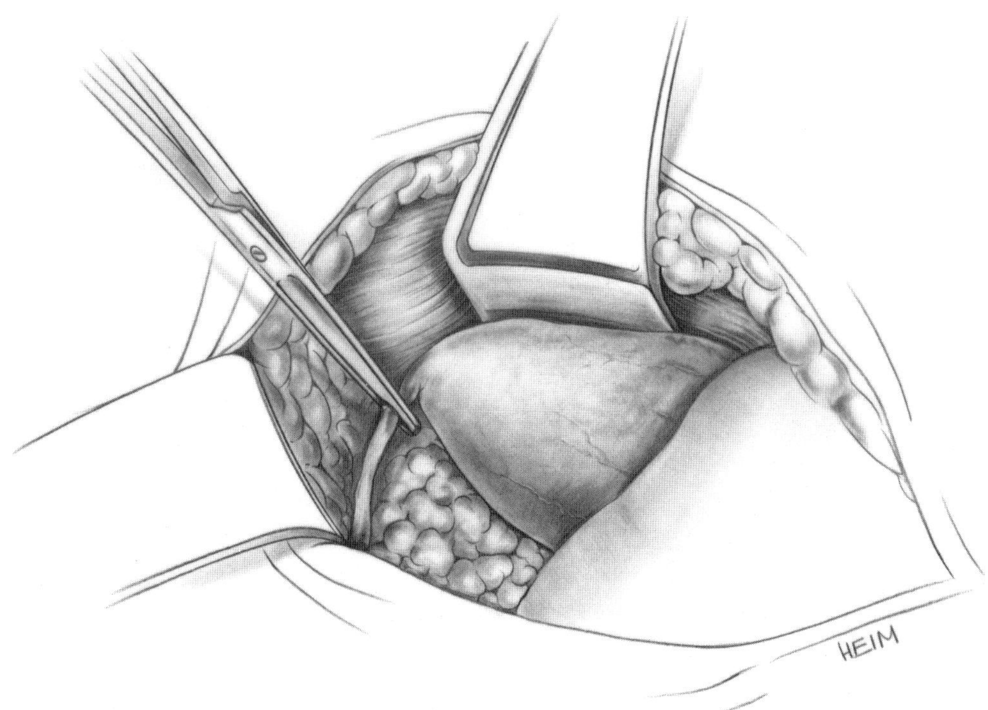

Figure 21.1. Mobilization of the entire pelvis and upper ureter should be done so that the ureteropelvic junction obstruction is identified. Care should be taken to leave adequate periureteral tissue to preserve blood supply to the upper ureter so that ischemia does not occur postoperatively. Under adequate exposure, the ureteropelvic junction obstruction is excised.

Figure 21.2. On the Pelvis, 4–0 chromic sutures are placed at the margins where excess pelvis will be excised. A small tacking suture is placed in the proximal end of the ureter to minimize handling and traumatic injury. The ureter is then incised for approximately 1–2 cm on the lateral portion of the ureter.

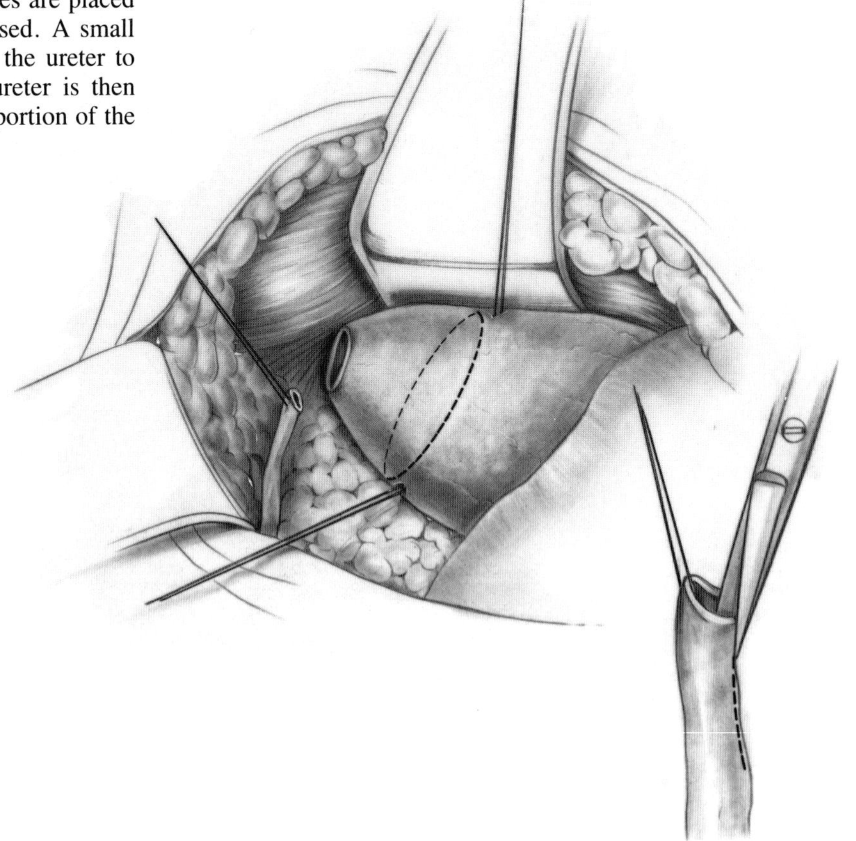

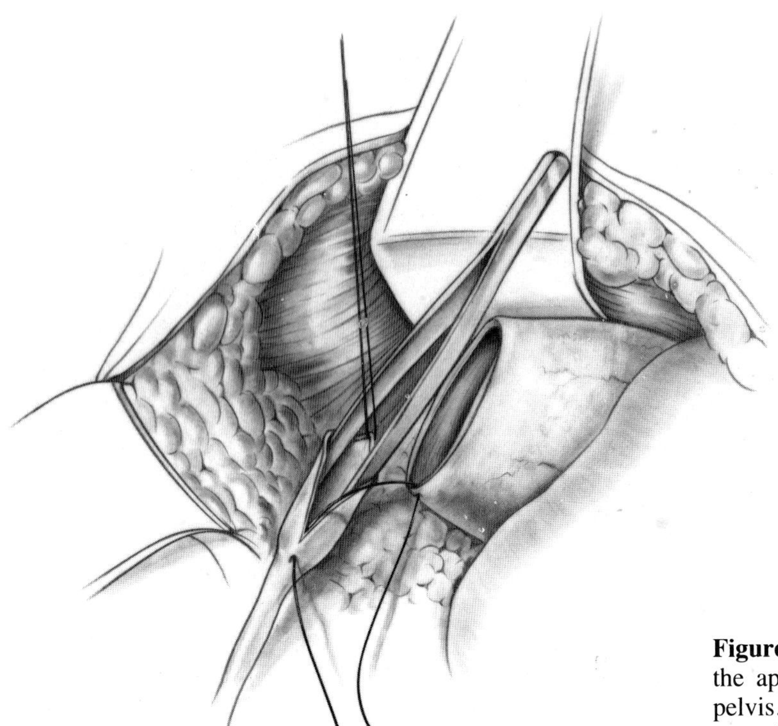

Figure 21.3. A 4–0 or 5–0 chromic suture is then placed at the apex of the incised ureter to the inferior portion of the pelvis. A pair of forceps is used to spread the internal diameter of the ureter to facilitate the placement of this suture.

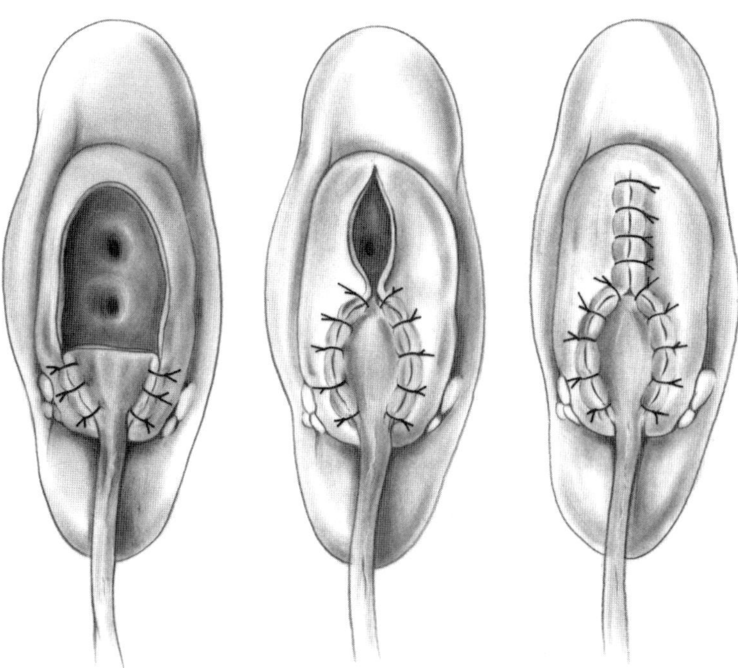

Figure 21.4. Interrupted absorbable sutures are then placed from the pelvis to the ureter for a mucosa-mucosa anastomosis. Care is taken to minimize the amount of ureteral tissue incorporated. The remaining pelvis is closed using either interrupted absorbable sutures or a simple running suture.

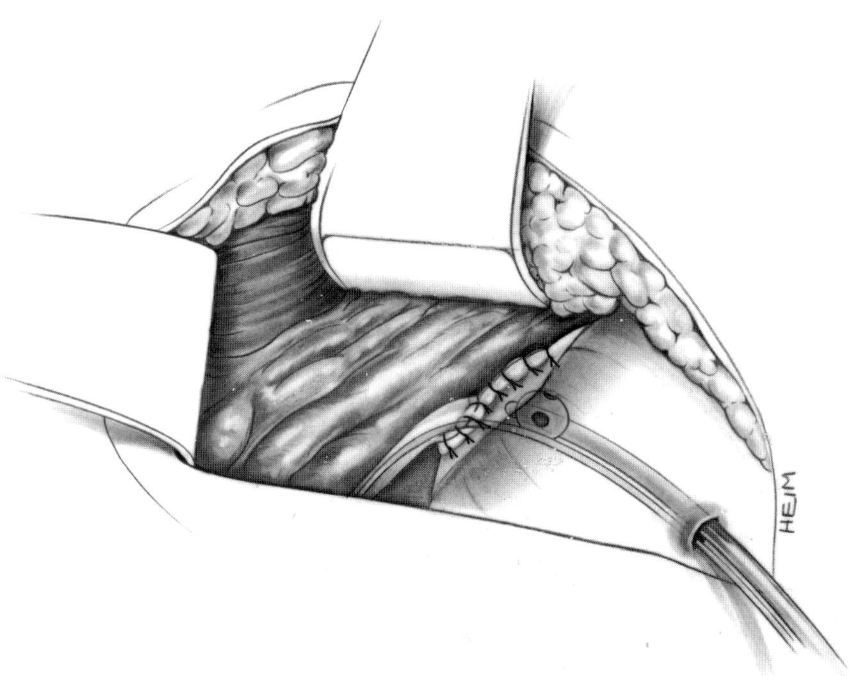

Figure 21.5. At the completion of the repair, the kidney is placed in its proper orientation in the renal bed. If one is using urinary diversion and ureteral stents as depicted here, they must be examined and irrigated for patency. A nephrostomy tube and stenting catheter are placed in the lower pole calix before the ureteropelvic anastomosis and left in place at the end of the procedure.

Figure 21.6. A ureteropelvic junction obstruction may be found with accessory vessels. A dismembered pyeloplasty is the procedure of choice in this fashion.

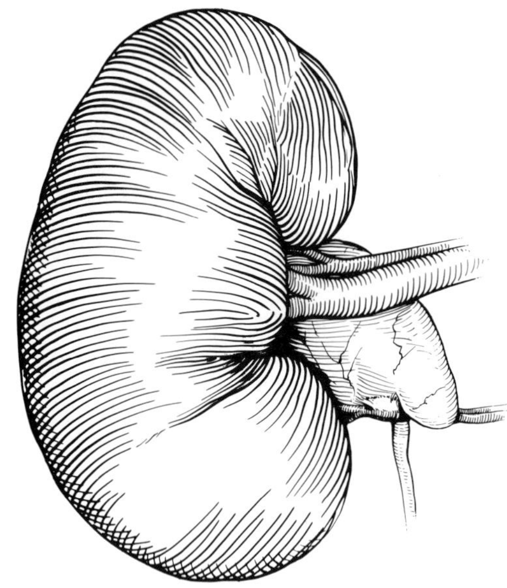

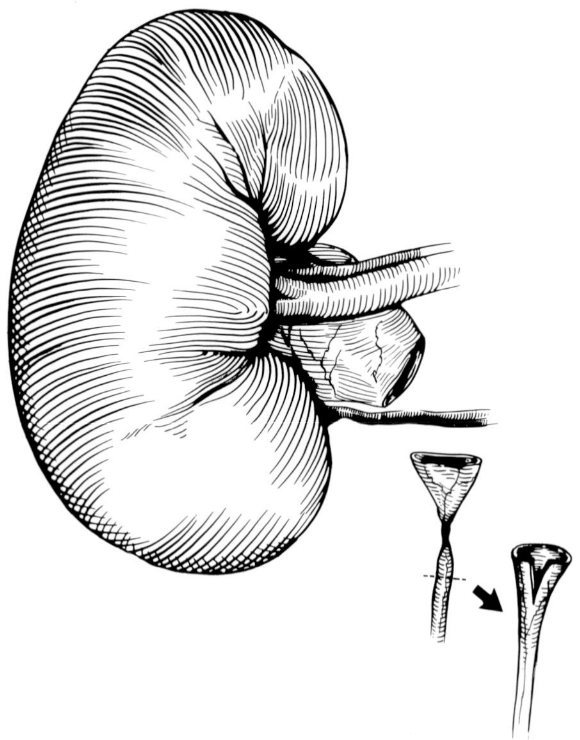

Figure 21.7. The lower pole vessels are mobilized free of the pelvis. The pelvis as well as the upper ureter are mobilized. The ureteropelvic junction is then excised so that the pelvis may be brought anterior to the vessels. The upper portion of the ureter is also excised with spatulation in the lateral aspect of the ureter as in a standard dismembered pyeloplasty.

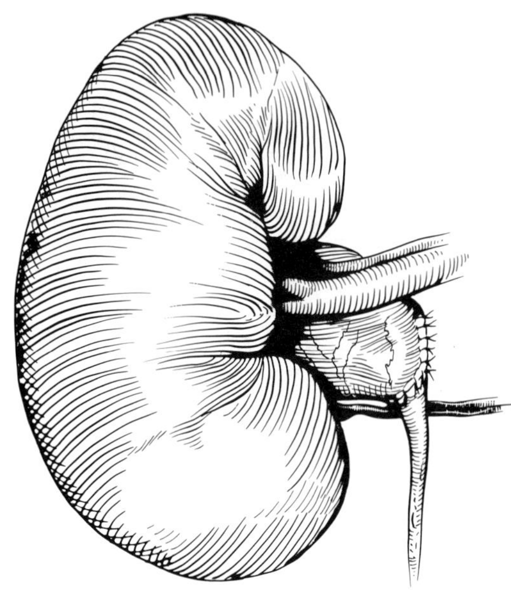

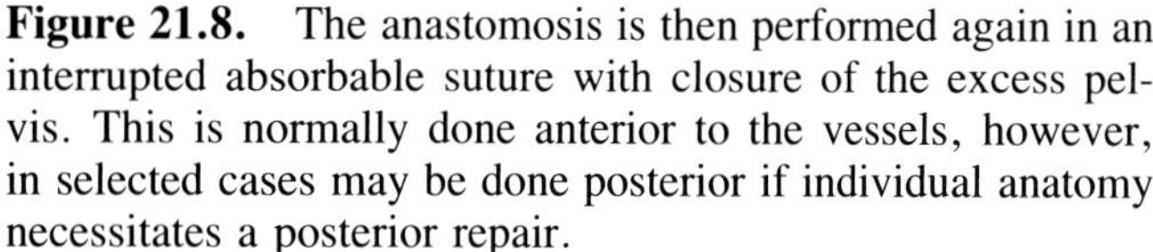

Figure 21.8. The anastomosis is then performed again in an interrupted absorbable suture with closure of the excess pelvis. This is normally done anterior to the vessels, however, in selected cases may be done posterior if individual anatomy necessitates a posterior repair.

Ureterocalicostomy

For revisions of pyeloplasty failures as well as intrarenal pelvic obstruction certain innovative techniques must be considered. Ureterocalicostomy is a technique that allows a complete dependent drainage of the kidney by using the lower pole calix. Most commonly, this is seen in revisions of pyeloplasties although any anatomic case in which there is difficulty approaching the pelvis or the kidney may be appropriate for a ureterocalicostomy.

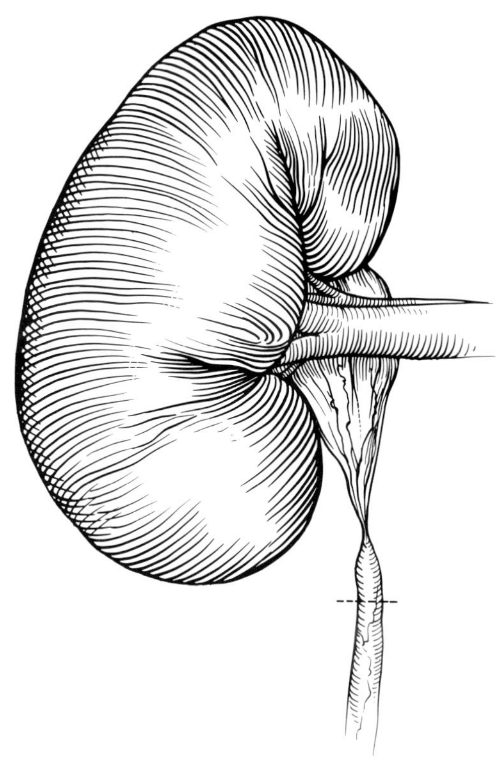

Figure 21.9. The ureter is traced inferiorly up to the kidney where fibrosis and blood supply necessitates ureterocalicostomy. The ureter is then excised at its superior viable position.

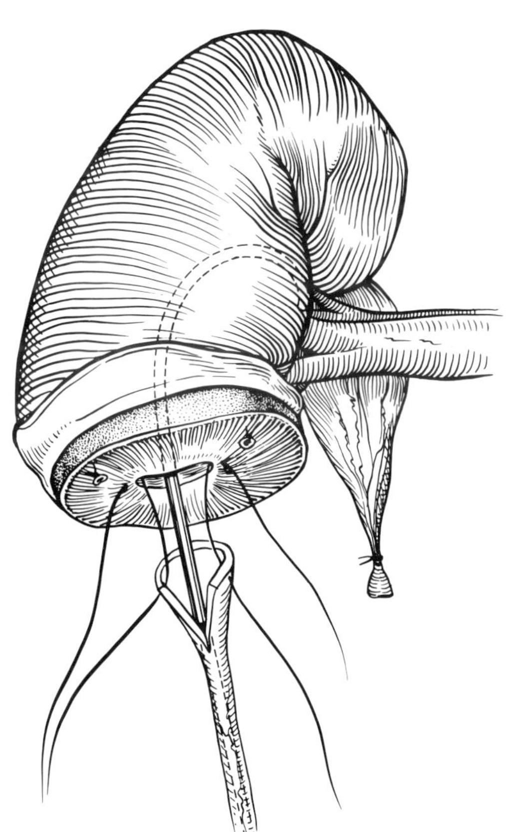

Figure 21.10. A lower pole heminephrectomy is performed. It is essential that an adequate amount of renal tissue be excised so that the lower pole calix is easily reached. To avoid strictures of the anastomosis, one must excise adequate amounts of renal tissue. The ureter is then spatulated on its lateral aspect as in a dismembered pyeloplasty. Absorbable sutures are then placed through the apex of the spatulation and it is brought through the mucosa of the calix. A suture is placed at 180° from the previous suture. A double J indwelling ureteral stent is placed to position itself within the pelvis and down to the bladder.

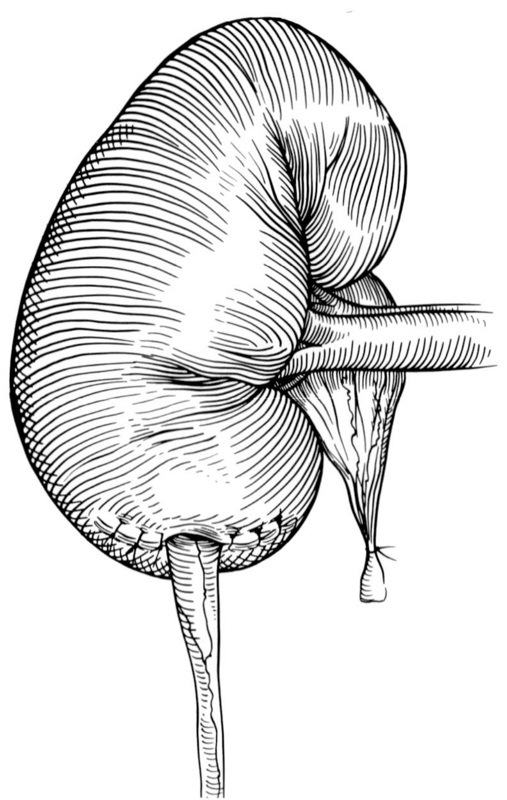

Figure 21.11. The remaining mucosa to mucosa anastomosis is performed using 5–0 absorbable interrupted sutures.

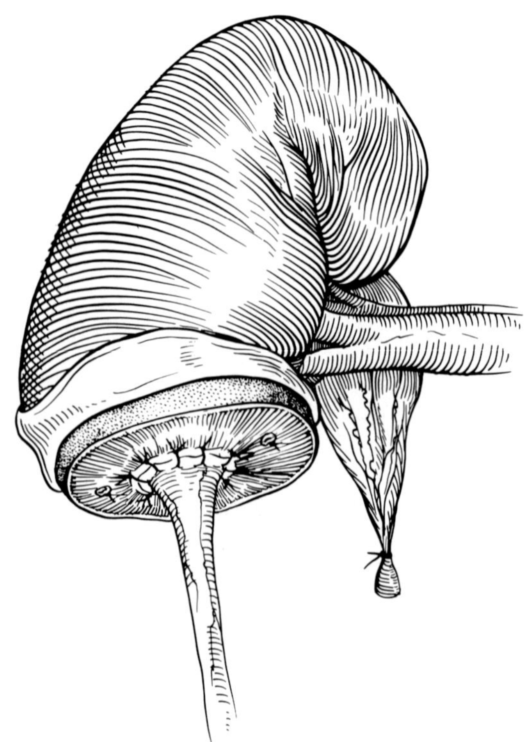

Figure 21.12. The capsule of the kidney is then closed over the previously resected parenchyma using interrupted 3–0 chromic with care being taken to avoid constricting the ureter. The indwelling stent is left for a minimum of 3 weeks and is then removed under local anesthesia.

Foley Y-V Plasty

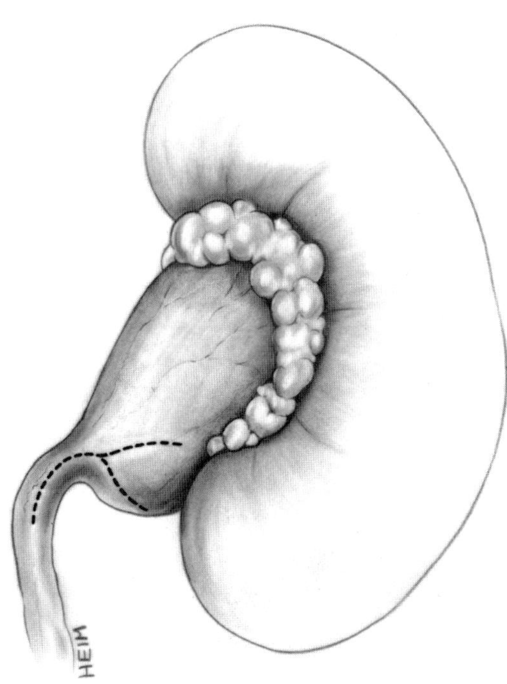

Figure 21.13. The Foley Y-V plasty (3) is indicated when ureteropelvic junction obstruction is associated with a high insertion of the ureter into the renal pelvis. A triangular flap is outlined in the dependent portion of the renal pelvis with its base arising from the medial aspect of the lower pole of the kidney and its apex at the point of the ureteropelvic junction obstruction. The future ureteral incision is carried for a distance of 2–3 cm on the anterior lateral surface of the ureter.

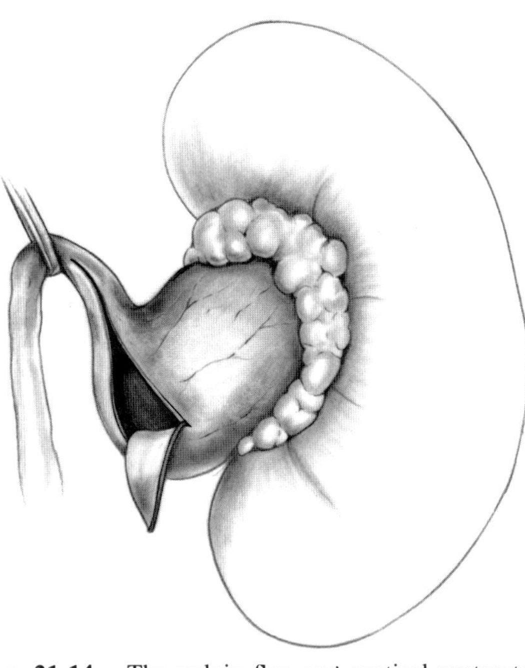

Figure 21.14. The pelvic flap and vertical ureterotomy is then developed with a scalpel and dissection scissors. Again, care must be taken to preserve the blood supply to the upper ureter and renal pelvis.

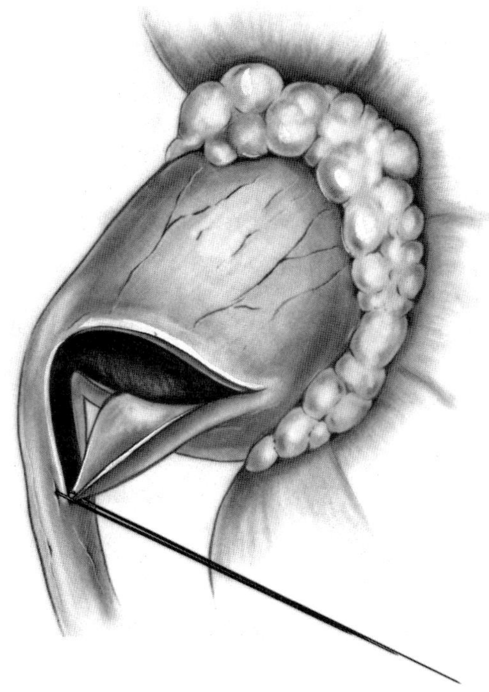

Figure 21.15. The apex of the pelvic flap is then brought to the apex of the ureterotomy incision with a stay suture of 5–0 chromic. It is wise to place the nephrostomy tube and ureteral stent at this time if one elects to use urinary diversion.

Figure 21.16. The posterior wall of the renal pelvis is then closed using interrupted 5–0 chromic with care being taken upon compromising the ureteral edge of the incision. Running sutures may be used, however, we prefer interrupted sutures.

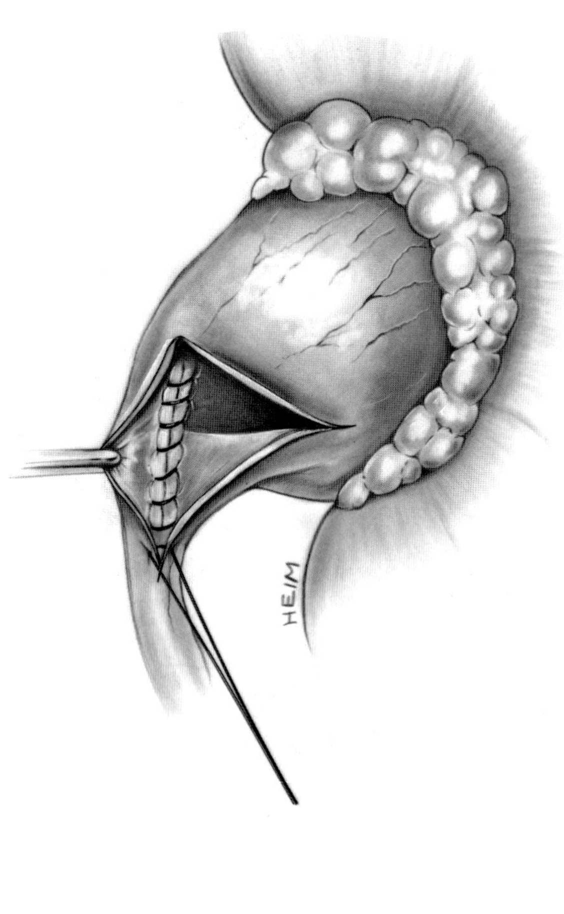

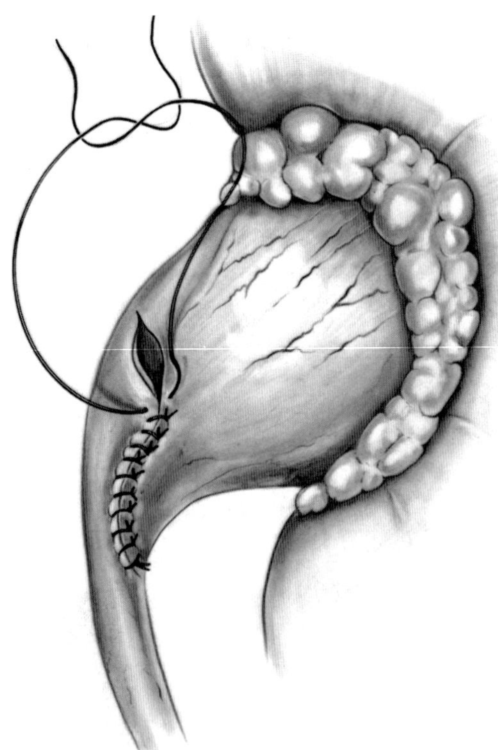

Figure 21.17. The anterior wall of the pelvic flap is anastomosed then using interrupted or running 5–0 chromic.

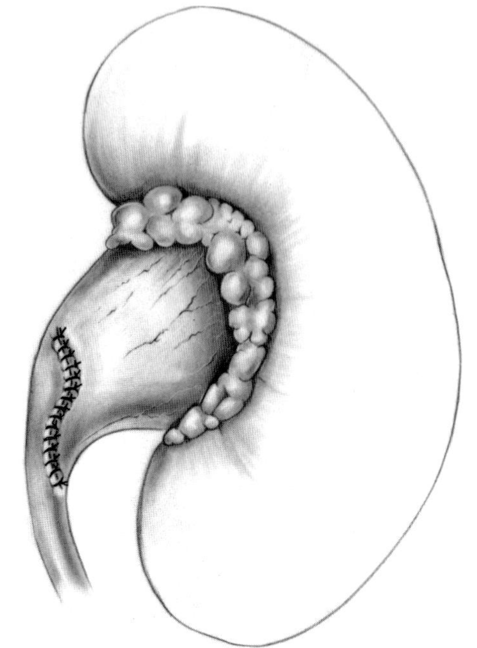

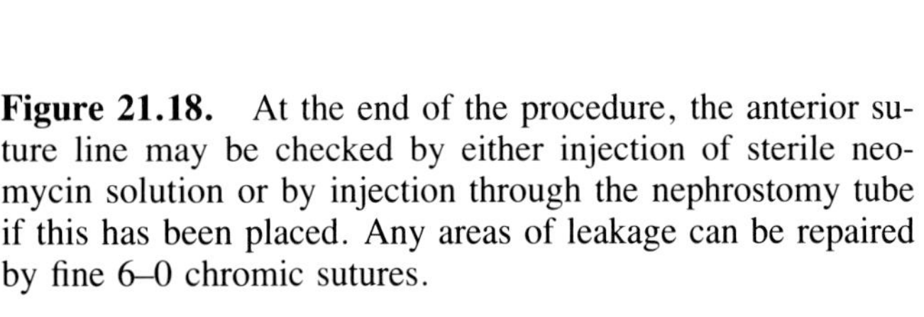

Figure 21.18. At the end of the procedure, the anterior suture line may be checked by either injection of sterile neomycin solution or by injection through the nephrostomy tube if this has been placed. Any areas of leakage can be repaired by fine 6–0 chromic sutures.

Procedures for Ureteropelvic Junction Obstruction

Standard Flap Techniques (Culp, Scardino)

The Culp spiral flap (2) and the Scardino vertical flap (4) pyeloplasties may be employed where the obstruction is accompanied by an already dependent ureteropelvic junction.

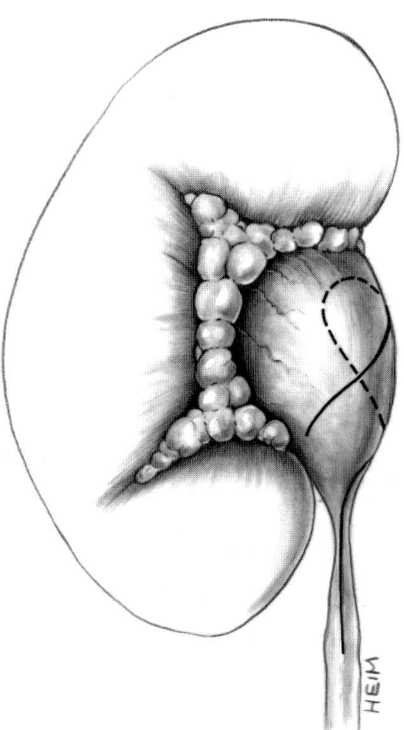

Figure 21.19. A spiral flap is outlined over the anterior medial surface of the renal pelvis with the lower limb being carried down the anterior surface of the ureter beneath the ureteropelvic junction obstruction. The flap is then opened by sharp dissection, again, preserving the blood supply to the renal pelvis and upper ureter.

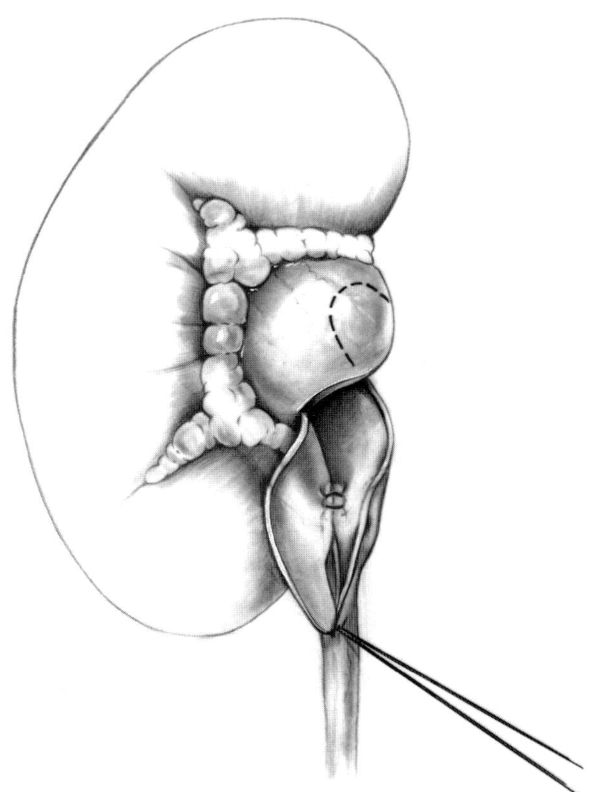

Figure 21.20. The apex of the spiral flap is then brought to the apex of the ureterotomy incision and secured with a stay suture of 5–0 chromic. The posterior anastomosis is then completed with interrupting or running 5–0 chromic suture.

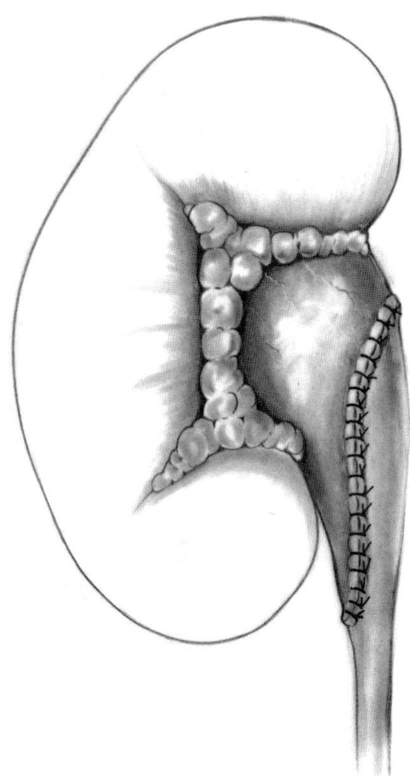

Figure 21.21. The anterior portion of the spiral flap is then anastomosed to the medial edge of the incised ureter completing the repair.

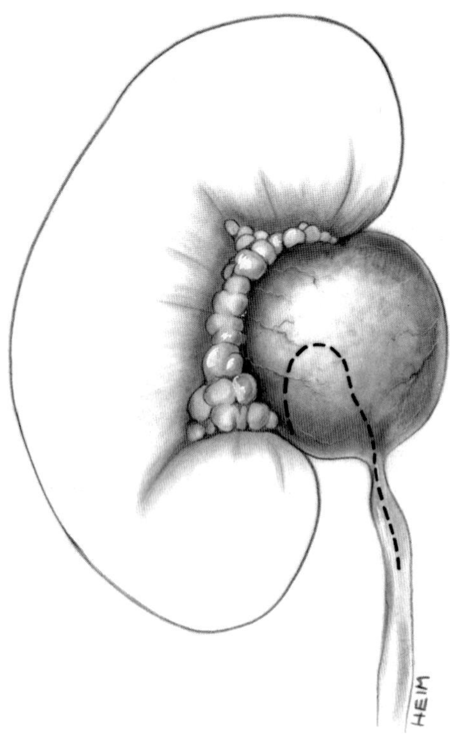

Figure 21.22. The Scardino vertical flap again is outlined over the anterior surface of the renal pelvis with the medial limb carried down the anterior ureteral wall to a point 1–2 cm below the ureteral obstruction.

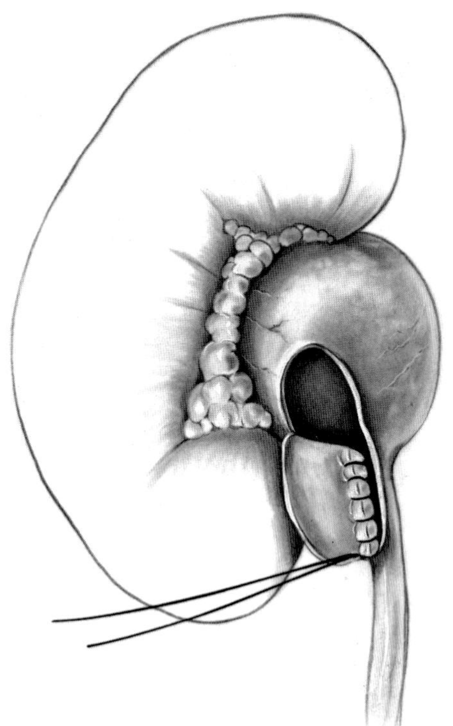

Figure 21.23. The apex of the vertical flap is brought to the apex of the ureterotomy incision and held by a stay suture of 5–0 chromic. The posterior anastomosis is completed with interrupted 4–0 or 5–0 chromic suture. This is secured bringing the medial aspect of the pelvic flap into apposition with the lateral edge of the ureterotomy incision.

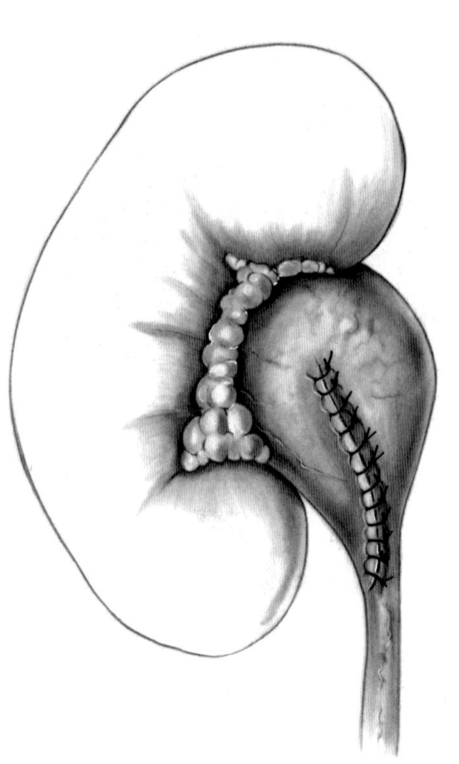

Figure 21.24. The anterior anastomosis is then completed by an interrupted 4–0 or 5–0 chromic suture of the lateral aspect of the vertical flap to the medial aspect of the ureterotomy incision. Again, the pelvis may be tested for leakage with either direct injectable neomycin solution or injection through a previously placed nephrostomy tube.

Intubated Ureterotomy (Davis)

The Davis intubated ureterotomy may be combined with one of the flap procedures or the dismembered pyeloplasty if an unusually long stricture is present in the upper ureter. Although rarely used today, the Davis intubated ureterotomy may be used as a definitive procedure.

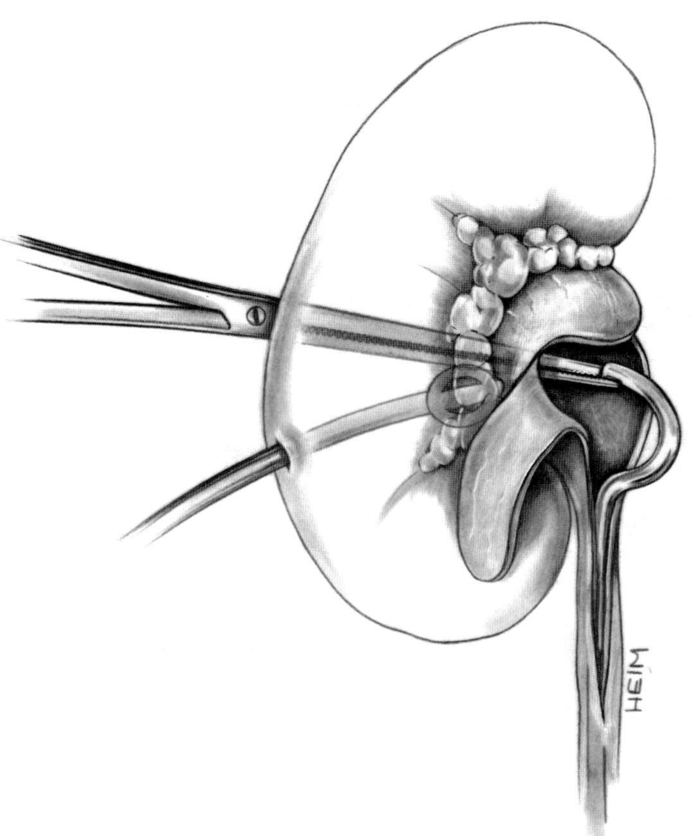

Figure 21.25. The incision is carried down the ureter through the strictured portion well into the normal ureter. Before the pyeloplasty is performed, a stenting catheter is passed down the ureter into the bladder and brought out laterally through the cortex of the kidney. A nephrostomy tube is also placed through the lower pole calix and anchored in place with a 3–0 chromic.

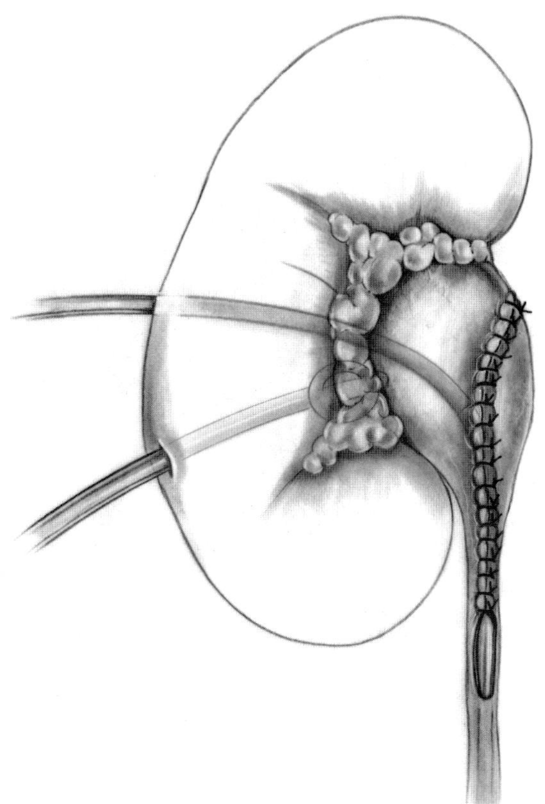

Figure 21.26. The pyeloplasty is then completed and the ureter is then left open over the stenting catheter. All tubes are left indwelling for a minimal period of 6 weeks after which the ureterostomy catheter is withdrawn. An antegrade pyelogram at this point is done to demonstrate patency of the ureter after which the nephrostomy tube is removed.

Capsule Flap Technique (Thompson)

The Thompson capsule flap pyeloplasty (6) is indicated when the renal pelvis has been damaged by disease or operative trauma such that an insufficient amount of pelvis is left for performance of a satisfactory pyeloplasty. This often occurs after removal of calculi through a small intrarenal pelvis that may be associated with fibrosis and inflammatory reaction. Depending upon the location and degree of pelvic destruction, the kidney may be approached either anteriorly or through a standard flank incision.

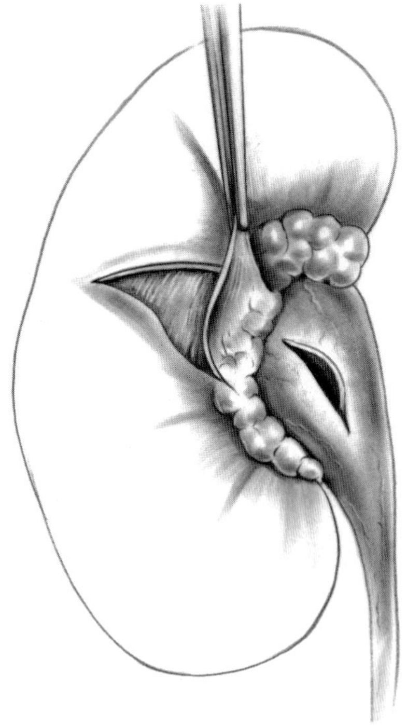

Figure 21.27. An incision is made through the ureteropelvic junction by sharp dissection. A triangular flap of adjacent kidney capsule is outlined and developed by sharp dissection.

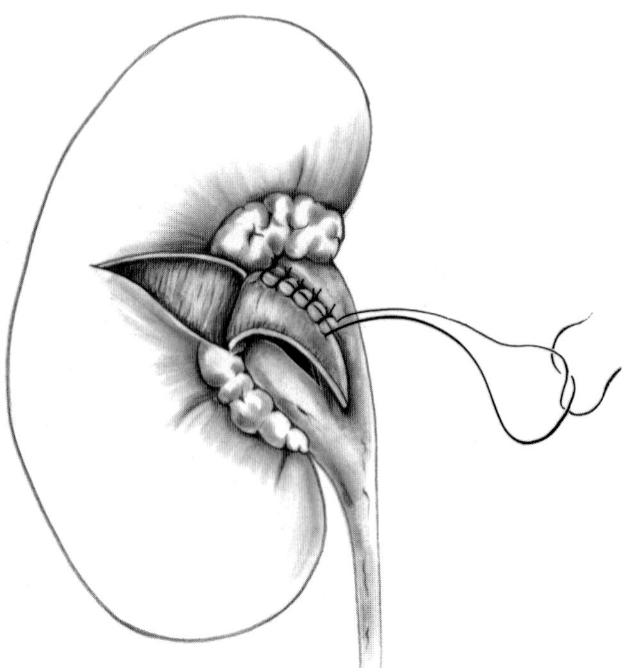

Figure 21.28. The flap is brought down to cover the pelvic and ureteral defect using interrupted 5–0 chromic suture.

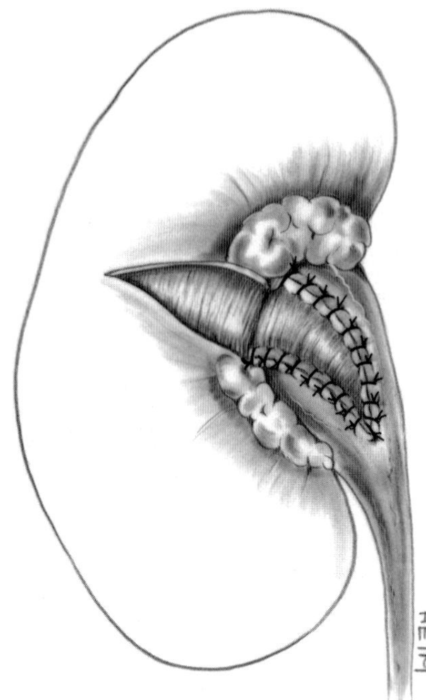

Figure 21.29. The anastomosis is then completed again in a watertight fashion with interrupted 4–0 or 5–0 chromic sutures. Again, in most cases requiring this type of procedure, a nephrostomy tube and stent is advised.

Postoperative Care

Postoperative care should include appropriate antibacterial therapy and adequate monitoring renal functions. The retroperitoneal space should be drained for a minimal of 7–10 days. In cases where stenting catheters and nephrostomy tubes are employed, the stent should be removed in 7–14 days depending upon the adequacy of repair and level of renal function. An antegrade pyelogram should then be performed. The nephrostomy tube may be clamped after adequate demonstration of the ureteropelvic junction integrity. If this is tolerated by the patient, it may be removed the following day. The indwelling double J Surgitek catheter stent may be left in place from 7–21 days or longer depending upon the individual case.

References

1. Anderson JC, Hynes W: Retrocaval ureter: A case diagnosed preoperatively and treated successfully by a plastic operation. *Br J Urol* 21:209, 1949.
2. Culp OS, DeWeerd JH: A pelvic flap operation for certain types of ureteropelvic obstruction: preliminary report. *Mayo Clin Proc* 26:483, 1951.
3. Foley FEB: New plastic operation for stricture at ureteropelvic junction. *J Urol* 38:643, 1937.
4. Scardino PL, Prince CL: Vertical flap ureteropelvioplasty—preliminary report. *South Med J* 46:325, 1953.
5. Schwyzer A: New pyelo-ureteral plastic for hydronephrosis. *Surg Clin North Am* 3:1441, 1923.
6. Thompson IM, Baker J, Robards VL Jr, Kovacsi L, Ross G Jr: Clinical experience with renal capsule flap pyeloplasty. *J Urol* 101:487, 1969.

Suggested Readings

Hawthorne NJ, Zincke H, Kelalis PP: Ureterocalicostomy: An alternative to nephrectomy. *J Urol* 115:583, 1976.

Hellstrom J: Aetiological and therapeutic experiences concerning kidney and ureteral stones. *Br J Urol* 21:9, 1949.

Murphy LJT: *The History of Urology*. Springfield, IL, Charles C Thomas, 1972, pp. 201–208.

CHAPTER 22

Surgery for Renal Trauma

JACK W. McANINCH

INDICATIONS FOR SURGERY

In his *Apologie and Treatise* of 1585, the French surgeon Ambrose Pare describes a patient with gross hematuria after a gunshot wound to the abdomen and thorax (1). This represents the first recorded evidence of penetrating renal injury. Even today, the presence of blood in the urine remains the single most important sign in the diagnosis of a renal injury. In 1884, Weir recommended nephrectomy for wounds of the kidney (2).

The resuscitation of the acutely injured patient is essential and initially includes control of hemorrhage and shock. The abdomen and chest should be examined carefully for evidence of injury. Flank contusions, lower rib fractures, and penetrating wounds of the upper abdomen, flank, and back should prompt suspicion immediately. Although hematuria is the best indicator of renal injury, major renal injuries have been reported without red blood cells being found in the urine.

Signs, symptoms, and laboratory findings that suggest renal injury should prompt immediate radiologic evaluation (3). This process of staging the injury begins with high-dose (2 ml/kg) excretory urography (IVP). Should the patient require immediate abdominal exploration, the IVP can be obtained in the operating suite. In some instances in which the patient is hemodynamically stable after resuscitation, the trauma surgeon may wish to evaluate the abdominal injury by computed tomography (CT) (4). In such cases, a renal CT should be done in lieu of IVP. Renal CT or arteriography should also be done when the injury is not clearly defined on IVP.

The indications for renal operation are based primarily upon clinical conditions, but the radiographic findings complement the urologic surgeon's knowledge by better defining the extent of injury. Absolute indications for renal exploration after trauma include an expanding retroperitoneal hematoma or a pulsatile hematoma (5). Relative indications are: urinary extravasation; nonviable renal tissue in association with a parenchymal laceration; and arterial injury. Many patients exhibit a combination of indications to prompt renal exploration. In certain situations, the trauma surgeon may choose to perform a laparotomy to manage an associated organ injury. This provides the urologic surgeon the opportunity to repair major renal injuries that might otherwise have been managed nonoperatively. This can be done with minimal risk of renal loss and can reduce the potential for late complications (6).

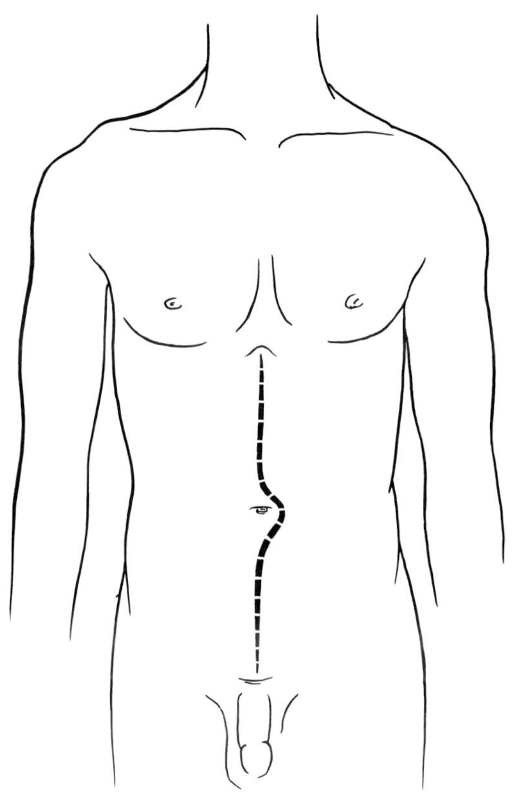

Figure 22.1. A transabdominal midline incision provides complete access to the intraabdominal viscera and vasculature at risk for injury. Major bleeding noted upon opening the abdominal cavity should be controlled immediately with laparotomy packs, followed by surgical control and repair (7). The bowel, liver, spleen, pancreas, and other organs should be inspected systematically and carefully.

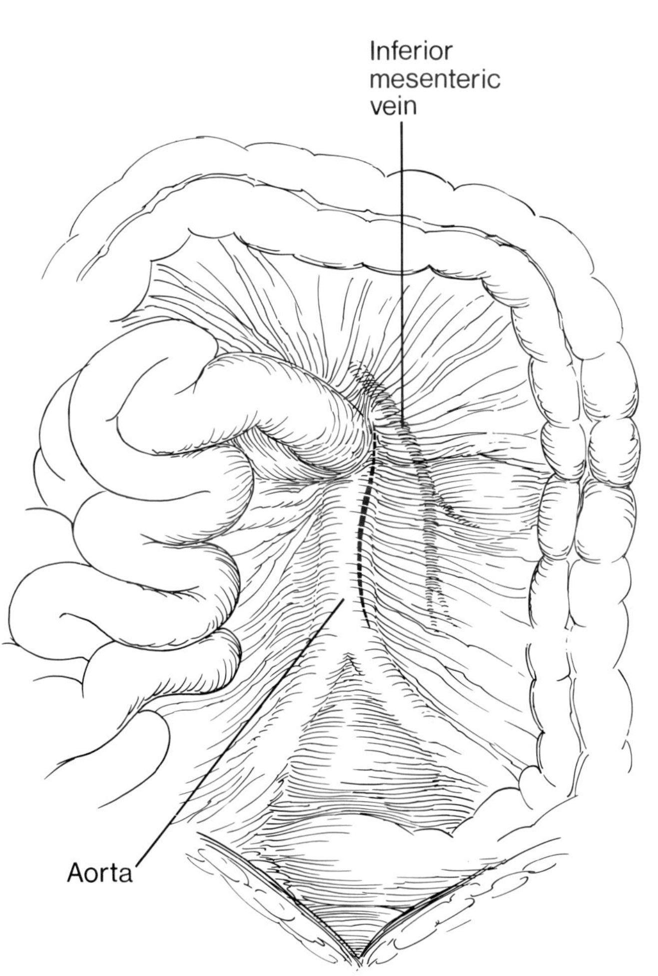

Figure 22.2. The surgical approach to the kidney can be performed easily through the transabdominal midline incision. The transverse colon is lifted from the abdomen superiorly and placed on moist laparotomy packs. The small bowel is then lifted on its mesentery superiorly and to the right to expose the retroperitoneum. An incision is made in the retroperitoneum just medial to the inferior mesenteric vein over the aorta. This incision should begin just above the bifurcation of the aorta and superior to the inferior mesenteric artery; it is extended superiorly up to the ligament of Treitz. Large retroperitoneal hematomas may be noted when the retroperitoneum is exposed and the aorta may not be palpable. The inferior mesenteric vein then becomes a key landmark in determining the site of the incision. Once the incision in the retroperitoneum has been made, one can dissect safely in this avascular plane down to the anterior surface of the aorta. When the aorta has been identified, its anterior surface should be dissected superiorly.

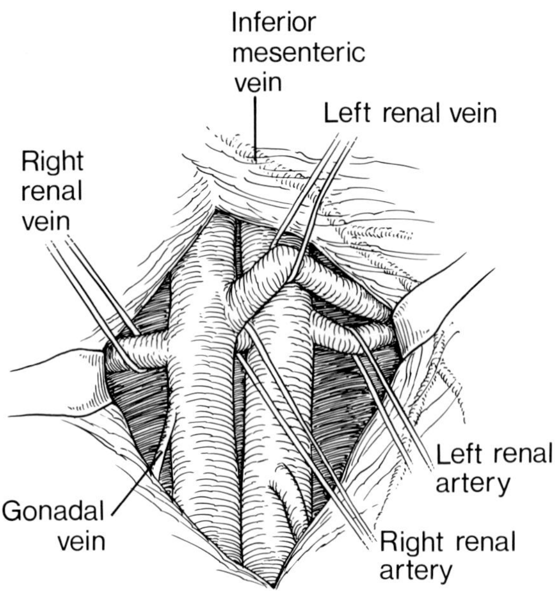

Figure 22.3. The first major vessel encountered will be the left renal vein crossing over the anterior aortic surface. This is a key anatomic landmark in locating the remaining renal vessels. The left renal artery will usually lie just superior and posterior to the left renal vein as it exits the aorta to the left kidney.

The right renal artery will also be superior to the left renal vein and exit the aorta medially behind the vena cava. The right renal vein can be isolated through this incision and usually enters the vena cava at about the same level as the left renal vein. Should the renal vein be difficult to isolate through this incision, the alternative approach is to mobilize the second portion of the duodenum over the vena cava to expose the vein. The vessels going to the involved kidney should be individually isolated with vessel loops. If bleeding is heavy, vascular clamps should be applied; otherwise, control with vessel loops will be adequate until the kidney has been exposed completely and the full extent of injury determined. By not clamping the vessels, renal perfusion is continuous and warm ischemia is avoided.

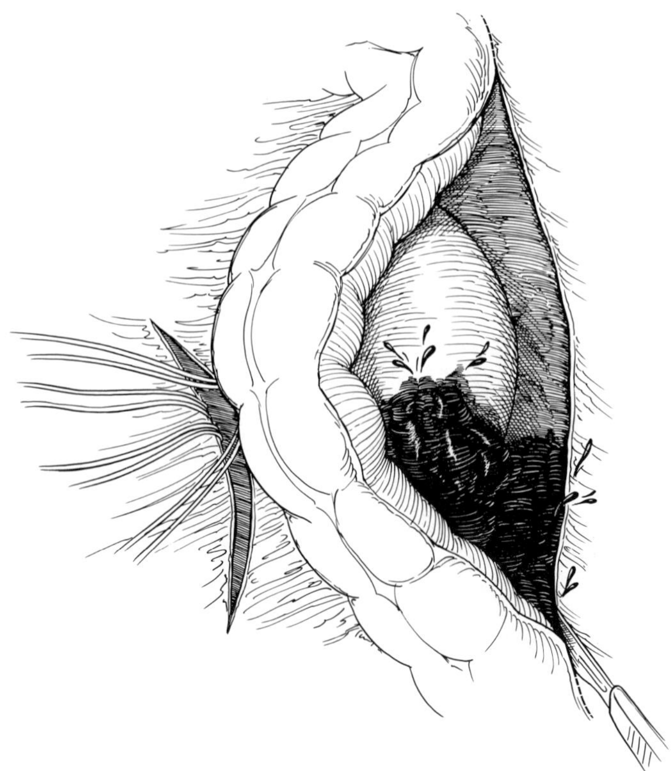

Figure 22.4. The colon is then reflected medially by an incision in the retroperitoneum just lateral to the colon. Dissection is carried out through the hematoma to expose the kidney and Gerota's fascia. The entire renal surface and vasculature must be exposed because often more than one injury has occurred: e.g., renal laceration and vascular injury. Should heavy bleeding be encountered, Rummel tourniquets can be applied to the vessel loops for vascular occlusion and control of bleeding.

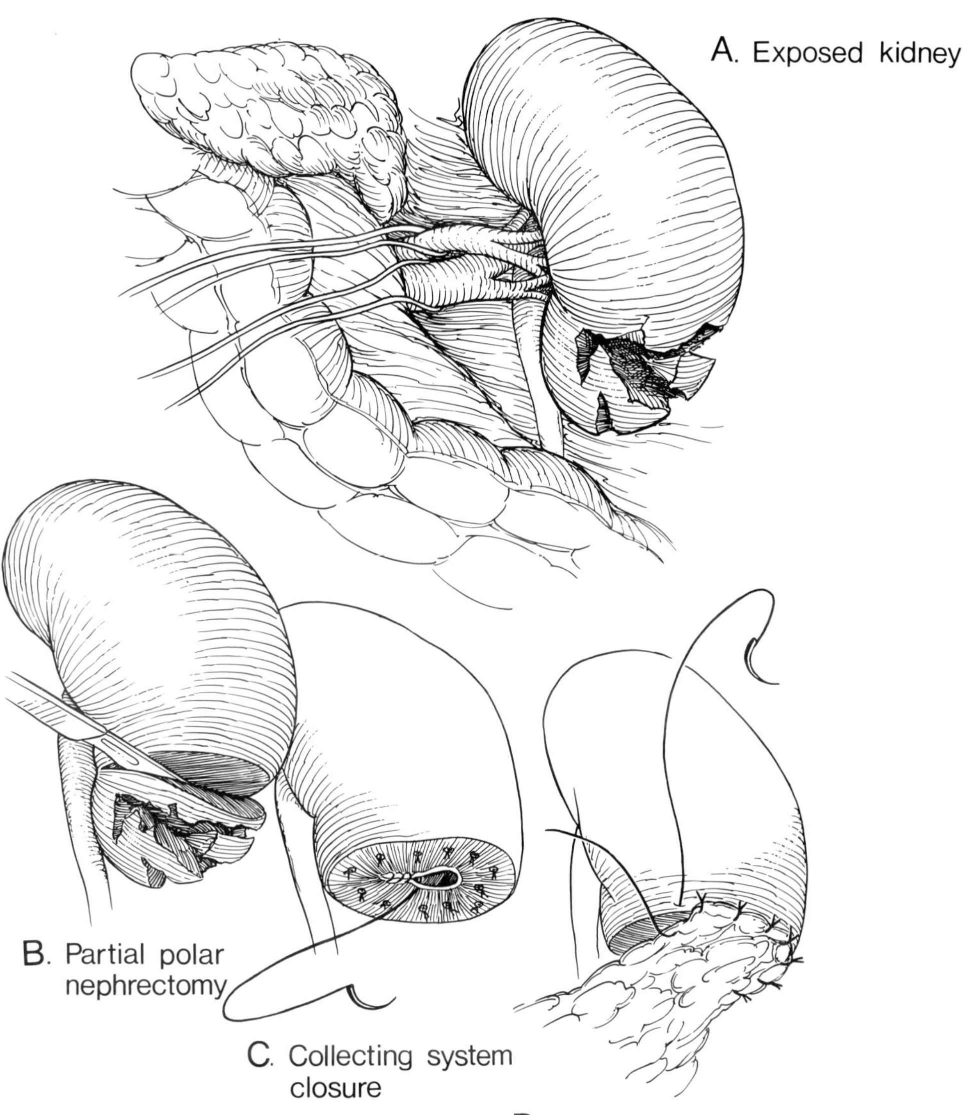

Figure 22.5. **A,** once the kidney is exposed, the sites of injury will become obvious. For major polar injury, partial nephrectomy offers the best management. If the renal capsule has not been destroyed by the injury, it should be preserved carefully. **B,** the injured area should be sharply dissected and debrided. If major bleeding occurs, the renal artery should be occluded, but not the renal vein. Should ischemia time in excess of 30 min be expected, the kidney should be cooled with slush ice.

After removal of all nonviable tissue, points of bleeding are individually suture-ligated with 4–0 chromic sutures. **C,** the collecting system is closed watertight with a running suture of 4–0 chromic. Absorbable gelatin sponge (Gelfoam) or microcollagen hemostatic material can be applied to the parenchymal surface to increase hemostasis. When sufficient capsule has been preserved, it is closed over the defect with a running suture. **D,** otherwise, an omental pedicle flap graft can be used to cover the existing parenchymal defect. The omentum can be brought through a window in the colon mesentery or brought over the colon laterally because of the defect. It is sutured into place with interrupted 4–0 chromic sutures, which should draw up only very small amounts of parenchyma and any existing capsule. The omental pedicle flap covers the defect with viable vascular tissue that has excellent lymphatic drainage to propagate wound healing.

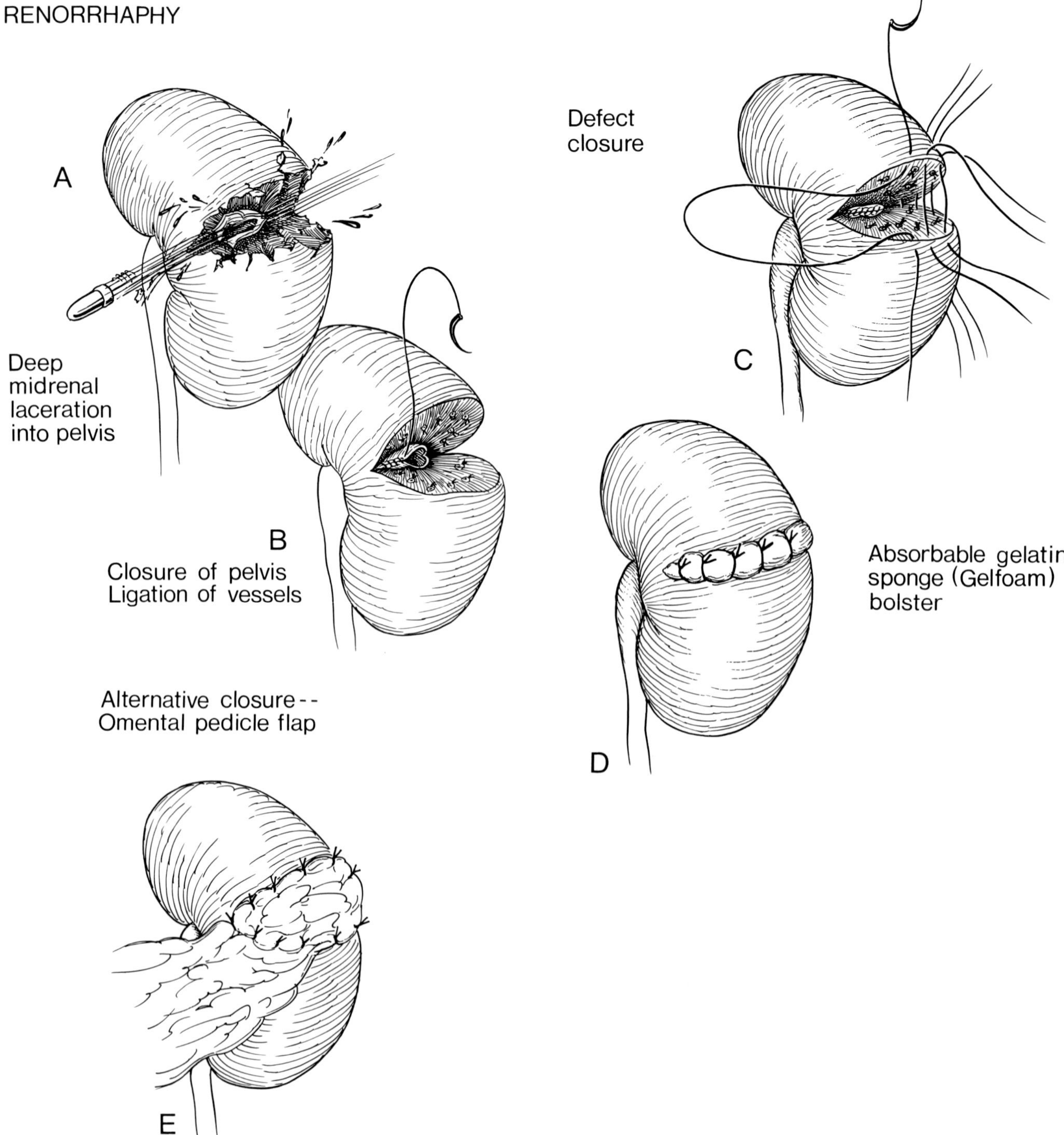

Figure 22.6. **A,** major injuries to the midportion of the kidney are more difficult to repair. The area must be completely debrided and all nonviable tissue removed. **B,** sites of bleeding should be individually ligated with a 4–0 chromic sutures and the collecting system closed watertight. Gelfoam or microcollagen hemostatic agents are again useful to control persistent vascular oozing and Gelfoam should be used in the closure when sufficient capsule is present. **C,** in the reconstruction, monofilament absorbable 3–0 sutures are placed in an interrupted fashion to include capsule and a small amount of parenchyma. The Gelfoam bolster is then placed over the sutures. **D,** as the individual sutures are tied, the bolster adds security to the reconstruction and seals the parenchymal defect effectively to prevent bleeding and urinary extravasation. **E,** if the defect is so extensive that the bolster method will not effect closure, an omental pedicle flap graft can be used.

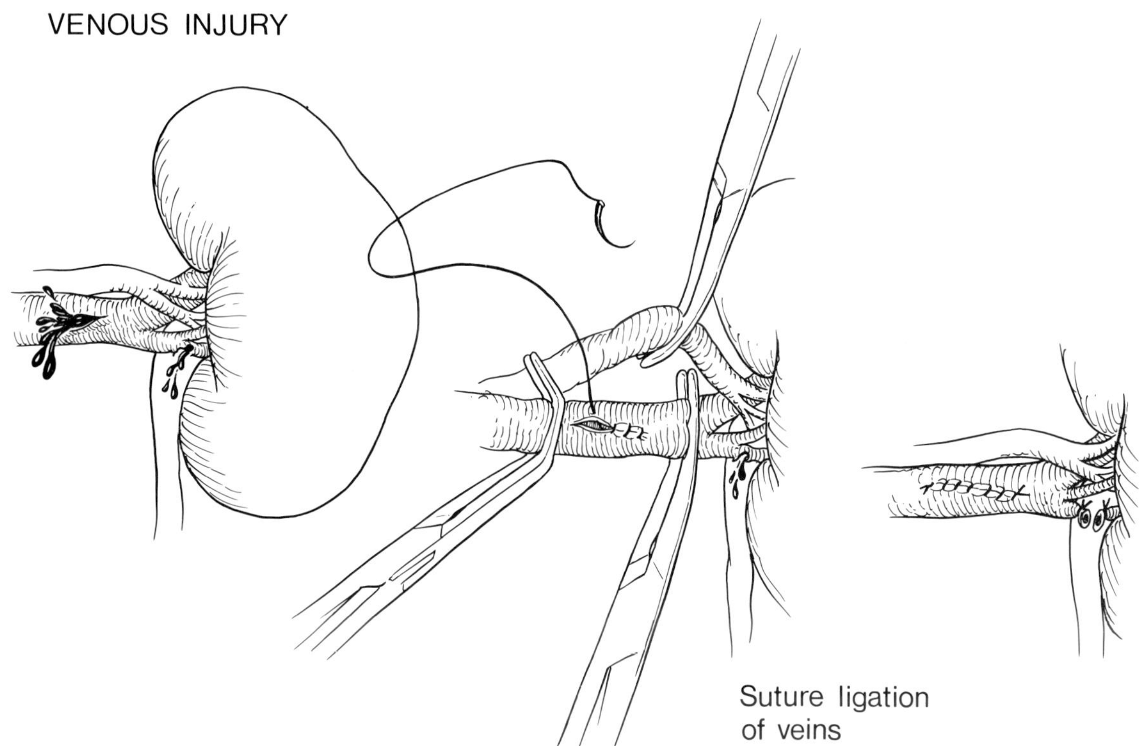

Figure 22.7. Renal vascular injuries are the major cause of renal loss. The techniques for renal arterial reconstruction are presented in other chapters. **A,** the venous system can be injured at the main renal vein or in the segmental vessels. Appropriate early control of the renal vessels will allow early and rapid access to the main renal vein. An occlusion clamp should be placed on the main renal artery to stop blood flow into the kidney. **B,** vascular clamps should then be applied proximal and distal to the venous laceration. A running suture of 5–0 vascular silk is then used to close the venous defect. **C,** lacerations in segmental renal veins can be managed by ligation of these vessels, which can be done without ischemic damage to the kidney because of the internal collateral circulation of the venous system.

Total nephrectomy is seldom necessary. In approximately 90% of cases, reconstruction is successful and can be undertaken despite fecal spillage from bowel injury, pancreatic injury, or other associated abdominal injuries. Drains should be left in the retroperitoneum when the abdominal cavity has been contaminated by fecal matter or when the potential for extravasation from the repaired collecting system exists. Nephrostomy drainage or internal stents are not used in the absence of associated ureteral injury.

POSTOPERATIVE CARE AND FOLLOW-UP

Urinary output should be monitored closely in the postreconstructive period. Gross blood in the urine usually clears within 24 hours. Fluid drainage from the flank drains should be checked for creatinine—a level equal to that of serum suggests peritoneal fluid rather than urine. Persistent drainage of urine through the flank drains is unlikely and these drains are usually removed within 48–72 hours. When left in place longer, they offer a source of infection to the retroperitoneal hematoma.

A radionuclide renal scan is usually obtained approximately 10 days and 3 months after reconstruction. An IVP or renal imaging study is done at about 3 months. These patients should have their blood pressure evaluated frequently in order to detect hypertension, and a 1-year follow-up IVP is recommended.

References

1. Keynes G: *The Apologie and Treatise of Ambrose Pare*. London, Falcon Books, 1951, pp. 54–61.
2. Meade RH: *An Introduction to the History of Surgery*. Philadelphia, WB Saunders, 1968.
3. Nicolaisen GS, McAninch JW, Marshall GA et al: Renal trauma: Reevaluation of the indications for radiographic assessment. *J Urol* 133:183, 1985.
4. Bretan PN Jr, McAninch JW, Federle MP, et al: Computerized tomographic staging of renal trauma: 85 consecutive cases. *J Urol* 136:561, 1986.
5. Carroll PR, McAninch JW: Operative indication in penetrating renal trauma. *J Trauma* 25:587, 1985.
6. Carlton CE Jr, Scott R Jr, Goldman M: The management of penetrating injuries of the kidney. *J Trauma* 8:1071, 1968.
7. McAninch JW, Carroll PR: Renal trauma: Kidney preservation through improved vascular control—a refined approach. *J Trauma* 22:285, 1982.

CHAPTER 23

Miscellaneous Renal Operations

MARK J. NOBLE

OPEN RENAL BIOPSY

Open renal biopsy sometimes is requested by an internist or nephrologist who requires a tissue diagnosis to aid in managing a patient's renal disease. It may also be helpful during a revascularization procedure if there is some question concerning chances for renal salvage. Open biopsy is usually preferred in patients with atypical anatomy, solitary kidney, mild coagulopathy, or other factors that predispose to risk with the percutaneous technique. More tissue is available for study with the open method, and complications such as arteriovenous fistula, perirenal hematoma, and gross hematuria are less likely as well. Although any anatomic approach may be utilized for this procedure, we prefer a posterior (dorsolumbotomy) incision as morbidity seems to be lower and patients are usually more comfortable postoperatively (1, 2). A general anesthetic is best, but in thin, cooperative patients, the procedure may be done under local anesthesia with little difficulty. Although a biopsy needle may be utilized once the kidney is exposed, bleeding is more difficult to control and less tissue can be sampled than by eliptical wedge biopsy. While either kidney (or both) may be biopsied by the posterior approach, the right is usually found to be in a more caudad direction on preoperative tomograms (or scan) and, thus, may be more easily exposed. The technique is illustrated below.

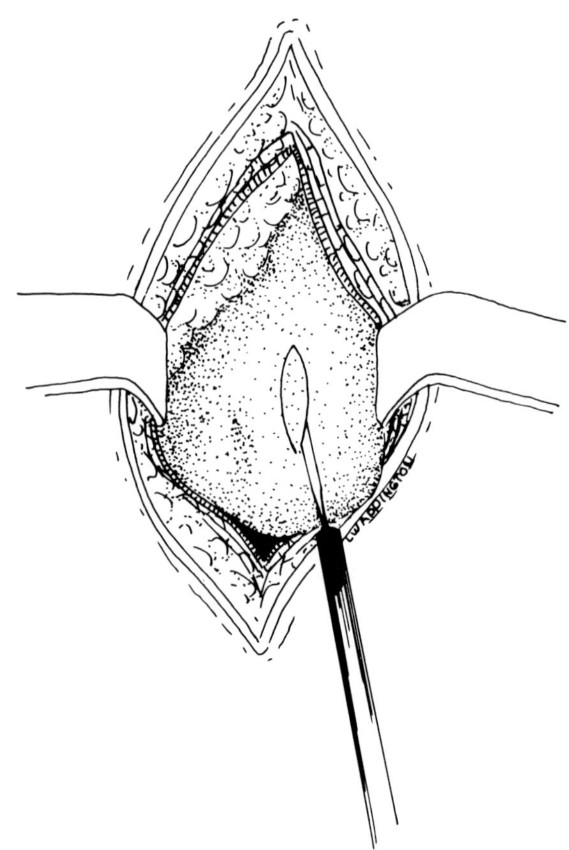

Figure 23.1. The posterior surface of the lower pole of the kidney is exposed. Care is taken to dissect perirenal fat off the capsular surface with minimal, meticulous use of cautery so as not to damage tissue in the area from which the specimen will be taken. It is sometimes helpful to pack this fat out of the field, or alternatively, it can be seized with a clamp and used to elevate the kidney more superficially into the wound. An elliptical incision is made in the renal capsule to define the size of the specimen, usually 1–2 cm long and 0.5–11.0 cm wide. The incision is then deepened on either side with a scalpel and bevelled so that the final wedge depth will include a generous segment of cortical tissue, usually at least 5–8 mm deep.

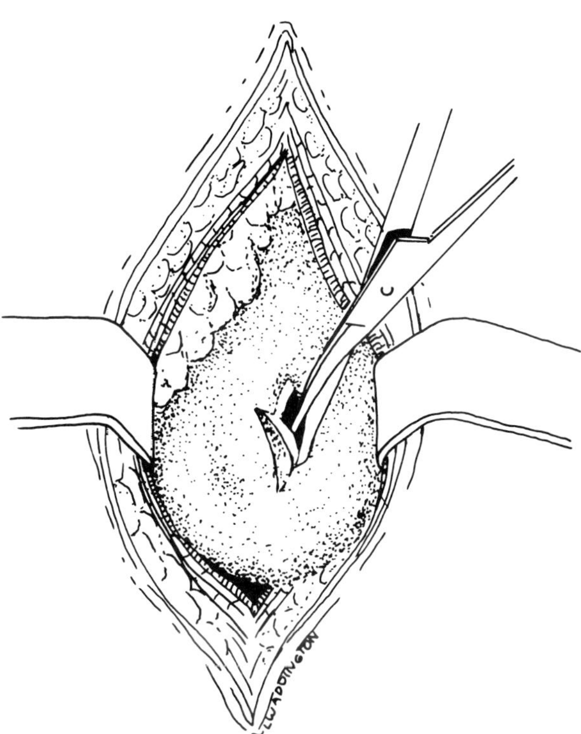

Figure 23.2. A fine Metzenbaum scissor is used to complete the transection of cortex at the bottom of the wedge and the tissue is then gently lifted out using the slightly spread scissor blades rather than a forceps (which might crush the specimen). Suction is avoided during this final maneuver to prevent loss of tissue into the suction tip. Tissue should be processed without delay by pathology to minimize autolysis and deterioration.

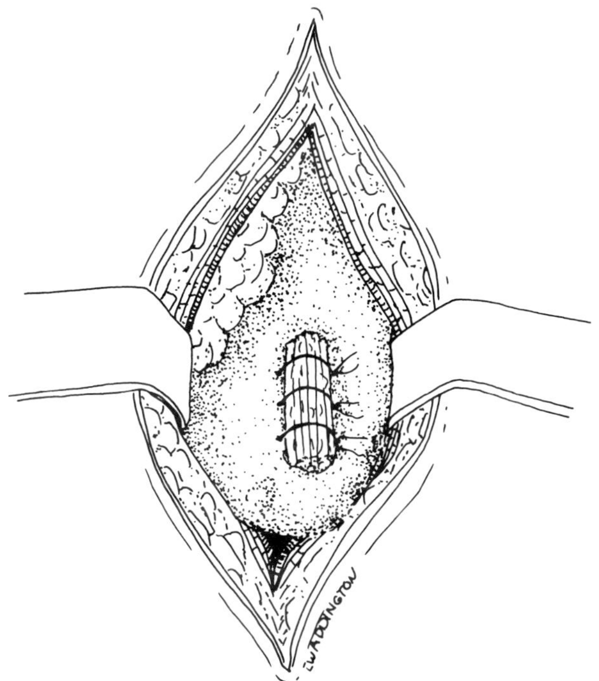

Figure 23.3. Absorbable 2–0 or 3–0 sutures are placed across the defect and gently tied over Oxycel or other absorbable, hemostatic material. No attempt is made to close the defect, as tight, large sutures necessary to accomplish this will necrose additional parenchyma and may rip. A "surgeon's" knot will keep the suture snug and hold the material onto the defect while the subsequent locking throws are being placed. By this method, pulling up on the suture will not be necessary and "tearing through" is avoided. Slight oozing at this point is easily controlled by pressure with a sponge-stick, and the area is then irrigated, reinspected, and the surgical wound closed in standard fashion without drainage.

SURGERY FOR RENAL CYSTS

In the past few years, widespread use of computed tomography (CT) to evaluate abdominal complaints has demonstrated that renal cysts are far more common than once thought, especially in the middle-to-older age groups. These cysts, when evaluated, nearly always turn out to be benign (3–5). Hence, routine percutaneous needle aspiration (or surgical exploration) is seldom needed and should be reserved for symptomatic cysts or cysts with atypical features. Any large renal cyst causing obstruction should be drained and open drainage with unroofing may prove more definitive than needle aspiration alone in preventing recurrence. The unsuspected cystic renal lesion encountered intraoperatively is sometimes best aspirated and unroofed because this is more cost-beneficial to the patient than risking a postoperative diagnostic workup and possible reexploration to clarify a questionable lesion. (Obviously, there will be circumstances where unroofing should not be carried out lightly, such as in the presence of a newly placed vascular prosthesis).

On occasion, a percutaneously drained cystic lesion will yield bloody fluid, positive cytology, or will otherwise appear suspicious for harboring neoplasm. The urologist must then weigh the evidence with regard to cancer risk and potential operative morbidity. Controversy still exists concerning this gray area, but in most cases where a potentially malignant lesion comes to surgical exploration, an anterior, transperitoneal approach (or other cancer incision) will be required and the lesion regarded as cancer until proved otherwise. The approach to a benign, simple cyst, on the other hand, is best via an extraperitoneal incision (posterior, flank, or anterior) so that any persistent drainage after the cyst's unroofing remains out of the peritoneal space. The technique is illustrated below.

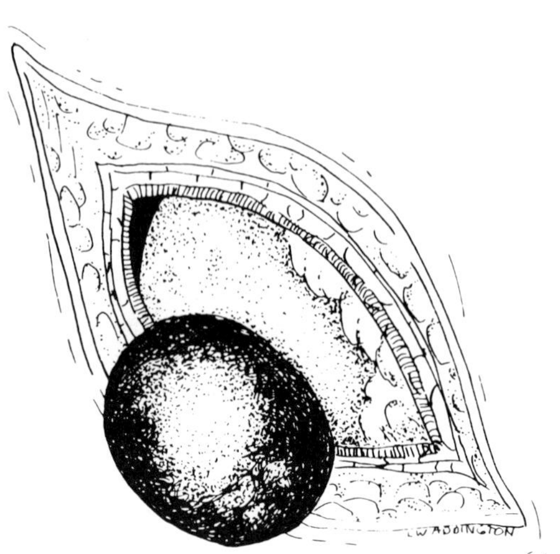

Figure 23.4. The cystic lesion is exposed by careful dissection of perirenal fat from the cyst and the adjacent renal cortex.

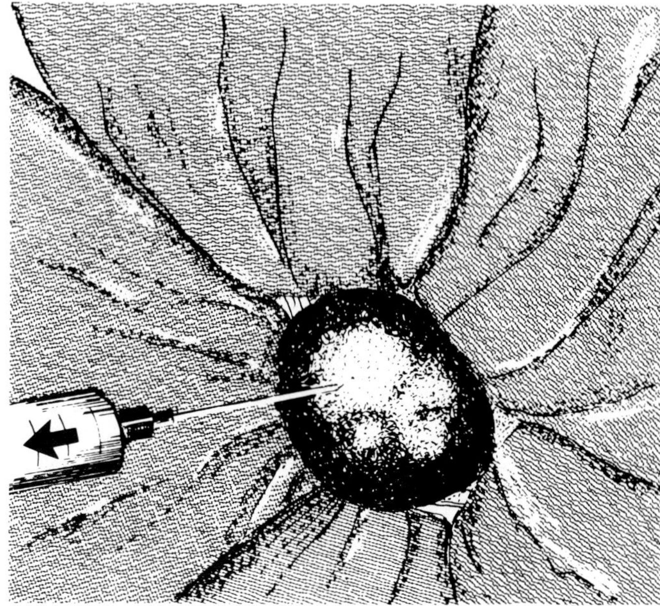

Figure 23.5. The surrounding area is packed off (to minimize spillage) and cyst fluid aspirated for diagnostic study (cytology, etc.).

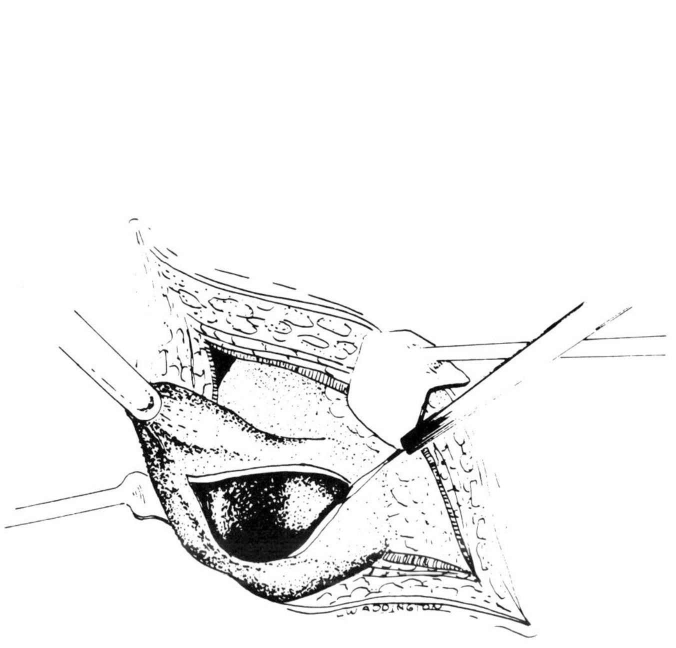

Figure 23.6. The cyst wall then is entered sharply and is resected near its junction with normal parenchyma. Excessive resection beyond this point results in heavy bleeding and is unnecessary. Any lesion within the cyst cavity is biopsied and sent with the cyst wall for frozen section examination. Rarely, unexpected neoplasm in a "normal-appearing" cyst wall is diagnosed and nephrectomy should be performed (opposite kidney being normal).

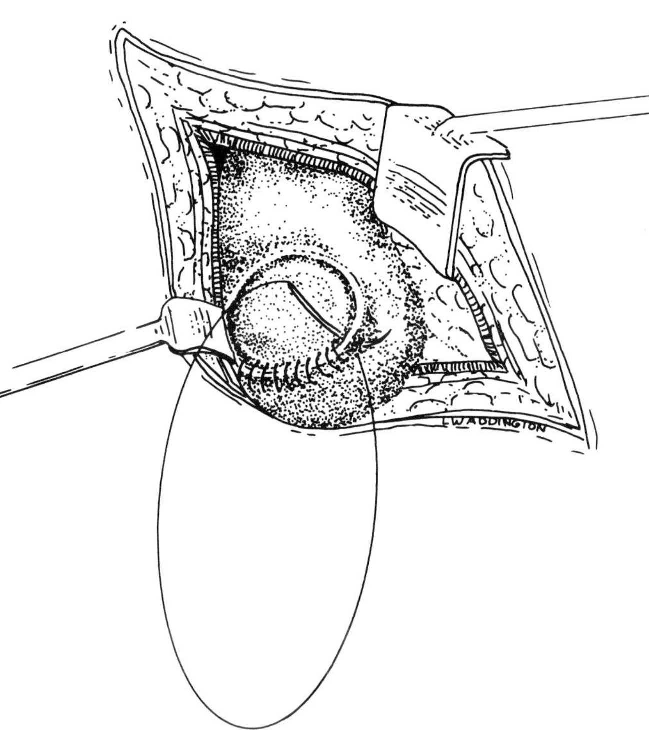

Figure 23.7. After unroofing, an absorbable suture (3–0 or 4–0) may be sewn in a running fashion around the perimeter of the cyst wall edge that remains so as to achieve hemostasis. Alternatively, the edge of the cyst wall may be cauterized and persistent bleeders controlled with figure-eight absorbable sutures. The bottom (renal side) of the cyst crater may lie adjacent to large intrarenal vessels and is best not unduly disturbed. A drain is placed in proximity to the cyst bed and brought extraperitoneally through a separate stab wound, the incision then being closed in layers in the usual fashion. The drain may be pulled when postoperative output is minimal (< 30 ml/24 hr).

DRAINAGE OF PERINEPHRIC AND CORTICAL ABSCESSES

Included in this section will be a discussion of both renal carbuncle and perinephric abscess. Renal carbuncle is a fusion of smaller parenchymal abscesses and is subcapsular in location. It is bounded by the capsular artery on arteriography, it indents the renal parenchyma as seen on intravenous pyelography (IVP) (if large), and it should be bounded by capsule and parenchyma on CT scan. Symptoms generally mimic those of acute pyelonephritis and the urine grows the identical organism to that of the abscess in a high percentage of cases, usually a Gram-negative rod (6). In some instances, this type of abscess will respond to medical therapy with high doses of appropriate antibiotics and the patient will be symptomatically improved and without fever after 48 hours. Treatment failure will require a drainage procedure along with correction of any anatomic defect or, in some cases, partial or total nephrectomy may be needed for cure (6).

Perinephric abscess may result from perforation of a carbuncle through the renal capsule into the perirenal fat (within Gerota's fascial envelope) or it may arise from pathology in other organs by direct or hematogenous spread. The term perinephric abscess should probably include all retroperitoneal infections in proximity to the kidney, including abscesses just anterior to Gerota's fascia but bounded by peritoneum (anterior retroperitoneal space) and abscesses posterior to Gerota's fascia but anterior to lumbodorsal fascia (posterior division of the posterior retroperitoneal space) (7). A perinephric abscess may or may not show abnormalities on IVP, but it should be detectable by sonography and, of course, CT scan. 111-Indium (labeled) leukocyte scan has been used in some centers but the time delay required for interpretation (48–72 hours) makes this study less practical than radiographic imaging techniques (6, 8). Often a urine culture will be negative and etiology of the lesion may be unclear, although hematogenous spread of cutaneous or other infection can explain *Staphalococcus aureus* or other less common organisms. Although perinephric abscess may be bilateral (perhaps due to communication of the fascial compartment across the midline in a few individuals), it is usually confined to one side and, thus, may be drained with one extraperitoneal incision.

With both renal carbuncle and perinephric abscess, antibiotic treatment failure (more likely in the latter situation) should lead rapidly to a drainage procedure. An increasing number of reports of successful treatment by percutaneous drainage make this method an attractive one, especially in an older, very ill patient who is a poor operative risk (6, 9). The percutaneous method may cure patients whose abscesses are not multilocular or it may allow improvement and lower the surgical risk. If symptoms and fever do not abate in 24–48 hours, an open procedure becomes imperative. This not only permits more complete drainage, it allows for possible correction of a predisposing factor (renal calculus, periappendiceal abscess, etc.) at the same time.

The surgical approach must be tailored individually and should take into account the anatomic location of the lesion and medical condition of the patient. Broad spectrum antibiotic coverage is important and, whenever possible, the abscess should be drained extraperitoneally. It is difficult to discuss all possible circumstances because almost any clinical situation may exist. If the anatomy is terribly distorted, options may be limited to drainage alone or with nephrectomy (subcapsular technique may be easiest, see chapter 20). Concomitant treatment of obstruction (stone removal, pyeloplasty, partial nephrectomy) may be possible or might need deferral until a period of drainage allows for partial decrease of inflammation. Ultimately, the surgeon must make the decision regarding salvage, taking all information including operative findings into consideration.

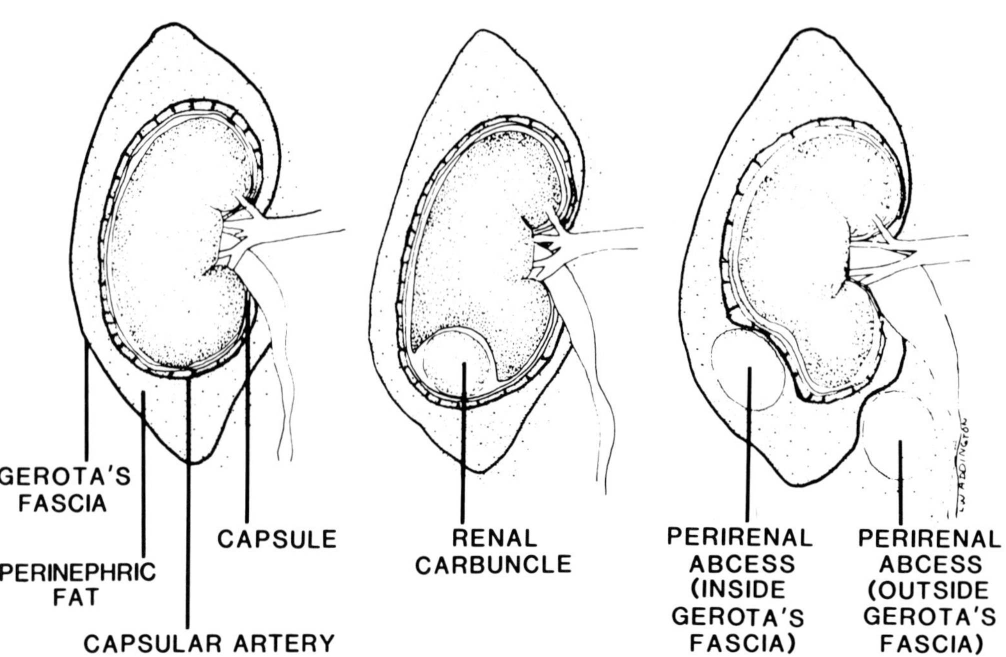

Figure 23.8. The anatomy is illustrated as normal *(left)*, abnormal with a renal carbuncle between capsular artery and parenchyma *(center)*, and abnormal with perinephric abscesses both inside and outside Gerota's fascia *(right)*. Note that a perinephric collection is capable of obstructing the ureter *(right drawing, lower right corner)*.

OPEN NEPHROSTOMY INSERTION

Nephrostomy can be an effective form of temporary or permanent supravesical diversion (10). Successful nephrostomy placement allows low pressure urinary drainage via a tube from the renal collecting system through the flank to a storage bag and it is indicated whenever the urine must be diverted above the level of the ureteropelvic junction. Nephrostomy also enables access to the upper urinary tract for percutaneous stone removal or other endourologic procedures (chapter 15), and it permits diagnostic procedures such as antegrade pyelography and Whittaker pressure-flow studies. (Some of the indications for nephrostomy placement have already been discussed in chapter 15, but for convenience a listing appears in Table 23.1).

Nephrostomy tube drainage is usually achieved by the percutaneous approach (chapter 14), but there are rare instances where encasement by tumor or other difficult anatomy plus a minimally dilated upper urinary tract can make percutaeous methods unsuccessful. Obviously, if an open surgical procedure is being performed for other reasons (anatrophic nephrolithotomy, pyeloplasty, ureterocalycostomy, etc.) then placement of a nephrostomy tube may be accomplished at that time and usually involves little additional morbitity. Whether the approach is percutaneous or open, complications may arise and are similar to those involving any renal operation. These include bleeding (and possible renal loss), damage to renal parenchyma, arteriovenous fistula, infection, obstruction (if the tube becomes malpositioned or dislodged), and stone encrustation (as with any foreign body in the urinary tract). Some patients will complain of chronic pain or encounter difficulty with care of the nephrostomy tube; thus, it may not be the best long-term solution to obstruction for some patients.

The technique for open nephrostomy insertion is illustrated below.

Table 23.1
Indications for Nephrostomy Insertion

Usually temporary
Reconstruction (pyeloplasty)
Lithotomy procedures
Endopyelotomy, other endourology procedures
Ureteral injuries
Antegrade studies (pyelography, Whittaker)
Irrigation therapy (stone dissolution)
Often permanent
Malignancy
Radiation, tuberculous, arteritis, or other damage not suitable for repair

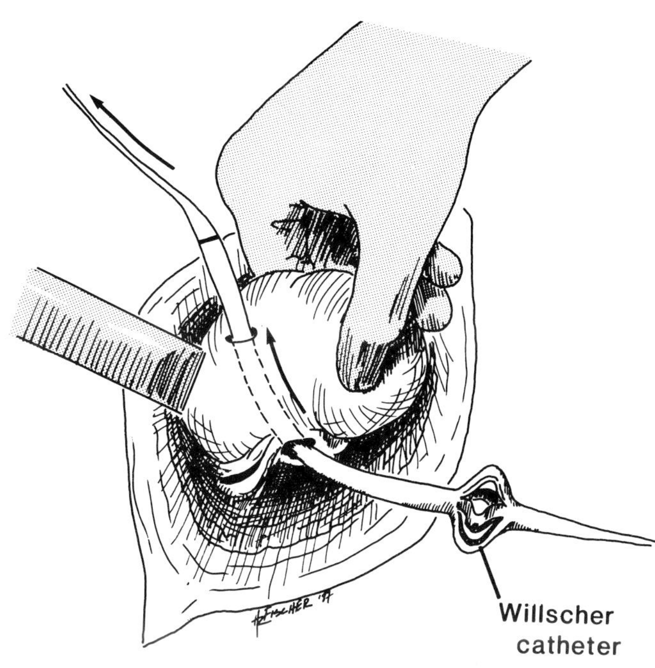

Figure 23.9. Tubes for open nephrostomy placement may be single, with a mushroom or flared end to inhibit dislodgment or they may be of the "circle" type where entry occurs through one portion of the cortex. A segment of tube lies within the collecting system (and usually has side-holes in it) and exits occur through a second area of cortex. The circle tube, thus, makes a "U" turn and requires two punctures through kidney (and flank). Some urologists prefer the circle type in that it may be easier to change than a single (straight) tube. Others find that the circle cuts or erodes into the parenchyma causing more trauma than a single tube. Some straight tubes (Willscher) have a hole placed in the tip to facilitate placement of a guidewire for replacement.

The Willscher tube (illustrated) is particularly simple to place because of a built-in malleable stylet within a smoothly tapered sheath. These catheters come in a range of sizes, but usually 18F or 24F is suitable, depending on the requirements. The kidney, exposed through an incision of the surgeon's choice, mobilized, and with the renal pelvis exposed, is examined for a "thin" spot in the cortex. The stylet of the Willscher catheter is bent to proper curvature, passed through a pyelotomy, and then used to puncture the cortex from within a calyx. Sometimes a small incision must be made through the capsule over the tip of the stylet to enable it to pass through with minimal trauma. This configuration of tube has a flared portion with wide openings (like a Malecot catheter) and then either a short or a long tip containing a guidewire hole. The long tip may be trimmed short or left long and used as a splint through the ureteropelvic junction, depending on the indication. The catheter is carefully pulled through the cortex until the flared "Malecot" portion lies in good position within the collecting system, usually in a calyx of a dependent portion of the kidney. A purse-string suture of 3–0 absorbable suture may be placed through the renal capsule and used to secure the nephrostomy tube if it does not seem adequately stable.

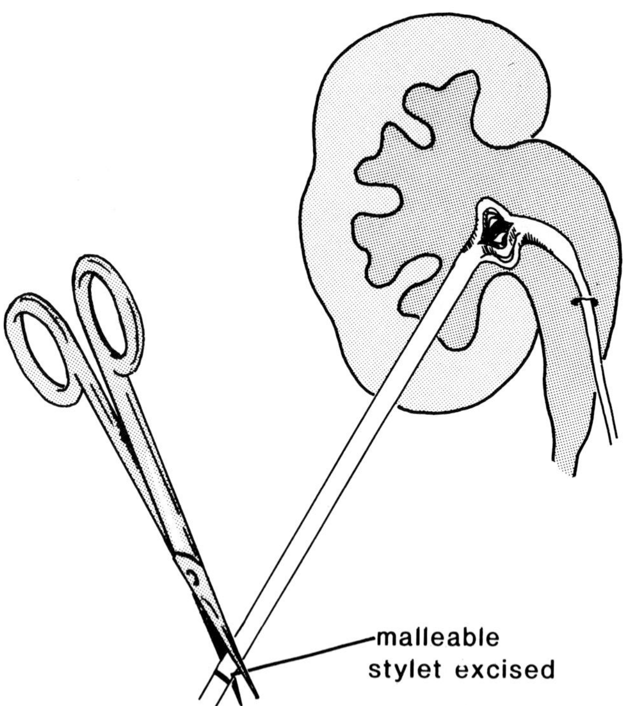

Figure 23.10. A suitable area on the patient's flank is chosen for proper alignment with the exit point of the tube from the kidney (based on the resting position of the kidney before mobilization). The stylet is passed through flank muscles, subcutaneum, and skin, if necessary, incising skin over the tip to help its passage. The kidney is placed carefully back into position during this maneuver, the stylet is excised, and the connector placed on the remaining end of the nephrostomy tube. Large (2–0 or larger) skin sutures may be used to secure the tube near the flank wall exit point to prevent inadvertant dislodgment.

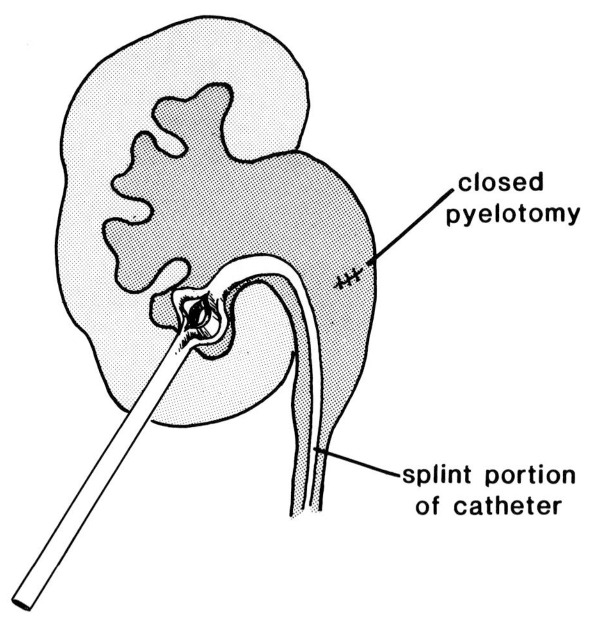

Figure 23.11. The redundant portion of the catheter splint, if not excised earlier, is now placed into the pyelotomy and through the ureteropelvic junction. The pyelotomy is closed with interrupted 3–0 or 4–0 absorbable suture and a drain is placed near the pyelotomy site (and near the cortical exit point of the nephrostomy tube as well). The drain is brought through a separate stab wound in the flank, it is sutured in place, and the incision is closed as per usual technique. Careful dressing is applied so as to prevent kinking of the tube, with adequate tape to again protect against tube dislodgment.

Circle tube placement (not illustrated) is performed in nearly the same way as straight tube insertion (these tubes usually have stylets for both ends). Once one end has been brought from inside to outside, as with the Willscher, the other end is simply used to create a similar puncture but through a calyx at the opposite pole. Markings on the tube usually aid in positioning the center (with the drainage side-holes) within the collecting system. The two ends (still with stylets) can then be used to puncture the flank wall from inside to outside, at spots again selected to align with the renal cortical exit points. The pyelotomy is then closed (and drained) as above.

Care of a nephrostomy tube is quite important and nursing protocols should include specific instructions regarding irrigation and dressing management. Excess pressure (greater than 15 cm H_2O) during irrigation or created by kinking of the drainage tubing may result in bacteremia or at least mechanical damage to the kidney. Drainage should be dependent and free-flowing. Dislodgment of the tube before establishment of a good tract (before 7 days) may result in inability to replace the tube and may require a secondary procedure to again establish drainage. No matter what type of care one employs, encrustation will probably require periodic replacement of a nephrostomy tube. This is usually not difficult under fluoroscopic guidance once a chronic tract has been established.

References

1. Novick AC: Posterior surgical approach to the kidney and ureter. *J Urol* 124:192, 1980.
2. Noble MJ, Mebust WK: Posterior approach to the kidney and upper ureter. In AUA Update Series, Houston, AUA Office of Education, 1987.
3. Allen TD: Renal cysts. In Glenn JF (ed): *Urologic Surgery*. Hagerstown, Harper & Row, 1975.
4. Steg A: Renal cysts—chemical and dynamic study of cystic fluid. *Eur Urol* 2:164, 1976.
5. Stanisic TH, Babcock JR, Grayhack JT: Morbidity and mortality of renal exploration for cyst. *Surg Gynecol Obstet* 145:733, 1977.
6. Cheinfeld J, Erturk E, Spataro RF, Cockett ATK: Perinephric abscess: Current concepts. *J Urol* 137:191, 1987.
7. Gerzoff SG, Gale ME: Computed tomography and ultrasonography for diagnosis and treatment of renal and retroperitoneal abscesses. *Urol Clin North Am* 9:185, 1982.
8. Carroll B, Silverman PM, et al: Ultrasonography and Indium-111 white blood cell scanning for the detection of intraabdominal abscesses. *Ultrasound* 140:155, 1981.
9. Finn DJ, Palestrant AM, DeWolf WC: Successful percutaneous management of renal abscess. *J Urol* 127:425, 1982.

SECTION 6

Renal Vascular Surgery

CHAPTER 24

Aortorenal Bypass

ANDREW C. NOVICK

There are two main categories of renal artery disease, atherosclerosis and fibrous dysplasia, which account for approximately 60% and 40% of all such lesions, respectively. Other unusual renal vascular disorders include an arterial aneurysm, arteriovenous fistula, neurofibromatosis, extrinsic obstruction of the renal artery, the middle aortic syndrome, and renal artery thrombosis or embolism. Revascularization of the kidney is indicated either to treat renovascular hypertension, to preserve renal function that is threatened by advanced vascular disease or, in a few cases, to prevent rupture of an arterial aneurysm.

There are currently two methods of intervention available for patients with renal arterial occlusive disease, namely, surgical revascularization and percutaneous transluminal angioplasty (PTA). PTA provides satisfactory treatment for most patients with main renal artery disease due to fibrous dysplasia or a nonostial atherosclerotic plaque and has become the initial therapeutic approach in such cases. Surgical revascularization remains the indicated treatment for patients with an ostial atherosclerotic plaque, branch renal artery disease, an arterial aneurysm, or patients in whom PTA has been unsuccessful.

Advances in surgical renovascular reconstruction have limited the role of total or partial nephrectomy in the management of patients with renal artery disease. These operations are occasionally indicated in patients with renal infarction, severe arteriolar nephrosclerosis, severe renal atrophy, and noncorrectable renovascular lesions. Nephrectomy may also be indicated in the elderly poor surgical risk patient with a normal contralateral kidney or after a failed revascularization procedure.

Although a variety of surgical revascularization techniques are available for treating patients with renal artery disease, aortorenal bypass with a free graft of autogenous saphenous vein or hypogastric artery is the preferred method in most cases. While an arterial autograft is theoretically advantageous, use of the hypogastric artery as a bypass graft is limited by its short length and frequent involvement with atherosclerosis. Therefore, autogenous saphenous vein is most often employed and excellent clinical results continue to be achieved with this type of bypass graft. It is important to note that the gonadal vein should never be used as a renal artery bypass graft. This vein is extremely friable and may either rupture postoperatively or undergo severe dilatation. Currently, aortorenal bypass with a synthetic material is indicated only when an autogenous vascular graft is not available, and polytetrafluorethylene has become the synthetic graft of choice in such cases.

All patients undergoing surgical renal revascularization are hydrated with 200 ml of 5% dextrose with half-normal saline, intravenously, for 12 hours before surgery. Because renovascular hypertension is associated with secondary hyperaldosteronism, potassium supplement and monitoring of serum potassium levels are needed to guard against hypokalemia. To further ensure optimal renal perfusion and an active diuresis intraoperatively, mannitol, 12.5 gm, is given intravenously before commencing the operation; equivalent doses of mannitol are subsequently given before revascularization, immediately after revascularization, and again in the recovery room.

Figure 24.1. In order to obtain a saphenous vein graft, an oblique groin incision is made just medial to the pulsation of the femoral artery. Care is taken not to overdistend the vein or to dissect periadventitial tissue injudiciously, both of which may cause devascularization of the graft. All venous tributaries are suture ligated with 4–0 silk, and a 4–6 cm segment of saphenous vein is removed. A bulldog clamp is placed on the cephalic end of the vein and the vein is gently distended with heparin solution. Because of the presence of valves in the saphenous vein, blood flow in the graft should always be directed toward the cephalic end, which will be anastomosed directly to the distal renal artery. A fine suture is placed in the cephalic end of the graft for identification purposes. After its removal, the graft is stored in chilled Ringer's lactate solution to which dilute heparin solution has been added.

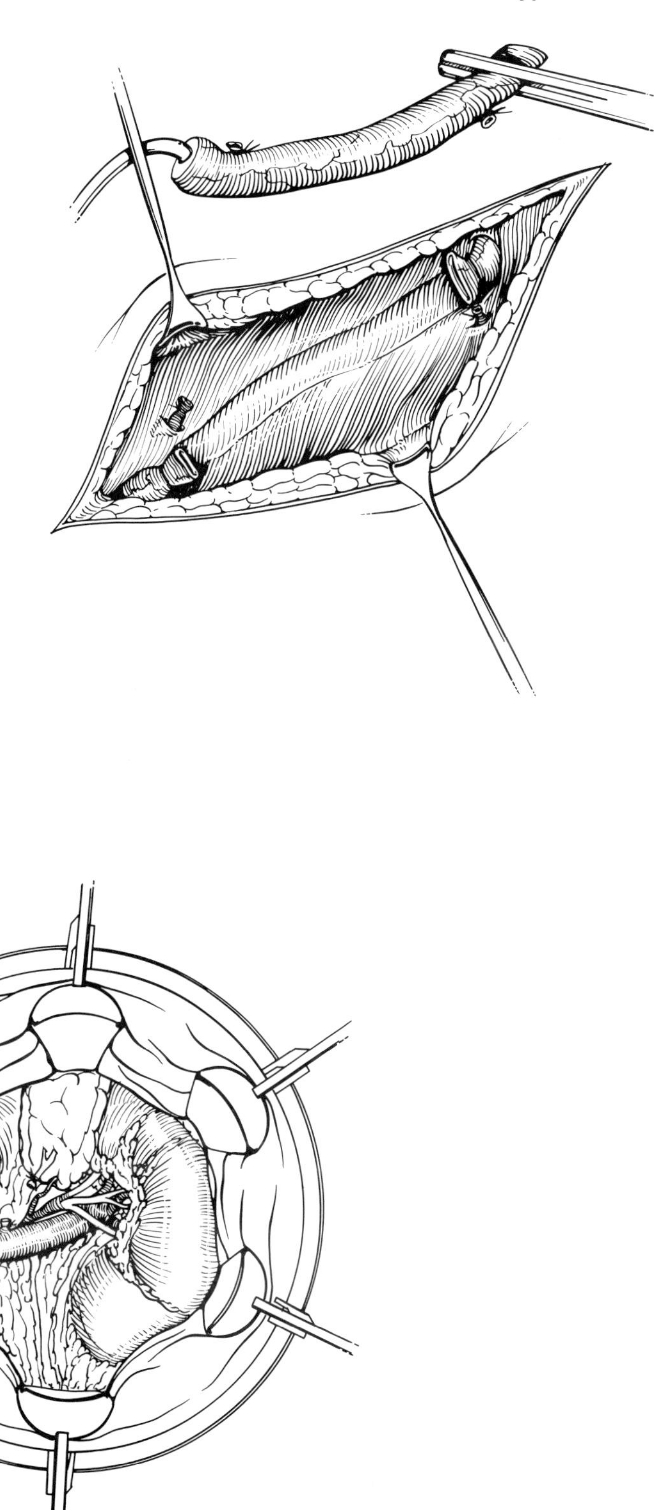

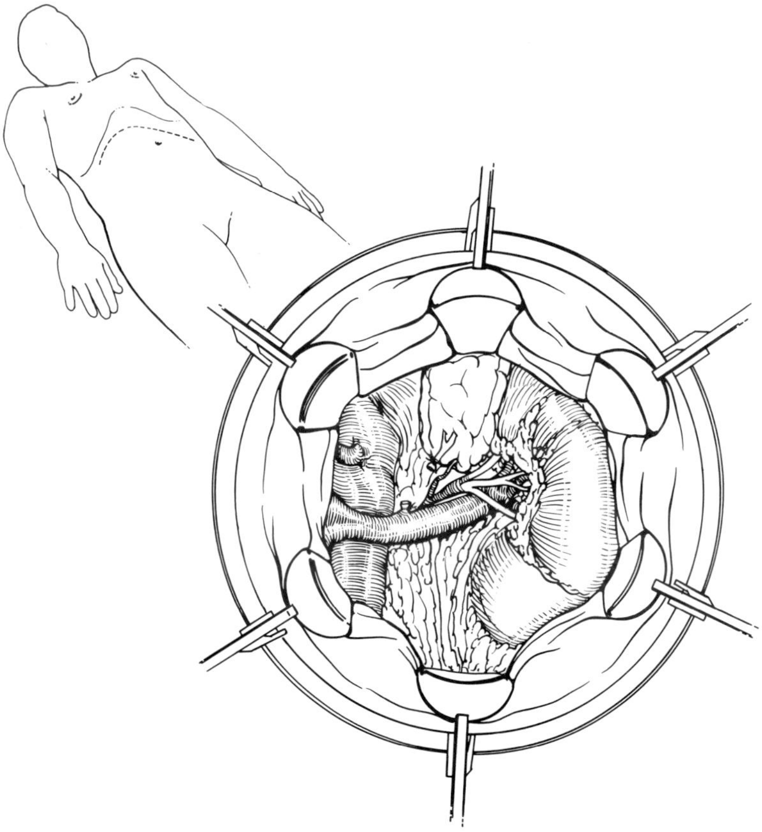

Figure 24.2. A transperitoneal subcostal incision is made, the medial end of which is curved across the midline. On the left side, the left colon and duodenum are reflected medially. The plane between Gerota's fascia and the pancreas is developed by blunt dissection, and the pancreas and spleen are gently retracted cephalad. The Buckwalter self-retaining ring retractor is then inserted, which provides excellent exposure and allows the operation to be performed comfortably by a surgeon and one assistant. Gerota's fascia is opened laterally over the lower pole of the kidney so that the color and consistency of the kidney can be observed throughout the revascularization procedure.

Figure 24.3. The left renal vein is mobilized and its adrenal and gonadal branches are ligated and divided. The left renal vein is then retracted upward to expose any lumbar tributaries on its posterior aspect, which are similarly secured. Ligation and division of additional small extrahilar renal venous branches can be done safely and is helpful in obtaining complete mobilization of the left renal vein. The immobilized renal vein then may be retracted upward or downward to expose the left main renal artery in its entirety, which now can be dissected from adjacent tissues and exposed under direct vision.

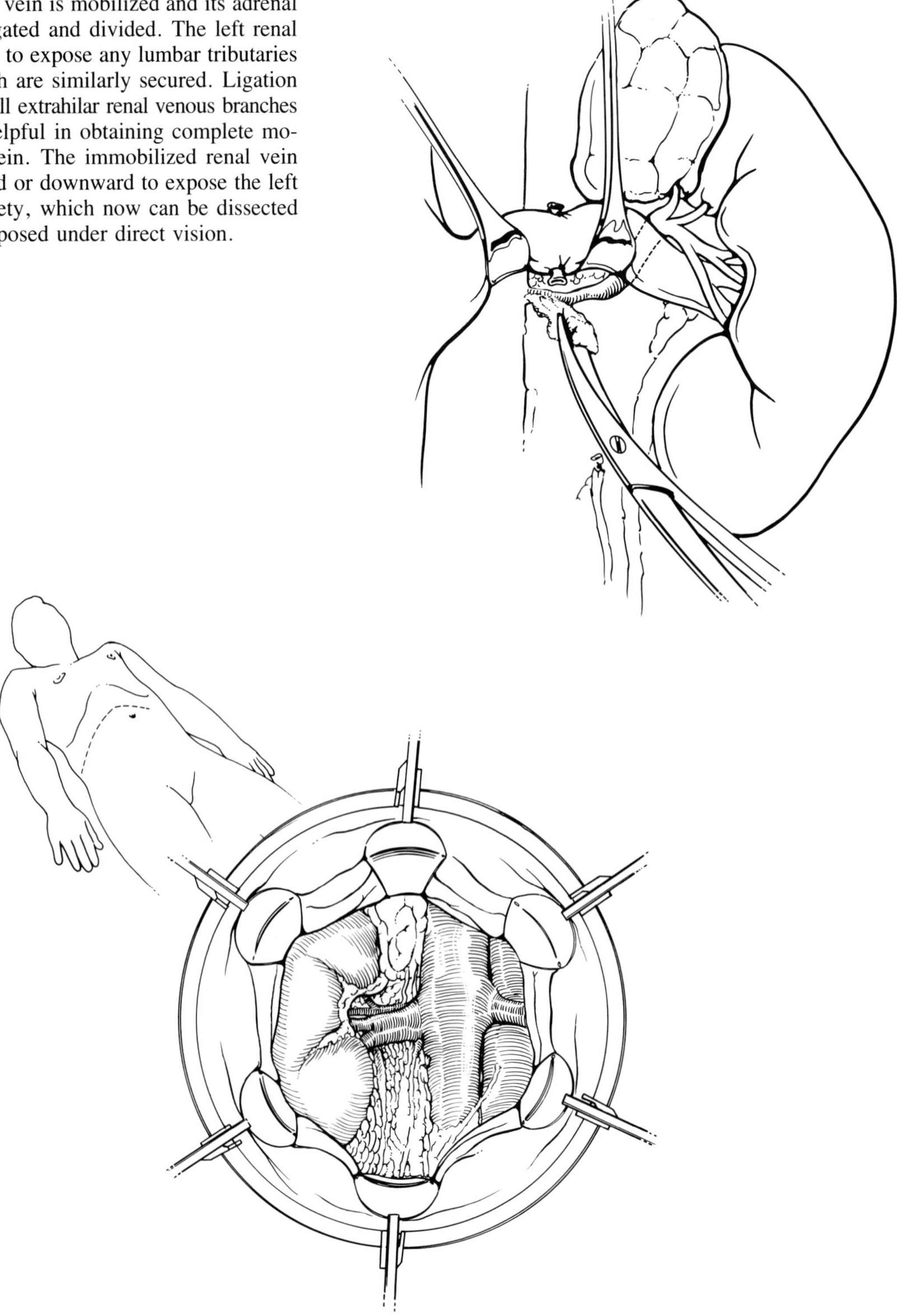

Figure 24.4. To perform an aortorenal bypass on the right side, the kidney is exposed by reflecting the ascending colon medially and using the Kocher maneuver on the duodenum. The liver and gallbladder are retracted upward taking care to protect the hepatic ligament with its vessels and common bile duct. Exposure of the right renal artery, right renal vein, inferior vena cava, and the aorta is thereby obtained. The Buckwalter self-retaining ring retractor is inserted to maintain exposure. Gerota's fascia is opened laterally to expose the surface of the kidney so that its color and consistency may be observed.

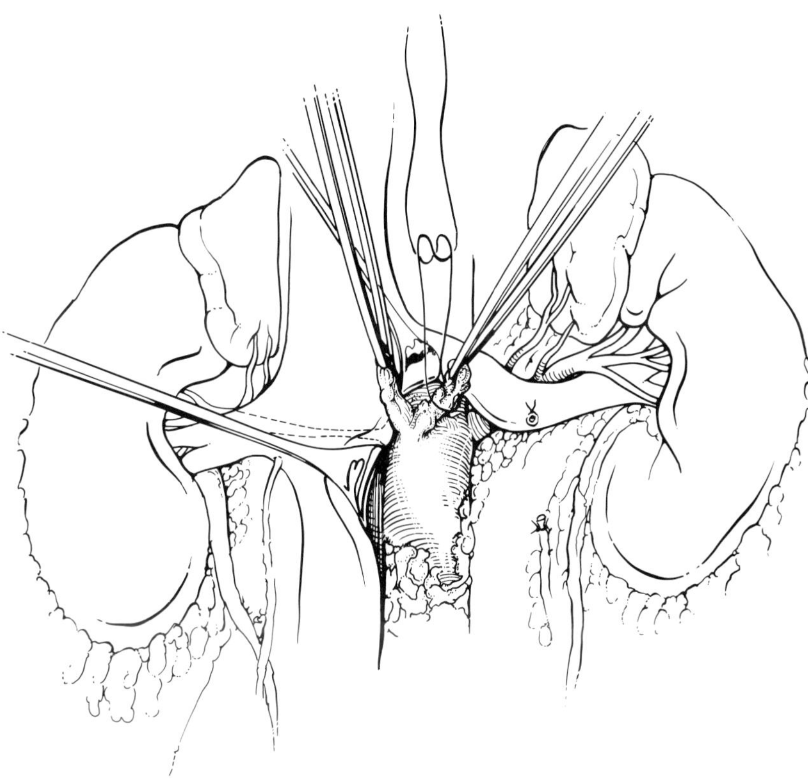

Figure 24.5. The aorta is exposed from the level of the left renal vein to the inferior mesenteric artery, ligating overlying lymphatic vessels and lumbar segmental branches as necessary to gain exposure. The proximal aspect of the right renal artery is exposed by mobilizing and retracting the vena cava laterally and the left renal vein superiorly, carrying the dissection along the anterolateral aspect of the aortic wall until the renal artery origin is encountered.

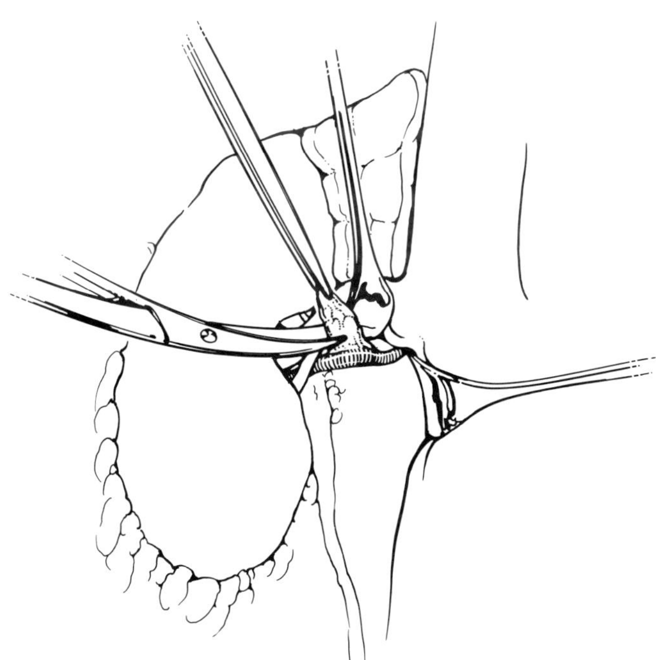

Figure 24.6. The distal two-thirds of the main right renal artery is exposed by retracting the mobilized vena cava medially and the right renal vein superiorly. To accomplish this, it is often necessary to secure and divide one or more lumbar veins entering the posterior aspect of the vena cava. There are generally no significant tributaries of the right renal vein. After exposure of the right renal artery, this is then mobilized from its attached and surrounding lymphatics and nerves. Small vessels and lymphatics are secured by light electrocautery or fine suture ligatures.

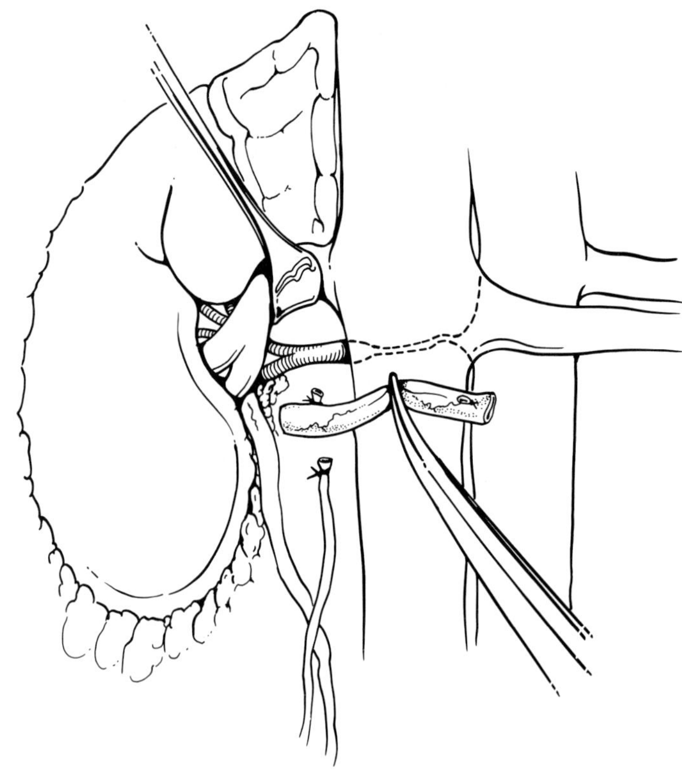

Figure 24.7. The bypass graft is placed along the lateral aortic wall to determine the best position for placement of the graft. At this point, the ring retractor blades are relaxed to allow the aorta to return to its normal position and to prevent distortion of an otherwise well-placed graft after the final retraction is released.

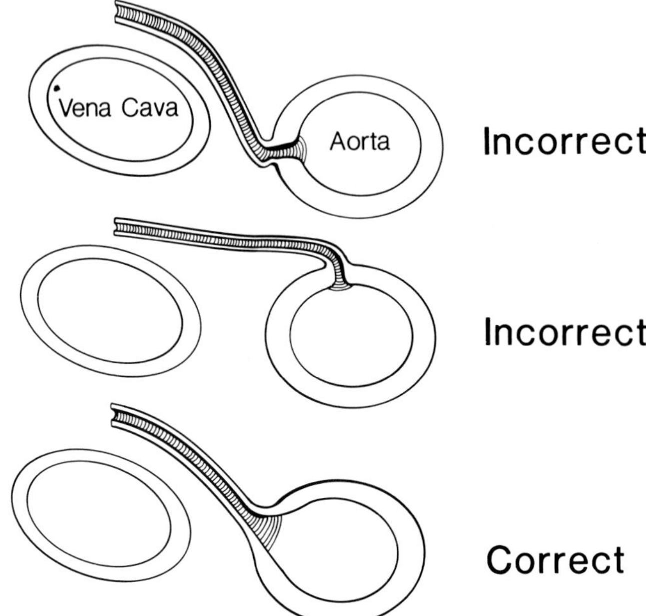

Figure 24.8. On the right side, it is important to bring the graft off the anterolateral aspect of the aortic wall to avoid kinking of the proximal anastomosis as the graft passes in front of the vena cava. If the aortotomy is made too far anteriorly or posteriorly, the graft may kink with subsequent development of stenosis or thrombosis. On the left side, the graft may be placed directly off the lateral aspect of the aorta.

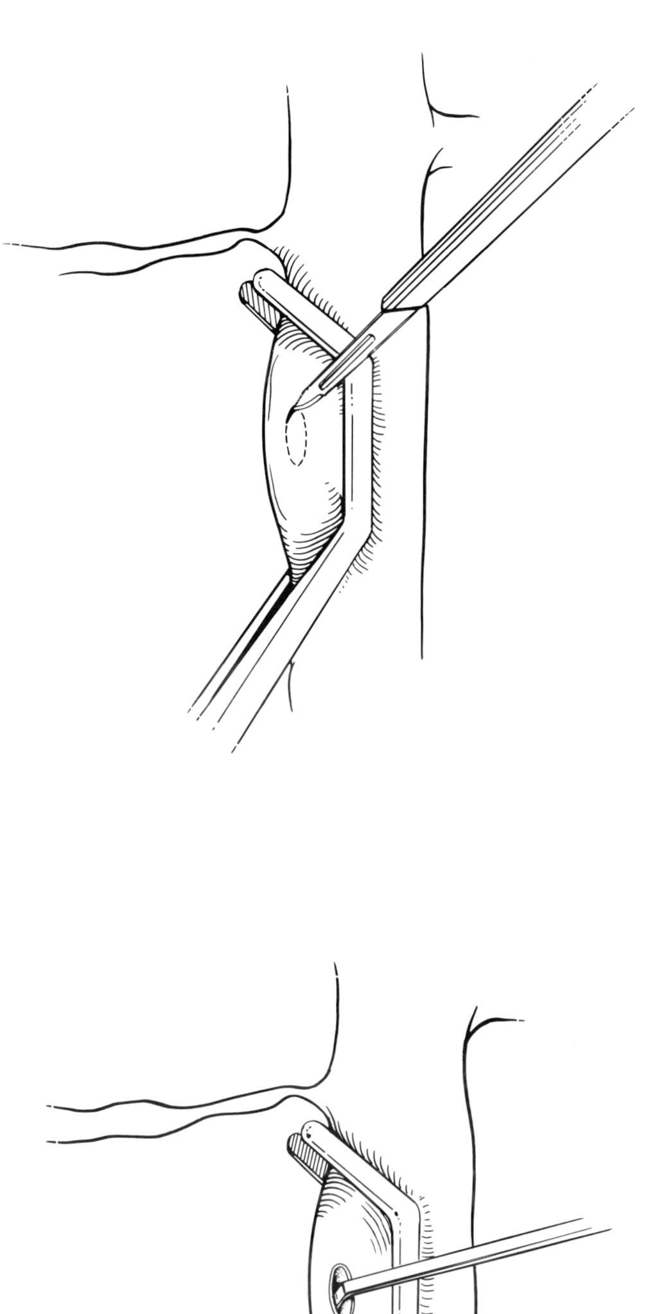

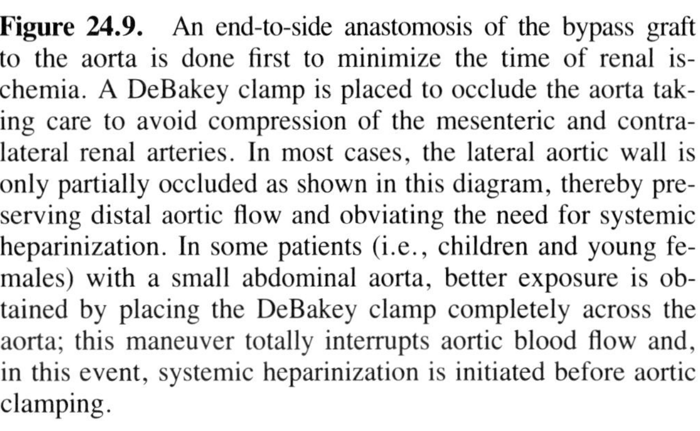

Figure 24.9. An end-to-side anastomosis of the bypass graft to the aorta is done first to minimize the time of renal ischemia. A DeBakey clamp is placed to occlude the aorta taking care to avoid compression of the mesenteric and contralateral renal arteries. In most cases, the lateral aortic wall is only partially occluded as shown in this diagram, thereby preserving distal aortic flow and obviating the need for systemic heparinization. In some patients (i.e., children and young females) with a small abdominal aorta, better exposure is obtained by placing the DeBakey clamp completely across the aorta; this maneuver totally interrupts aortic blood flow and, in this event, systemic heparinization is initiated before aortic clamping.

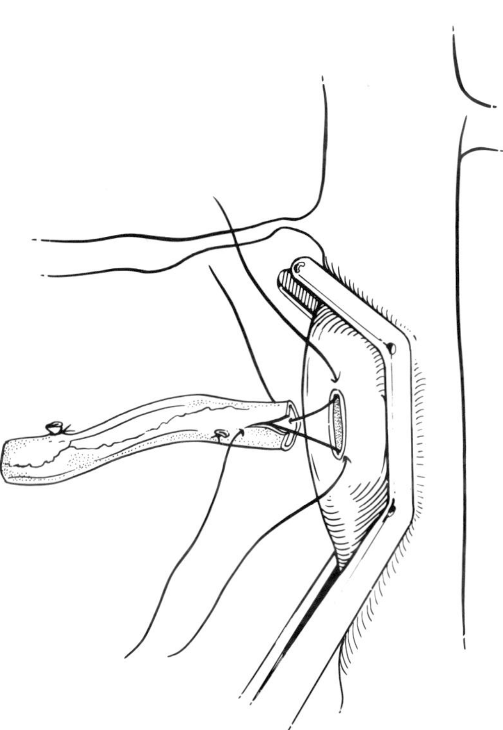

Figure 24.10. An oval aortotomy is made on the anterolateral wall of the aorta. If significant atherosclerosis of the perirenal aorta is present, a local endarterectomy is performed to remove atheromatous plaque from the region of the anastomosis.

Figure 24.11. The bypass graft is spatulated for a short distance and, if length permits, the apex of the spatulation is generally placed at the caudal end of the aortotomy so that the graft can follow a gentle curve as it emerges from the aorta. If the aortotomy is located a significant distance below the distal renal artery or if the graft is short, as on the left side, then the apex is reversed cephalad to avoid kinking of the aortorenal bypass graft. Two corner sutures of 6–0 silk are inserted 180° apart to begin the anastomosis.

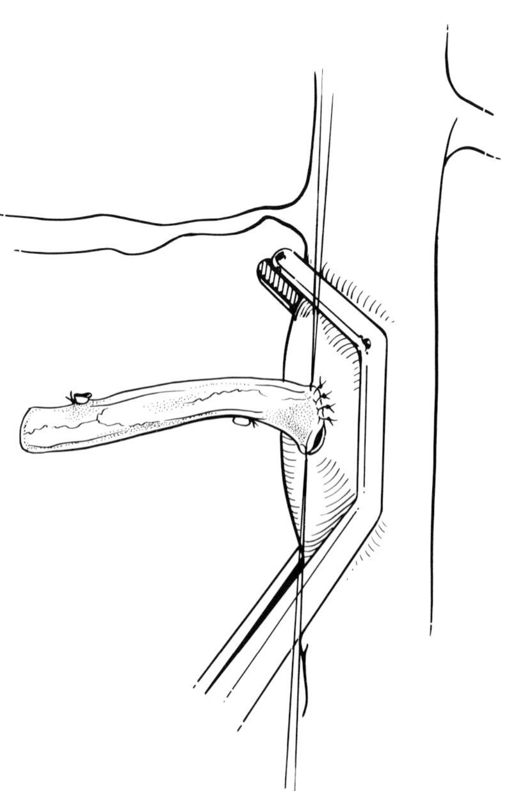

Figure 24.12. The anastomosis is performed with interrupted 6–0 arterial sutures and the anterior wall of the anastomosis is completed first.

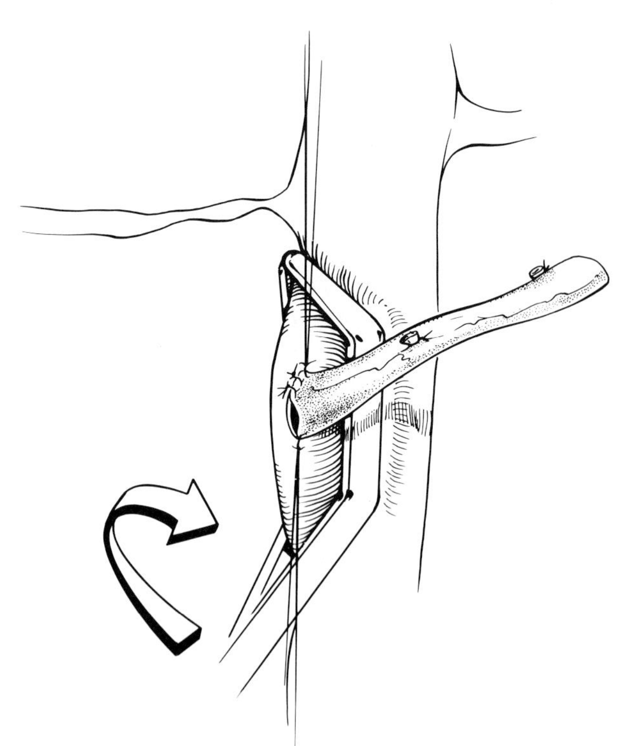

Figure 24.13. The aorta is rotated anteriorly to expose the posterior wall of the anastomosis, which is similarly completed with interrupted 6–0 arterial sutures.

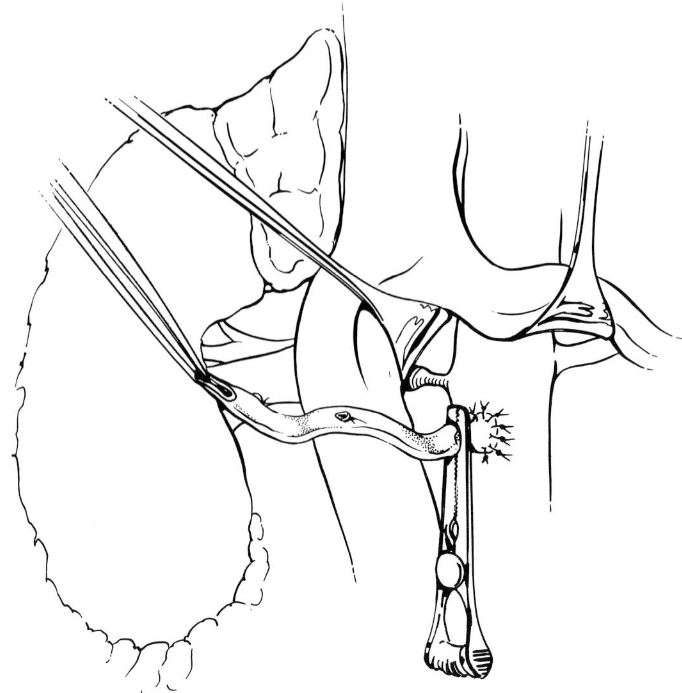

Figure 24.14. The graft is occluded beyond its origin with a bulldog clamp and the aortic clamp is gently released. An arterial leakage is corrected at this time with additional sutures as needed. The bulldog clamp is intermittently released to ensure good blood flow and to flush the graft free of any atherosclerotic fragments. The graft distal to the clamp is then irrigated with heparin solution.

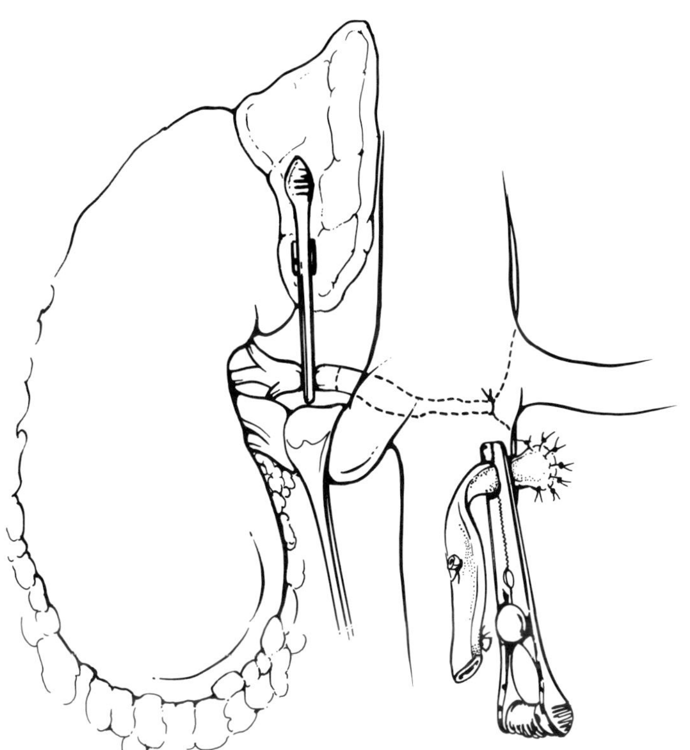

Figure 24.15. The main renal artery is then mobilized in its entirety, if this has not already been done. The renal artery is ligated proximally, a bulldog clamp is placed distally, and the diseased arterial segment is excised and sent for pathologic examination. Before the distal anastomosis is performed, 10 ml of dilute heparin solution are instilled into the distal renal artery.

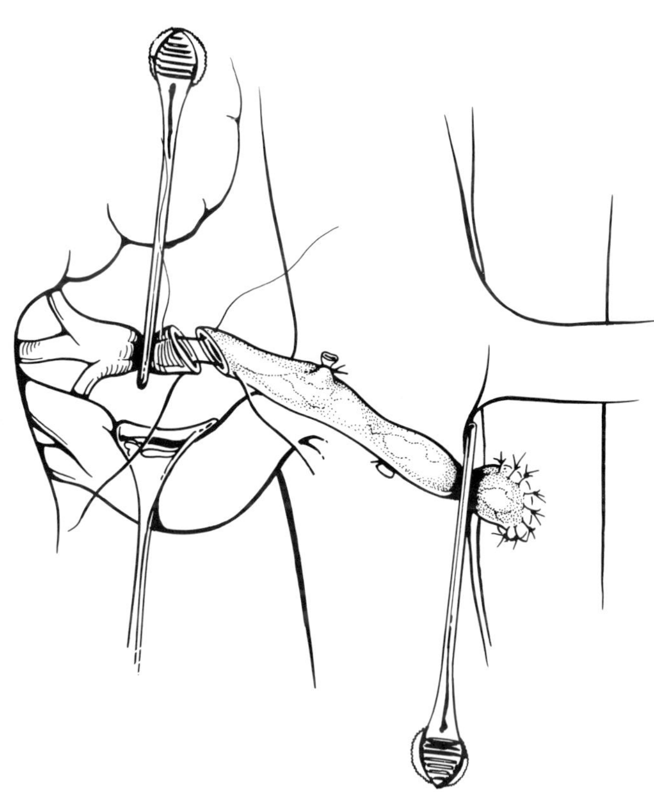

Figure 24.16. The bypass graft is brought anterior to the vena cava to lie in proximity to the distal renal artery. The graft is trimmed as necessary to allow a tension-free end-to-end anastomosis with no redundancy in the length of the graft. The graft and distal renal artery are spatulated to create a wider anastomosis, which minimizes the possibility for subsequent stenosis. The anastomosis is performed with 6–0 arterial sutures. Stay sutures, 180° apart, are placed in the cephalic and caudal margins of the anastomosis. An end-to-end anastomosis of the graft to the renal artery is preferred over an end-to-side technique because this provides better flow rates, is easier to perform, and allows removal of the diseased renal arterial segment for pathologic study.

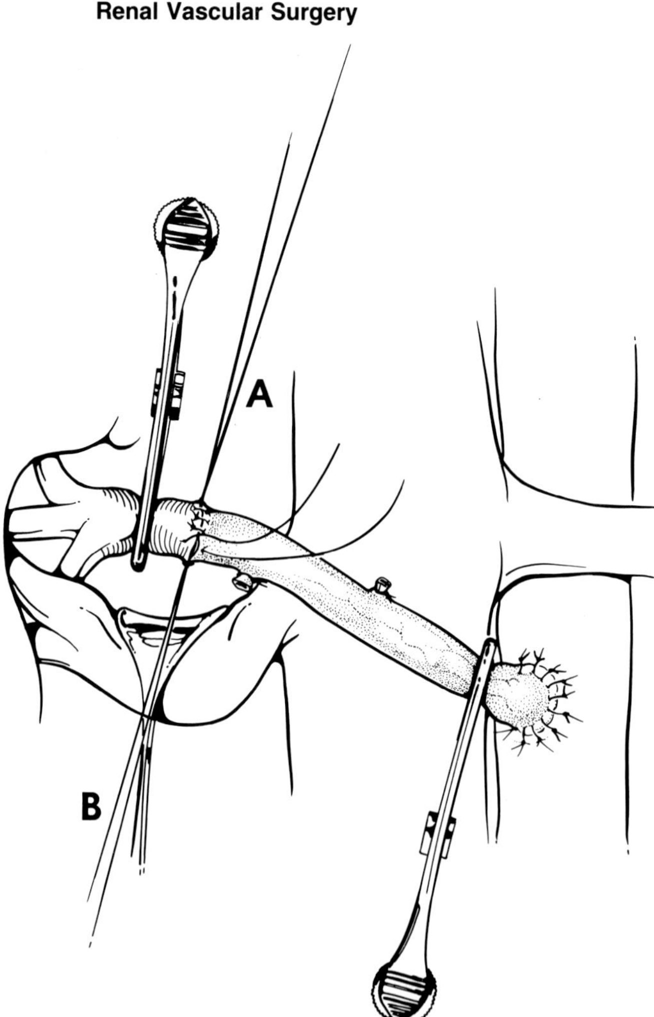

Figure 24.17. The anastomosis is performed with interrupted 6–0 arterial sutures and the anterior wall is completed first.

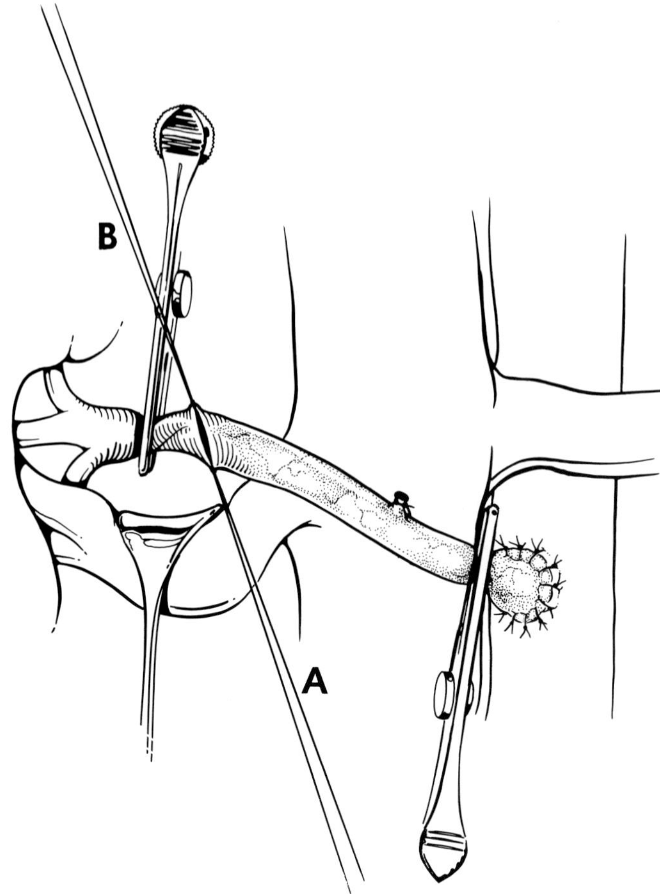

Figure 24.18. The caudal stay suture, **B,** is then rotated up anteriorly and the cephalic stay suture, **A,** is rotated down posteriorly to expose the posterior wall of the anastomosis.

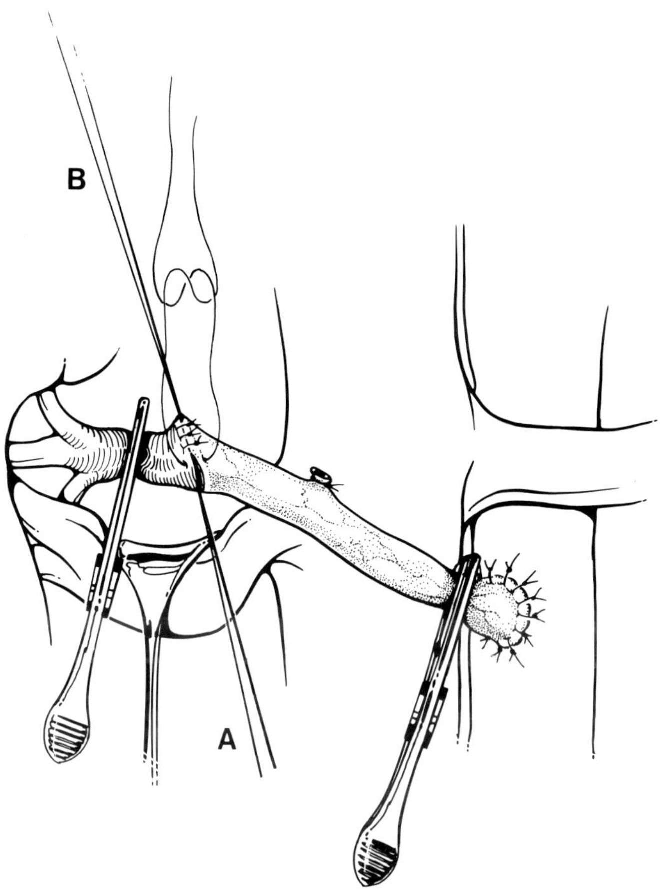

Figure 24.19. The posterior wall of the distal anastomosis is then completed with interrupted 6–0 arterial sutures.

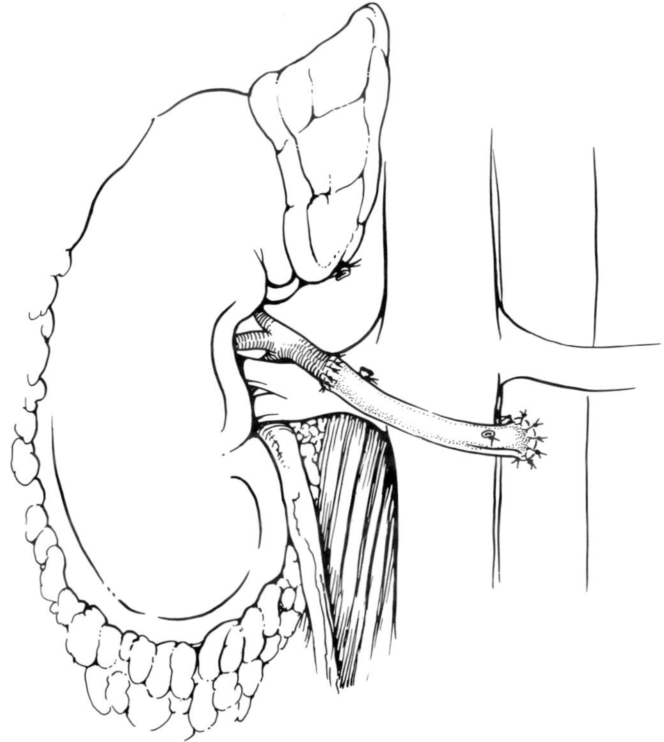

Figure 24.20. The proximal and distal bulldog clamps are released and circulation to the kidney is restored. Adequate renal perfusion is verified by palpating the pulse in the distal renal artery and by visual inspection of the renal surface. Arterial anastomotic leakage, if present, is controlled with Oxycel cotton and/or additional 6–0 interrupted arterial sutures. This drawing illustrates the completed aortorenal bypass operation.

AORTORENAL BYPASS FOR BRANCH RENAL ARTERY DISEASE

Surgical revascularization is more complicated when the disease extends into the branches of the renal artery or when vascular reconstruction is required for a kidney supplied by multiple renal arteries. When disease-free distal arterial branches occur outside the renal hilus, an aortorenal bypass operation can usually be done in situ. The size of the involved vessels is not a significant factor because, utilizing microvascular instruments and optical magnification, vessels as small as 1.5 mm diameter can be repaired in situ. There are several variations of the standard aortorenal bypass technique, described earlier in this chapter, which may be used to repair branch renal artery disease. Because the bypass graft must be sufficiently long to reach the renal artery branches, autogenous saphenous vein is the graft of choice in these cases.

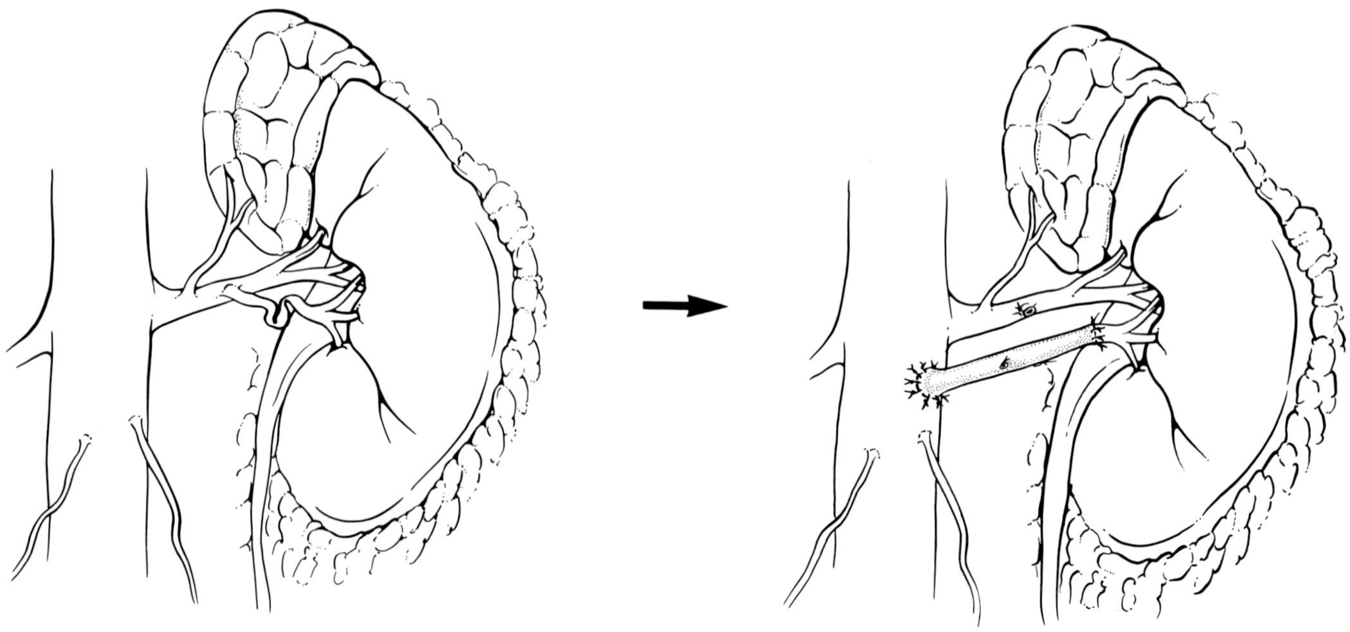

Figure 24.21. In patients with disease confined to a single major renal artery branch, aortorenal bypass may be done exclusively to the disease-free distal branch, leaving the main renal artery and its remaining branches intact.

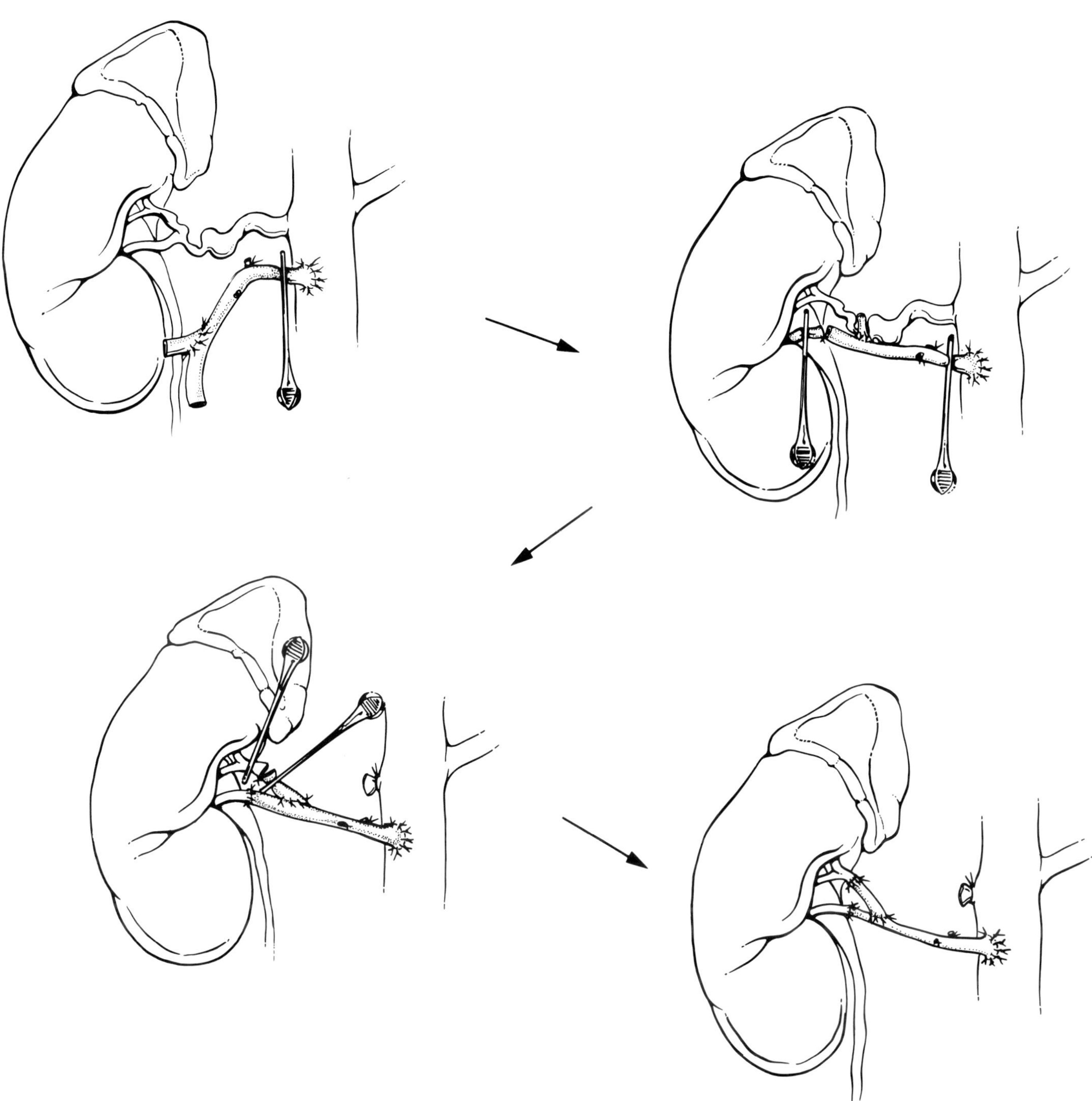

Figure 24.22. In patients with disease involving two or more renal artery branches, the author has found that aortorenal bypass with a branched vascular graft offers the most useful and versatile technique for in situ vascular reconstruction. Although the hypogastric artery may be removed intact with its branches, this type of graft is invariably too short to reach from the aorta to the renal artery branches. In these cases, a branched saphenous vein graft is fashioned by attaching one or more side-arms of vein to the main graft. These end-to-side anastomoses are done with interrupted 7–0 arterial sutures and lead to creation of a multibranched graft that can be used to replace several diseased renal artery branches. After insertion of the proximal graft into the aorta, direct end-to-end anastomosis of each graft branch to a renal artery branch is done. During performance of each individual branch anastomosis, the remainder of the kidney continues to be perfused and overall renal ischemia, thus, is limited to the time required for completion of a single end-to-end anastomosis (approximately 15–20 min), which is an important advantage.

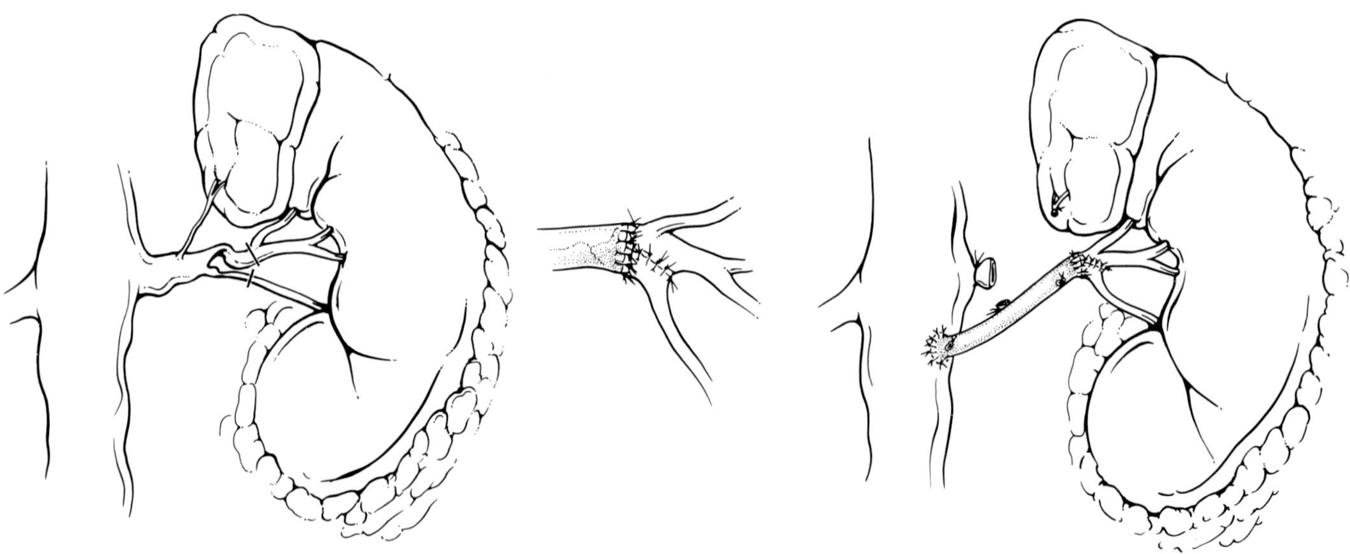

Figure 24.23. Another alternative in these cases is aortorenal bypass to the conjoined distal branches of the renal artery. The limitations of this technique are that it is not readily applicable when disease extends into more than two arterial branches and it also involves a longer period of in situ renal ischemia.

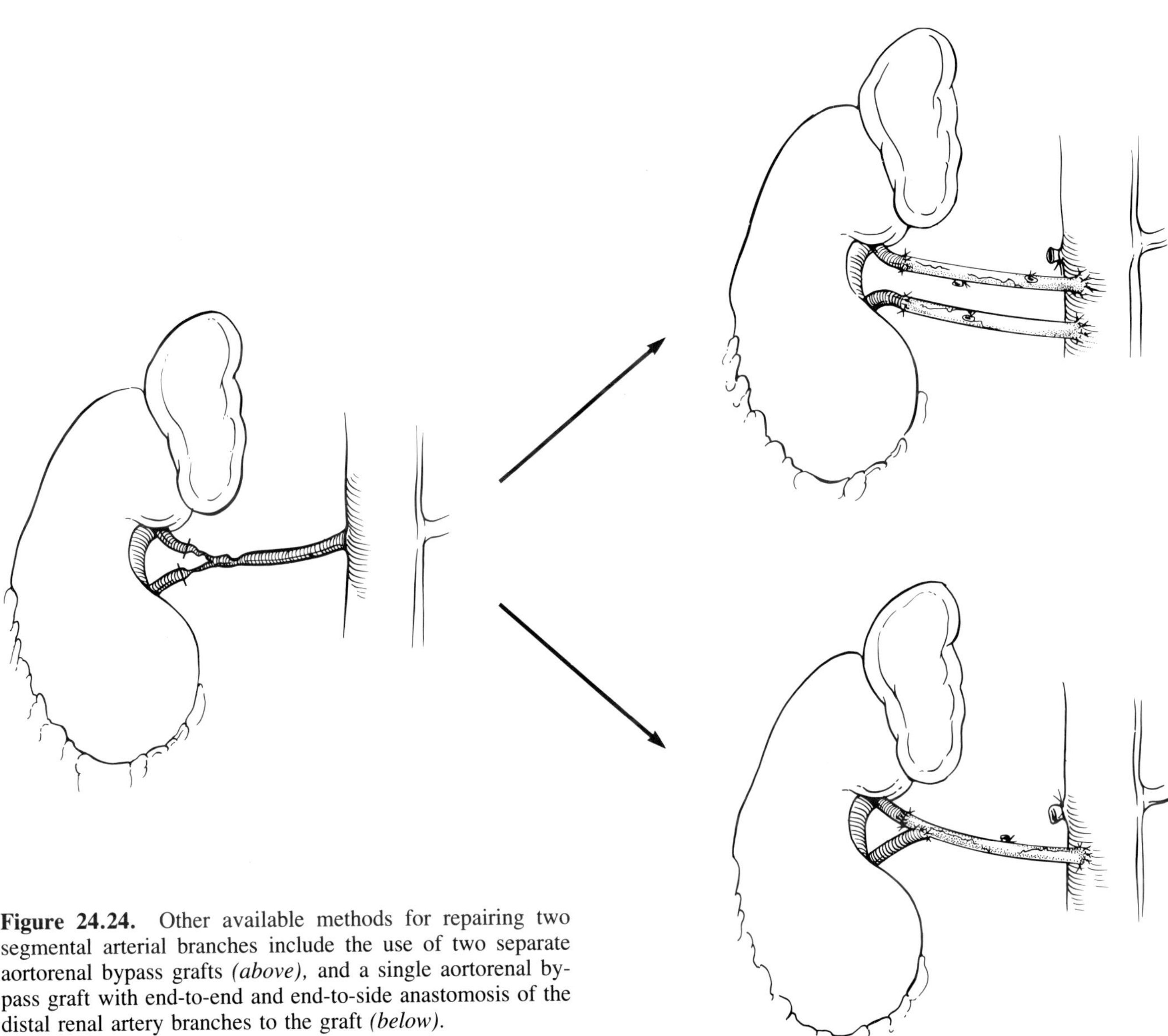

Figure 24.24. Other available methods for repairing two segmental arterial branches include the use of two separate aortorenal bypass grafts *(above)*, and a single aortorenal bypass graft with end-to-end and end-to-side anastomosis of the distal renal artery branches to the graft *(below)*.

AORTORENAL REIMPLANTATION

Aortorenal reimplantation occasionally may be used to repair short lesions of the proximal renal artery such as atherosclerosis or intimal fibroplasia. Because an adequate amount of disease-free distal renal artery is a prerequisite for performance of this operation, it is particularly well-suited to the anatomical variant presented by an anomolous high origin of the renal artery. The advantage of aortorenal reimplantation is that it involves only a single vascular anastomosis and obviates the need for a bypass graft. Although the indications for its use are limited, it can provide satisfactory revascularization for a few patients with renal artery disease.

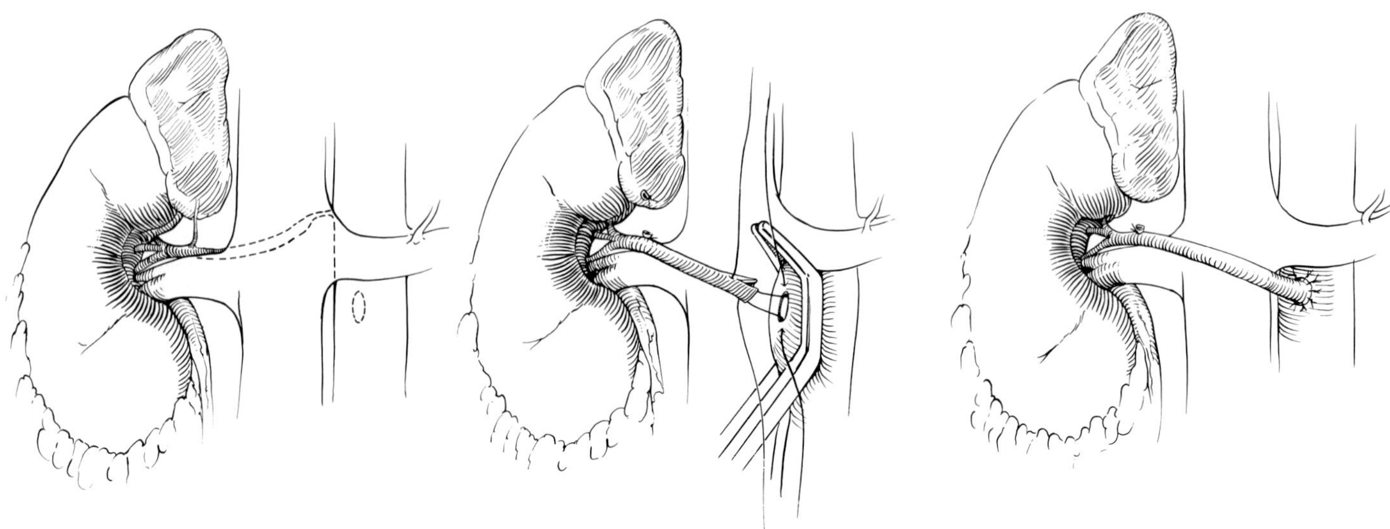

Figure 24.25. Mobilization and exposure of the aorta and right renal artery are performed as described for an aortorenal bypass. The aorta is partially occluded over its lateral aspect with a DeBakey clamp and an oval aortotomy is made laterally. For repairs on the right side, retrocaval reimplantation is performed because this enables maximum utilization of distal renal artery length; a precaval anastomosis may result in angulation of the renal artery. The renal artery is reimplanted end-to-side into the aorta, suturing the posterior wall initially with a continuous 6–0 arterial suture. Extra care must be taken in performing the posterior layer since, once the anastomosis is complete, it is difficult to control hemorrhage from the posterior wall. The anterior wall of the anastomosis may be completed with interrupted sutures.

REPAIR OF RENAL ARTERY ANEURYSM

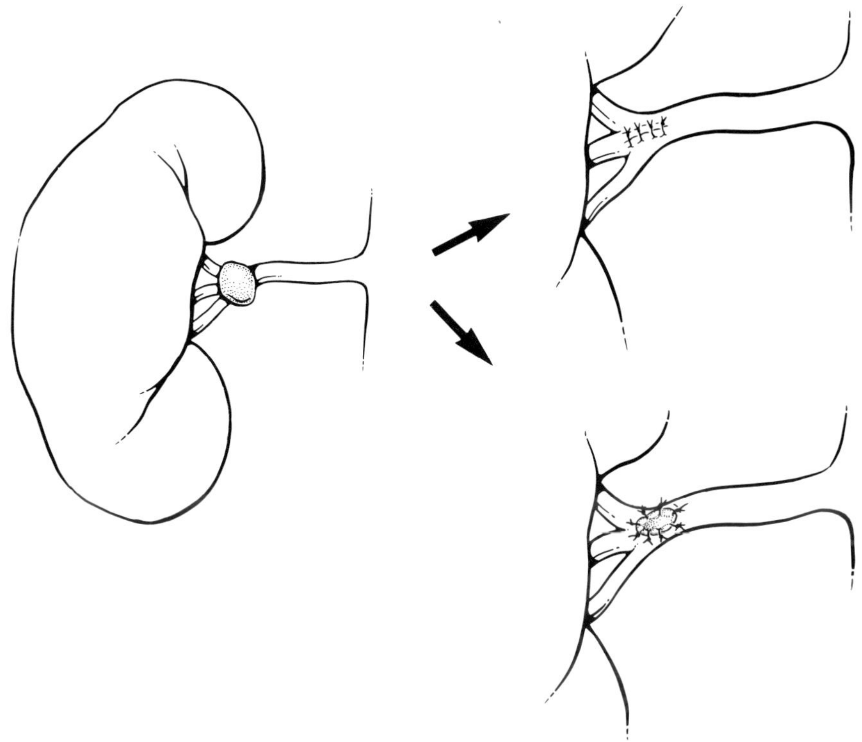

Figure 24.26. Renal artery aneurysms have a variable presentation and vascular involvement may be focal or diffuse. Saccular aneurysms are the most commonly encountered type of renal artery aneurysm and these are often located at the initial bifurcation or trifurcation of the main renal artery. When the aneurysm is located outside the renal hilus, in situ excision may be done. If the renal artery wall at the base of the aneurysm is intact, aneursymectomy with either primary closure *(above)* or patch angioplasty with a segment of saphenous vein *(below)* can be performed as shown on this diagram. If the entire circumference of the renal artery wall is diseased, then aortorenal bypass with a branched autogenous vascular graft is done as described earlier in this chapter.

POSTOPERATIVE CARE

Patients undergoing surgical renal revascularization may experience wide fluctuations in blood pressure in the early postoperative period, with either hypotensive or hypertensive episodes that may predispose to graft thrombosis or bleeding from vascular anastomotic sites, respectively. Therefore, these patients are placed in the intensive care unit for monitoring the central venous pressure, urine output, pulse rate, and serum levels of hemoglobin and creatinine. During this period, the diastolic blood pressure is maintained between 90 and 100 mm Hg to ensure satisfactory renal perfusion. If hypertensive episodes occur, they are managed with intravenous infusion of sodium nitroprusside. Within the first 24 hours postoperatively, a technetium renal scan is obtained to verify perfusion of the revascularized kidney. If clear evidence of the latter is not present, then arteriography should be done immediately to visualize the repaired renal artery directly.

If the patient's condition is stable, the nasogastric tube, central venous line, arterial line, and urethral catheter are removed 48 hours postoperatively and intensive care monitoring is discontinued. Before discharge from hospital, if there is no contraindication to the administration of contrast material, an intravenous digital subtraction angiogram is obtained. This provides an excellent noninvasive method for evaluating the arterial supply of the revascularized kidney. Subsequent patient follow-up is performed by periodic evaluation of the blood pressure, serum creatinine level and/or glomerular filtration rate, and technetium renal scanning.

Suggested Readings

Dean RH: Late results of aortorenal bypass. *Urol Clin North Am* 11:425, 1984.

Ernst CB, Stanley JC, Marshall FF, Fry WJ: Autogenous saphenous vein aortorenal grafts: A 10-year experience. *Arch Surg* 105:855, 1972.

Khauli RB, Novick AC, Coseriu GV: Renal revascularization with polytetrafluorethylene graft. *Cleve Clin Quart* 51:365, 1984.

Noble MJ, Novick AC, Straffon RA, Stewart BH: Aortorenal reimplantation in treatment of renovascular hypertension. *Urology* 14:566, 1979.

Novick AC, Stewart BH, Staffon RA: Autogenous arterial grafts in the treatment of renal artery stenosis. *J Urol* 118:919, 1977.

Novick AC, Ziegelbaum M, Vidt DG, Gifford RW, Pohl MA, Goormastic M: Trends in surgical revascularization for renal artery disease: Ten year's experience. *JAMA* 257:498, 1987.

Novick AC, Straffon RA, Stewart BH: Surgical management of branch renal artery disease: In situ versus extracorporeal methods of repairs. *J Urol* 123:311, 1980.

Novick AC: Microvascular reconstruction of complex branch renal artery disease. *Urol Clin North Am* 11:465, 1984.

Ortenberg J, Novick AC, Straffon RA, Stewart BH: Surgical treatment of renal artery aneurysm. *Br J Urol* 55:341, 1983.

Straffon RA, Siegel DF: Saphenous vein bypass graft in the treatment of renovascular hypertension. *Urol Clin North Am* 2:337, 1975.

Streem SB, Novick AC: Aortorenal bypass with a branched saphenous vein graft for in situ repair of multiple segmental renal arteries. *Surg Gynecol Obstet* 155:885, 1982.

Wylie EJ: Endarterectomy and autogenous arterial grafts in the surgical treatment of stenosing lesions of the renal artery. *Urol Clin North Am* 2:351, 1975.

Zabbo A, Novick AC: Digital subtraction angiography for non-invasive imaging of the renal artery. *Urol Clin North Am* 11:409, 1984.

CHAPTER 25

Hepatorenal Bypass

JOHN A. LIBERTINO
MICHAEL J. MALONE

Hypertension, a relatively virulent disease, affects an estimated 50 million persons in the United States and predisposes them to the potentially fatal complications of myocardial infarction, stroke, and renal failure. The cause is unknown in most patients and is considered to be essential hypertension. Renal disease is thought to be the responsible mechanism in 5–10% of patients with hypertension; renal hypertension may be of vascular origin or secondary to renal parenchymal disease. Renovascular hypertension, once thought to be uncommon, affects nearly one-half million Americans and surgical intervention has now been shown to rectify the clinical course of this disease.

Freeman and associates (1) in 1954 demonstrated that renal thromboendarterectomy could cure renovascular hypertension. Since that time, a variety of surgical procedures have been described to correct the hypertension caused by renal artery stenosis or occlusion and to improve deteriorating renal function.

At the Lahey Clinic, we have performed 350 surgical procedures for renovascular hypertension and compromised renal function since 1970. Aortorenal bypass with either saphenous vein or, less commonly, a prosthetic graft has become the preferred surgical procedure. However, with the expansion of the indications for renal revascularization in an older, referred patient population with prior abdominal aortic surgery, severe atherosclerosis of the abdominal aorta, small asymptomatic abdominal aortic aneurysms, or complete occlusion of the abdominal aorta, alternative surgical procedures have been necessary for renal artery revascularization (2, 3).

Since 1970, we have performed more than 100 alternative bypass procedures, including 60 splenorenal and 38 hepatorenal bypass procedures. Alternative bypass procedures included the use of superior mesenteric, inferior mesenteric, colic, and iliac circulations as well as the use of auto-transplantation, all with favorable results. This chapter focuses on the use of the hepatic circulation, including the gastroduodenal artery, for renal artery revascularization and presents the indications for, surgical technique of, and results of surgical intervention of viable alternative.

INDICATIONS FOR SURGERY

Patients with renal artery stenosis or occlusion and patients with diffuse atherosclerosis make renal revascularization a high-risk procedure. Originally, indications for operation included age of less than 50 years, the presence of mural dysplasia rather than atherosclerosis, and hypertension of short duration. Currently, surgical intervention is frequently recommended for patients 50 years of age and older even with atherosclerotic disease. Operation is also recommended for patients with azotemia to improve deteriorating renal function, revascularization of the totally occluded renal artery, and concomitant renovascular hypertension and aortic disease performed as a two-stage procedure, that is, renal revascularization followed by the abdominal aortic procedure.

Although the number of patients with complex disease being referred for renal revascularization has increased and more patients are found to be candidates for operation, the underlying indications for renal revascularization have not changed. Clearly, the indications for surgical intervention are poor control of hypertension after aggressive, appropriate drug therapy; poor patient compliance; total renal artery occlusion or dissection; deterioration of renal function as manifested by an elevation of the blood urea nitrogen and creatinine levels; radiographic evidence of renal parenchymal loss; angiographic evidence of progressive renal artery disease or loss of function demonstrated on renal scan; severely symptomatic or accelerated hypertension; anuria from arterial occlusion in a solitary kidney; and any combination of these factors (4).

Preoperative and Intraoperative Preparation

Patients with renovascular hypertension may present with the complex problems associated with systemic atherosclerosis and the effect this hypertension has on the vasculature of other organs. All distal arterial pulses and bruits in the neck and extremities need to be documented by careful preoperative recording for baseline reference. A detailed history of the cardiovascular and cerebrovascular circulations is obtained, including past history of transient ischemic attacks, stroke, angina, myocardial infarctions, and peripheral vascular disease. A history positive for any of these factors may require further evaluation before a major renal revascularization procedure is performed because the perfusion pressure of the heart and brain will be reduced greatly by successful renal revascularization. The resultant decrease in diastolic pressure can cause myocardial injury and the overall decrease in systemic pressure can result in cerebral injury.

Metabolic derangements, such as hypokalemia from diuretic therapy or secondary hyperaldosteronism, should be corrected before administration of general anesthesia with its myocardial depressant and arrhythmogenic potentials. Acute pyelonephritis is treated for a minimum of 3 weeks before operation and the urine must be sterile, especially if a prosthetic graft is necessary. Severe hypertension can be controlled with short-acting agents up to the time of operation, and then nitroprusside can be given intravenously intraoperatively and continued postoperatively.

Continuous cardiac monitoring is of paramount importance. As with major abdominal aortic procedures, continuous electrocardiographic monitoring is required with use of an arterial line and a Swan-Ganz catheter. Familiarity with the various vasopressors and vasodilators is essential. Continuous monitoring of central venous pressure, pulmonary artery and pulmonary capillary wedge pressures, and the cardiac output index make renal revascularization a safer procedure.

Even without laboratory or radiographic evidence of deterioration in renal function, the effects of ischemia on the renal parenchyma can be minimized by the judicious use of mannitol and furosemide (Lasix) while the renal vessels are clamped. Systemic anticoagulation by intravenous administration of 5000 units of heparin 20–30 min before clamping the renal and hepatic vessels minimizes local and systemic thromboembolic complications.

Hepatic and Gastroduodenal Renal Artery Bypass

Stenosis of the right renal artery in association with previous abdominal aortic operation or diffuse abdominal aortic atherosclerosis precludes performing an aortorenal bypass operation. We (5) first described use of the hepatic circulation for the management of right renal artery stenosis in 1976. This work was confirmed 3 years later both experimentally and clinically by Novick and associates (6, 7) at the Cleveland Clinic as well as in a combined report from both institutions showing favorable results in 36 patients undergoing hepatorenal bypass procedures (3).

The hepatic circulation is unique in that it has a portal system with portal venous and hepatic artery inflow. The liver receives 28% (1500 ml/min) of the cardiac output in resting adults: 80% through the portal vein and 20% through the hepatic artery. The hepatic artery flow is 300 ml/min and is sufficient to maintain adequate renal perfusion. The mean pressure in the hepatic artery branches that converge on the sinusoids and the liver is approximately 90 mm Hg. The curve that describes renal circulatory autoregulation demonstrates that when the kidney is perfused at pressures between 90 mm Hg and 250 mm Hg, the renovascular resistance varies with the pressure so that a relatively constant renal blood flow is maintained (Fig. 25.1). The hepatic circulation has the proper blood flow and pressure profile to maintain adequate renal circulation.

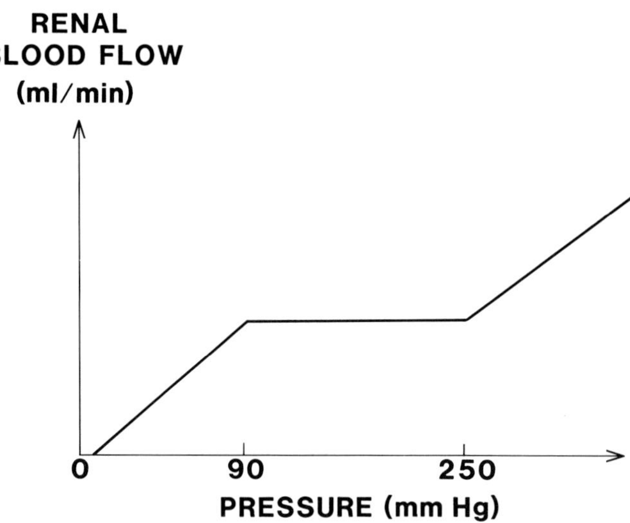

Figure 25.1. Renal circulatory autoregulation. (From Libertino JA, Zinman L, Breslin DJ, Swinton NW Jr.: Hepatorenal artery bypass in the management of renovascular hypertension. *J Urol* 115:371, 1976. © Williams & Wilkins, 1976.)

The hepatic artery (Fig. 25.2) originates from the celiac axis, runs along the upper border of the pancreas, and divides into the ascending and descending limbs at the portal vein. The ascending limb, the continuation of the main artery upward within the lesser omentum, lies anterior to the portal vein and to the left of the biliary tree. The descending limb becomes the gastroduodenal artery. The hepatic artery divides into the right and left hepatic arteries in the porta hepatis.

During preoperative abdominal aortography, it is essential to outline anatomic variations of the hepatic circulation and concomitant abnormalities of the visceral circulation. The location of the right hepatic artery is more variable than that of the left hepatic artery. It may be anterior (24%) or posterior (64%) to the common bile duct and may originate from the superior mesenteric artery 12% of the time (Fig. 25.3). The left hepatic artery arises from the left gastric artery 11.5% of the time. The anatomy of the hepatic circulation of each patient will determine whether the common hepatic, right or left hepatic, or the gastroduodenal artery will be used as a source for renal revascularization.

The patient, having already received intravenous fluid hydration, intravenous antibiotics on call to the surgical suite, and placement of a Foley catheter for monitoring urine output, is placed in the supine position with the arms at the sides.

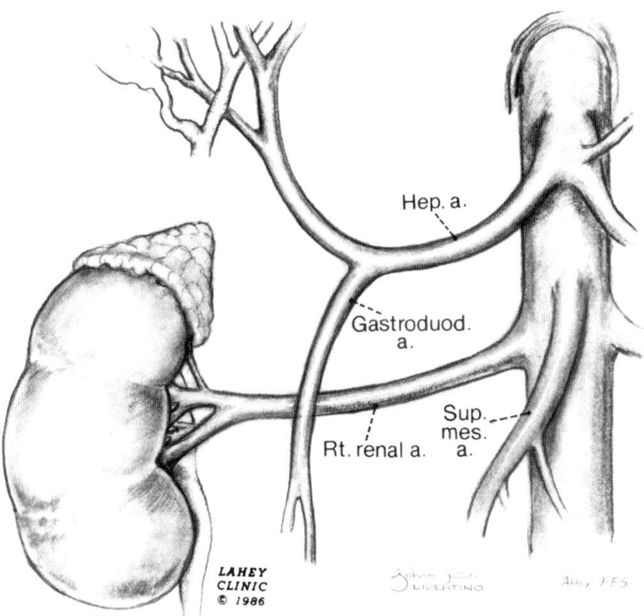

Figure 25.2. Normal hepatic artery anatomy. (By permission of Lahey Clinic.)

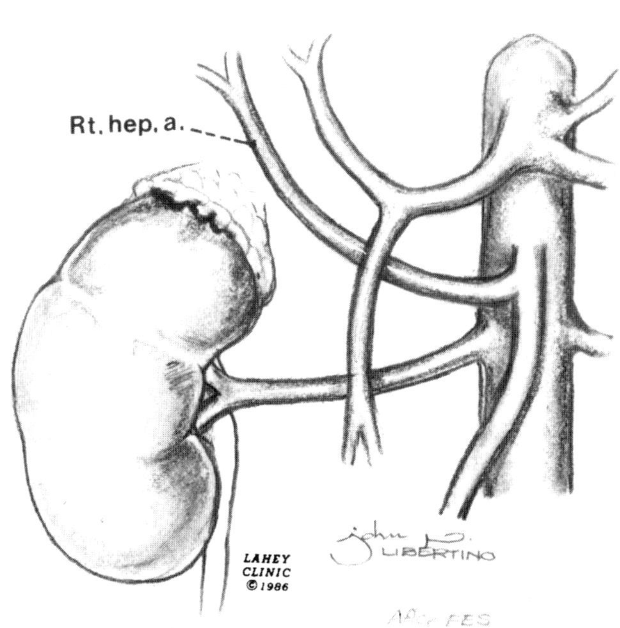

Figure 25.3. Right hepatic artery originating from the superior mesenteric artery. (By permission of Lahey Clinic.)

The skin of the chest, abdomen, and both legs is prepared and draped so that both lower extremities as well as the abdomen and lower part of the chest are exposed.

The surgical approach to the hepatic circulation and the right renal artery is through a transverse chevron incision extending from the tip of the right 11th rib to the lateral border of the left rectus muscle. The hepatic flexure and the duodenum are mobilized, exposing the right renal circulation (Fig. 25.4). The porta hepatis is carefully dissected enabling exposure of the common hepatic, gastroduodenal, and right and left hepatic arteries. Vessel loops are placed around these arteries where applicable and the common bile duct and portal vein are identified. The stenotic or occluded right renal artery is then dissected (Fig. 25.5).

Microvascular clamps are placed on the common hepatic and gastroduodenal arteries. The gastroduodenal artery is transected and ligated distally (Fig. 25.6). The hepatic artery is mobilized carefully and completely on its inferior surface from the underlying portal vein and common bile duct (Fig. 25.7). A 10- to 12-mm arteriotomy is made in the common hepatic artery beginning at the point of origin of the gastroduodenal artery. A reversed autogenous saphenous vein graft

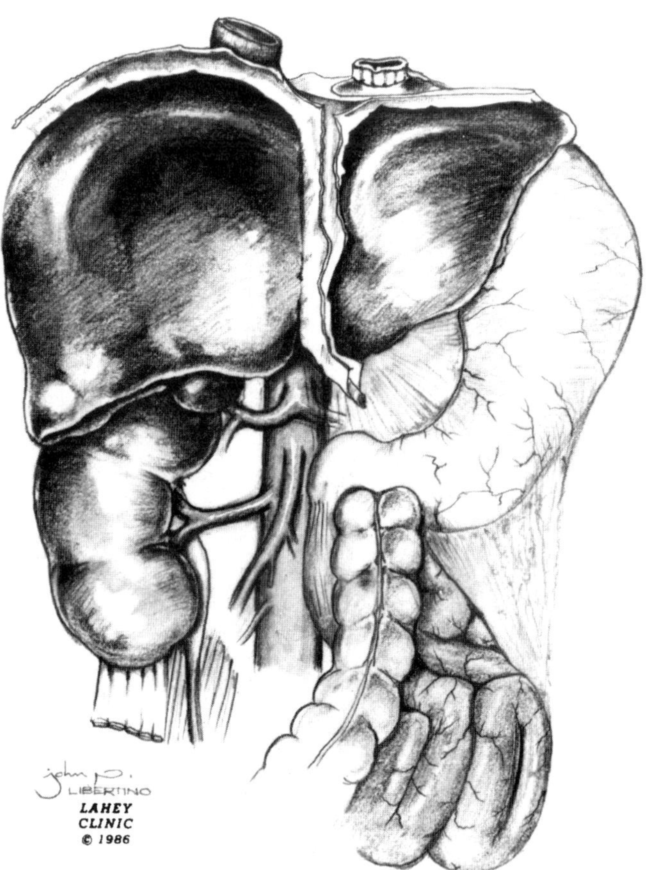

Figure 25.4. The hepatic and right renal arterial circulation exposed by mobilization of the hepatic flexure of the colon and the duodenum. (By permission of Lahey Clinic.)

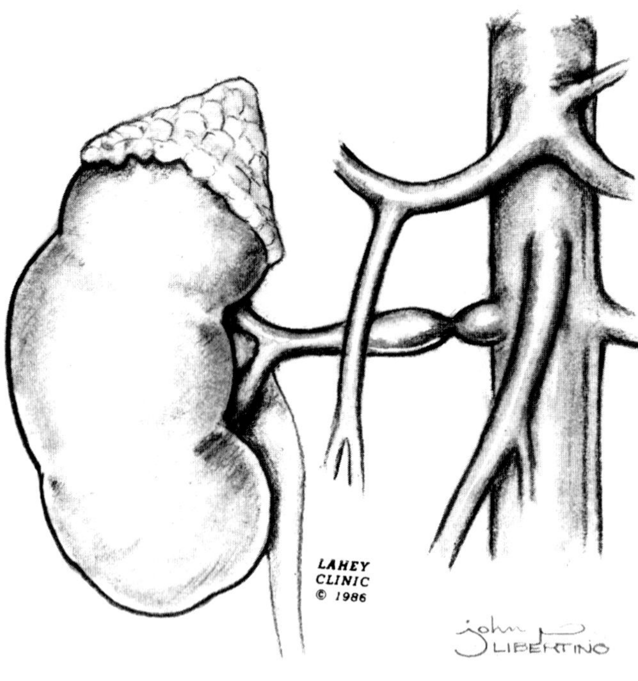

Figure 25.5. Stenosis of the right renal artery. (By permission of Lahey Clinic.)

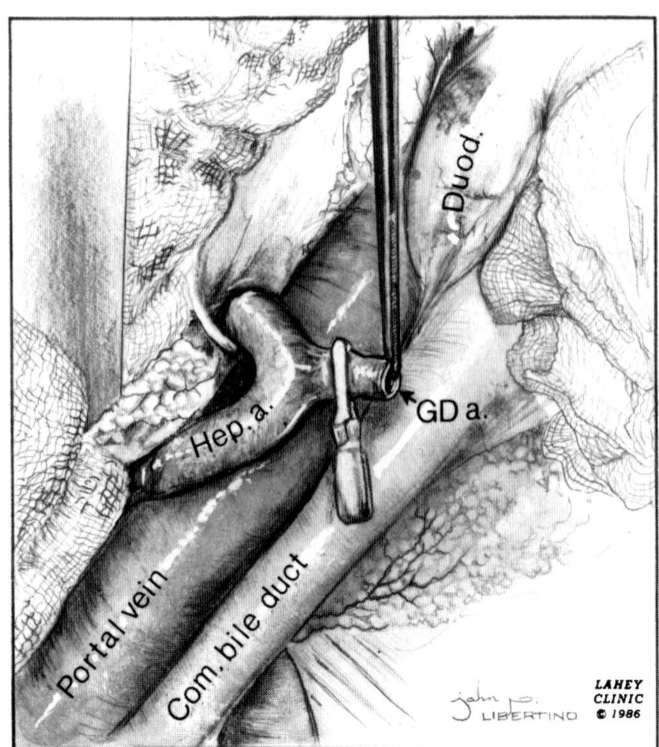

Figure 25.6. Mobilization of the anterior surface of the common hepatic artery. (By permission of Lahey Clinic.)

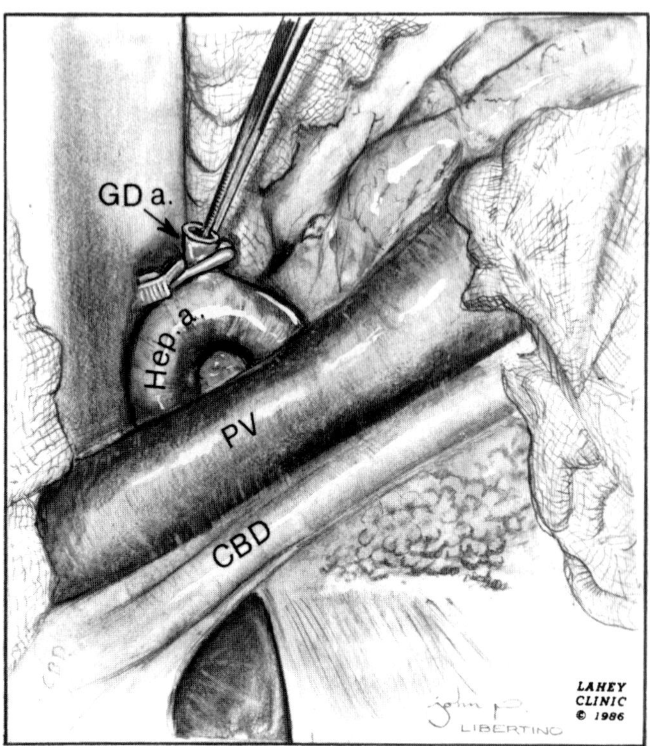

Figure 25.7. Mobilization of the posterior surface of the common hepatic artery. (By permission of Lahey Clinic.)

is inserted by an end-to-side anastomosis to the common hepatic artery. A microvascular clamp is placed on the vein graft after filling it with heparin solution and obtaining the proper alignment and length for the renal artery anastomosis. The clamps are removed from the hepatic artery and are placed on the proximal and distal ends of the renal artery. The vein graft is anastomosed to the right renal artery at a suitable site beyond the disease process in either an end-to-side or end-to-end fashion (Fig. 25.8). The microvascular clamps are removed and the pulse through the graft and the right renal artery is assessed. Occasionally, when clinically indicated, completion arteriography is performed to evaluate the possibility of a technical error.

In some patients, the common hepatic artery cannot be used for hepatorenal revascularization either because of an anatomic variation in which either hepatic lobar artery has a variant origin or because of an early bifurcation into the right and left lobar branches. In this situation, the right and left hepatic arteries may each be of insufficient caliber to maintain adequate perfusion to both the liver lobe and the right kidney. A direct end-to-end anastomosis can be accomplished between either of the major hepatic branches and the distal right renal artery, usually without an interposition saphenous vein graft. Direct end-to-end gastroduodenal-to-right renal artery bypass can also be performed if the gastroduodenal artery has sufficient flow (Fig. 25.9).

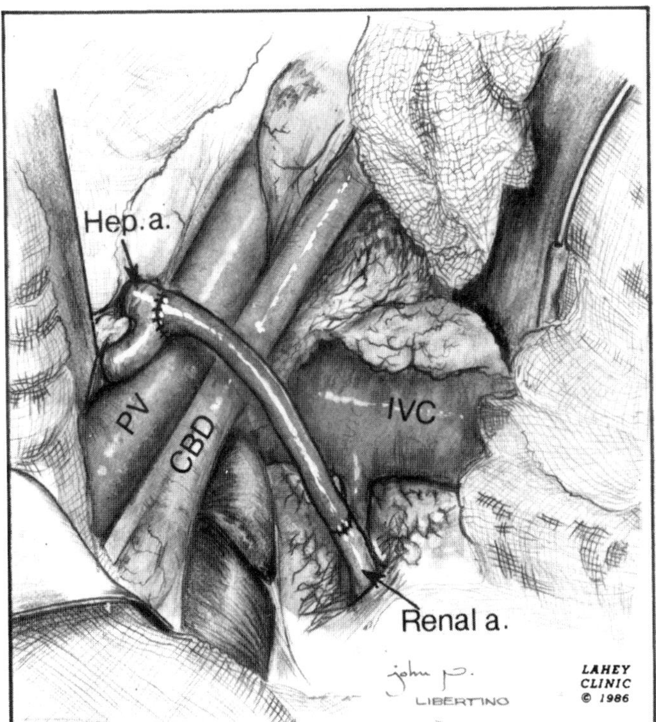

Figure 25.8. Anastomosis of the hepatic artery to the right renal artery using reversed saphenous vein graft. (By permission of Lahey Clinic.)

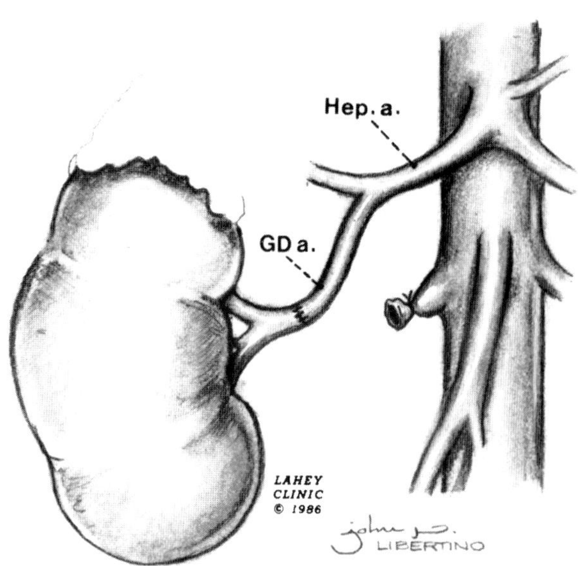

Figure 25.9. Renal artery-to-gastroduodenal artery end-to-end anastomosis. (By permission of Lahey Clinic.)

RESULTS

The major advantage of using the hepatic circulation as an alternative to aortorenal revascularization is its extensive collateral circulation that protects the liver should the bypass graft thrombose and a clot propagate into the hepatic circulation. Two patients in our series undergoing renal revascularization by all methods had postoperative graft thrombosis, but retrograde propagation of clot into the hepatic artery did not occur. Even in Novick's and associates' (6, 7) series, when an end-to-end anastomosis was constructed with either of the major hepatic branches, which results in hepatic devascularization, no patient had abnormal liver function tests.

Total or lobar hepatic artery ligation is compatible with life and has been performed frequently in conjunction with chemotherapy in the management of hepatic neoplasms. However, when the right hepatic artery is anastomosed end-to-end to the right renal artery, the gallbladder is more susceptible to ischemic damage than the liver and may undergo necrosis when the blood supply from the right hepatic artery is interrupted. In the series by Novick and associates (7), two patients exhibited this complication; one patient died, and the other patient recovered uneventfully from an emergency cholecystectomy. We prefer the end-to-side hepatic artery anastomosis. If an end-to-end anastomosis with the right hepatic artery must be performed, a prophylactic cholecystectomy should be considered.

Of our 38 patients who underwent renal revascularization using the hepatic circulation, 20 were men and 18 were women ranging in age from 12–75 years. Thirty-five patients (92%) had atherosclerotic lesions, while three patients (8%) had mural dysplasia. Thirty-five patients (92%) had right renal artery stenosis and three patients (8%) had total occlusion of the right renal artery. Twenty-nine patients (76%) had bilateral renal artery disease.

In 33 patients (86%), an hepatic artery-to-right renal artery reversed saphenous vein bypass was performed; five patients (13%) underwent gastroduodenal artery-to-right renal artery bypass. The operative morbidity was 18% (seven of 38 patients); complications included two postoperative thrombosed grafts, two myocardial infarctions, a splenic injury requiring splenectomy, a bleeding duodenal ulcer treated nonoperatively, and a hemoperitoneum requiring reexploration. Long-term complications within the first postoperative year included three graft failures as evidenced by recurrent hypertension and one death from a myocardial infarction.

Operative mortality (30 days) in this high-risk population was 2.6% (one of 38 patients) with this death being secondary to a myocardial infarction. This is less than the operative mortality of 5.7% as seen in the overall series of our last 123 patients undergoing 152 consecutive renal revascularizations (unpublished data).

Postoperatively, the 31 patients having hepatic artery or gastroduodenal artery-to-right renal artery bypass grafting followed up for more than 1 year were evaluated for reduction of blood pressure and improvement in renal function when either or both of these factors were surgical indications. Digital subtraction angiography or renal perfusion scan (earlier cases) was ordered to assess patency of the graft. Digital subtraction angiography is now exclusively utilized as a more reliable and less invasive method of delineating renal artery perfusion and anatomy after renal revascularization.

The criteria used to evaluate the effect of renal revascularization on the blood pressure response were those of Kaufman and Maxwell (8). Patients were considered cured if the blood pressure remained at or below 140/90 mm Hg for 1 year after operation without any antihypertensive medication. Improvement of hypertension was defined as a reduction in diastolic blood pressure of 15 mm Hg or more or maintenance of systemic blood pressure at or below 140/90 mm Hg with less antihypertensive medication than required preoperatively. The surgical result was considered to be a failure if either of these two criteria were not met.

Of the 31 patients followed up for more than 1 year and operated on primarily for uncontrollable hypertension, 12 patients (38.7%) were cured, 15 patients (48.4%) were improved, and four patients (12.9%) failed to obtain any benefit from renal revascularization. The combined rate of cure and improvement was 87.1%. Two patients improved after revascularization of the left renal artery. All patients with mural dysplasia had patent grafts and were cured of hypertension 1 year or more after surgery.

Of the eight patients (26%) operated on primarily for renal failure, seven patients (87.5%) had improved renal function with one of the eight patients (12.5%) having stabilization of renal function.

Eight patients (26%) had a combination of uncontrollable hypertension and deterioration of renal function. A cure or improvement of hypertension and improvement in renal function were obtained in seven patients (87.5%). In only one of the eight patients (12.5%) was the result considered a failure because the criteria of both cure or improvement of hypertension combined with improvement of renal function were not met.

Stenosis or occlusion of the right renal artery with resultant hypertension in a patient with a contraindication to the use of the abdominal aorta can be corrected readily and safely by the hepatic artery method. Our results indicate that this choice of surgical intervention will continue to be a viable alternative to aortorenal saphenous vein bypass with reduced morbidity and mortality in this high-risk patient population.

References

1. Freeman NE, Leeds FH, Elliott WG, Roland SI: Thromboendarterectomy for hypertension due to renal artery occlusion. *JAMA* 156:1077, 1954.
2. Libertino JA, Selman FJ Jr: Alternatives to aortorenal revascularization. *J Cardiovasc Surg* 23:318, 1982.
3. Chibaro EA, Libertino JA, Novick AC: Use of the hepatic circulation for renal revascularization. *Ann Surg* 199:406, 1984.
4. Libertino JA, Zinman L: Surgery for renovascular hypertension. In Breslin DJ, Swinton NW Jr, Libertino JA, Zinman L (eds): *Renovascular Hypertension*. Baltimore, Williams & Wilkins, 1982, pp. 166–212.
5. Libertino JA, Zinman L, Breslin DJ, Swinton NW Jr: Hepatorenal artery bypass in the management of renovascular hypertension. *J Urol* 115:369, 1976.
6. Novick AC, Palleschi J, Straffon RA, Beven E: Experimental and clinical hepatorenal bypass as a means of revascularization of the right renal artery. *Surg Gynecol Obstet* 148:557, 1979.
7. Novick AC, McElroy J: Renal revascularization by end-to-end anastomosis of the hepatic and renal arteries. *J Urol* 134:1089, 1985.
8. Kaufman JJ, Maxwell MH: Surgery for renovascular hypertension: Analysis of 67 cases. *JAMA* 190:709, 1964.

EDITORIAL COMMENT

Doctor Libertino and his colleagues have made a major contribution to the field of renovascular surgery through their initial description and subsequent large experience with the technique of hepatorenal saphenous vein bypass. I agree completely that this operation is the treatment of choice for patients with a surgically difficult aorta who require right renal revascularization. We use the technique described in this chapter with the exception of leaving the gastroduodenal artery (GDA) intact and performing end-to-side anastomosis of the saphenous vein graft to the common hepatic artery just beyond the origin on the GDA. This is done to obviate the theoretical risk of a devascularization injury to the duodenum that may, perhaps, be associated with transection of the GDA. I agree that the end-to-side hepatic artery anastomosis should be used whenever possible because this preserves distal hepatic arterial flow and thereby prevents ischemic damage to the gallbladder.

Andrew C. Novick, M.D.
Chairman, Department of Urology
Cleveland Clinic Foundation

CHAPTER 26

Splenorenal Bypass

ANDREW C. NOVICK

Aortorenal bypass, as outlined in chapter 24, is well established as the preferred vascular reconstructive technique for patients with renal artery disease. Nevertheless, in some patients, involvement of the abdominal aorta with severe atherosclerosis, aneurysmal disease or dense fibrosis from a prior operation may render an aortorenal bypass technically difficult and potentially hazardous to perform. Simultaneous aortic replacement and renal revascularization has been associated with high operative mortality rates and should only be considered in patients with a significant aortic aneurysm or symptomatic aortoiliac occlusive disease. Alternative surgical approaches, which allow renal revascularization to be accomplished safely and effectively while avoiding operation on a badly diseased aorta, are preferable in such cases.

At the Cleveland Clinic, splenorenal bypass has become the preferred vascular reconstructive technique for patients with a troublesome aorta who require left renal revascularization. For patients in this category who require right renal revascularization, our approach is to perform a hepatorenal bypass. The requisite conditions for this operation and the technique for its performance are described in chapter 25. The problem of a troublesome aorta that precludes performance of an aortorenal bypass most often presents in patients with evidence of generalized atherosclerosis. The use of alternative effective methods of revascularization, such as splenorenal and hepatorenal bypass, has been an important strategy toward minimizing operative morbidity and mortality in these high risk patients.

For splenorenal bypass to be employed as a method of renal revascularization, certain requisite conditions must be met. The stenotic renal arterial lesion must be on the left side and of the type that a bypass may be performed safely distal to the diseased segment. Transposition of the splenic artery by retroduodenal passage for right renal revascularization has been unsatisfactory and is not recommended. Another requirement for performing splenorenal bypass is the demonstration on preoperative aortography, with both anteroposterior and lateral views, of widely patent celiac and splenic arteries. The splenic artery must also be carefully examined intraoperatively for intramural atheromatous disease, which may be minimally occlusive and, therefore, not apparent on angiography but significant nonetheless. This problem, which is more commonly observed in women than in men, also mitigates against use of the splenic artery for renal revascularization.

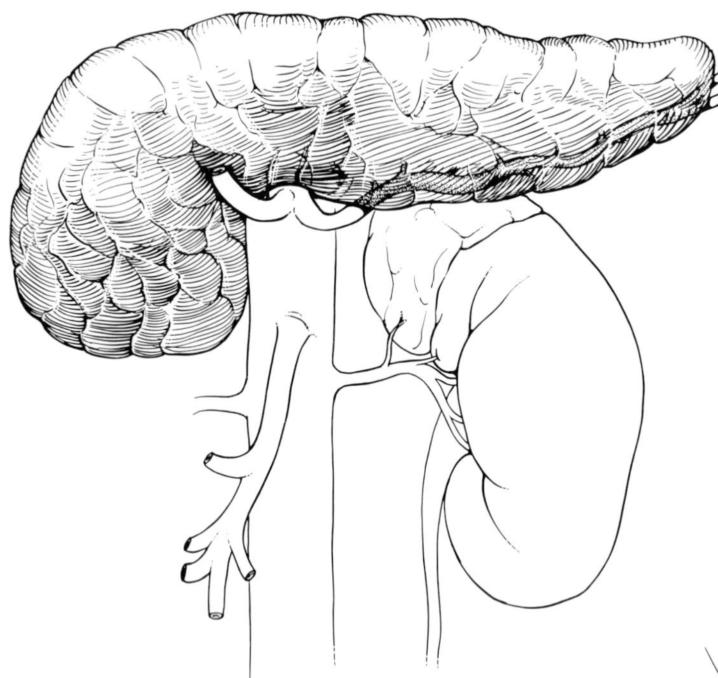

Figure 26.1. The normal anatomic relationships of the splenic and renal vessels are shown in this illustration. To perform splenorenal bypass, an extended left subcostal transperitoenal incision is made, and the left colon and duodenum are reflected medially. The plane between Gerota's fascia and the pancreas is developed by blunt dissection, and the pancreas and spleen are gently retracted cephalad. The Buckwalter self-retaining ring retractor is inserted to maintain exposure. Gerota's fascia is opened laterally over the lower pole of the kidney, so that the color and consistency of the kidney can be observed throughout the operation.

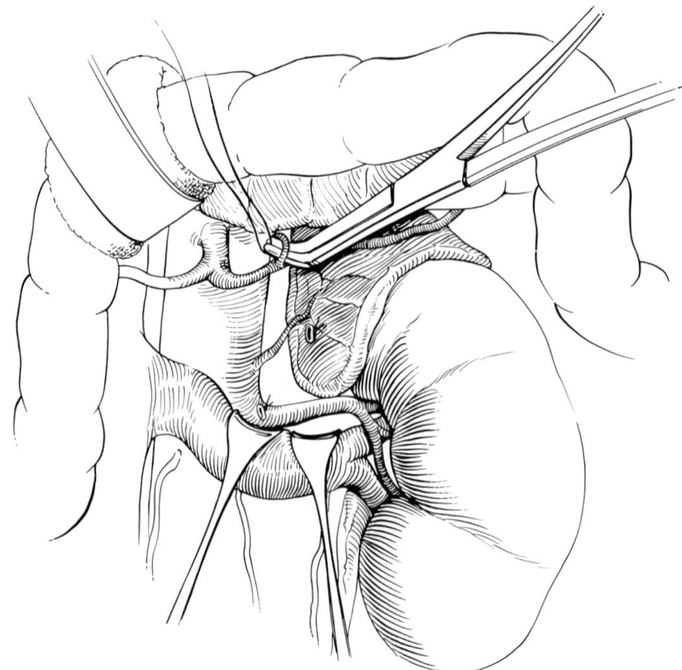

Figure 26.2. The left renal vein is mobilized and its adrenal and gonadal branches are ligated and divided. The left renal vein is then retracted inferiorly to expose the origin and the entire length of the main left renal artery. Dissection and mobilization of the infrarenal aorta are not required at any stage during the operation.

The pancreas is gently retracted upward to permit access to the splenic vessels. The splenic artery may be palpated posterior and superior to the splenic vein, and that portion lying closest to the distal aspect of the renal artery is chosen for mobilization. Small pancreatic arterial branches are divided and secured with fine silk sutures. The splenic artery may be quite tortuous and should be mobilized proximally as close to the celiac artery as possible, where the vessel wall is thicker and the luminal diameter larger. A tape may be passed around the splenic artery to aid in its mobilization.

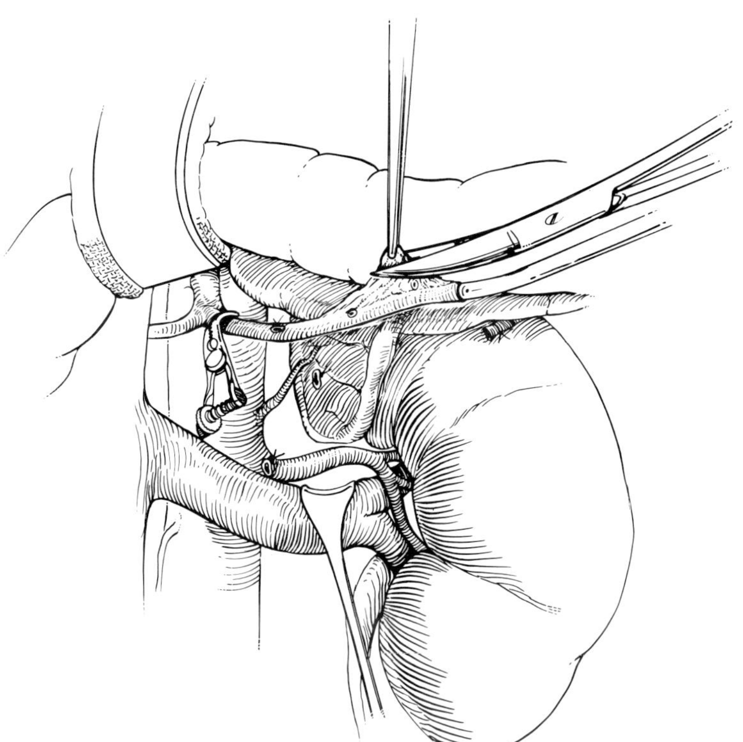

Figure 26.3. After its mobilization, the splenic artery is occluded proximally with a bulldog clamp, ligated distally with a 2–0 silk suture, and transected. It is not necessary to remove the spleen, which receives adequate collateral supply from the short gastric and gastroepiploic vessels to maintain its viability. After transection, the splenic artery is often observed to be in severe spasm with a considerably reduced luminal size. After irrigation of the lumen with dilute heparin solution, this spasm can be relieved by gentle dilation of the splenic artery with graduated sounds. This technique also facilitates removal of the periadventitial adhesions that may cause kinking or angulation of the graft.

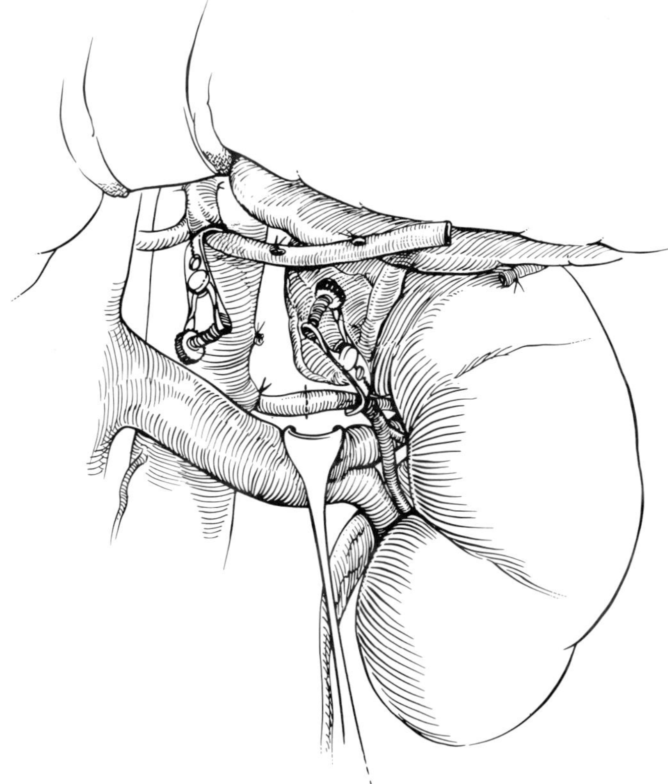

Figure 26.4. The left main renal artery is mobilized in its entirety, if this has not already been done. The renal artery is doubly ligated proximally, a bulldog clamp is applied distally, and the artery is transected beyond the area of disease. The diseased portion of the artery beyond the proximal ligature is resected and sent for pathologic examination. The bulldog clamp is temporarily released to allow instillation of 10 ml of dilute heparin solution into the distal renal artery.

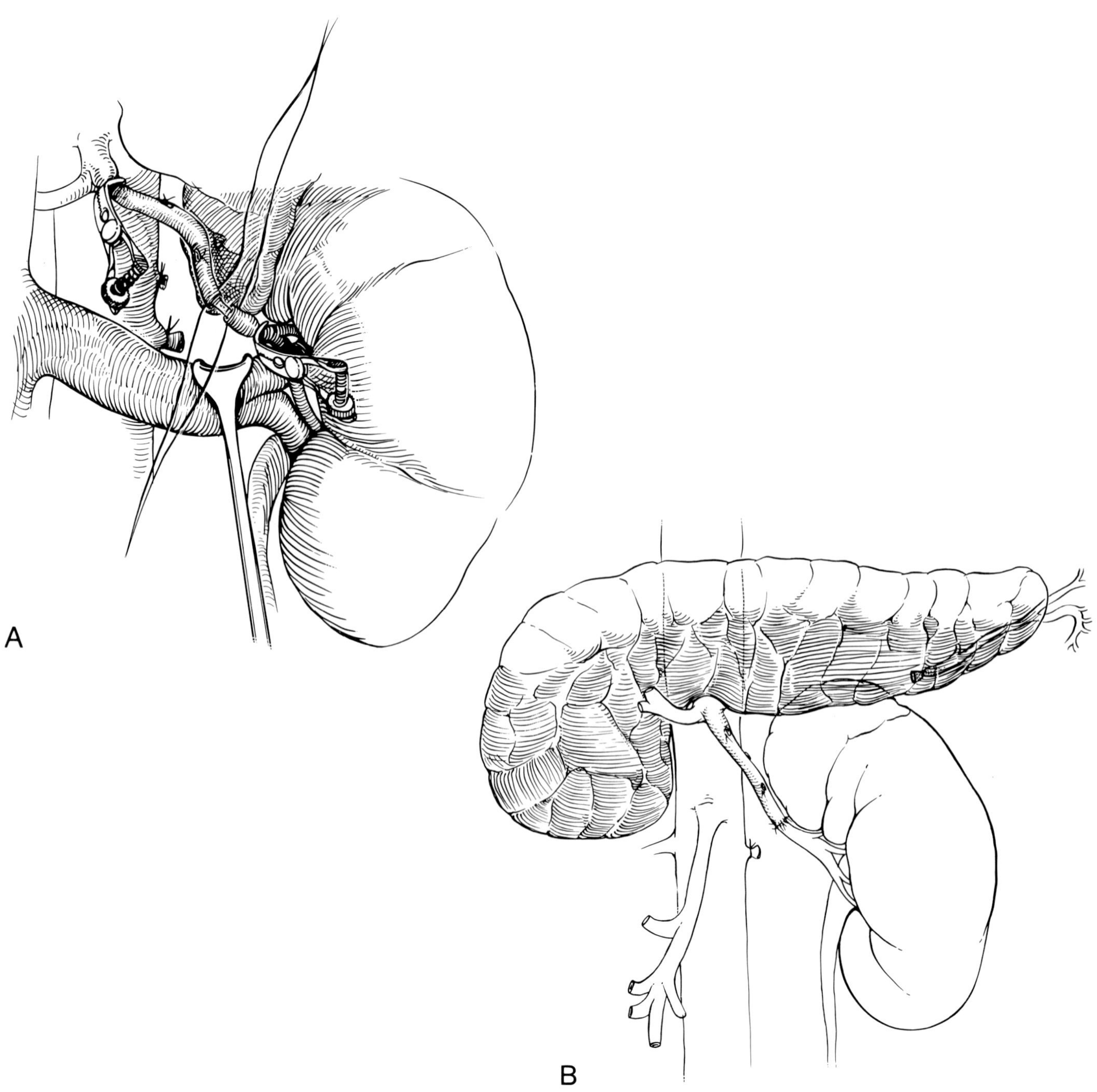

Figure 26.5. A and B, in general, there is no significant disparity in the caliber of the splenic and renal arteries and a direct end-to-end anastomosis is performed. We prefer this type of anastomosis because it provides better flow, is easier to perform, and allows removal of the diseased arterial segment for pathologic study. The anastomosis is performed with interrupted 6–0 arterial sutures. With this technique, the renal ischemia time is minimal and generally does not exceed 20 min. After completion of the anastomosis, all vascular clamps are removed and the kidney is observed for satisfactory perfusion.

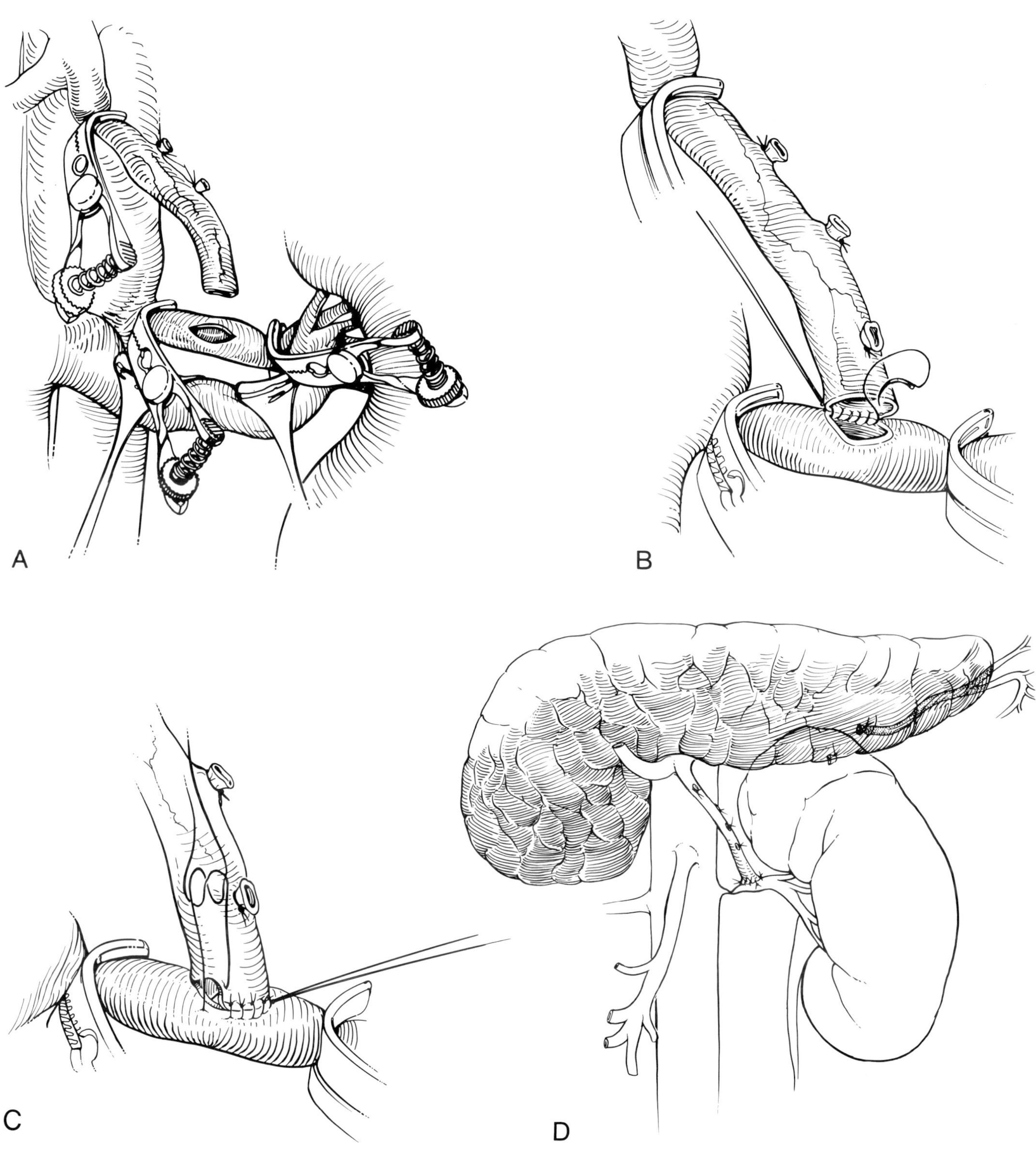

Figure 26.6. **A-D,** an alternative method for performing splenorenal bypass involves end-to-side anastomosis of the splenic artery to the distal disease-free renal artery. We have only employed this technique in the unusual event of a significant disparity in the caliber of the splenic and renal arteries.

The advantages of the splenorenal bypass technique are that the operation is done well away from the abdominal aorta, only a single vascular anastomosis is necessary, and revascularization is accomplished with an autogenous vascular graft. In properly selected patients, splenorenal bypass is an excellent method for performing vascular reconstruction of the left kidney.

Suggested Readings

Brewster DC, Darling RC: Splenorenal arterial anastomosis for renovascular hypertension. *Ann Surg* 189:353, 1979.

Kaufman JJ: Dacron grafts and splenorenal bypass in the surgical treatment of stenosing lesions of the renal artery. *Urol Clin North Am* 2:365, 1975.

Khauli R, Novick AC, Ziegelbaum M: Splenorenal bypass in the treatment of renal artery stenosis: Experience with 69 cases. *J Vasc Surg* 2:547, 1985.

Novick AC, Banowsky LH, Stewart BH, Straffon RA: Splenorenal bypass in the treatment of stenosis of the renal artery. *Surg Gynecol Obstet* 144:891, 1977.

Novick AC, Banowsky LH, Stewart BH, Straffon RA: Renal revascularization in patients with atherosclerosis or a previous operation on the abdominal aorta. *Surg Gynecol Obstet* 144:211, 1977.

Novick, AC, Straffon RA, Stewart BH et al: Diminished operative morbidity and mortality following revascularization for atherosclerotic renovascular disease. *JAMA* 246:749, 1981.

Novick, AC, Khauli RB, Vidt DG: Diminished operative risk and improved results following revascularization for atherosclerotic renovascular disease. *Urol Clin North Am* 11:435, 1984.

CHAPTER 27

Iliorenal and Mesenterorenal Bypass

ANDREW C. NOVICK

An important measure toward limiting surgical morbidity and mortality after renal revascularization in patients with generalized atherosclerosis has been the utilization of techniques that obviate operation on a badly diseased abdominal aorta. The two preceding chapters have described the preferred alternatives to aortorenal revascularization in such cases, namely, splenorenal and hepatorenal bypass. These methods are attractive because of their efficacy, relative simplicity, and the fact that they do not jeopardize the sole blood supply to an organ. Although these approaches are suitable for many patients, they cannot be employed when the celiac, splenic, and/or hepatic arteries are themselves involved with atherosclerotic occlusive disease. Iliorenal and mesenterorenal bypass are alternative approaches that, occasionally, can be employed in such cases to accomplish safe and effective renal revascularization while avoiding operation on a troublesome aorta.

ILIORENAL BYPASS

Iliorenal bypass is a useful technique for revascularization in patients with severe aortic atherosclerosis, provided there is satisfactory flow through the diseased aorta and absence of significant iliac disease. As mentioned above, our approach is to consider this operation only when a splenorenal or hepatorenal bypass cannot be done due to disease involving the celiac, splenic, or hepatic arteries. This philosophy is based on the fact that aortic atherosclerosis may continue to progress in these patients and, if so, this process is more likely to involve the infrarenal aorta. Such a development might then compromise flow to a revascularized kidney whose blood supply is derived exclusively from one of the iliac arteries. The suprarenal aorta from which the celiac artery originates is more often spared from progressive atherosclerosis, hence, our preference for splenorenal or hepatorenal bypass.

In patients with good flow through a severely atherosclerotic aorta and a relatively healthy common iliac artery, renal autotransplantation has also been employed as a method of achieving renal revascularization. In general, we prefer an iliorenal bypass in such cases for several reasons. When compared to renal autotransplantation, an iliorenal bypass involves a shorter period of renal ischemia and, because mobilization of the kidney is not required, the collateral renal arterial supply is preserved. An iliorenal bypass also requires less operative time, which is an important consideration in patients with generalized atherosclerosis.

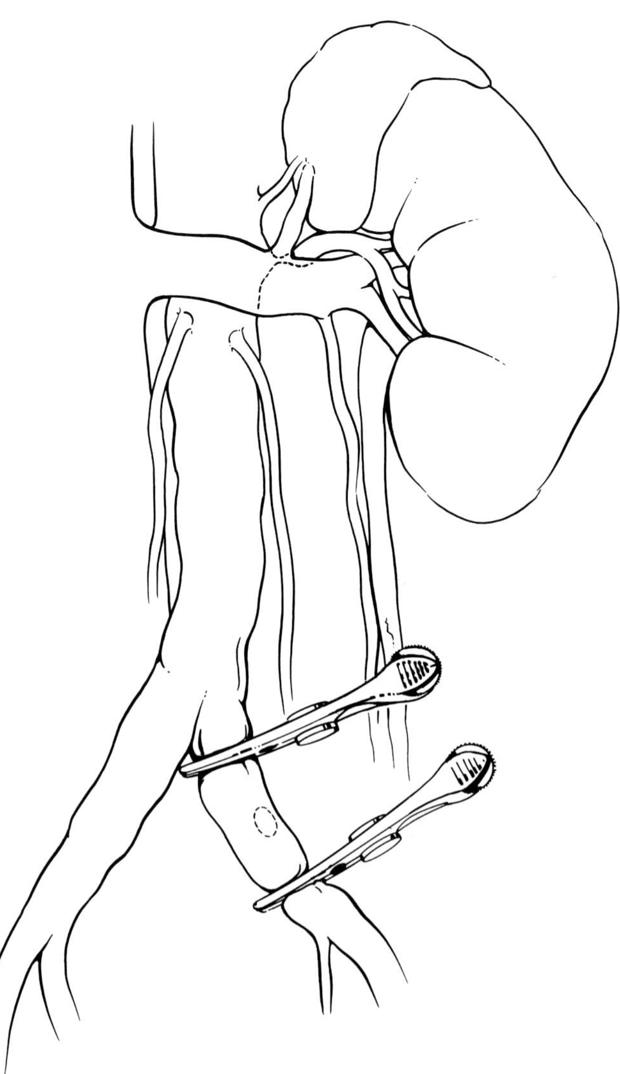

Figure 27.1. Iliorenal bypass is performed through a midline transperitoneal incision after harvesting a long saphenous vein graft. The colon is reflected medially to obtain simultaneous exposure of the ipsilateral common iliac and renal arteries. The common iliac artery is occluded proximally and distally with bulldog clamps. An oval arteriotomy is made on the anterolateral aspect of the common iliac artery. The distal clamp is temporarily released to enable 20 ml of dilute heparin solution to be instilled into the distal iliac and femoral arteries. Systemic heparinization is not routinely employed.

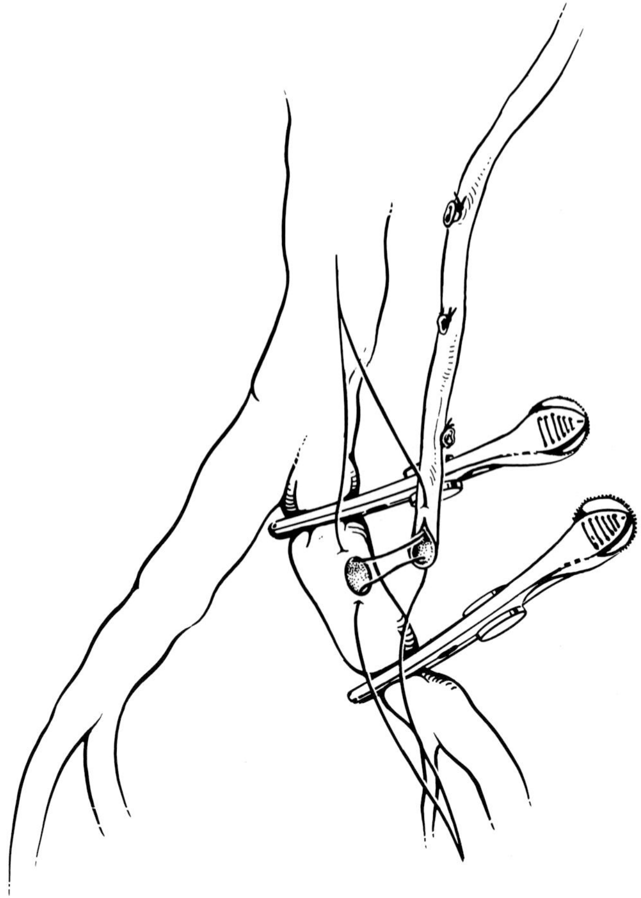

Figure 27.2. The proximal end of the saphenous vein graft is spatulated and the apex of the spatulation is placed at the cephalic end of the arteriortomy. Stay sutures are placed in both cephalic and caudal margins of the anastomosis, which is then completed with interrupted 6–0 arterial sutures.

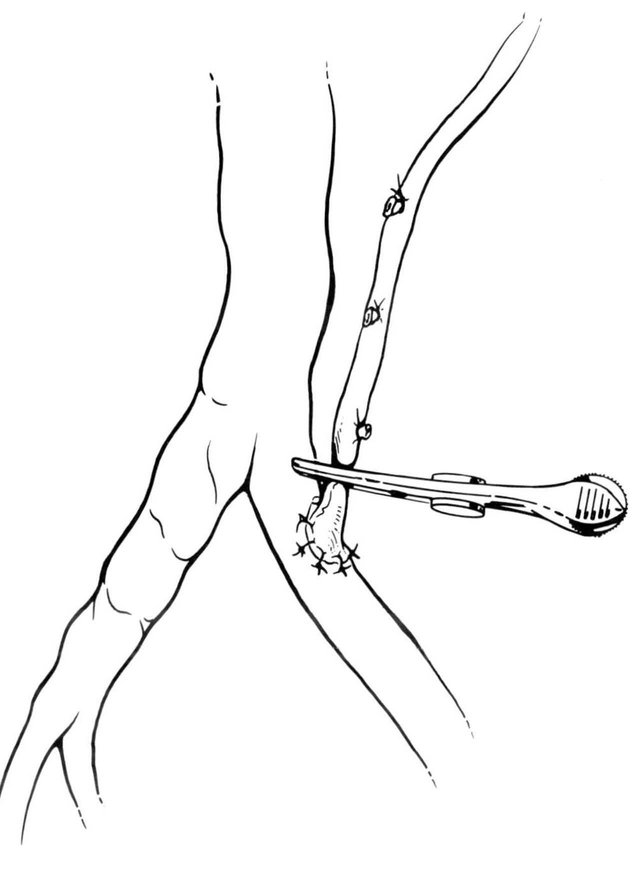

Figure 27.3. A bulldog clamp is placed across the proximal portion of the vein graft and the iliac clamps are removed restoring circulation to the lower extremity. The saphenous vein graft follows a direct cephalad course toward the ipsilateral renal artery between the aorta medially and the ureter laterally.

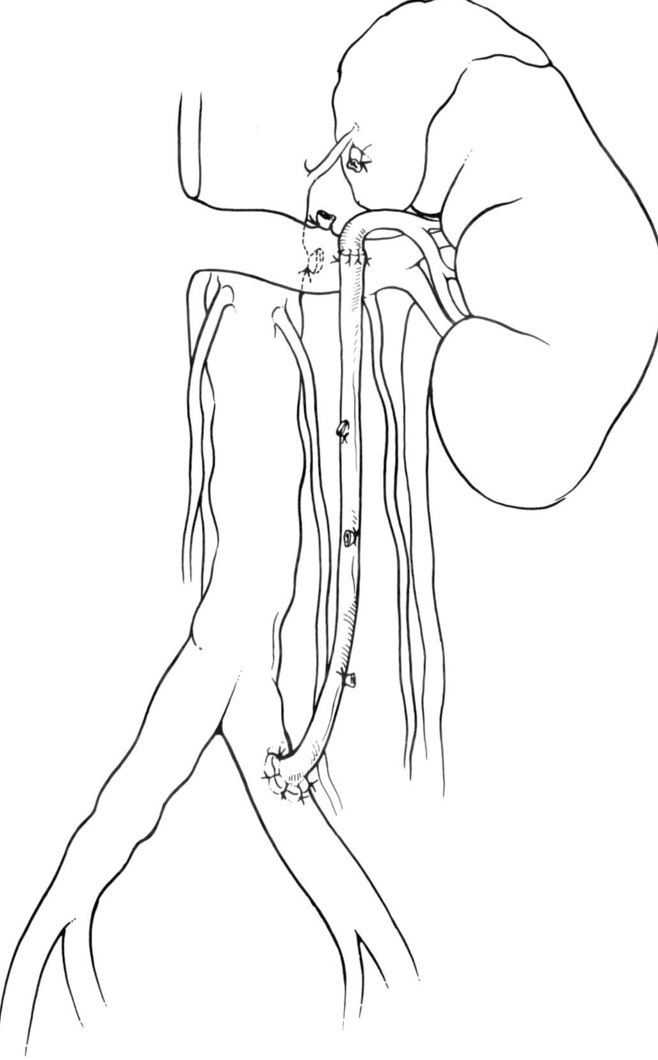

Figure 27.4. An end-to-end anastomosis of the saphenous vein graft to the distal disease-free renal artery is then performed with interrupted 6–0 arterial sutures. The graft is positioned to allow a tension-free distal anastomosis while avoiding angulation or kinking of the renal artery.

Figure 27.5. In general, iliorenal bypass is performed using the ipsilateral iliac artery because this simplifies exposure of the operative field. This is a relatively minor consideration and use of the contralateral common iliac artery (as shown in this diagram) is also satisfactory, particularly if this is less diseased than the ipsilateral counterpart.

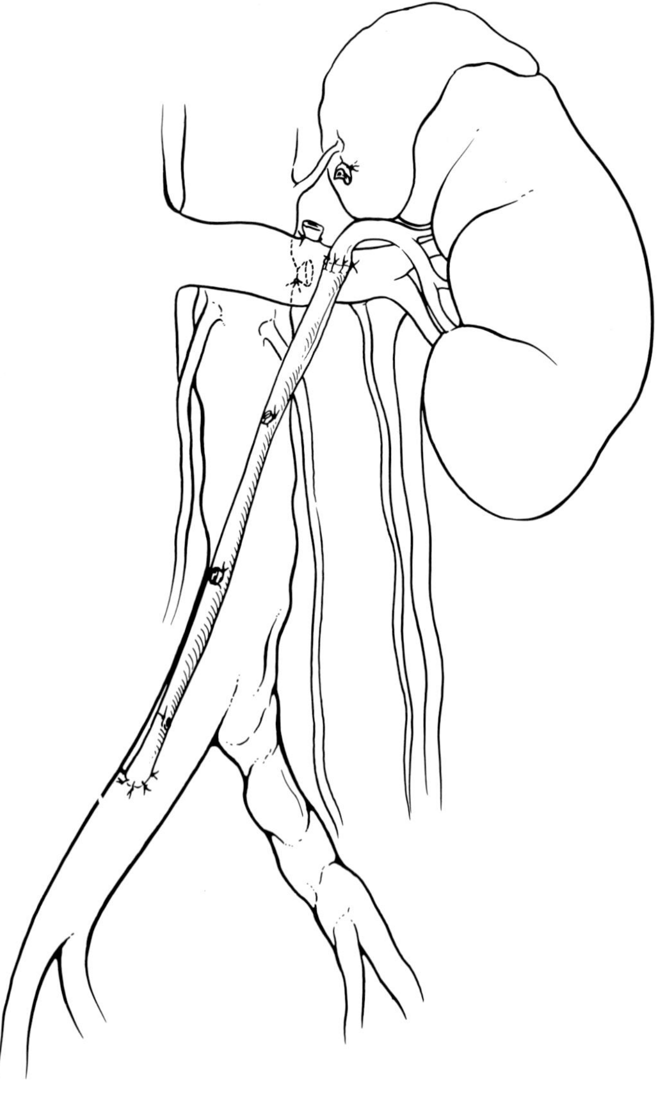

MESENTERORENAL BYPASS

In unusual cases, aortography reveals an enlarged superior mesenteric artery (SMA) that may then be employed for visceral arterial bypass to either kidney. We have employed the superior mesenterorenal bypass technique in patients with a troublesome aorta in whom a bypass to the kidney from the celiac or iliac arteries is not possible. The finding of an enlarged and widely patent SMA is most often observed in patients with total occlusion of the infrarenal aorta. In such cases, the SMA has a wider caliber than normal because it is supplying collateral vessels to areas ordinarily vascularized from the infrarenal aorta, i.e., the large bowel, pelvis, and lower extremities. Use of such an enlarged SMA for performance of a mesenterorenal bypass has been well tolerated with no compromise of intestinal blood flow. We have been reluctant to use this approach in patients with a normal-sized SMA and cannot comment on its efficacy in this setting.

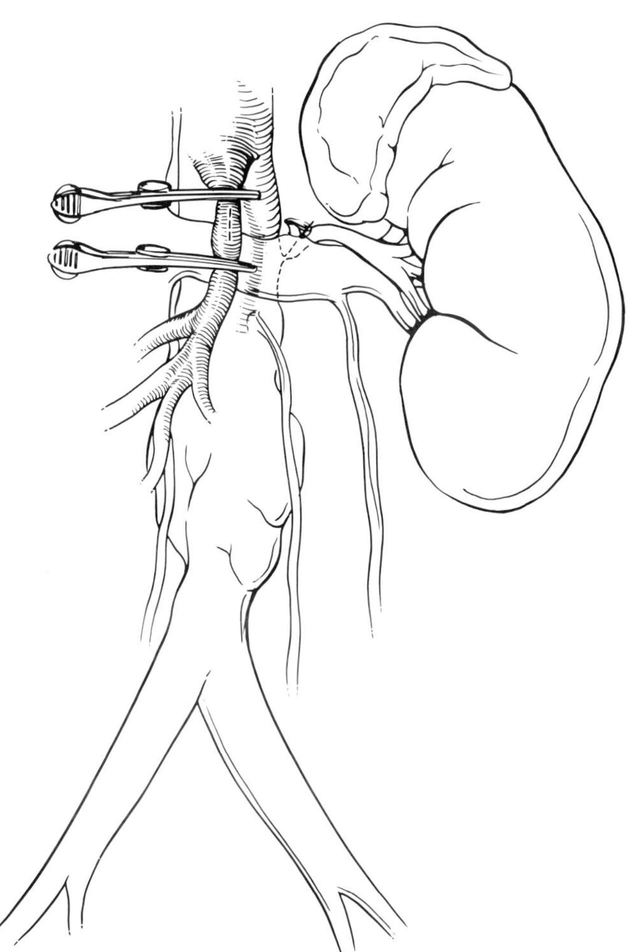

Figure 27.6. To perform mesenterorenal bypass, the abdomen is entered with a midline incision. In revascularization of the left kidney, the descending colon and splenic flexure are reflected medially and a plane of dissection is developed between the pancreas and Gerota's fascia. Exposure of the suprarenal aorta is obtained by gently retracting the pancreas and the first portion of the jejunum cephalad while reflecting the mesocolon medially. If necessary, additional exposure may be obtained by mobilizing and eviscerating the right colon and small bowel as is commonly done to perform retroperitoneal lymphadenectomy. The SMA can be palpated at its origin from the aorta approximately 1–2 cm above the level of the renal arteries. This vessel lies against the neck of the pancreas as it courses between the neck and the uncinate process. It then crosses the third part of the duodenum to enter the large bowel mesentery where it lies posterior and to the left of the superior mesenteric vein. The SMA is mobilized for a distance of 2–3 cm beyond its origin where it is most accessible and without branches. The patient is systemically heparinized using 5000 units of intravenous heparin solution. The SMA is occluded proximally and distally with small bulldog clamps and a short lateral arteriotomy is made.

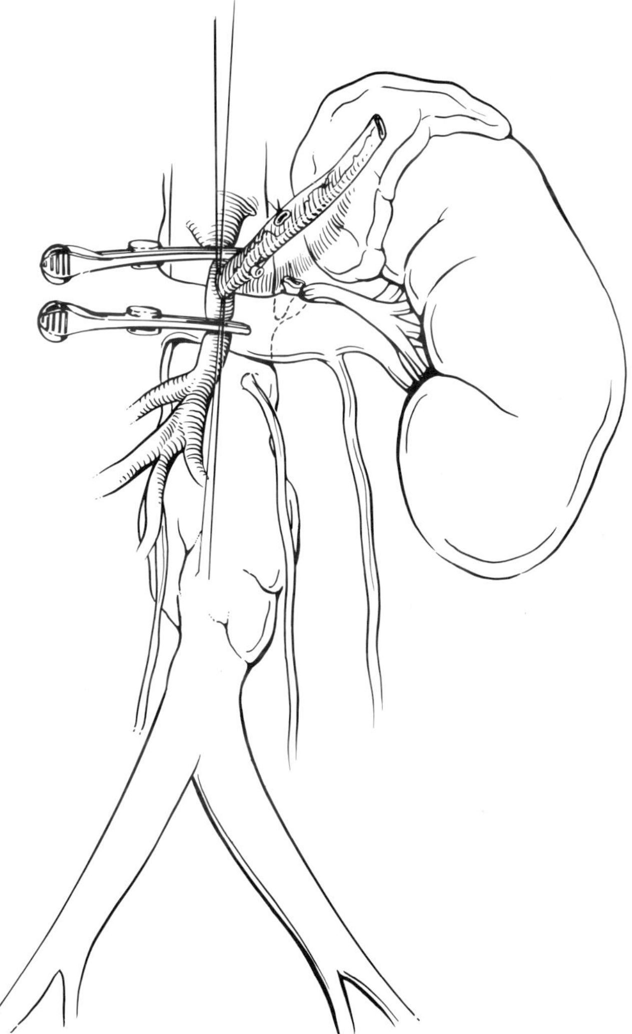

Figure 27.7. A reversed segment of saphenous vein is anastomosed end-to-side to the lateral aspect of the SMA using interrupted 6–0 arterial sutures. After completion of this anastomosis, which generally takes 15–20 min, blood flow through the SMA is immediately restored and the saphenous vein graft is temporarily occluded.

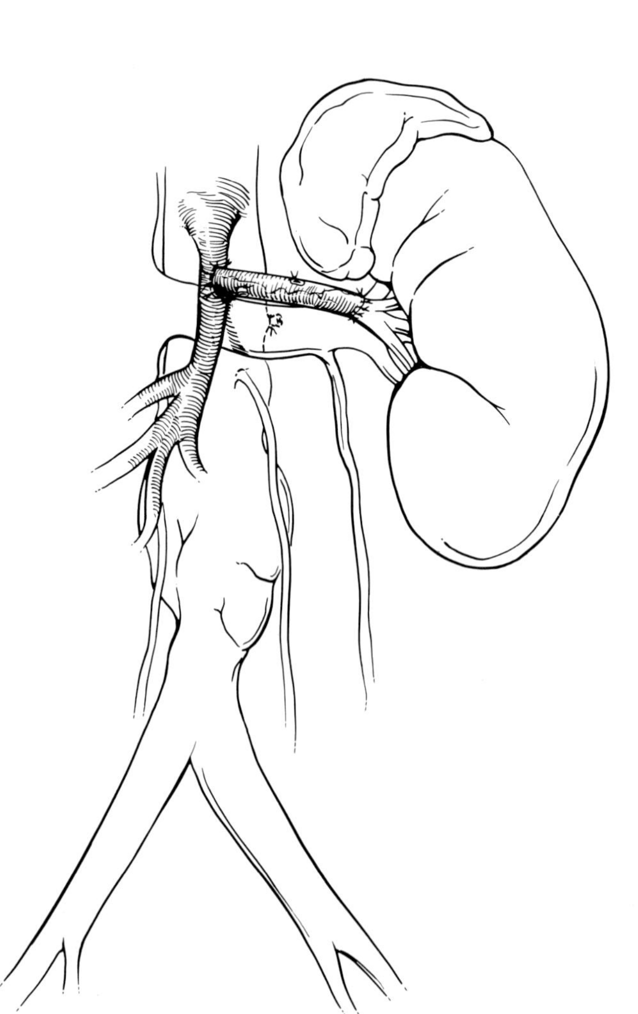

Figure 27.8. End-to-end anastomosis of the vein graft to the distal left renal artery is then done with interrupted 6–0 arterial sutures. A relatively short vein graft can be used for left renal revascularization and this diagram shows the completed operation.

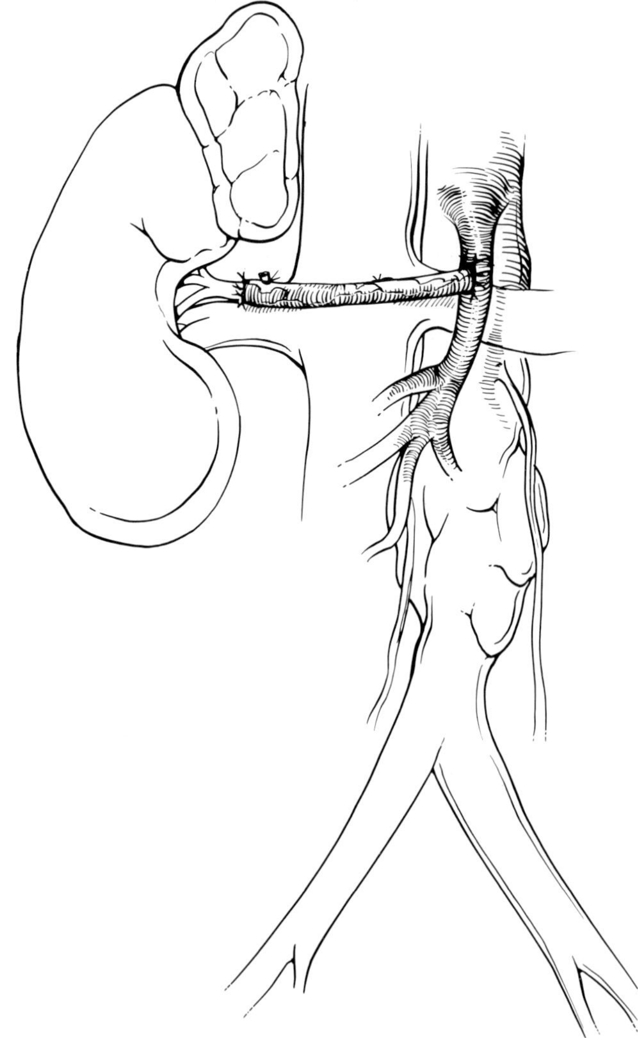

Figure 27.9. In performing mesenterorenal revascularization of the right kidney, the ascending colon and duodenum are reflected medially to gain exposure of the aorta and the right renal artery. The ascending colon and small bowel are then rotated back to their normal position and the SMA is palpated where it crosses the third portion of the duodenum; it is mobilized and isolated in this location for a distance of 3–4 cm. A saphenous vein graft is sutured end-to-side to this portion of the SMA and the graft is then passed through a tunnel in the root of the small bowel mesentery, following a gentle curve as it crosses the third portion of the duodenum to enter the right retroperitoneum. End-to-end anastomosis of the graft to the right renal artery is performed to complete the operation.

Suggested Readings

Khauli R, Novick AC, Coseriu G, Beven E, Hertzer N: Superior mesenterorenal bypass for renal revascularization in patients with infrarenal aortic occlusion. *J Urol* 133:188, 1985.

Novick AC, Banowsky LH, Stewart BH, Straffon RA: Renal revascularization in patients with atherosclerosis or a previous operation on the abdominal aorta. *Surg Gynecol Obstet* 144:211, 1977.

Novick AC, Banowsky LH: Iliorenal saphenous vein bypass: Alternative for renal revascularization in patients with surgically difficult aorta. *J Urol* 122:243, 1979.

Novick AC, Straffon RA, Stewart BH, et al: Diminished operative morbidity and mortality following revascularization for atherosclerotic renovascular disease. *JAMA* 246:749, 1981.

CHAPTER **28**

Extracorporeal Microvascular Branch Renal Artery Reconstruction

ANDREW C. NOVICK

Vascular disease involving the branches of the renal artery is most often caused by one of the fibrous dysplasias, namely, intimal, medial, or perimedial fibroplasia. Other causes of branch disease include an arterial aneurysm, arteriovenous malformation, Takayasu's arteritis, neurofibromatosis, trauma, and, rarely, atherosclerosis. In such cases, the task of renovascular reconstruction is considerably more complicated because this necessitates multiple vascular anatomses to renal artery branches that may be difficult to expose and are small in caliber. For these reasons, many patients in this category formerly were considered either inoperable or candidates for total or partial nephrectomy. However, technical advances during the past decade have improved this outlook, and successful vascular reconstruction is now possible in most patients. This evolution primarily has been due to the incorporation of microvascular and extracorporeal techniques into the armamentarium of the renovascular surgeon.

Branch renal artery lesions can often be repaired in situ with an aorto-renal bypass (see chapter 24) when distal branches free of disease are present outside the renal hilus. Extracorporeal branch arterial repair and autotransplantation are indicated primarily when preoperative arteriography, with oblique views, demonstrates intrarenal extension of renovascular disease. The advantages of employing an extracorporeal surgical approach include optimum exposure and illumination, a bloodless surgical field, greater protection of the kidney from ischemia, and more facile employment of microvascular techniques and optical magnification. Removing and flushing the kidney also causes it to contract in size, thereby enabling more peripheral dissection in the renal sinus for mobilization of distal arterial branches. Finally, the completed branch anastomoses can be tested for patency and integrity before autotransplantation.

In evaluating patients for extracorporeal revascularization and autotransplantation, preoperative renal and pelvic arteriography should be performed to define renal arterial anatomy, to ensure disease-free iliac vessels, and to assess the hypogastric artery and its branches for use as a reconstructive graft. Autotransplantation of kidneys involved by severe renal parenchymal and/or small vessel disease should be avoided. Such kidneys generally flush poorly after their removal, often leading to irreversible ischemic damage and nonfunction postoperatively.

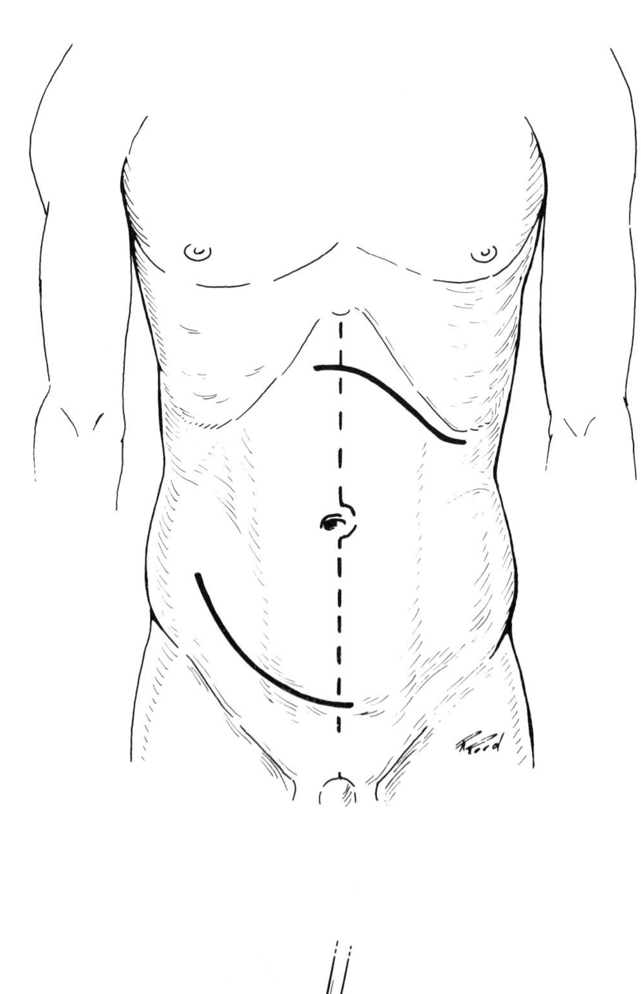

Figure 28.1. Extracoropreal revascularization and autotransplantation are generally performed through an anterior subcostal transperitoneal incision combined with a separate lower quadrant transverse semilunar incision. For nonobese patients, a single midline incision extending from the xyphoid process to the symphysis pubis may be used. The same intraoperative measures are taken as in live-donor nephrectomy for allotransplantation to ensure minimal renal ischemia and immediate function after revascularization. These include prevention of hypotension during anesthesia, administration of mannitol, minimal surgical manipulation of the kidney, and rapid flushing and cooling of the kidney after its removal. Systemic heparinization before nephrectomy is unnecessary.

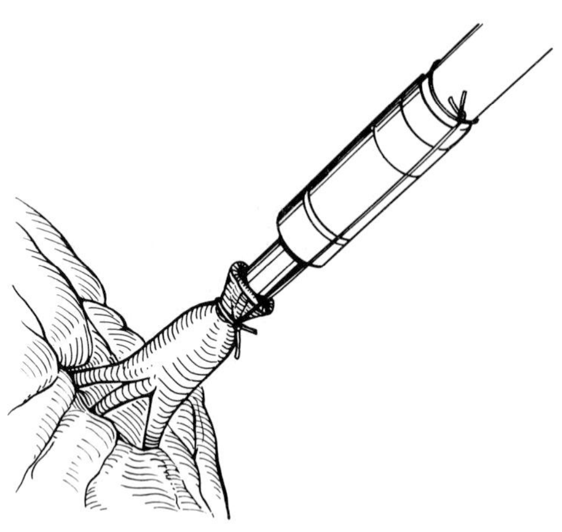

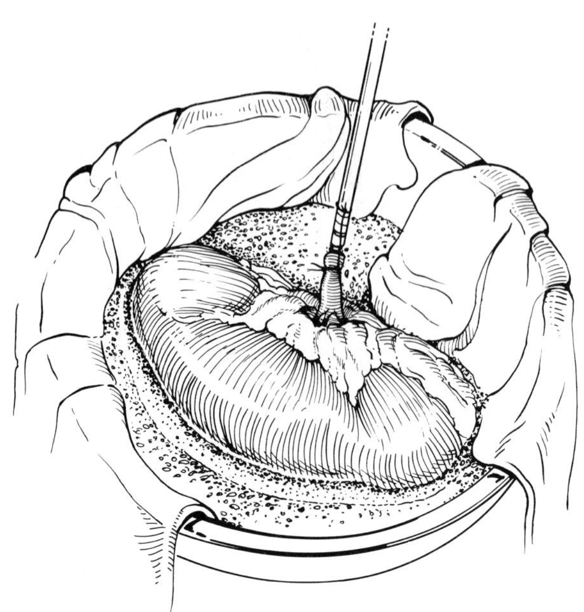

Figure 28.2. Immediately after its removal, the kidney is flushed intraarterially with 500 ml of chilled Collins intracellular electrolyte solution and is then submerged in a basin of ice slush saline to maintain hypothermia. The extracorporeal operation is completed under ice slush surface hypothermia and, if there has been minimal warm renal ischemia, the kidney can be preserved safely in this manner for many more hours than are needed to perform even the most complex renal repair. In performing extracorporeal revascularization, we have found it cumbersome to work on the abdominal wall with the ureter attached. It is preferable to divide the ureter and place the kidney on a separate workbench. This provides better exposure for the extracorporeal operation and allows a second surgical team to prepare the iliac fossa simultaneously. This approach is also justified by the low incidence of complications after ureteroneocystostomy in renal allotransplantation.

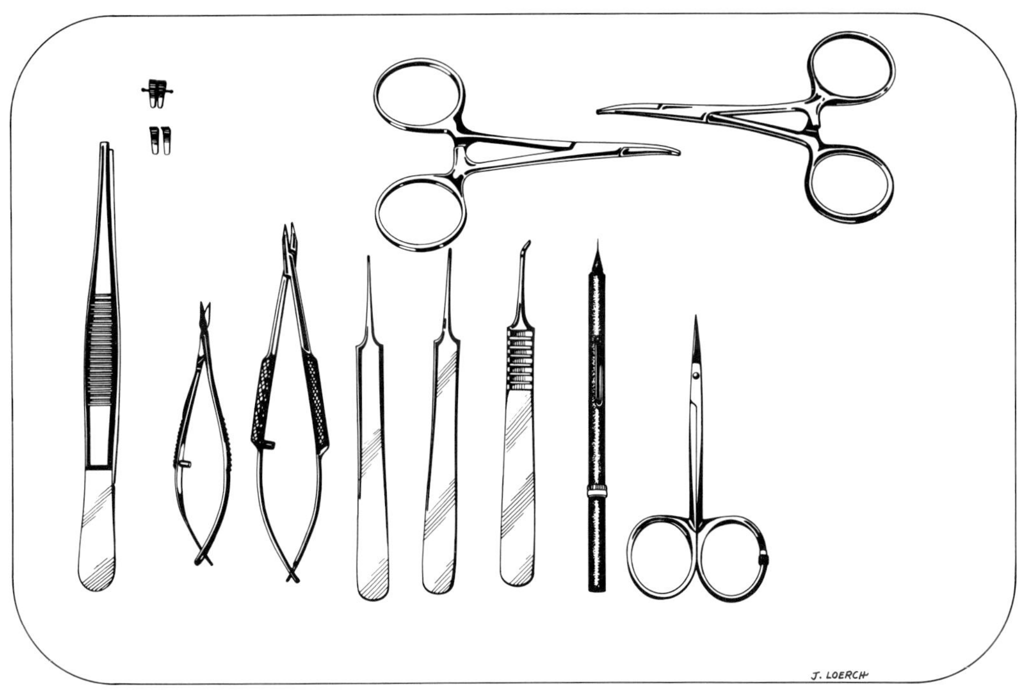

Figure 28.3. Extracorporeal branch arterial reconstruction is performed with microvascular instruments, 7–0 to 9–0 suture material, and optical magnification with loupes (3.5 × or 6.0 ×) or an operating microscope. The basic instruments required for microvascular surgery include a microneedle holder, microscissors, fine jeweler's forceps, small vessel dilators, microvascular clamps, and a 10-ml syringe with a 27-gauge blunt needle for irrigation.

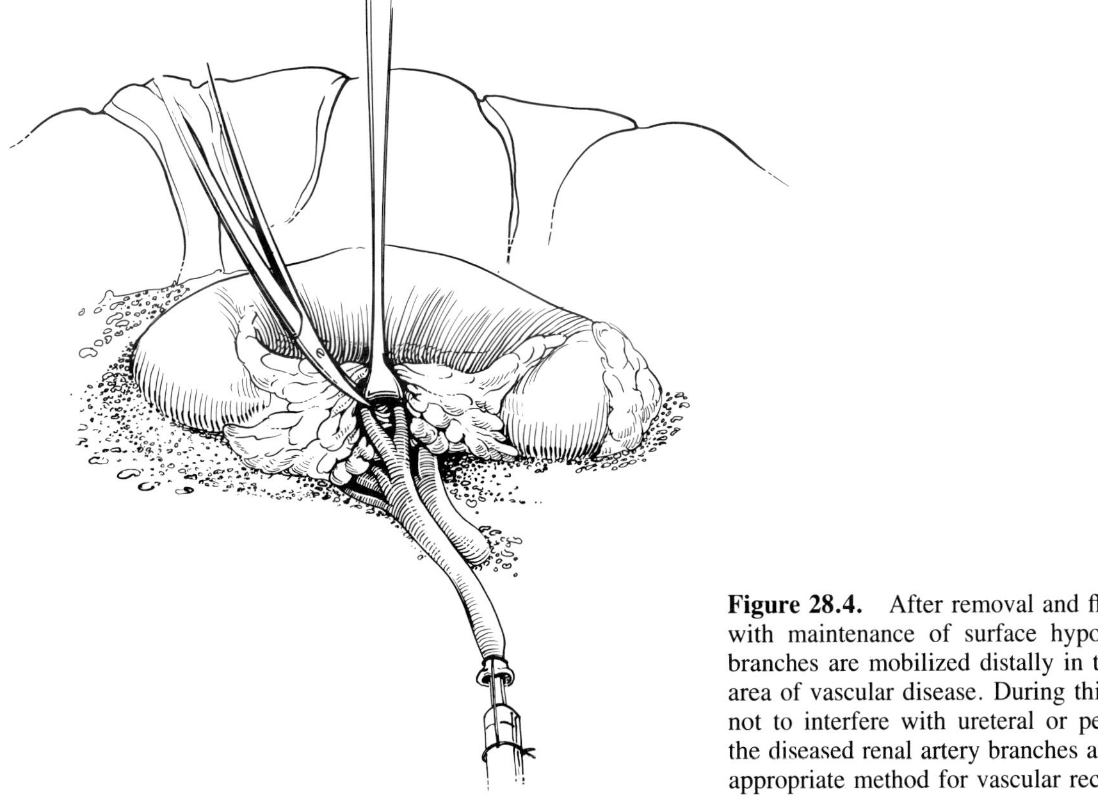

Figure 28.4. After removal and flushing of the kidney, and with maintenance of surface hypothermia, the renal artery branches are mobilized distally in the renal sinus beyond the area of vascular disease. During this dissection, care is taken not to interfere with ureteral or pelvic blood supply. When the diseased renal artery branches are completely exposed, an appropriate method for vascular reconstruction is selected.

Figure 28.5. The optimum method for extracorporeal branch renal arterial repair involves the use of a branched autogenous vascular graft. This technique permits separate end-to-end microvascular anastomosis of each graft branch to a distal renal artery branch. A hypogastric arterial autograft is the preferred material for vascular reconstruction because this vessel may be obtained intact with several of its branches.

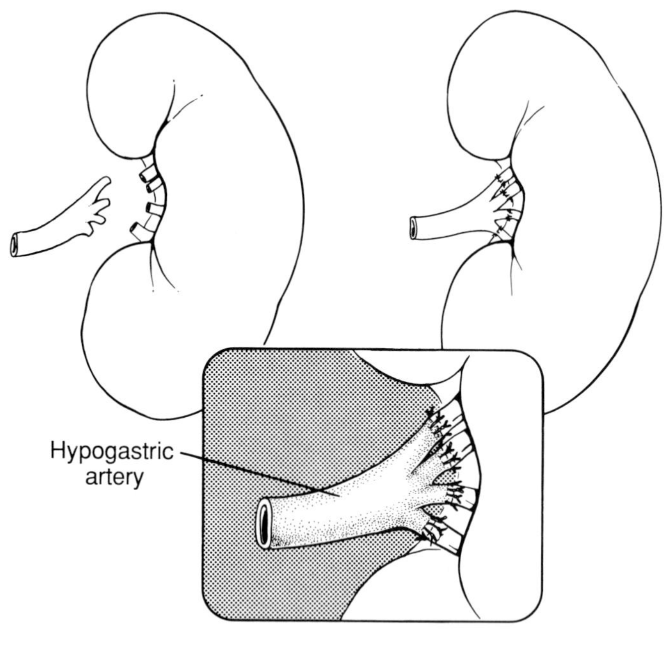

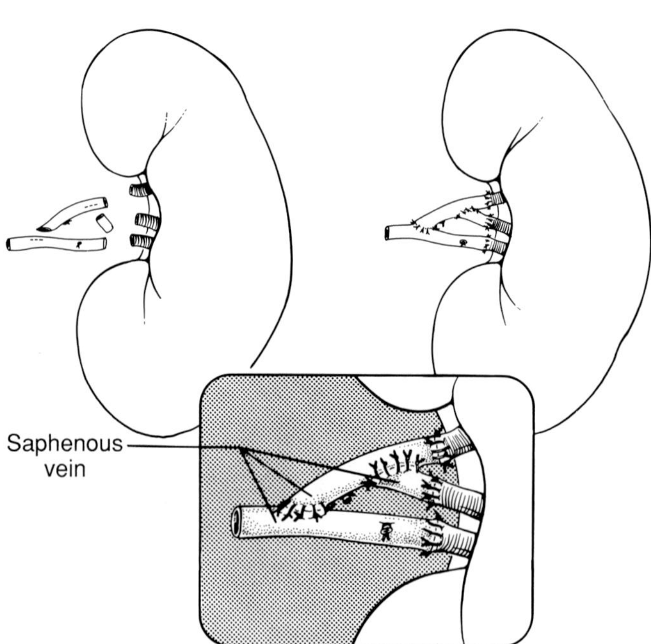

Figure 28.6. Occasionally, the hypogastric artery is not suitable for use as a reconstructive graft because of atherosclerotic degeneration. When this occurs, a long segment of saphenous vein can be harvested and, employing sequential end-to-side microvascular anastomoses, a branched graft can be fashioned from this vessel. This branched graft is then used in a similar manner to achieve reconstruction of the diseased renal artery branches.

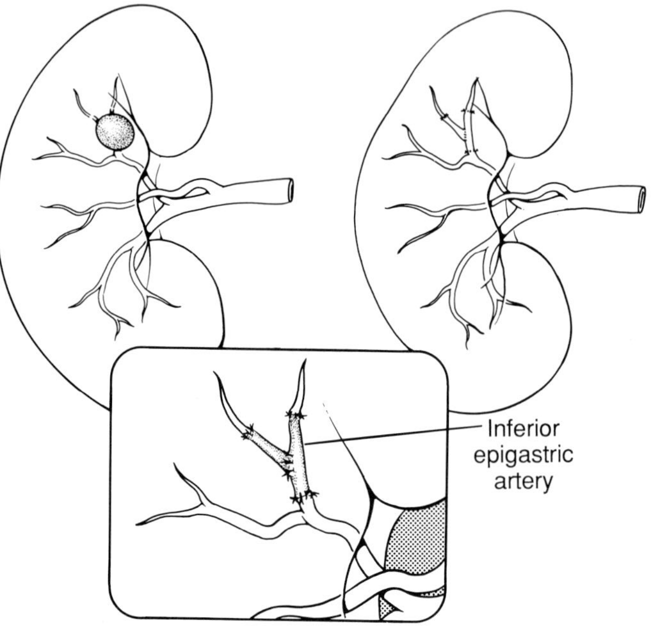

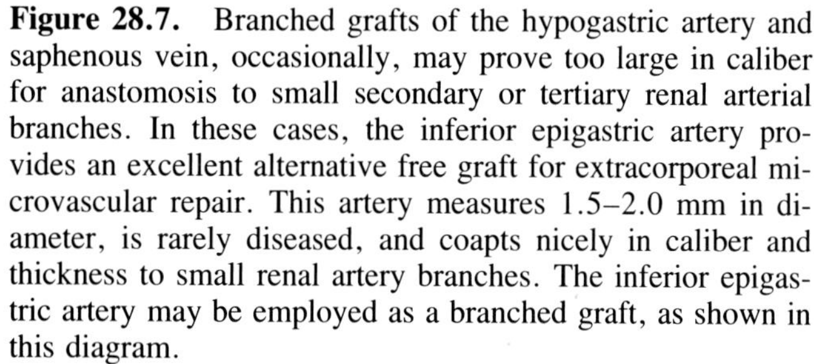

Figure 28.7. Branched grafts of the hypogastric artery and saphenous vein, occasionally, may prove too large in caliber for anastomosis to small secondary or tertiary renal arterial branches. In these cases, the inferior epigastric artery provides an excellent alternative free graft for extracorporeal microvascular repair. This artery measures 1.5–2.0 mm in diameter, is rarely diseased, and coapts nicely in caliber and thickness to small renal artery branches. The inferior epigastric artery may be employed as a branched graft, as shown in this diagram.

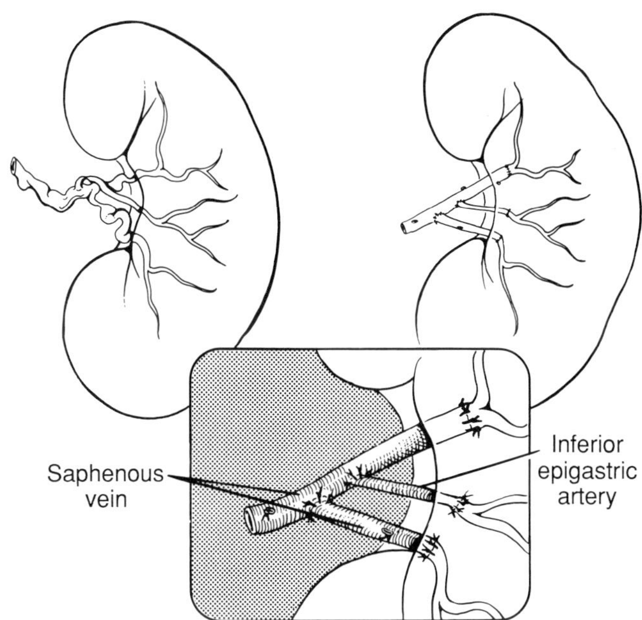

Figure 28.8 The inferior epigastric artery may also be used as a branched graft in conjunction with a segment of saphenous vein, as shown in this diagram, to repair multiple branches of varying caliber.

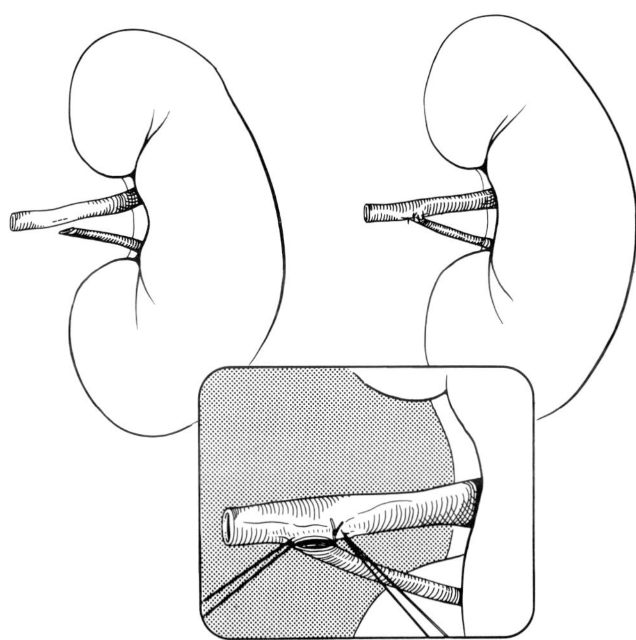

Figure 28.9. Although use of a branched autogenous vascular graft provides a simple, versatile, and effective method for branch renal arterial reconstruction, other techniques occasionally are preferable depending upon the extent of vascular disease. In some patients with localized segmental intrarenal branch lesions, there may be other arterial branches that are either uninvolved or have more proximally located vascular disease. Such branches with longer disease-free distal segments may be anastomosed end-to-side either into a larger arterial branch or into the reconstructive vascular graft.

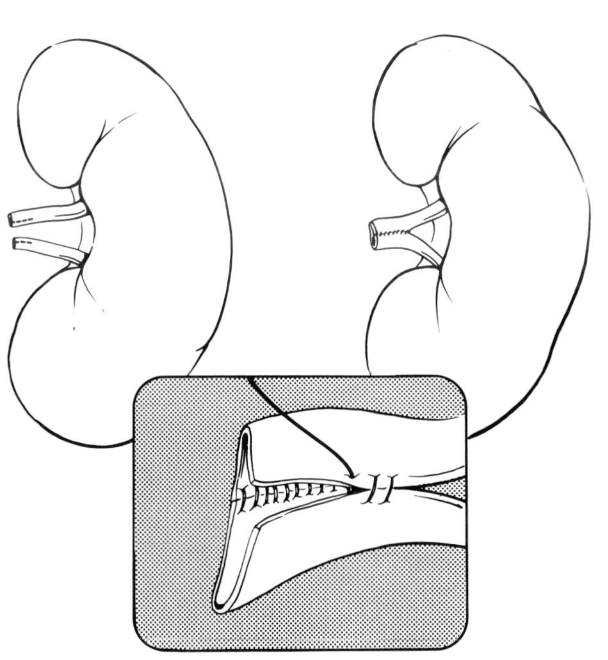

Figure 28.10. Occasionally, two distal arterial branches of similar diameter and free of disease are found adjacent to one another. When this occurs, the two adjacent branches can be conjoined (with a continuous suture) and then anastomosed end-to-end to a single limb of the branched graft.

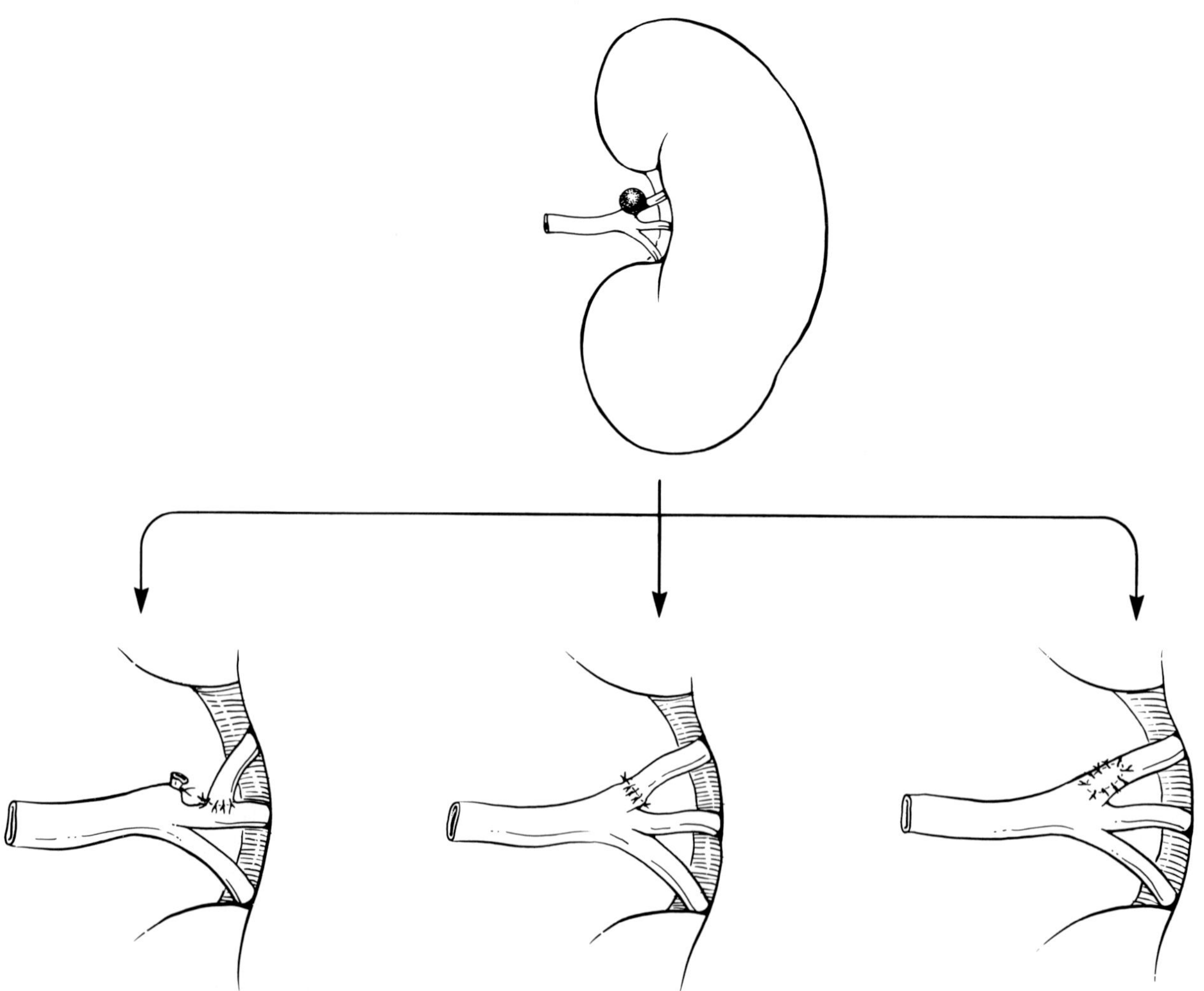

Figure 28.11. Renal artery aneurysms have a variable presentation and the method of extracorporeal repair is determined by whether renovascular involvement is focal or diffuse. If the renal artery wall at the base of an aneurysm is intact, aneurysmectomy with patch angioplasty *(right)* can be performed. Aneurysms with short focal involvement of renal artery branches may also be simply resected with end-to-end branch reanastomosis *(middle)* or end-to-side reimplantation into an adjacent branch *(left)*. In other cases, with more extensive vascular disease, aneurysmectomy and revascularization with a branched autogenous graft are indicated.

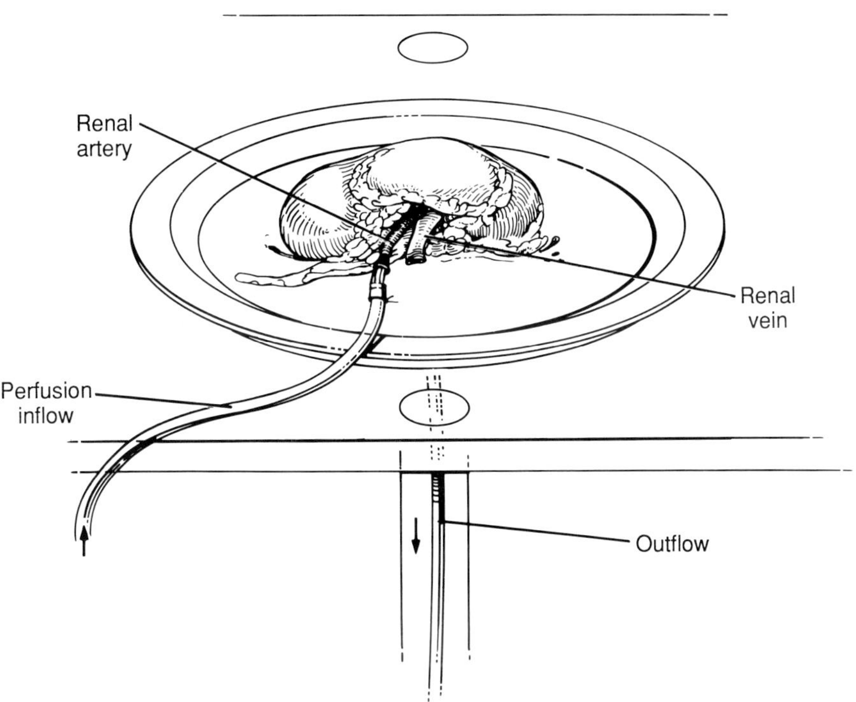

Figure 28.12. These extracorporeal vascular techniques are all performed with interrupted sutures, except for the conjoined anastomosis where a continuous suture is used. When revascularizing multiple arterial branches, one must anticipate the position that the various branches will assume in relation to one anther upon completion of the repair. Individual branch anastomoses are then done with careful attention to avoid subsequent malrotation, angulation, or tension. In all cases, extracorporeal repair leads to creation of a single main renal artery so that autotransplantation may be performed with one arterial anstomosis and no increase in the revascularization time. When extracorporeal revascularization has been completed, the kidney is placed on the hypothermic pulsatile perfusion unit to verify patency and integrity of the repaired branches. Renal autotransplantation into the iliac fossa is then performed (see chapter 32), with anastomosis of the renal vessels to the iliac vessels and restoration of urinary continuity by ureteroneocystostomy.

Suggested Readings

Kaufman JJ: Renal autotransplantation and ex vivo surgery for renovascular hypertension. *Urol Clin North Am* 6:295, 1979.

Novick AC, Stewart BH, Straffon RA: Extracorporeal renal surgery and autotransplantation: Indications, techniques and results. *J Urol* 123:806, 1980.

Novick AC: Management of infrarenal branch arterial lesions with extracorporeal microvascular reconstruction and autotransplantation. *J Urol* 126:150, 1981.

Novick AC: Use of inferior epigastric artery for extracorporeal microvascular branch renal artery reconstruction. *Surgery* 89:513, 1981.

Novick AC: Extracorporeal renal surgery and autotransplantation. In Novick AC, Straffon RA (eds): *Vascular Problems in Urologic Surgery*. Philadelphia, WB Saunders, 1982.

Novick AC: Renal hypothermia: in vivo and ex vivo. *Urol Clin North Am* 10:637, 1983.

Novick AC: Microvascular reconstruction of complex branch renal artery disease. *Urol Clin North Am* 11:465, 1984.

Salvatierra O, Olcott C, Stoney RJ: Ex vivo renal artery reconstruction using perfusion preservation. *J Urol* 119:16, 1978.

SECTION 7

Renal Transplantation

CHAPTER 29

Cadaver Donor Nephrectomy

JOHN M. BARRY

CADAVER KIDNEY RETRIEVAL

Kidney transplantation is the preferred treatment for most patients with end-stage renal disease. The need for cadaver kidneys has increased because suitable, living, related kidney donors are unavailable for most patients, and more patients with failed kidney grafts are presenting for retransplantation. Cadaver organs for transplantation are becoming more available because of brain-death legislation, required request laws, public education, education and organization of health care professionals, and kidney sharing among transplant centers. However, the supply still does not satisfy the need. The successful transplantation of livers, hearts, pancreata, and heart-and-lung preparations have made it necessary to develop combined organ retrieval teams, and for kidney retrieval surgeons to be aware of technique modifications for multiple organ retrievals.

Generally acceptable medical criteria for cadaver kidney donors are age 18 months to 55 years and normal renal function by urinalysis, blood urea nitrogen, and serum creatinine. The lower age limit is primarily because of delicate ureteral blood supply. Concerns about cyclosporine nephrotoxicity when a pediatric kidney is transplanted into an adult have prompted some kidney transplant teams to transplant both kidneys from a pediatric donor en bloc when the donor is under 7 years of age. For this reason, these small kidneys should be left as an en bloc specimen until the desires of the transplanting team are known. The upper age limit is based on the probability of nephrosclerosis in the aging donor. Kidneys from donors recovering from acute tubular necrosis on the basis of declining serial serum creatinine levels can provide satisfactory renal function after transplantation. Malignant disease outside the brain or superficial skin, intestinal perforation, and generalized infection including hepatitis, syphillis, tuberculosis, or acquired immune deficiency syndrome are considered contraindications to organ donation.

DONOR PREPARATION

The goals of donor preparation are restoration of intravascular volume, elimination of vasopressors and the establishment of a diuresis. A central venous line is helpful for managing fluid administration. Adult donor blood pressure and urinary output goals during the initial resuscitation are 90 mm Hg and 0.5 ml/kg/hr, respectively. The prospective donor can be fluid-challenged by the intravenous administration of at least 30 ml/kg/hr of Ringer's lactate solution, then matching the urinary volume with intravenous Ringer's lactate solution or 0.25 normal saline containing 20 mEq potassium/liter. Serum electrolytes should be checked every 2–4 hr to maintain electrolyte balance. If the central venous pressure is greater than 15 cm H_2O and vasopressors cannot be discontinued, a dopamine infusion of less than 50 μ/kg/min is preferred. Higher doses can cause renal vasoconstriction. A dobutamine infusion of less than μ/kg/minute is preferred by many retrieval teams. An isoproterenol infusion up to 0.07 GK μ/kg/min is an acceptable substitute, but ventricular arrhythmias may occur. If volume expansion and vasopressors have been unsuccessful in initiating a diuresis, furosemide, 1 mg/kg, or mannitol 0.5–1.0 gm/kg may be infused. Diabetes insipidus is best managed by matching intravenous fluid to urinary output and maintaining serum electrolyte balance. If that is not possible, pitressin can be administered. Intravenous methylprednisolone 30 mg/kg, within 4 hours of kidney retrieval may reduce the incidence of posttransplant acute tubular necrosis when cold storage time is prolonged. For histocompatibility testing, 100 ml of blood can be drawn to allow tissue typing and crossmatching before organ retrieval.

TECHNIQUE OF CADAVER DONOR NEPHRECTOMY

The major steps in the operating room are the administration of fluid and drugs, exposure of the critical anatomy, control and cannulation of major blood vessels, in situ organ perfusion, removal and separation of the en bloc nephrectomy specimen, and removal of histocompatibility testing specimens.

The cerebrally dead cadaver organ donor receives at least 30 ml/kg/hr of crystalloid every hour the abdomen is open and 1 gm/kg mannitol intravenous push with the skin incision. Colloid or blood administration may be necessary to improve organ perfusion. The surgical goals are minimal warm ischemia time, preservation of multiple or anomalous renal vessels, preservation of the inferior vena cava with the right kidney, and preservation of ureteral blood supply. All of these goals are achieved with in situ flushing followed by en bloc nephrectomy and separation of the specimen by splitting the aorta and transecting the left renal vein at its junction with the inferior vena cava.

A total midline incision between the suprasternal notch and pubis adequately exposes not only the kidneys, but also the liver, pancreas, and heart (Fig. 29.1). The incision is deepened with the electric knife to the sternum and into the peritoneal cavity. A plane is developed under the sternum and a Lebsche knife and mallet or a sternal saw is used to split the sternum in the midline. Self-retaining retractors are placed in the chest and abdomen, the liver is retracted inferiorly, and the diaphragm is incised to allow proximal aortic control or retraction of the intestines into the chest.

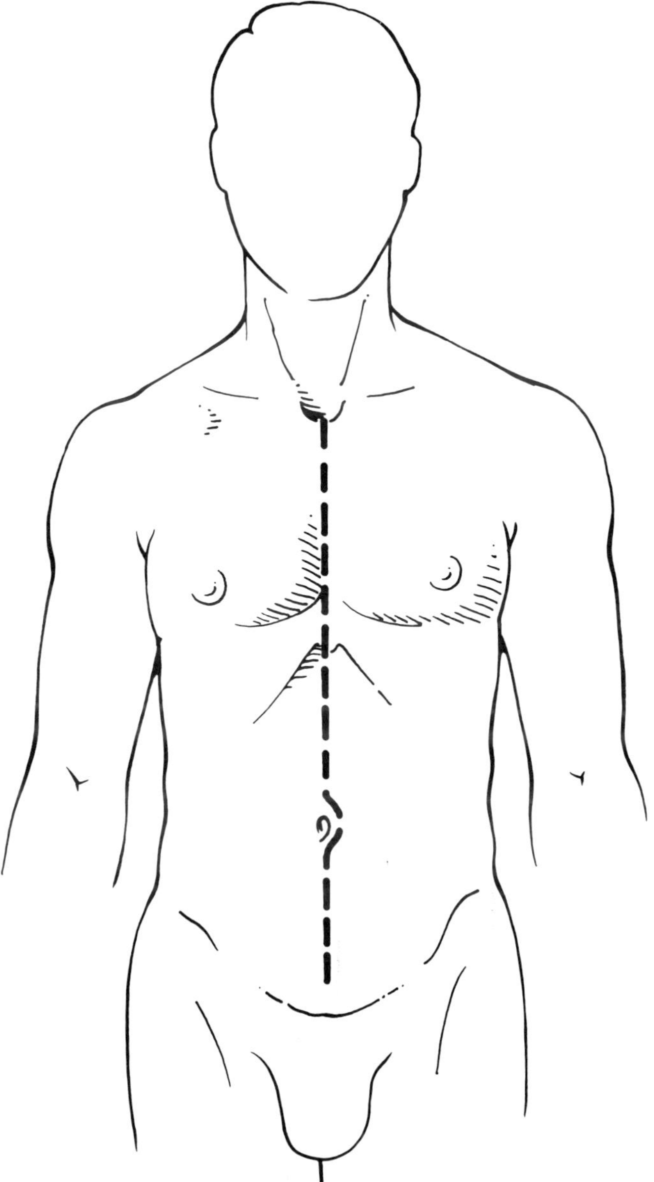

Figure 29.1. Total midline incision, including sternal and diaphragm splitting, exposes all potentially transplantable organs in the chest and abdomen.

The intestines are retracted to the left. In a thin individual, this exposes the kidneys, abdominal aorta, and inferior vena cava. The posterior peritoneum is opened to the inferior mesenteric vein, which is usually divided between ligatures (Fig. 29.2). If a liver retrieval is contemplated, this vessel may be ligated distally and cannulated proximally for hepatic flushing through the portal venous system. If a pancreas retrieval is contemplated, the inferior mesenteric venous cannula may vent the pancreatic circulation if the portal vein is occluded in the portal triad. The inferior mesenteric artery is divided between ligatures. Some retrieval teams place the aortic flush cannula through the stump of this artery. The distal abdominal aorta is controlled with an umbilical tape that will be converted to a Rumel tourniquet. This procedure is repeated with the distal inferior vena cava. In preparation for cannulation, 0-silk ligatures are passed twice around the distal abdominal aorta and inferior vena cava proximal to the controlling tapes. Following the left renal vein medially leads one to the superior mesenteric artery that is just medial to the left adrenal vein. The superior mesenteric artery is divided between ligatures unless a liver or whole pancreas retrieval is also being performed. In the former situation, the superior mesenteric artery must be left intact until it is certain that the right hepatic artery does not arise from it. In the latter situation, it is divided at

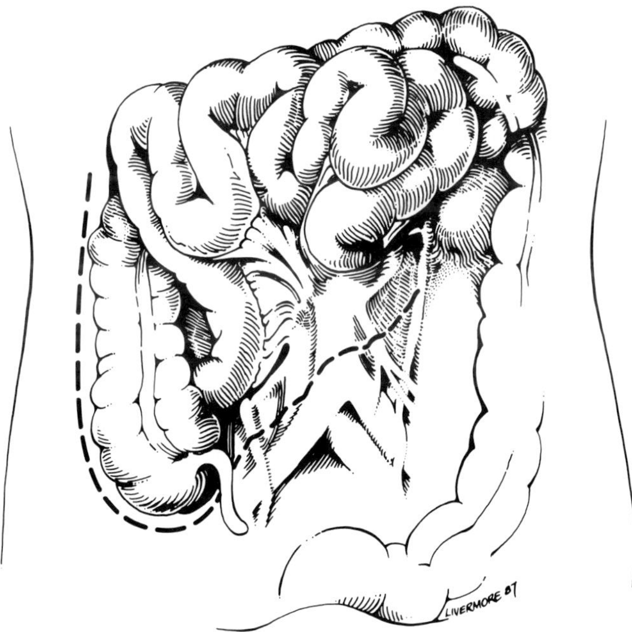

Figure 29.2. Opening the posterior peritoneum from the hepatic flexure around the cecum to the inferior mesenteric vein exposes the great vessels and kidneys in the retroperitoneum.

the inferior margin of the pancreas. The plane under the proximal inferior vena cava is gently developed with the index finger and proximal control is obtained with an umbilical tape between the liver and the renal veins. This will also be converted to a Rumel tourniquet. If the liver is being removed, this step can be omitted. Cutting the crura of the diaphragm allows excellent exposure of the proximal abdominal aorta above the superior mesenteric artery and, if necessary, above the celiac axis. Minor bleeding from the phrenic and adrenal arteries is controlled with suction. An umbilical tape is passed around the proximal abdominal aorta and this is converted to a Rumel tourniquet (Fig. 29.3). If the liver or pancreas is being retrieved, proximal abdominal aortic control is obtained in the chest. Heparin, 100–400 units/kg, is administered intravenously immediately before cannulation to prevent clotting within the cannulas. The distal abdominal aorta is occluded with a Rumel tourniquet. The aorta is occluded between the thumb and forefinger of the nondominant hand just below the previously placed 0-silk ligature, and the anterior surface of the aorta is incised between the tourniquet and thumb and forefinger. A cannula is inserted, the 0-silk ligature is pulled taut and, if a Foley catheter has been used as the cannula, 3 ml is injected to inflate the balloon, and the silk ligature is tied. If the vena cava is to be vented distally, the cannulation procedure is repeated (Fig. 29.4). With hepatectomy, the vena cava will be vented in the chest by incising it where it joins the right atrium. At this time the ice cold intracellular electrolyte flush solution is connected to the tubing, flow is assured, and it is connected to the previously occluded aortic cannula and clamped. When only the subdiaphragmatic organs are being removed, an α-blocker, usually chlorpromazine, 1 mg/kg, is administered intravenously at this time. When the blood pressure decreases dramatically, intraaortic flushing is initiated, the proximal aorta is crossclamped, and the vena cava is vented. Once flushing is initiated, further dissection of the en bloc specimen is carried out. The gonadal vessels are ligated lat-

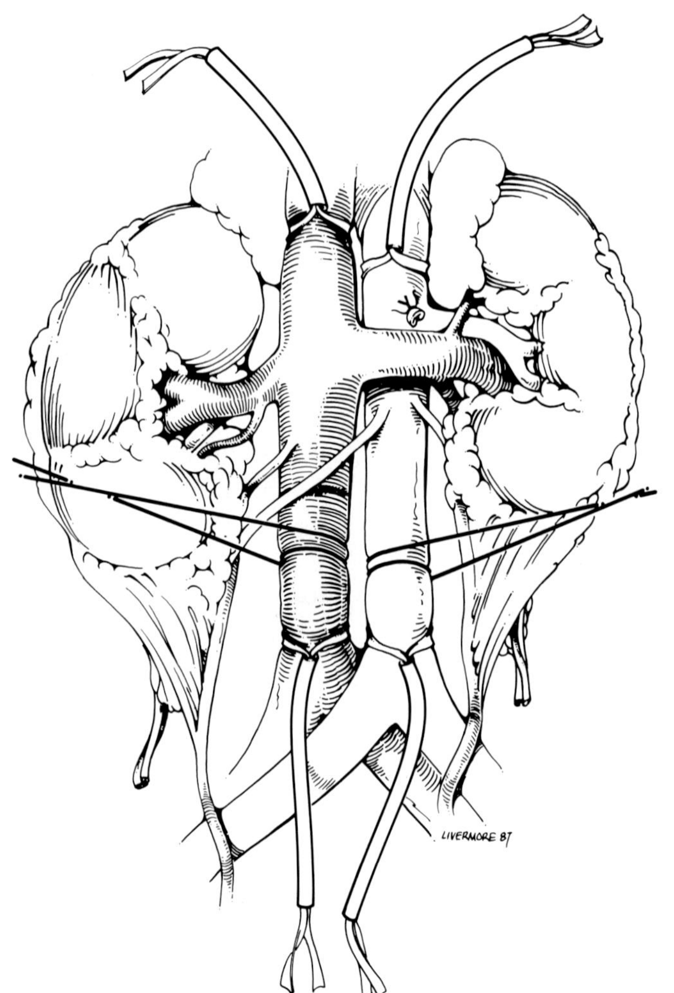

Figure 29.3. The aorta and inferior vena cava are controlled above and below the renal vessels and prepared for cannulation.

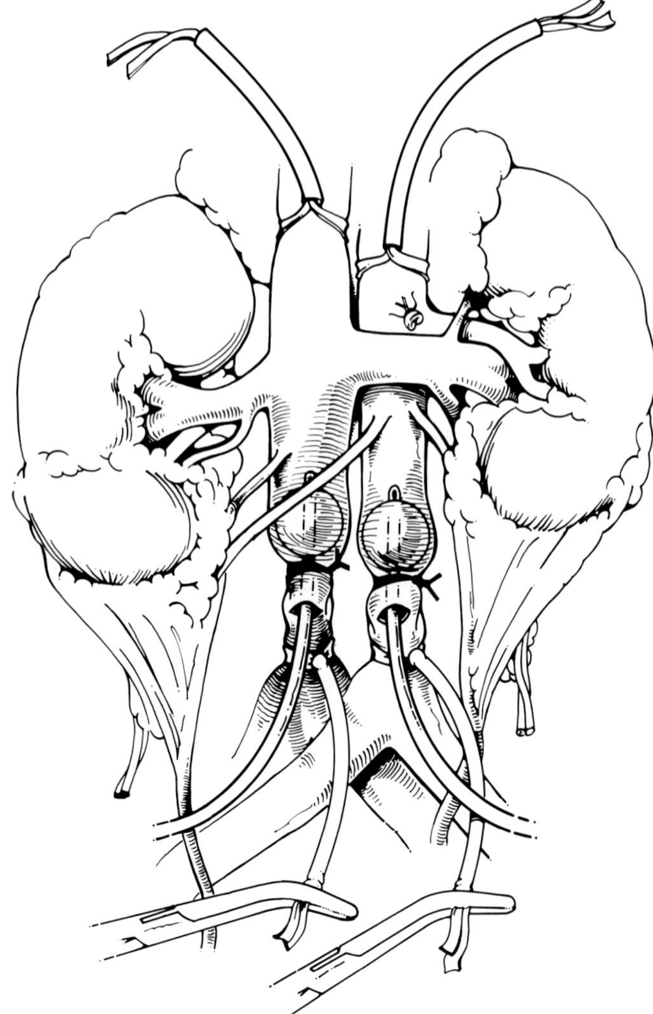

Figure 29.4. Cannulation of distal aorta and inferior vena cava.

eral to the ureters. The ureters are divided deep within the pelvis. Gerota's fascia is entered lateral to both kidneys. The kidneys are dissected free of the adrenals, if convenient, or this step is done during separation of the en bloc specimen at the back table. The kidneys are lifted out of their respective beds in the retroperitoneum. A lumbar vein commonly joins the left renal vein posteriorly and this is divided between ligatures. The distal aorta and inferior vena cava are transected distal to the cannulas and retracted anteriorly. This exposes the lumbar arteries that are clipped on the aortic side and divided to prevent rapid run-off the intraaortic flush solution. The lumbar veins may be transected without controlling them, but this will obscure the field with a mixture of blood and flush solution. The proximal abdominal aorta is clamped and transected. The vena cava is transected between the liver and the renal veins, the ureters are transected deep within the true pelvis, and the en bloc specimen consisting of the kidneys, ureters, gonadal vessels, inferior vena cava, and aorta is taken to the back table where they are placed in an ice cold electrolyte solution bath and flipped over. The aorta is opened posteriorly between the lumbar arteries (Fig. 29.5). This exposes the ostia of the renal arteries that may be reflushed at this time if there has been concern about the in situ flushing. Next the anterior surface of the aorta is split. The fibrolymphatic and autonomic nervous tissue is separated at the posterior surface of the left renal vein where it joins the inferior vena cava. The left renal vein is then divided where it joins the inferior vena cava, thus, separating the kidneys. If not done immediately upon opening the posterior surface of the aorta, the kidneys are now reflushed to be certain they are clear of blood.

Fifteen lymph nodes and 30 gm of spleen are removed for histocompatibility testing. If the number of mesenteric lymph nodes is inadequate, retroperitoneal lymph nodes can be dissected from the renal specimens.

The kidney specimens are now packaged. If the en bloc specimen has not been separated, it is placed in a sterile plastic container containing ice cold electrolyte solution for kidney preservation. This container is sealed and placed within another sterile container containing more of the electrolyte solution and those two containers are placed within a sterile plastic bag, which his twisted shut and occluded with a ligature or rubber band. The specimen containers are now packed in ice for transportation to the transplant center.

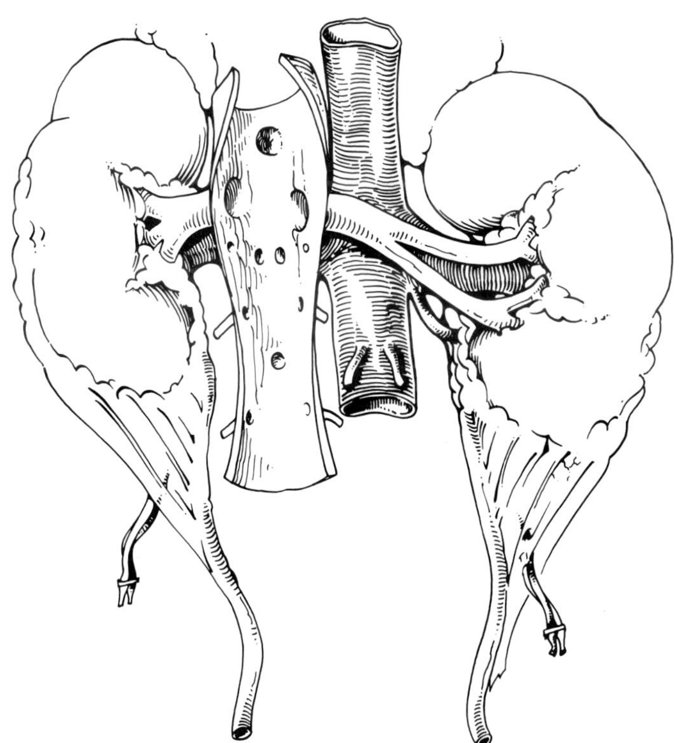

Figure 29.5. Splitting the aorta posteriorly between the lumbar arteries exposes the renal artery and superior mesenteric artery ostia. This also assures identification of all renal arteries and prevention of damage to renal veins.

ALTERNATIVE SURGICAL TECHNIQUES FOR THE REMOVAL OF CADAVER KIDNEYS

The goals of cadaver kidney retrieval can be achieved by removing the kidneys separately or en bloc with ex situ intraaortic flushing. If the surgeon is unfamiliar with the total midline incision, kidney retrieval can take place via a vertical midline incision, a chevron incision, or a cruciate abdominal incision (Fig. 29.6).

When the kidneys are removed separately, the left kidney is usually removed first. The retroperitoneum is opened as previously described. The left adrenal vein is divided between ligatures. The left renal vein is dissected to the medial surface of the inferior vena cava and a 0-silk ligature is passed around it. The left gonadal vein is left with the ureter to assure ureteral blood supply. The left renal vein and gonadal vein are retracted anteriorly to search for a left lumbar vein draining into the posterior aspect of the left renal vein. If present, it is divided between ligatures, taking care not to occlude the periarterial tissue and compromise the lumen of the renal artery. The renal artery or arteries are identified at the aorta and encircled with 0-silk ligatures. The kidney is freed from the retroperitoneum and left adrenal gland with sharp and blunt dissection. Adrenal arteries arising from the renal artery are divided between fine silk ligatures. The ureter is transected deep within the pelvis and, once it is certain that the diuresis is continuing, intravenous heparin is administered, the renal artery or arteries are ligated, the renal vein is ligated, those vessels are transected, and the kidney removed and immediately placed in an ice cold bath. The renal artery is cannulated and an ice cold intracellular electrolyte solution is flushed through the renal artery until the venous effluent is clear. The procedure is repeated for the right kidney except that the inferior vena cava is removed with the specimen to allow extension of the short right renal vein (Fig. 29.7).

En bloc nephrectomies with ex situ flushing follows the same procedure as described for in situ flushing except that the aorta is cannulated after the en bloc specimen has been removed and placed in an ice cold solution at a back table.

Table 29.1
Commonly Used Intracellular Electrolyte Flush Solutions

	Gm/Liter		mEq/Liter
Basic Components of Both Solutions			
KH_2PO_4	2.05	K^+	115
		Na^+	10
$K_2HPO_4 \cdot 3H_2O$	9.7	Cl^-	15
		HCO_3^-	10
KCL	1.12	$HPO_4^=$	85
$NaHCO_3$	0.84	$H_2PO_4^-$	15
Specific Additives (Gm/Liter)			
	EuroCollins		Collins 2
$MgSO_4 \cdot 7H_2O$	0.00		7.38
Glucose	35.00		25.00
pH at 20° C	7.33		7.00
Osmolarity (mosm/liter)	355		320

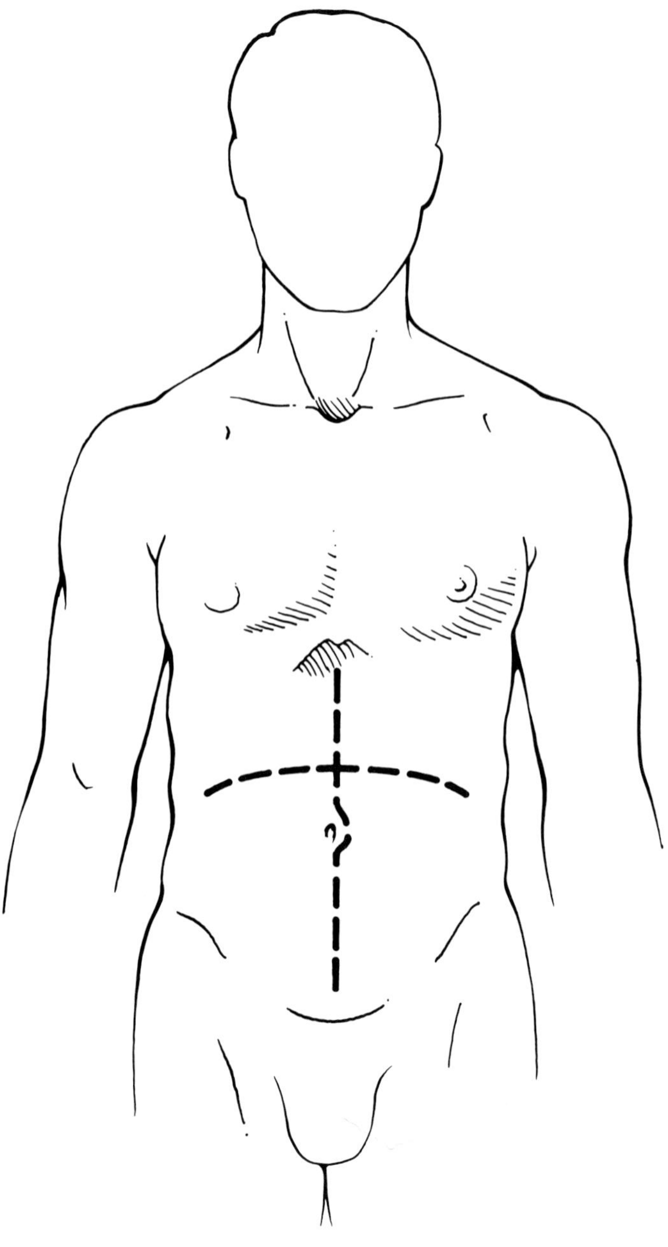

Figure 29.6. Cruciate abdominal incision adequately exposes intraabdominal organs for retrieval. The wound edges can be towel-clipped to the chest and thighs to eliminate the need for a self-retaining retractor.

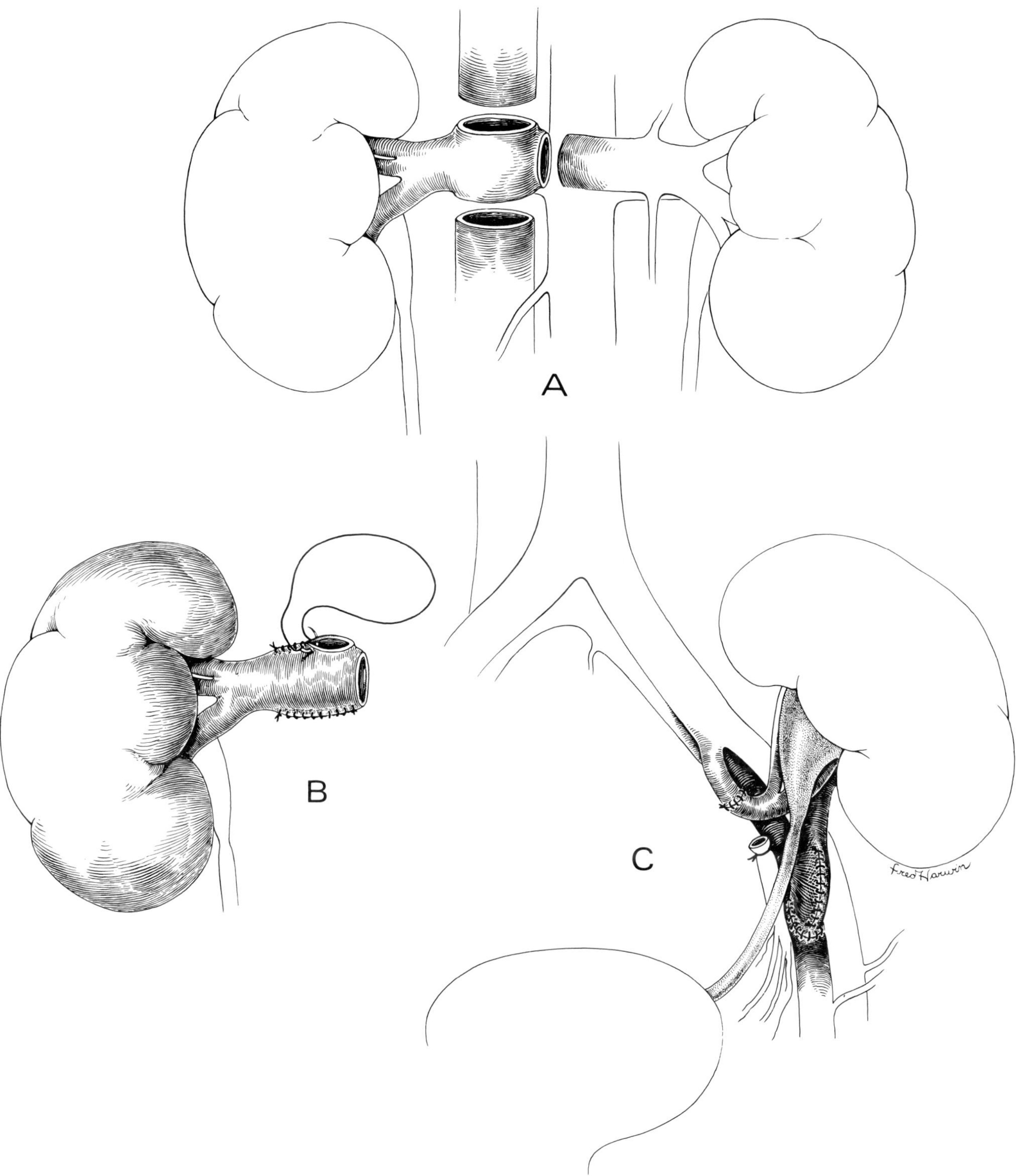

Figure 29.7. Principle of inferior vena cava modification to extend the right renal vein. (From Barry JM, Fuchs EF: Right renal vein extension in cadaver kidney transplantation. *Arch Surg* 113:300, 1978.)

Renal Transplantation

Suggested Readings

Barry JM, Fuchs EF: Right renal vein extension in cadaver kidney transplantation. *Arch Surg* 113:300, 1978.

Barry JM, Lieberman S, Wickre C, Lieberman C, Fischer S, and Craig D: Human kidney preservation by intracellular electrolyte flush followed by cold storage for over 24 hours. *Transplantation* 32:485, 1981.

Collins GM, Barry JM, Maxwell JG, Sampson D, VanderWerf BA: The value of magnesium in flush solutions for human cadaveric kidney preservation. *J Urol* 131:220, 1984.

Linke CA, Linke CL, Davis RS, Frid CW: Cadaver donor nephrectomy. *Urology* 66:133, 1975.

Physician's Deck Reference. Oradell, NJ, Medical Economics Company, 1985, pp. 1143, 1510, 2201–2202.

Starzl T, Hakala TR, Shaw BW Jr, Hardesty RL, Rosenthal TJ, Griffith BP, Iwatsuki S, Bahnson HT: A flexible procedure for multiple cadaveric organ procurement. *Surg Gynecol Obstet* 158:223, 1984.

CHAPTER 30

Extracorporeal Renal Preservation

PETER N. BRETAN, JR.

For the past 20 years, kidneys have been preserved extracorporeally for as long as 3 days. This has contributed to more regional and national organ sharing. All aspects of clinical renal transplantation have progressed tremendously in the past 34 years since the first successful renal transplant was performed (1). Currently, with cyclosporine, we are noting an 80% 1-year allograft survival (a 20% increase over that of conventional therapy), however, we seem to lose this advantage with increasing preservation times (Table 30.1) (2). Thus, in today's cyclosporine era, better preservation maneuvers are essential for optimal allograft survival, not just to diminish the detrimental effects of prolonged preservation times, but also to prevent the occurrence of delayed graft function that is associated with further graft loss using cyclosporine before the complete resolution of post renal transplant acute tubular necrosis (3–5). Much progress in research has been made in understanding cellular mechanisms as well as in developing new preservation maneuvers for keeping kidneys viable, not only during cold storage, but also after revascularization and reperfusion of these organs. In this chapter, we will review current extracorporeal renal preservation techniques that help minimize the ischemic damage to the kidney during cold storage and preview future maneuvers that may preserve viability in the organs immediately after transplantation.

Table 30.1
Effect of Increasing Preservation Times on 1-Year Allograft Survival[a]

Preservation Time (hr)	Cyclosporine (n = 600)	Pred/AZA (n = 2700)
0–24	87%	64%
25–36	72%	64%
37–48	66%	69%

[a] From Opelz G: Multicenter impact of cyclosporin on cadaver kidney graft survival. *Prog Allergy* 38:329, 1986.

HISTORIC ASPECTS

Attempts to maintain isolated organs extracorporeally in a functional and viable state have been made for more than a century. Early investigators were mainly interested in studying physiologic characteristics of isolated organs. Their methods allowed only very short observation periods before the organs suffered irreversible ischemic damage. In 1938, Carrel and Lindbergh contributed substantially to our knowledge of organ preservation by showing that kidneys could be kept viable extracorporeally for a limited time by using a special blood perfusion apparatus (6). Later, profound hypothermia was found to prolong the period in which tissues could tolerate ischemia. Successful cadaver kidney transplantation in the early 1960s greatly stimulated further work in the field of renal preservation. In 1963, Humphries and coworkers reimplanted dog kidneys after 24 hours of extracorporeal hypothermic perfusion with diluted serum or plasma (7). Belzer and colleagues, in 1967, achieved a very significant breakthrough by preserving dog kidneys for as long as 72 hours using hypothermic pulsatile perfusion with cryoprecipitated plasma (8). This was very quickly followed by consistently successful human cadaver kidney preservation using Belzer's method. Subsequently, Johnson et al. transplanted canine kidneys preserved with pulsatile perfusion but employing plasma protein fraction as the perfusate (9), while Claes and associates introduced 4.6% human albumin solution as a kidney preservation perfusate (10). In 1969, Collins and colleagues further simplified the preservation technique by showing that ample storage of dog kidneys in ice slush after immediate initial flushing with an intracellular electrolyte solution was successful in preserving the kidney for as long as 30 hr (11). Today, both simple cold storage and continuous pulsatile perfusion are used in clinical renal transplantation, either separately or in combination. Simple cold storage is used more extensively because it is generally accepted that a human cadaver kidney can be preserved safely by the simple cold storage method when the kidney has sustained only minimal ischemia and can be implanted within 40 hr. Otherwise, hypothermic pulsatile perfusion has been recommended.

The ability to preserve the kidney successfully for as long as 72 hr has been of immense benefit to cadaver renal transplantation. This had provided sufficient time for both histocompatibility testing of the donor and sensitive crossmatch testing for performed cytotoxic antibodies in the recipient or for organ sharing between transplant centers.

BASIC PRINCIPLES

To understand renal preservation techniques and their rationales, we must first understand what occurs at the cell level during periharvest warm ischemia, subsequent hypothermic storage, and reperfusion, such as diminished metabolic activity as well as cessation of cell membrane function that leads to cell swelling and acidosis. Concurrent with this there is a continued loss of intracellular energy stores that subsequently generate toxic free radicals, contributing to further endothelial damage or ''reperfusion'' injury after revascularization. Preservation maneuvers can be divided so far into four categories (Table 30.2) in which to counteract specific pathologic processes, such as: *(a)* the hypothermia effect; *(b)* cold flush solution effect; *(c)* preservation of intracellular high energy metabolites; and *(d)* free radical scavengers. (FRS).

The main function of hypothermia (4–8°C) is to slow metabolic activity by a factor of 10–20, extending the 1-hr normothermic (37°C) limit to 3 hr of cold. This is the main rationale for in situ cooling without flushing. Preservation can be extended further to 24–48 hr of cold storage with the help of specific flush solutions, which prevents cell swelling and loss of intracellular ions from passive diffusion. Other flush solutions and new additives support future clinical considerations (to be discussed later) that may diminish subsequent endothelial damage that occurs after revascularization. The mechanisms in which these additives work may help clarify pathways that contribute to the reperfusion injury that occurs after cold storage. These basic preservation maneuvers will now be discussed separately in greater detail.

Hypothermia

Hypothermia, as previously stated, extends our limits of preservation by a factor of 10–20 (Table 30.3). In 1959, Levy (12) (also subsequently verified by Schirmer and Walton in 1964 [13]) showed that hypothermia will slow metabolic activity and intracellular respiration by the same amount (a factor of 10–20), accounting for all of this effect. However,

Table 30.2
Basic Renal Preservation Maneuvers

Maneuver	Preservation Limit
Hypothermia	13 hr
Cold intracellular solution flush	24–48 hr
Preservation of intracellular energy metabolites	>48 hr
Free radical scavengers	>48 hr
Regeneration of intracellular energy metabolites in combination of above	Possibly 3–6 days

Table 30.3
Hypothermic Effect

	Preservation Limits	Respiration	Total Adenine Nucleotide
Normothermic (37°C)	1–2 hr	9.09 ml/mg/hr[a] 100%[b]	2.74 mM/kg[c] at 30 min
Hypothermic 4–8°C	12–24 hr	0.61 ml/mg/hr[a] 5%[b]	2.83 mM/kg[c] at 24 hr
Ratio	12	15–20	50

[a]From Shirmer HKA, Walton KN: The effect of hypothermia upon respiration and anaerobic glycolysis of dog kidney. *Invest Urol* 1:604, 1964.
[b]From Levy MN: Oxygen consumption and blood flow in the hypothermic perfused kidney. *Am J Physiol* 197:1111, 1959.
[c]Net weight, renal tissue, from Buhl MR, Jorgensen J: Breakdown of 5′-adenine nucleotides in ischemic renal cortex estimated by oxypurine excretion during perfusion. *Scand J Clin Lab Invest* 35:211, 1975.

measurement of intracellular high energy metabolites (total adenine nucleotides) by Buhl and Jorgenson (14) in 1975, showed a loss of 50 times the energy stores in 24 hr of cold storage compared to 30 mins of warm ischemia. Thus, there is much room for improvement with respect to preservation of these metabolites despite adequate hypothermia. New considerations in this area will be discussed later in this chapter.

Intracellular Flush Solution Effect

The electrolyte flushing solutions used for simple cold storage may be either extracellular or intracellular in composition. Ringer's lactate and isotonic saline solutions are extracellular flushing solutions and allow safe renal preservation for only short periods of up to 4 hr. Thus, extracellular solutions may be used in the living renal donor transplant setting, however, longer periods are not advised. For example, in our laboratory, we have observed severe histologic ischemic damage and subsequent nonfunction in dog kidneys preserved for 5 hr by cold storage after flushing with Ringer's lactate solution.

The intracellular electrolyte solution developed by Collins and associates offers several advantages (11). Table 30.4 shows the ingredients of the Collins solution (solution C2) most commonly used today. The rationale for using this flushing solution for simple cold storage is based on the fact that profound cooling of the kidney depresses the action of the cell membrane sodium pump or the (NA^+, K^+) -adenosine tri-

Table 30.4
Composition of Collins Solution (Solution C2)

KH_2PO_4	2.05 gm/liter
$K_2HPO_43H_2O$	9.70 gm/liter
KCl	1.12 gm/liter
$NaHCO_3$	0.84 gm/liter
Glucose	25.00 gm/liter
$MgSO_47H_2O$	7.38 gm/liter
Heparin	5,000 U/liter

phosphatase (ATPase). This leads to the passive diffusion of sodium and water into the cell and potassium loss from the intracellular space. The high concentrations of potassium and magnesium in Collins solution, thus, prevents the loss of intracellular potassium by passive diffusion. Collectively, the osmotic actions of these ions that prevent cell swelling are known as the flush solution effect. The magnesium has an added beneficial effect as a metabolic inhibitor, as well as inhibiting calcium binding (which may cause activation of a phosphorylation cascade that is detrimental to intracellular metabolism) (15). Euro-Collins solution does not contain magnesium; despite this, multiple studies have shown equivalent preservation using both types of Collins' flush solutions during simple hypothermic storage (16–20). The exact mechanism of action and the significance of the ionic composition of the intracellular flushing solution have been disputed. Belzer and Downes performed interesting laboratory experiments comparing Collins solution and hyperosmolar Ringer's lactate solution, and concluded that cellular potassium loss during cold storage is not as critical to subsequent renal function as is the prevention of water gain (21). These authors also suggested that the osmotic effect of a high glucose content in Collins solution was more important than were the high potassium and magnesium concentrations. Nevertheless, it is well accepted that these phosphate buffer solutions are quite effective in preventing cell swelling and acidosis during simple hypothermia storage as previously discussed.

Proponents of simple cold storage with Collins or other comparable flush solutions, for renal preservation, have long maintained that this method provides equivalent initial renal function and graft survival as does pulsate perfusion. In the past, it has been suggested that perfusion injury to the preserved kidney may cause pathologic changes that can compromise graft function or even enhance the antigenicity of the kidney (22, 23). Past studies in our laboratory were unable to demonstrate any difference in canine renal allograft survivals whether simple cold storage with Collins' solution or pulsatile perfusion was used for 24 hr of renal preservation (24). The weight of available experimental and clinical data suggests that both methods can be employed usefully, either separately or in combination, to achieve successful preservation of human cadaver kidneys (25).

Simple Cold Storage

Simple cold storage combines the hypothermic and flush solution effects to decrease metabolic activity and prevent subsequent cell swelling and acidosis and is accomplished by rapidly cooling the kidney immediately after harvesting by flushing the renal vasculature with chilled electrolyte solution and then placing the kidney in ice slush. Cannulation of the renal artery can be done by use of a tapered catheter that is trimmed to the size of the artery or with variously sized cannulas similar to those used during pulsatile preservation. The core temperature is kept between 0 and 4°C by placing the sterile-sealed kidney container in ice, where it is kept until the cadaver transplant procedure can be performed. This method of preservation is also employed for most extracorporeal renal operations.

Continuous Hypothermic Pulsatile Perfusion

Simple cold storage methods have offered consistently successful preservation of kidney viability up to 48 hr (25). This time period becomes more critical if the cadaver donor was poorly prepared before donor nephrectomy or if the kidney has sustained a period of warm ischemia. In these situations, hypothermic pulsatile perfusion is the preferred method of renal preservation. An advantage of this method is a longer safe preservation period, in some cases as long as 72 hr. Most transplantation centers are employing human cadaver kidneys that have been preserved for longer periods than in the past, due to an increase in regional and national organ sharing. These kidneys can be transported readily in a portable pulsatile renal preservation unit such as that shown in Figure 30.1. Compared to simple hypothermia, pulsatile perfusion (Fig. 30.2) is technically more complex and more costly (26), however, it does seem to offer more reliable preservation in the 48- to 72-hr range. Thus, this type of preservation is often used for questionably viable kidneys obtained from inadequately prepared cadaveric donors or rare (blood group) AB kidneys, which may travel through several centers before matching with an appropriate recipient. It is important to note that the lower incidence of postoperative dialysis has not translated to an increase in graft survival (27–29). Thus, taking these factors into consideration, common sense dictates that in a living related donor setting, ex vivo flush followed by brief simple hypothermia is preferred. Pulsatile perfusion also offers the ability to perform viability testing of kidneys and, thereby, to identify those that may be unsuitable for transplantation (the accuracy of these parameters will be discussed later). In extracorporeal renovascular surgery, pulsatile perfusion further allows the patency and integrity of complicated vascular repairs to be tested before implantation.

PERFUSION CONSIDERATIONS

Technique

In the chapter by Dr. Barry (chapter 29), the importance of in situ flush, followed by en bloc removal of kidneys during harvest is emphasized. This effectively reduces or eliminates any warm ischemia that may be incurred during this procedure. In addition, this enables subsequent en bloc perfusion, if preferred, such as for kidneys from pediatric donors or those donors with multiple arteries. In these settings, the arteries are often too small to cannulate individually; in addition, the preservation of the Carrel patch often is desired. However, most adult kidneys have single renal arteries and these can be separately cannulated (Fig. 30.3) and placed on a preservation machine. The kidney is flushed immediately after its removal with chilled Ringer's lactate solution or Collins solution until the effluent is clear of blood. This will achieve rapid cooling and thereby prevent warm ischemic damage. The flushing solution enters the kidney through a perfusion cannula of proper size that has been inserted into the renal artery taking great care not to damage the vessel's intima. After initial flushing, the kidney is placed in the preservation machine, which has already been primed with the selected perfusate. When the kidneys have been removed en bloc with a

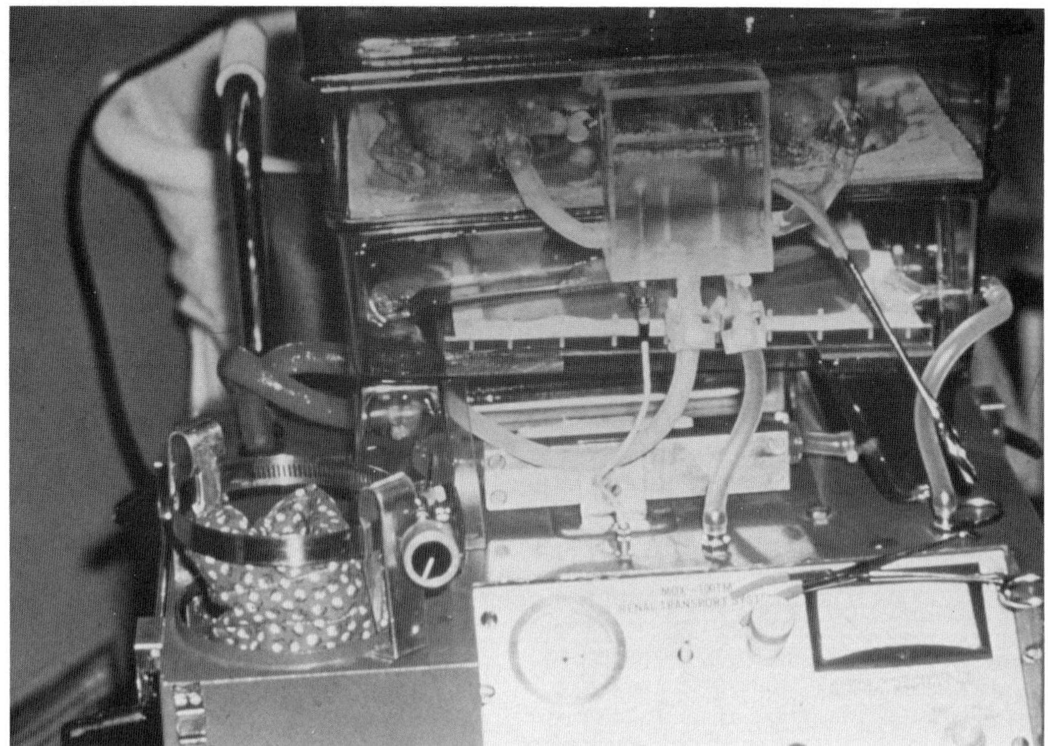

Figure 30.1. The MOX TM-100 portable renal preservation machine.

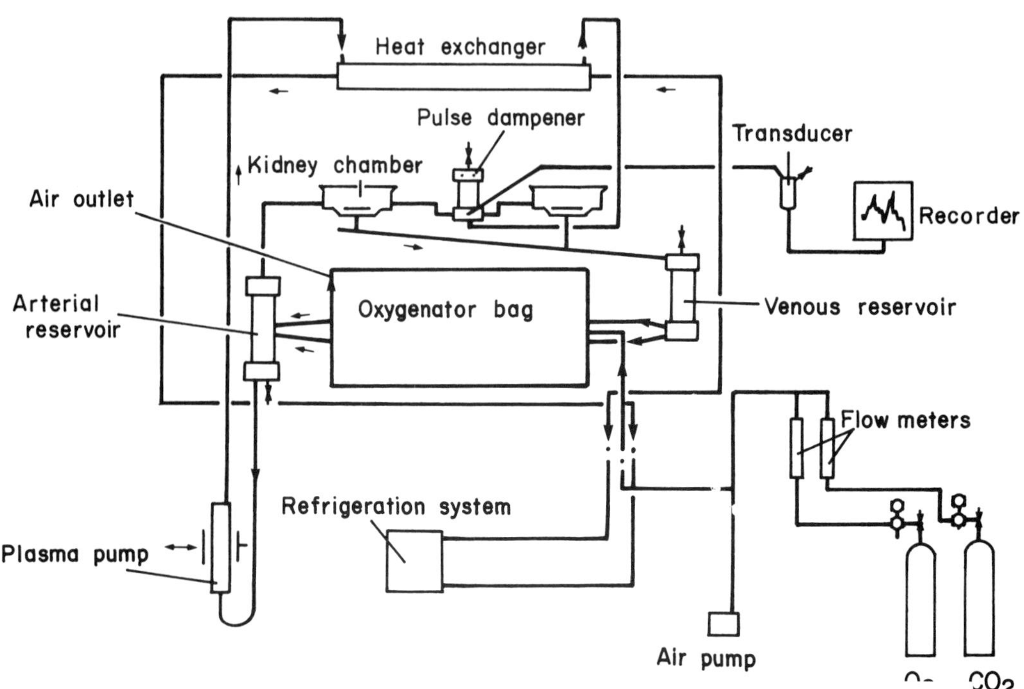

Figure 30.2. Schematic drawing of a typical renal preservation perfusion system.

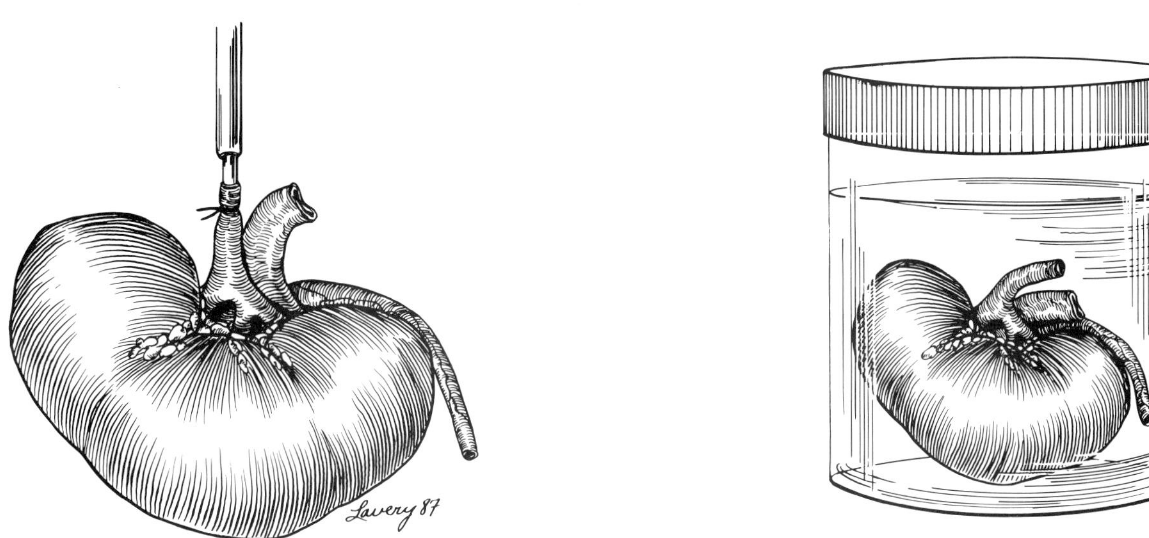

Figure 30.3. Ex vivo cannulation for cold flushing and simple hypothermic storage of kidney.

section of the aorta, it is very important to ascertain that no twisting of the renal vessels has occurred, which might impede perfusate flow to the kidney. These are kidneys attached to perfusion cannulus in the disposable cassette portion of the MOX-100 preservation machine (Fig. 30.4). Circulation of a cold perfusate through the kidneys enables toxic wastes to be removed, but in addition, the different flow (Table 30.5) parameters can be monitored as possible indexes for viability. As a general rule, the perfusion pressure is set at 60 mm Hg. A higher pressure is likely to initiate tissue swelling that may damage the kidney and also may lead to increased vascular resistance and poor perfusion. Kidneys that have been properly harvested from a suitable well-prepared donor will invariably show a drop in pressure during the first hour with a

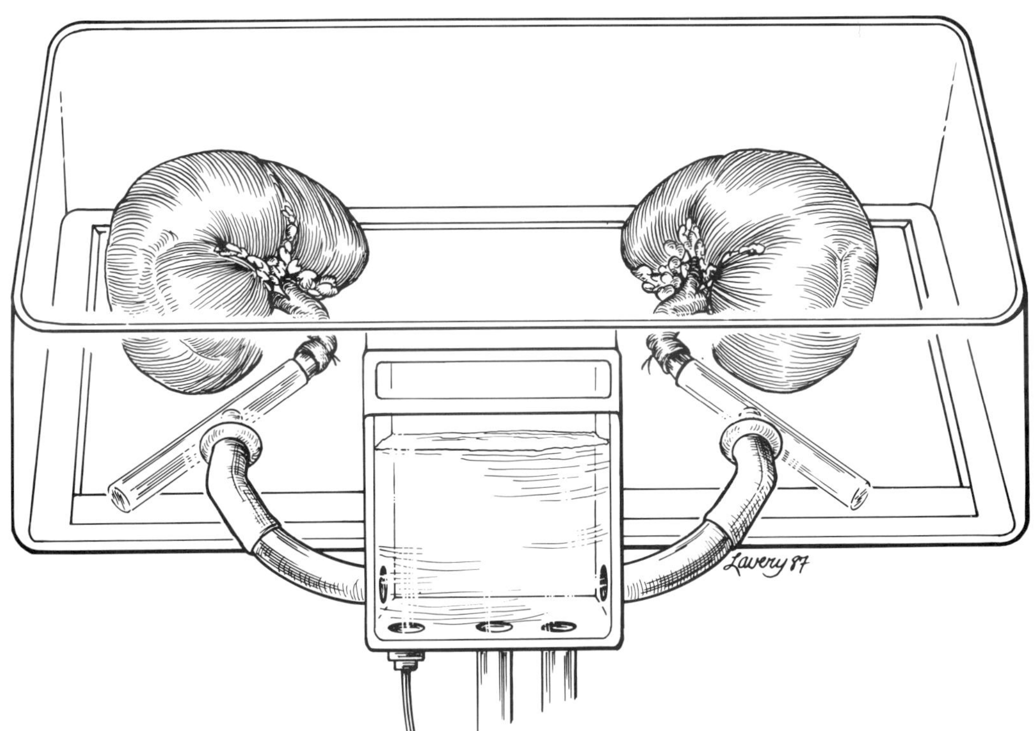

Figure 30.4. Separately cannulated kidneys perfused in the MOX TM-100 cassette.

Table 30.5
Favorable Hypothermic Pulsatile Perfusion Viability Parameters

1. Flow >1.0 ml/min/gm renal tissue >100 ml/min for most adult kidneys
2. Systolic pressure <60 mm Hg
3. Differential pressure >10 mm Hg
4. Diastolic pressure <45 mm Hg

concomitant increase in flow. Close observation of perfusion characteristics during the first couple of hours is important to detect any change that may reflect the viability of the kidney.

Perfusates

Extracorporeal hypothermic perfusion preservation of kidneys requires specially prepared perfusates. Whole or diluted blood is not suitable for this purpose because of the unphysiologic environment to which the organ is exposed. Tissue culture media that can sustain the life of isolated cells are seldom able to maintain the functional viability of a whole organ such as the kidney. The perfusate should contain the proper concentration of nutrients and possess the ability to neutralize toxic waste products. Prefusates available today are all either albumin or plasma derivatives that have produced similar experimental and clinical results in organ preservation in the hands of different investigators. For plasma to be employed successfully as a perfusate, low density β-lipoproteins must be cryoprecipitated and removed to prevent formation of harmful denatured aggregates. the plasma fibrinogen level is also lowered by cryoprecipitation. Disadvantages of using plasma include the possibility of transmission of infective viruses (i.e., hepatitis) and the potential for cytotoxic antibody-induced damage to the perfused kidney. In the past, preparation of the cryoprecipitated plasma (CPP) has been tedious and time-consuming. More recent studies have shown that plasma protein fraction and albumin solutions are as effective as perfusates as is CPP. These are presently in widespread use. Their main advantage over CPP is a matter of convenience inasmuch as cryoprecipitation is not needed and they can be stored on the shelf until used.

To improve the properties of the perfusate, various constituents are usually added. Mannitol increases perfusate osmolality and, because it crosses cell membranes poorly, it prevents cellular swelling. In addition, mannitol may act as an FRS. This potential effect will be discussed later in this chapter. Magnesium is added to the perfusate to substitute for the low level of ionized calcium, to improve ATPase activity and oxygen consumption, and for its membrane-stabilizing effect. The practice of adding a vasoactive drug (e.g., phenoxybenzamine, phentolamine, chlorpromazine, or papaverine) to the perfusate in an attempt to block intrarenal vasoconstriction has been unrewarding because hypothermia modifies the responses to drugs. Pharmacologic dosages of methylprednisolone are avoided and have been shown to cause both precipitation of eosinophilic material from the perfusate and glomerular damage. Propranolol, when added to the perfusate in dog experiments, provided a protective effect against ischemia, possible by membrane stabilization (30).

Perfusion Machines

Although hypothermic perfusion preservation has been performed with a variety of machines, two types are in use today. These are the MOX TM 100 (Fig. 30.1) and the Belzer machines, both of which are transportable models but can also be used as stationary units. In both of these machines, circuitry (Fig. 30.2) consists of an organ chamber, a pulsatile pump, a membrane oxygenator, arterial and venous blood reservoirs, a heat exchanger, and gauges for monitoring pressures and flow. When in transit, the machine runs by a self-contained battery and cooling is supplied by ice slush pumped through the heat exchanger. In our laboratory, we now use only the MOX TM 100 model, which has been very reliable and easy to operate. With this machine, sterile interchangeable cassettes are available; these are inserted after priming with the proper perfusate.

VIABILITY TESTING

Assessment of the viability of a kidney is one of the more difficult problems in renal preservation. Kidneys removed from donors with suboptimal blood pressures, inadequate diuresis, elevated serum creatinine levels, and prolonged ischemia times are of particular concern in this regard. The assessment of functional viability during perfusion preservation can be divided into two groups of tests, hemodynamic and metabolic. In considering the former, the pressure-flow relationship was initially described by Belzer et al. to be a reliable indicator of function after transplantation (8). The viability criteria proposed by Belzer were normal renal function at the time of harvesting, minimal warm renal ischemia, and a systolic pressure of 60 mm Hg or less during perfusion with a flow rate of 100 ml/min or more (Table 30.5). Abouna et al. subsequently demonstrated that perfusion pressures as high as 80–100 mm Hg could be compatible with good function (31). Stowe and associates further showed, using the xenon-washout technique, that the vascular filling and perfusion pattern within a kidney could not be predicted from the pressure-flow relationship of the kidney (32). In spite of these shortcommings, the pressure-flow relationship remains a simple method for evaluating the viability of preserved kidneys. A rising perfusion pressure and a decrease in flow generally indicate a failing kidney, especially when these are associated with an increase in swelling of the organ.

The release of various intracellular cytoplasmic enzymes into the perfusate as an indication of cell damage has also been used to predict viability. Elevations of lactic dehydrogenase and serum glutamic oxalacetic transaminase can be helpful in this regard and generally reflect severe ischemic renal damage. Measurements of perfusate pH changes and lactic acid accumulation during the first hours of perfusion are also useful tools in viability monitoring. Until recently, there has been no single, uniformly reliable test for renal viability available. Decisions of whether to use a given kidney were based on several difficult to assess factors. These include the clinical condition of the donor, prenephrectomy renal function, the warm ischemia time, the technical efficacy of the harvesting operation, and the ease of initial flushing of the kidney, combined with the perfusion characteristics mentioned previously. However, most of these parameters are difficult to quantify, or are invasive and not practical for the clinical setting of renal transplantation.

Phosphorous-31 magnetic resonance spectoscopy (31P-MRS) is a noninvasive, nondestructive technique in which intracellular metabolites can be quantified for use as accurate viability parameters. Bretan et al. (1985) developed this technique for routine use in the United States (33) for assessment of cadaveric renal viability pretransplantation by identification of specific 31P-MRS viability parameters. This technique has enabled us to study cadaveric kidneys routinely (Fig. 30.5A and B) to determine their viability (34). The transplant kidney can be studied noninvasively using a superconducting (> 1.4 Tesla) magnetic resonance imager as a spectrometer (Fig. 30.5B), without removal from its sterile container or interruption of hypothermia (Fig. 30.5A), using the magnetic characteristics of intracellular phosphorus. Thus, intracellular energy metabolites can be monitored for renal metabolic integrity. Although a detailed description of 31P-MRS and its potential is not possible in this discussion, studies (33–35) have supported that MRS can be a powerful tool for the assessment of renal transplant viability. In addition, precise preservation experiments are now possible.

PHARMACOLOGIC CONSIDERATIONS

Reperfusion Injury and Free Radical Scavengers

Many types of preservation additives work through modulation of different ischemic renal metabolic pathways, separate from that of hypothermia and the flush solution effects. We shall now present current rationales and the postulated mechanisms of action of these additives, such as calcium entry blockers (CEB), xanthine oxidase (XO) inhibitors, ATP, inosine, prostaglandins (PGs), and FRS.

To review briefly, with ischemia, ATP is degraded to hypoxanthine and because of further degradation with XO (present in vascular endothelial cells) during reperfusion and reoxygenation, supraoxide (O_2^-) is produced (Fig. 30.6) (36, 37). This O_2^- free radical can induce hydroxyl ion free radical (OH^-) formation, a very toxic ion that can break down cell membranes. Normally, the cytochrome oxidase complex can supply enzymes such as supraoxide dismutase and catalase (SOD + CAT) to scavenge these free radicals and rid the cell of these toxins by further degradation. However, with ischemia, these are not sufficient and additional FRS may be required to prevent further injury (36, 38–41) after reperfusion. Thus, it is not only important to understand what is going on in the kidney during cold storage, but also to assess what occurs in the immediate reperfusion period after renal transplant. The crucial period appears to be 0–2 hr after revascularization (42, 43).

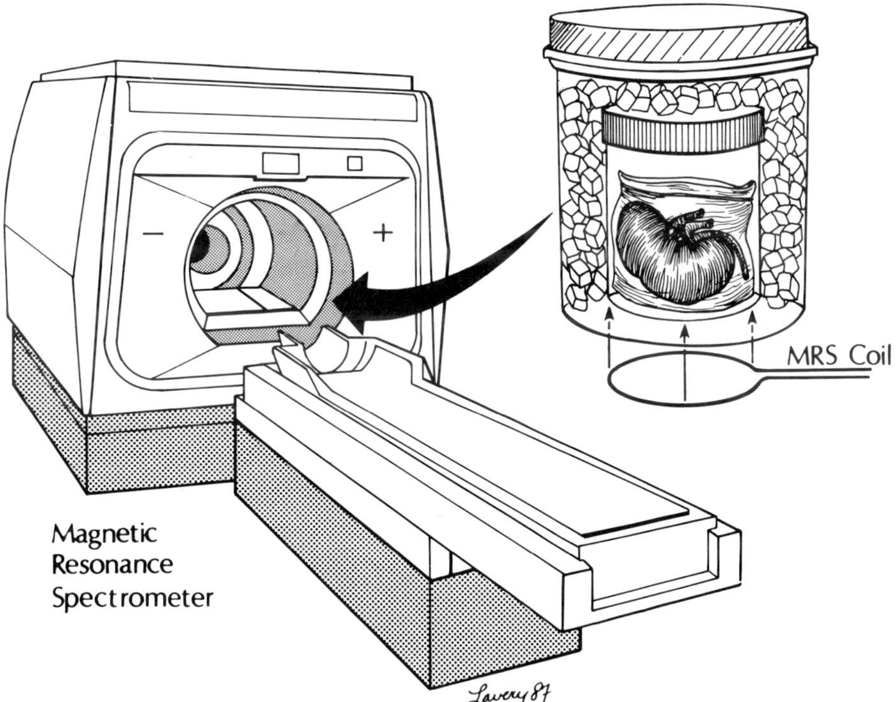

Figure 30.5. **A,** cadaveric kidney in sterile hypothermic storage container with external MRS coil below. **B,** cold storage container positioned within a super conducting magnet bore (2.0 Tesla).

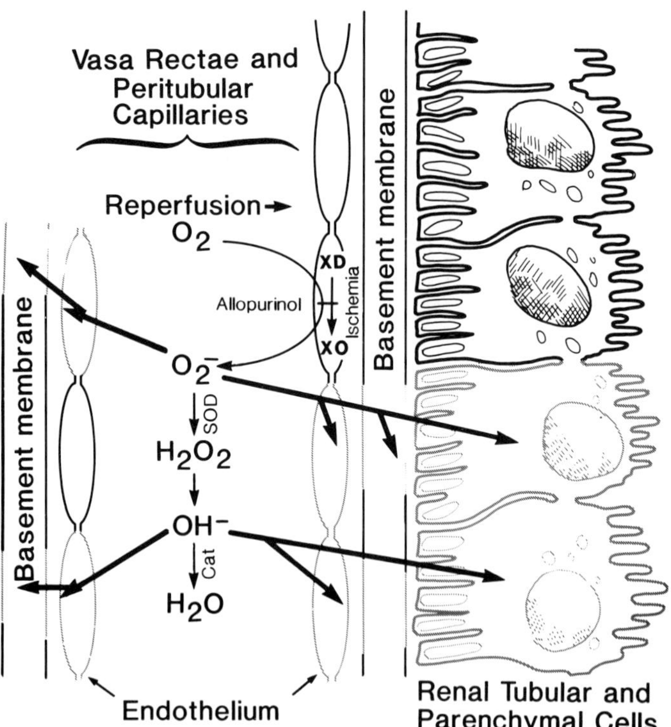

Figure 30.6. Mechanism of renal reperfusion injury after transplant revascularization. See text for full discussion.

In the clinical setting of renal transplantation, much controversy exists because there has been no prior definition for this reperfusion injury. Toledo-Pereyra (1987) recently attributes this skepticism to the secondary parenchymal damage caused by this phenomenon, which may occur concurrently with the primary parenchymal damage direclty related to cold ischemia (44). Thus, it would be impossible to separate all these effects in a clinical setting. Nevertheless, many laboratory studies (45) have greatly supported its existence by showing that the associated maneuvers to prevent this progressive ischemic damage have been very successful (37–40, 45–50).

ATP Mg Cl_2 and Inosine

Since 1976, there have been numerous animal studies supporting the use of ATP Mg Cl_2 (51–56), AMP Mg Cl_2 (55) or inosine (47), as protective additives in flush or perfusate solutions. These additives are associated with improvement in postreperfusion microcirculation and subsequent regeneration of intracellular ATP (57). It is postulated that these additives do not actually "recharge" the intracellular energy stores of renal cells, but they either slow the degradation of energy stores or supply substrate during the immediate reperfusion period enabling prevention of cell swelling of intrarenal vascular endothelia cells, thus, minimizing other aspects of the reperfusion injury. As mentioned earlier in this chapter, hypothermia slows the ischemic induced degradation of ATP (57) and adenosine to hypoxanthine by a factor of 20; by adding ATP Mg Cl_2 or inosine, this process may be slowed even more, generating even less hypoxanthine. With less hypoxanthine, less O_1^- is generated during reperfusion and the cytochrome oxidase complex can now deal more efficiently with degradation of free radicals.

The improved posttransplant microcirculation that was first noted in clinical renal transplant settings using Belzer perfusate (51) (containing ATP, Mg Cl_2) in 1984 has been reproduced by many centers and has been associated with a significantly higher immediate function rate compared to perfusates containing silicate gel (58).

Calcium Entry Blockers

There has been much controversy about the role of calcium overload in cells after ischemia has been thought to be a secondary process (59–61). Nevertheless, there have been many studies that have supported the salutary effects of calmodulin (59, 62–64) inhibitors and CEB in renal transplant settings. These beneficial effects in renal preservation are independent of blood flow effects (65, 66) and seem to work when administered to the kidney during cold storage (66–69). Currently used CEBs are verapamil (19, 65, 66, 70–73) nifidipine (68), and diltiazem (74, 75). It is postulated that these CEBs work by inhibiting calcium-induced phospholipases (61, 70, 71, 73) (also inhibited by chlorpromazine). These phospholipases can start a cascade of reactions that amplifies the destructive effects of ischemia (Fig. 30.7). In addition, verapamil pretreatment has been shown to modify the immune response and to reduce postischemic cyclosporine nephrotoxicity (74). Currently, these effects are poorly understood. Most studies (75, 76) successful in decreasing postoperative acute tubular necrosis require loading of CEBs in the recipient patient just before revascularization, as well as 2 days postoperatively.

Prostaglandins

There has been much debate over the clinical significance of renal PG in the recovery of the kidney from ischemia. Bulkley (77) postulates that PGs may play a primary role in predicting the body's response to injury and other noxious stimuli, however, this may not be the case for an individual organ such as the kidney. For example, under ordinary physiologic conditions, renal function is not dependent on the integrity of PG synthesis, as inhibition of PG synthesis in normal animals and humans does not induce a significant decline of renal functions (78). Pgs do have a significant effect on renal vascular resistance, as acute PG inhibition will reduce renal blood flow substantially, however, renal function is largely unaffected (79). Chronic nonsteroidal anti-inflammatory drugs also do not seem to alter measurable renal function. Thus, the vascular effect of PG may be overriden easily by other regulatory mechanisms, such as mediated by adrenergic tone, renin secretion, dopamine, and adenosine (80). All these evidences support the idea that PG may be responsible for the fine tuning of the homeostatic mechanisms needed to optimize long-term renal function. However, its role in the acute setting, such as for renal preservation, may be negligible. For example, Klintmalm and coworkers (81) studied 26 renal allografts and found no evidence that PGs are involved in the

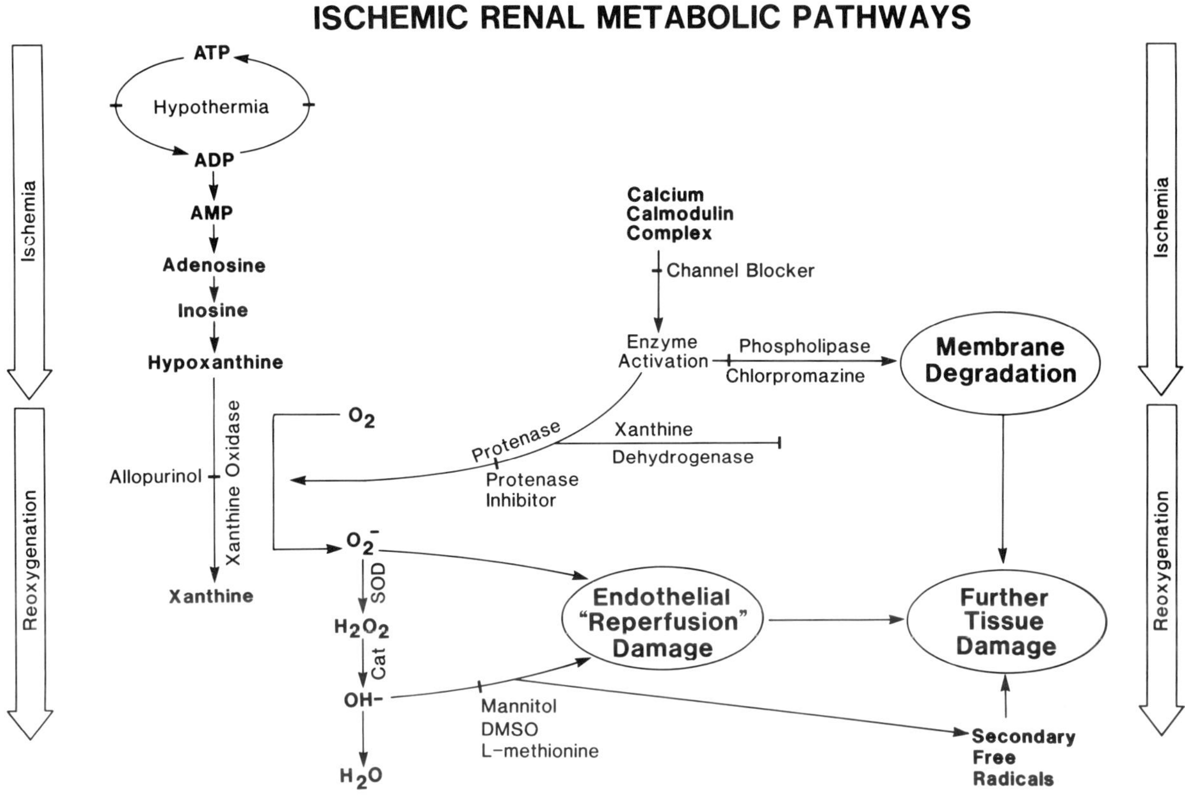

Figure 30.7. Proposed metabolic pathways involved in renal transplant preservation. See text for discussion of this model.

regulation of blood flow to these kidneys. On the other hand, recent preliminary studies by Bradley and coworkers (82) have showed prostacyclin (Flolan) pretreatment of five cadaveric renal donors (specifically, PGI_2) was encouraging. These PGs possess strong vasodilatary effects (causing an increased renal blood flow and maintenance of glomerular filtration rate), as well as inhibitory effects on platelet aggregation. Subsequently, only two of five recipients required hemodialysis in the first 5 days after transplantation. The 3-month graft survival was 88%. An explanation of these contrary results is that evaluation of PG use in a transplant setting is complicated by the effect of these compounds on the immune system. Shelby and associates (83) studied the role of PG in the inductive phase of transfusion-induced immunosuppression and found (in rats) that the splenic suppressor cells produced in this setting can down-regulate normal graft versus host responsiveness via a PG-dependent pathway. In addition to this PG suppressor cell effect, PGE_2 has been shown to inhibit effectively the function of cloned T-cells (84). Thus, it may be difficult to separate subtle PG-induced alterations in renal preservation from immunologic ones.

ISCHEMIC RENAL METABOLIC PATHWAY

A major breakthrough in preservation contributing to a greater insight of cellular ischemic processes is our ability to differentiate ischemic renal damage at the endothelial versus parenchymal levels. It is important to note that there are many studies that have isolated the reperfusion injury (Fig. 30.6) to the level of the endothelial cells that line the fine microcirculation of the kidney Thus, one of the primary ischemic injuries is not a whole organ injury, but an endothelial injury (45). Nevertheless, this reperfusion injury can cause severe secondary (Figs. 30.6 and 30.7) parenchymal damage from further ischemia induced by disruption of the microcirculation of the kidney. The complex puzzle of the many interrelated ischemic renal metabolic pathways is slowly being completed.

Briefly to review the proposed schema of ischemic metabolic pathways (Fig. 30.7), it is postulated that, during cold ischemia, ATP degredation to hypoxanthine is slowed by hypothermia and ATP (ATP Mg Cl_2) as well as other precursor substitutes (AMP Mg Cl_2 and inosine). In addition, calmodulin inhibitors and CEBs block the subsequent activation of calcium-dependent phospholipases, which can trigger a cascade responsible for cell membrane degradation. Chlorpromazine (47, 50) has been noted also to inhibit phospholipase-induced cell membrane degradation. During reperfusion and reoxygenation, xanthine dehydrogenase with the help of a proteinase generates XO (this conversion can be inhibited by a proteinase inhibitor). XO, in turn, generates O_2^-, but can be inhibited by allopurinol (45) or oxypurinol (both XO inhibitors). O_2^- can generate OH^- by the Haber-Weiss reaction (46), leading to endothelial reperfusion damage. FRS, such as SOD and CAT can degrade O_2^- and OH^- to nontoxic products. In addition, OH^- can also be deactivated furher by mannitol (50) dimethyl sulfoxide (48), and L-methionine (48). Both the reperfusion injury of the renal microcirculation and increasing OH^- ion levels (via generation of secondary free radicals) can lead to more severe tissue damage.

With more precise understanding of these pathways, more specific and rational maneuvers during extracorporeal hypothermic renal preservation can be instituted, taking into consideration what occurs at the parenchymal and endothelial cell levels.

FUTURE CONSIDERATIONS AND SUMMARY

All preservation maneuvers presented thus far work by reducing cellular metabolic degradation processes that are associated with renal ischemia. In terms of future prospects, regeneration of ATP during hypothermic storage has been supported just recently by normothermic blood perfusion using the technique of Rijkman etal. (85). Briefly, 3 hr of 37°C blood perfusion is given to a cold-stored kidney after being stored by simple hypothermia for 3 days. These investigators noted consistently extended cold storage capabilitites from 3–6 days in canine kidneys. More recent data have supported the "recharging" of intracellular energy stores in these kidneys by preservation studies using 31P-MRS by Bretan and coworkers (35), using a similar canine model.

As previously discussed 31P-MRS is a noninvasive and nondestructive method in which to monitor the bioenergetics of cells. MRS, being similar in technique to magnetic resonance imaging, has enabled us to "look" inside cells by monitoring specific phosphorous metabolites. Thus, the energy degradation pathways we have reviewed that are associated with ischemia can be studied more precisely so that further delineation of these biochemical pathways can be mapped out enabling institution of more rational preservation maneuvers.

In summary, not only have we come a long way in renal transplantation, but also in renal preservation. More improvement in the latter should help us increase graft survival and perhaps decrease cyclosporine toxicity. In addition, the knowledge and therapies gained may be extrapolated to preservation of other organs, such as the heart, lung, liver, and pancreas.

References

1. Merrill JP, Murry JE, Harrison JH, et al: Successful homotransplantations of the human kidney between identical twins. *JAMA* 160:277, 1956.
2. Opelz G: Multicenter impact of cyclosporine on cadaver kidney graft survival. *Prog Allergy* 38:329, 1986.
3. Bia MJ, Tyler KA: Effect of cyclosporine on renal ischemic injury. *Transplantation* 43:800, 1987.
4. Canafax DM, Torres A, Fayd DS, et al: The effect of delayed function on recipients of cadaveric renal allografts. *Transplantation* 41:177, 1986.
5. Kanazi G, Stowe N, Steinmuller D, et al: Effect of cyclosporine upon the function of ischemically damaged kidneys in the rat. *Transplantation* 41:782, 1986.
6. Carrel A, Lindbergh CA: *The Culture of Organs*. New York, Paul B. Hoeber, Inc., 1938.
7. Humphries AL, Russell R, Ostafin J, et al: Successful reimplantation of canine kidney after twenty-four hour storage. *Surgery* 54:136, 1963.
8. Belzer OF, Ashby BS, Dunphy JE: Twenty-four hour and seventy-two hour preservation of canine kidneys. *Lancet* 2:536, 1967.
9. Johnson RWG, Anderson M, Flear CTG, et al: Evaluation of a new perfusion solution for kidney preservation. *Transplantation* 13:270, 1972.
10. Claes G, Ahimen J, Gelin LE, et al: Albumin as perfusate in continuous perfusion for renal preservation. *Fourth International Transplant Conference*. New York, Grune & Stratton, 1972, p. 46.
11. Collins GM, Bravo-Sugarma M, Terasaki P: Kidney preservation for transplantation. *Lancet* 2:1219, 1969.
12. Levy MN: Oxygen consumption and blood flow in the hypothermic perfused kidney. *Am J Physiol* 197:1111, 1959.
13. Schirmer HKA, Walton KN: The effect of hypothermia upon respiration and anaerobic glycolysis of dog kidney. *Invest Urol* 1:604, 1964.
14. Buhl MR, Jorgenson J: Breakdown of 5'-adenine nucleotides in ischemic renal cortex estimated by oxypurine excretion during perfusion. *Scand J Clin Lab Invest* 35:211, 1975.
15. Collins GM, Barry JM, Maxwell JG, et al: The value of magnesium in flush solutions for human cadaveric kidney preservation. *J Urol* 131:220, 1984.
16. Barry JM, Farnsworth MA, Bennett WM: Human kidney preservation by flushing with intracellular solution and cold storage. *Arch Surg* 113:830, 1978.
17. Collins GM, Halasz NA: Forty-eight hour ice storage of kidneys—importance of cation content. *Surgery* 79:432, 1976.
18. Downs G, Hoffman R, Huang J. Belzer OF: Mechanism of action of washout solutions for kidney preservation. *Transplantation* 16:46, 1973.
19. Sacks SA, Woo YC, Smith RB, et al: Magnesium—not essential for renal preservation by initial perfusion and hypothermic storage. *Transplant Proc* 10:287, 1978.
20. Squifflet JP, Pirson Y, Gianello P, et al: Safe preservation of human renal cadaver transplants by Euro-Collins' solution up to 50 hours. *Transplant Proc* 13:693, 1981.
21. Belzer OF, Downes GL: *Organ Preservation for Transplantation*. Boston, Little, Brown & Co., 1974.
22. Fantini GA, Zadeh BJ, Chiao J, et al: Effect of hypothermia on cellular membrane function during low-flow extracorporeal circulation. *Surgery* 102:132, 1987.
23. Spector D, Limas C, Forst JL, et al: Perfusion nephropathy in human transplants. *N Engl J Med* 295:1217, 1976.
24. Magnusson M, Stowe N, Loening S, et al: The effect of two different renal preservation methods on canine renal allograft survival. *Urol Res* 6:65, 1978.
25. Halasz NA, Collins GM: Forty-eight hour kidney preservation—a comparison of flushing and ice storage with perfusion. *Arch Surg* 111:175, 1976.
26. Alijani MR, Cutler JA, DelValle CJ, et al: Single-donor cold storage vs. machine perfusion in cadaver kidney preservation. *Transplantation* 40:659, 1985.
27. Barry JM, Metcalfe JB, Farnsworth MA, et al: Comparison of intracellular flushing and cold storage to machine perfusion for human kidney preservation. *J Urol* 123:14, 1980.
28. Gregg CM, Cos LR, Saraf P, et al: Recovery of glomerular and tubular function in autotransplanted dog kidneys preserved by hypothermic storage or machine perfusion. *Transplantation* 42:453, 1986.
29. Halloran P, Aprile M: A randomized prospective trial of cold storage versus pulsatile perfusion for cadaver kidney preservation. *Transplantation* 43:827, 1987.
30. Stowe N, Emma J, Magnusson M, et al: Protective effect of propranolol in the treatment of ischemically damaged canine kidneys prior to transplantation. *Surgery* 84:265, 1978.
31. Abouna GM, Lim F, Cook JS, et al: Three-day canine kidney preservation. *Surgery* 71:736, 1972.
32. Stowe N, Wolterink LF, Lewis AE, et al: Intrarenal hemodynamics during hypothermic perfusion of cadaver kidneys. Dialysis, transplantation nephrology. *Proc Eur Dial Transplant Assoc Eur Ren Assoc* 10:493, 1973.
33. Bretan PN, Vigneron DB, Hricak H, et al: Assessment of clinical renal preservation by 31P-MRS. *J Urol* 137:146, 1987.
34. Bretan PN, Vigneron DB, Hricak H, et al: Pretransplant assessment of renal viability of phosphorus-31 MRS—preliminary clinical experience. *Proc Soc Magn Reson Med* 1:1015, 1987.
35. Bretan PN, Vigneron DB, Hricak H, et al: Assessment of renal preser-

vation by phosphorus 31 magnetic resonance spectroscopy—*in vivo* normothermic blood perfusion. *J Urol* 136:1356, 1986.
36. Ratych RE, Chuknyiska RS, Bulkley GB, et al: The primary localization of free radical generation after anoxia/reoxygenation in isolated endothelial cells. *Surgery* 102:122, 1987.
37. Hansson R, Jonsson O, Lundstam S, et al: Effects of free radical scavengers on renal circulation after ischemia in rabbits. *Clin Sci* 65:605, 1983.
38. Atalla SL, Toldeo-Pereyra LH, Mackenzie GH, et al: Influence of oxygen-derived free radical scavengers on ischemic livers. *Transplantation* 40:584, 1985.
39. Baker GL, Curry RJ, Autor AP: Oxygen free radical induced damage in kidneys subjected to warm ischemia and reperfusion—protective effect of superoxide dismutase. *Ann Surg* 202:628, 1985.
40. Koyama I, Bulkley GB, Williams GM, et al: The role of oxygen free radicals in mediating the reperfusion injury of cold-preserved ischemic kidneys. *Transplantation* 40:590, 1985.
41. McEnroe CS, Pearce FJ, Ricotta JJ, et al: Failure of oxygen-free radical scavengers to improve post ischemic liver function. *J Trauma* 26:892, 1986.
42. Green CJ, Healing G, Lunec J, et al: Evidence of free-radical-induced damage in rabbit kidneys after simple hypothermic preservation and autotransplantation. *Transplantation* 41:161, 1986.
43. Spragg RG, Hinshaw DB, Hyslop PA, et al: Alterations in adenosine triphosphate and energy charge in cultured endothelial and P388D cells after oxidant injury. *J Clin Invest* 76:1471, 1985.
44. Toledo-Pereyra LH: Definition of reperfusion injury in transplantation. *Transplantation* 43:931, 1987.
45. Parks DA, Bulkley GB, Granger DN, et al: Role of oxygen free radicals in shock, ischemia, and organ preservation. Surgery 94:428, 1983.
46. Del Maestro RF: An approach to free radicals in medicine and biology. *Acta Phys Scand* (Suppl) 492:153, 1980.
47. Frega WS, et al: Ischemic renal injury. *Kidney Int* 10:517, 1976.
48. Hansson R, Gustafsson B, Jonsson S, et al: Effect of xanthine oxidase inhibition of renal circulation after ischemia. *Transplant Proc* 14:51, 1982.
49. Jellinek M, Castanēda M, Garvin PJ, et al: Oxidation-reduction maintenance in organ preservation. *Arch Surg* 120:439, 1985.
50. Pavlock GS, Southard JH, Lutz MF, et al: Effects of mannitol and chlorpromazine pretreatment of rabbits on kidney mitochondria following in vivo ischemia and reflow. *Life Sci* 29:2667, 1981.
51. Belzer FO, Hoffman RM, Miller DT, et al: A new perfusate for kidney preservation. *Transplant Proc* 16:161, 1984.
52. Belzer FO, Hoffman RM, Rice MJ, et al: Combination perfusion-cold storage for optimum cadaver kidney function and utilization. Transplantation 39:118, 1985.
53. Guadio KM, Ardito TA, Reilly HF, et al: Accelerated cellular recovery after ischemic renal injury. *Am J Pathol* 112:338, 1983.
54. Siegel NJ, Auison MJ, Reilly JR, et al: Enhanced recovery of renal ATP with post ischemic infusion of ATP-Mg Cl_2 determined by 31P-NMR. *Am J Physiol* 245:F530, 1983.
55. Stromski ME, Cooper K, Thulin G, et al: Postischemic ATP-Mg Cl_2 provides precursors for resynthesis of cellular ATP in rats. *AM J Physiol* 250:F834, 1986.
56. Sumpio BE, Chaudry IH, Clemens MG, et al: Accelerated functional recovery of isolated rat kidney with ATP-Mg Cl_2 after warm ischemia. Am J Physiol 247:R1047, 1984.
57. Stromski ME, Cooper K, Thulin G, et al: Chemical and functional correlates of post ischemic renal ATP levels. *Proc Natl Acad Sci* 83:6142, 1986.
58. Henry ML, Sommer BG, Ferguson RM: Improved immediate function of renal allographs with Belzer perfusate. *Proc Am Soc Transplant Phys* 1:70, 1987.
59. Anaise D, Waltzer WC, Rapaport FT, et al: Metabolic requirements for successful extended hypothermic kidney preservation. *J Urol* 136:345, 1986.
60. Cheung JY, Bonventure JV, Malis CD, et al: Calcium and ischemic injury. *N Engl J Med* 314:1670, 1986.
61. Humes HD: Role of calcium in the pathogenesis of acute renal failure. *Am J Physiol* 250:F579, 1986.
62. Anaise D, Bachvaroff RJ, Sato K, et al: Enhanced resistance to the effects of hypothermic ischemia in the preserved canine kidney. *Transplantation* 38:570, 1984.
63. Anaise D, Lane B, Waltzer WC, et al: The protective effect of calcium inhibitors and of Captopril on the microcirculation during reperfusion. *Transplantation* 43:128; 1987.
64. Schwertschlag U, Schrier RW, Wilson P, et al: Beneficial effects of calcium channel blockers and calmodulin binding drugs on in vitro renal cell anoxia. *J Pharm Exp Ther* 238:119, 1986.
65. Harris DCH, Hammond WS, Burke TJ, et al: Verapamil protects against progression of experimental chronic renal failure. *Kid Int* 31:41, 1987.
66. Shapiro JI, Cheng C, Itabashi A, et al: The effect of verapamil on renal function after warm and cold ischemia in the isolated perfused rat kidney. *Transplantation* 40:596, 1985.
67. Burke TS, Arnold PE, Gordon JA, et al: Protective effect of intra renal calcium membrane blockers before or after renal ischemia. *J Clin Invest* 74:1830, 1984.
68. Hertle L, Garthoff B: Calcium channel blocker nisoldipine limits ischemic damage in rat kidney. *J Urol* 134:1251, 1985.
69. Mills S, Chan L, Schwertschlag U, et al: The protective effect of (−) Emopamil on renal function following warm and cold ischemia. *Transplantation* 43:928, 1987.
70. Blank W, Unni-Mooppan MM, Chhajwani B, et al: Effects of verapamil on preservation of renal function after ischemia—functional and ultrastructural study. *J Urol* 131:992, 1984.
71. Danon A, Zenser TV, Thomasson DL, et al: Effect of verapamil on prostaglandin E2 synthesis by hydronephrotic rabbit cortical interstital cells in primary culture. *J Pharm Exp Ther* 238:125, 1986.
72. Ishigami M, Magnusson MO, Stowe NT, et al: The salutary effect of verapamil and d-propranolal in ischemically damaged kidneys. *Transplant Proc* 16:40, 1984.
73. Schrier RW, Arnold PE, Vicki J, et al: Cellular calcium in ischemic acute renal failure—role of calcium entry blockers. *Kid Int* 32:313, 1987.
74. Sumpio B, Bave AE: Treatment with verapamil and adenosine triphosphate Mg Cl_2 reduces cyclosporine nephrotoxicity. *Surgery* 101:315, 1987.
75. Wagner K, Neumayer HH: Prevention of delayed graft function in cadaveric kidney transplants by Diltiazem. *Lancet* 2:1555, 1985.
76. Wagner K, Albrecht S, Neumayer HH: Prevention of delayed graft function in cadaveric kidney transplantation by a calcium antagonist—preliminary results of two prospective randomized trials. *Transplant Proc* 28:510, 1986.
77. Bulkley GB: The role of oxygen free radicals in the human disease processes. *Surgery* 94:407, 1983.
78. Dunn MJ: Nonsteroidal anti-inflammatory drugs and renal function. *Ann Rev Med* 35:411, 1984.
79. Terragno NA, Terragno DA, McGiff JC: Contribution of prostaglandins to the renal circulation in conscious, anesthetized and laparotomized dogs. *Circ Res* 40:590, 1977.
80. Dunn MJ: Renal prostaglandins. In Dunn MJ, (ed): *Renal Endocrinology*. Baltimore, Williams & Wilkins, 1983, pp. 1–74.
81. Klintmalm GBG, Cronestrand R, Wennmaln A, et al: Human renal allograft blood flow, oxygen extraction, prostaglandin release: the bearing on graft function. *Surgery* 95:427, 1984.
82. Bradley JW, Grossman SH, Atwood BF, et al: Flolan (prostacyclin) pretreatment of kidney donors: a pilot study. *Transplant Proc* 28:447, 1986.
83. Shelby J, Marushak MM, Nelson EW: Prostaglandin production and suppressor cell induction in transfusion-induced immune suppression. *Transplantation* 43:113, 1987.
84. Jordan ML, Hoffman RA, Debe EF, et al: Prostaglandin E2 mediates subset-specific effects on the functional responses of allosensitized T lymphocyte clones. *Transplantation* 43:117, 1987.
85. Rijkman BG, Buurman WA, Koostra G: Six-day canine kidney preservation. *Transplantation* 37:130, 1984.

CHAPTER 31

Live Donor Nephrectomy

STEVAN B. STREEM

A successful renal transplant is the optimal form of management for end-stage renal disease and, at the present time, this is best achieved using living, related donors. Further justification for the use of such donors and, in selected cases, living, nonrelated donors, such as well-motivated spouses is based on the low morbidity and mortality consistently documented after live donor nephrectomy and the chronic shortage of suitable cadaver kidneys

DONOR EVALUATION

When a potential living-related donor is identified on the basis of ABO (blood type) compatibility, human lympocyte antigen tissue typing, and preliminary crossmatching, an extensive evaluation is undertaken to assess both the general health and renal function and structure of the donor. A complete history and physical examination is performed and initial laboratory studies are obtained. These include at least a complete blood count; test for syphilis (VDRL), serum electrolytes and creatinine, blood urea nitrogen, SMA-12 or similar general profile, clotting parameters, and fasting blood sugar. Where indicated, glucose tolerance test, urinalysis and culture, glomerular filtration rate, chest x-ray, and electrocardiogram should also be assessed. A screening for hepatitis and determination of human T cell lymphotrophic virus (HTLV), cytomegalovirus, and herpes simplex virus antibody titers may also be performed at this time. Upon completion of the preliminary investigation, an excretory urogram and renal angiogram are performed.

When both kidneys have single arteries and ureters, the left one is generally selected for donation because its longer renal vein will facilitate implantation in the recipient. If multiple renal arteries or an uncomplicated duplication anomaly is present, the contralateral kidney should be taken. If a duplication anomaly or multiple vessels are found bilaterally, the left kidney again generally would be chosen for donation. Although other minor abnormalities found in one kidney would not necessarily preclude donation, the donor must always be left with the unaffected unit.

PHYSIOLOGIC PREPARATION OF THE DONOR

Several measures must be taken to minimize ischemic injury to the donor kidney, thereby ensuring its prompt and optimal function in the recipient. Adequate hydration of the donor begins the night before surgery with an intravenous infusion of 5% dextrose and one-half normal saline at a physiologic rate. Fluids are increased in the morning so that at least 1 liter is given in the hour just before surgery and mannitol, 12.5 gm, is infused just after induction of anesthesia. Intravenous fluids are then given at a minimum rate of 10–15 ml/kg/hr, with hypotension scrupulously avoided during the operation. Throughout the procedure, the severed ureter is monitored for urine output and appropriate adjustments made should that drop below 1 ml/min from the operated side. After dissection of the ureter and vessels, the kidney is replaced in its bed and an additional 12.5 gm of mannitol is given. Actual removal of the kidney is deferred until any possible vasospasm has resolved and a vigorous sustained diuresis is evident. After its removal, the kidney is flushed with a chilled electrolyte solution and the donor intravenous rate is reduced to maintenance levels.

OPERATIVE TECHNIQUE

The multiple operative approaches to live donor nephrectomy that have been described are all variations of either thoracoabdominal, flank, or anterior subcostal incisions. In earlier years at the Cleveland Clinic, it had been the policy to perform all living donor nephrectomies through an anterior subcostal transperitoneal approach. For the past 5 years, however, we have exclusively used an extraperitoneal flank approach with a subperiosteal rib resection. The advantages of this approach are several. The postoperative stay has been reduced by almost 50%. Whereas donors had been hospitalized for 7–10 days after an anterior transperitoneal nephrectomy, they are currently discharged only 4–6 days postoperatively. At the same time, both short- and long-term morbidity has been further improved and well-documented potential complications such as "incidental splenectomy" and late bowel obstruction have been eliminated entirely. Finally, the excellent exposure to the vessels that this procedure allows is documented by an incidence of acute tublar necrosis or ureteral fistula formation in less than 3% of the kidneys.

Figure 31.1 The retroperitoneum is entered through a modified flank incision with a subperiosteal rib resection. For a left nephrectomy, the 11th rib is generally chosen. The incision is carried medially off the tip of the rib and then gently curved downward ultimately to allow exposure of the ureter where it crosses the iliac vessels.

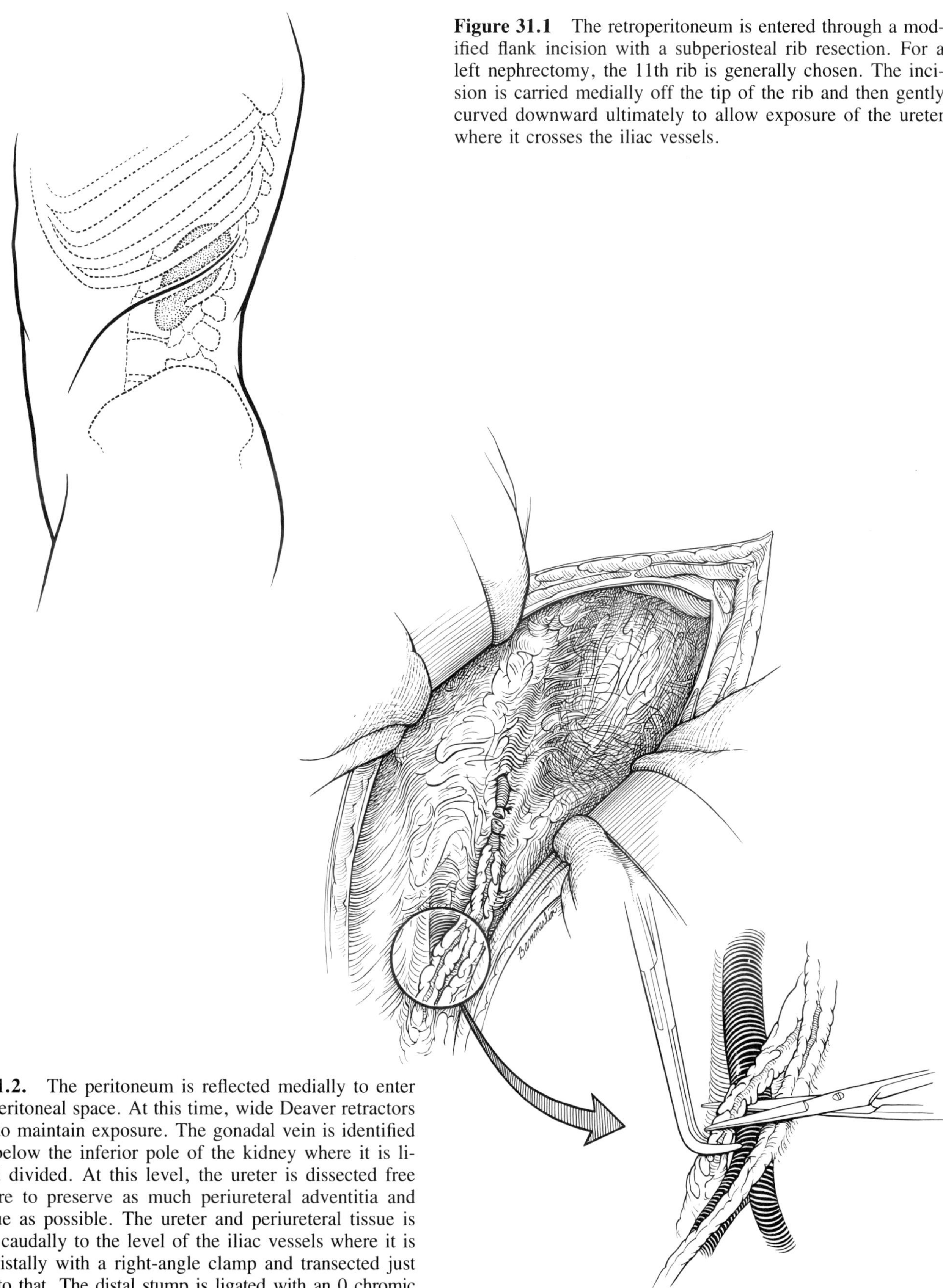

Figure 31.2. The peritoneum is reflected medially to enter the retroperitoneal space. At this time, wide Deaver retractors are used to maintain exposure. The gonadal vein is identified 2–3 cm below the inferior pole of the kidney where it is ligated and divided. At this level, the ureter is dissected free taking care to preserve as much periureteral adventitia and fatty tissue as possible. The ureter and periureteral tissue is dissected caudally to the level of the iliac vessels where it is secured distally with a right-angle clamp and transected just proximal to that. The distal stump is ligated with an 0 chromic ligature.

Figure 31.3. The ureter is followed back cephalad again preserving as much periureteral tissue as possible. As the ureteral dissection proceeds upward, the small vascular and lymphatic tributaries between the ureter and lateral wall of the aorta are spot fulgurated and transected. Laterally, the dissection is carried upward to the point where periureteral fatty tissue merges with the perirenal fat covering the lower pole of the kidney. The dissection is kept medial to the gonadal vein from the point where it was ligated and divided as it crossed the ureter up to where it enters the renal vein. The anterior surface of the renal vein is exposed at this time.

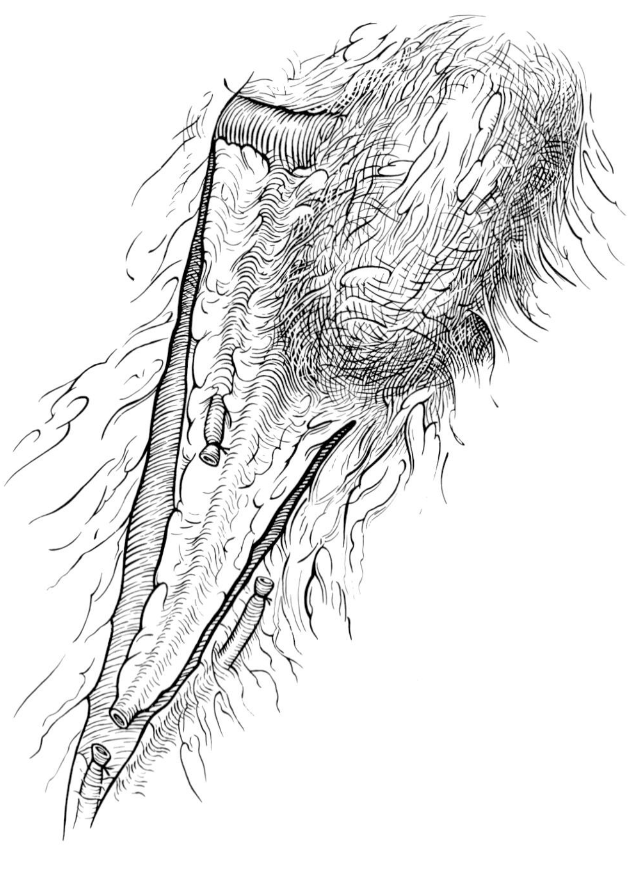

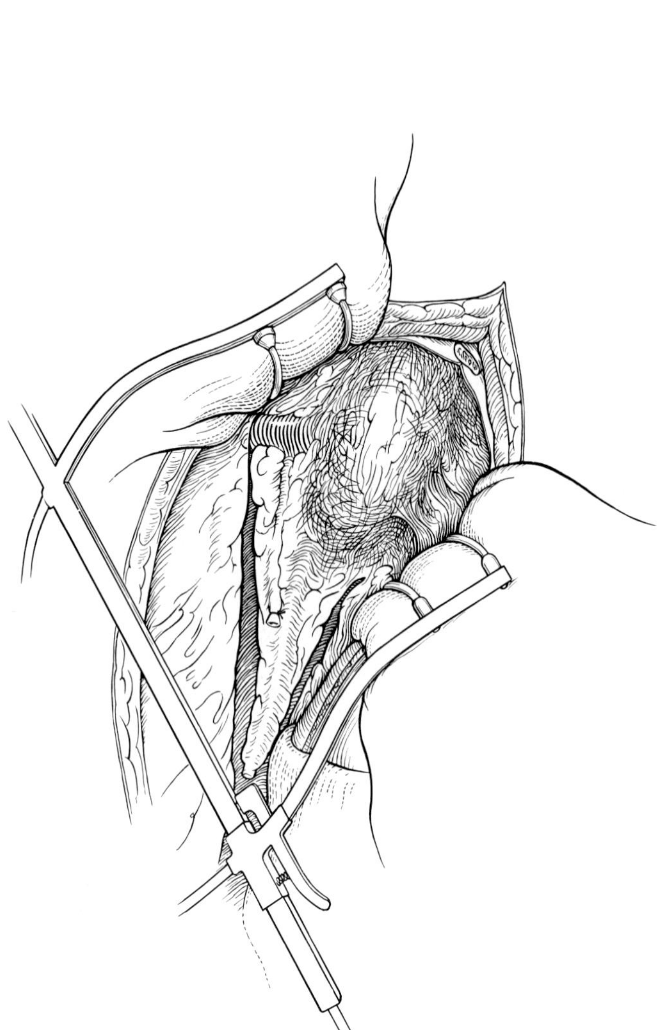

Figure 31.4. The Deaver retractors are replaced with a self-retaining Forder retractor. This affords constant exposure for the remainder of the dissection.

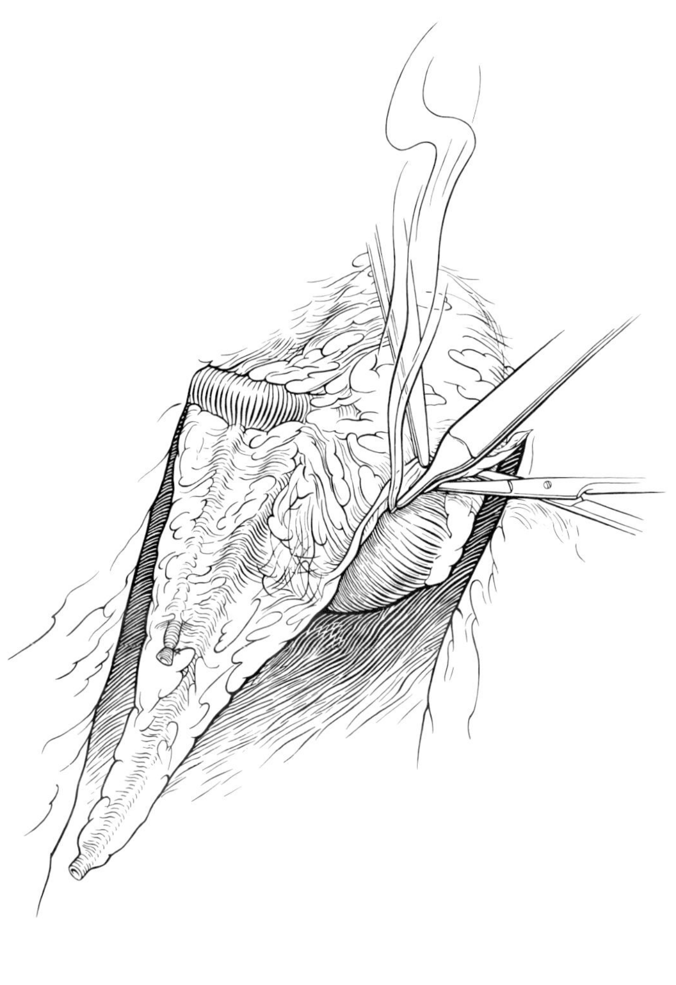

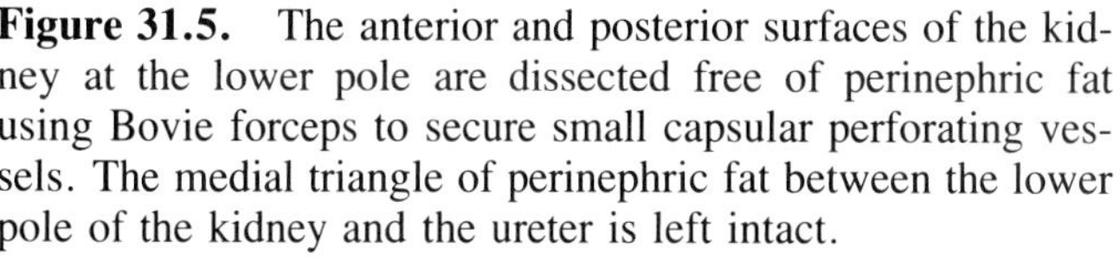

Figure 31.5. The anterior and posterior surfaces of the kidney at the lower pole are dissected free of perinephric fat using Bovie forceps to secure small capsular perforating vessels. The medial triangle of perinephric fat between the lower pole of the kidney and the ureter is left intact.

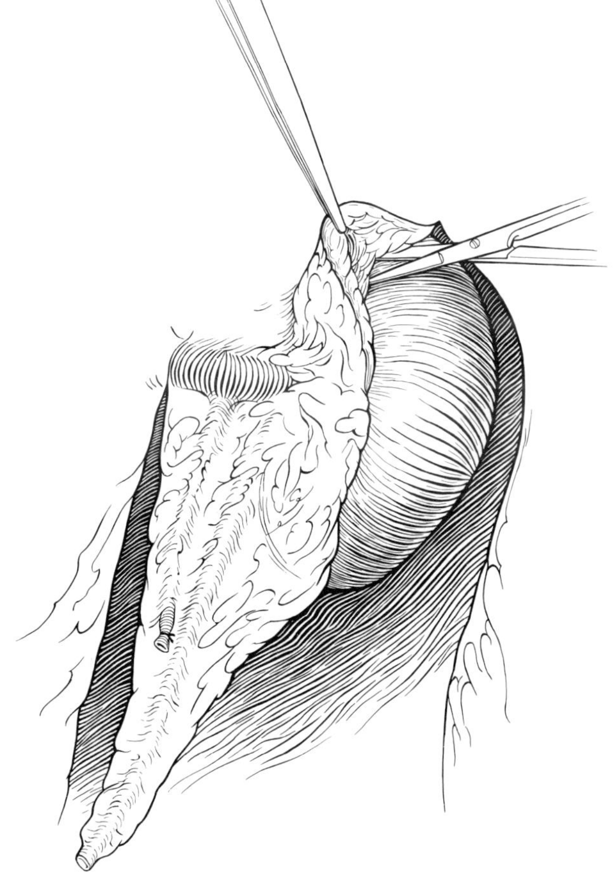

Figure 31.6. Clearing of the perinephric fat continues upward, care being taken not to carry the dissection closer than 2–3 cm to the renal hilus. The perinephric fat is dissected off up to the medial aspect of the upper pole of the kidney, at the level where the lower lateral margin of the adrenal gland comes into view.

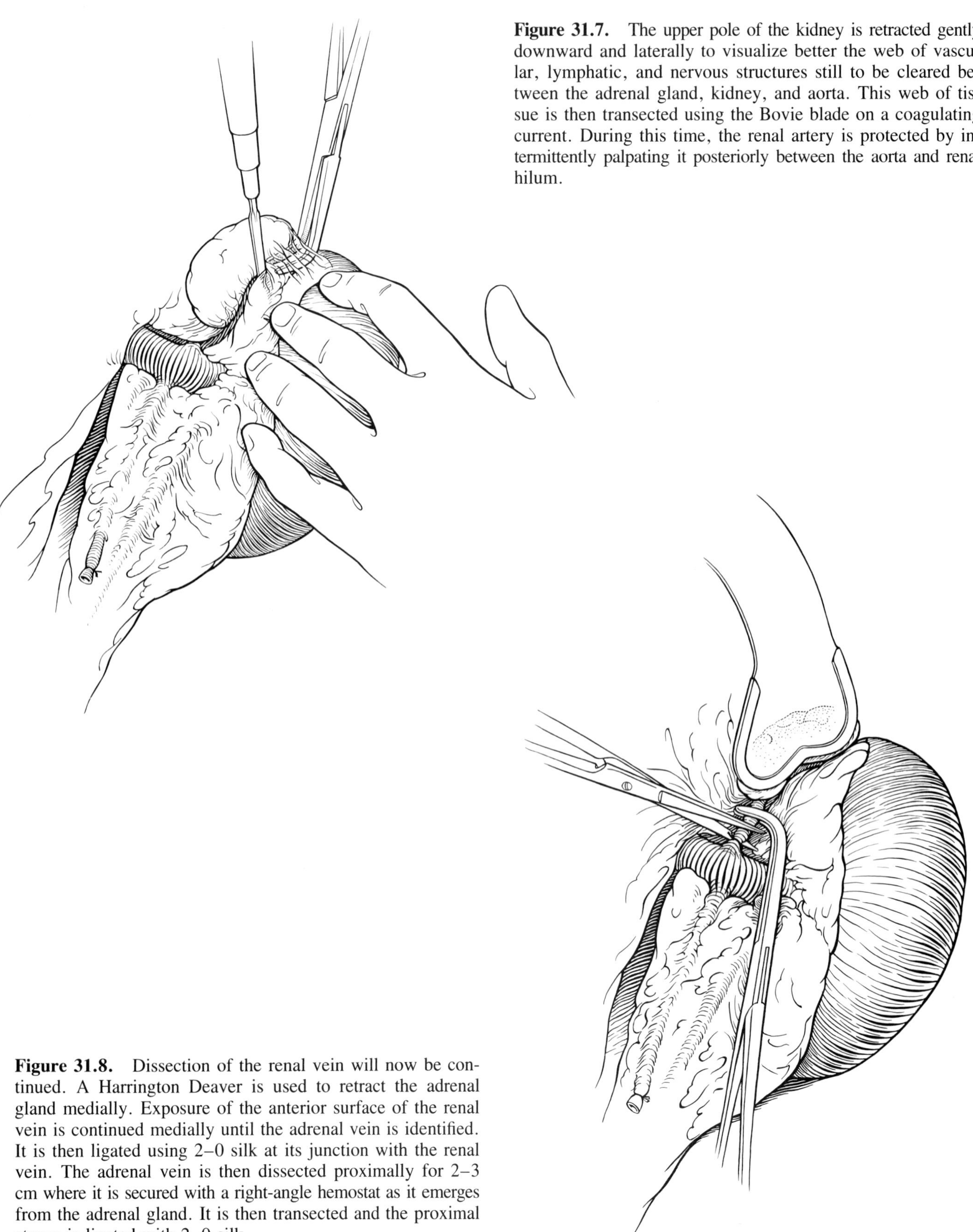

Figure 31.7. The upper pole of the kidney is retracted gently downward and laterally to visualize better the web of vascular, lymphatic, and nervous structures still to be cleared between the adrenal gland, kidney, and aorta. This web of tissue is then transected using the Bovie blade on a coagulating current. During this time, the renal artery is protected by intermittently palpating it posteriorly between the aorta and renal hilum.

Figure 31.8. Dissection of the renal vein will now be continued. A Harrington Deaver is used to retract the adrenal gland medially. Exposure of the anterior surface of the renal vein is continued medially until the adrenal vein is identified. It is then ligated using 2–0 silk at its junction with the renal vein. The adrenal vein is then dissected proximally for 2–3 cm where it is secured with a right-angle hemostat as it emerges from the adrenal gland. It is then transected and the proximal stump is ligated with 2–0 silk.

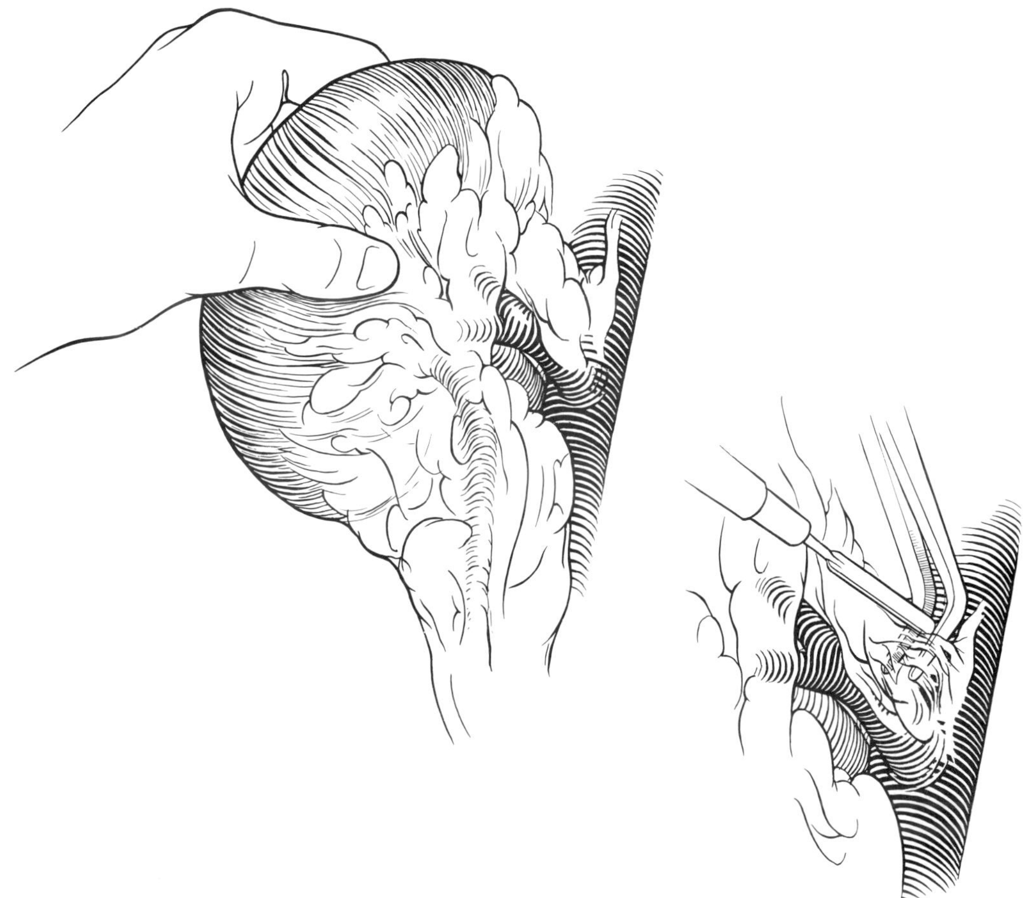

Figure 31.9. The kidney is reflected medially to gain exposure to the posterior hilar area. The renal artery is now identified easily by visual inspection and palpation. At this time, the artery is still surrounded by a few lymphatic and nervous structures. These are dissected off the artery with a right-angle clamp and divided using a Bovie blade and coagulating current, freeing the renal artery near its origin on the aorta. There is no need to isolate the artery more distally by further dissection into the hilum because this might compromise ureteral blood supply.

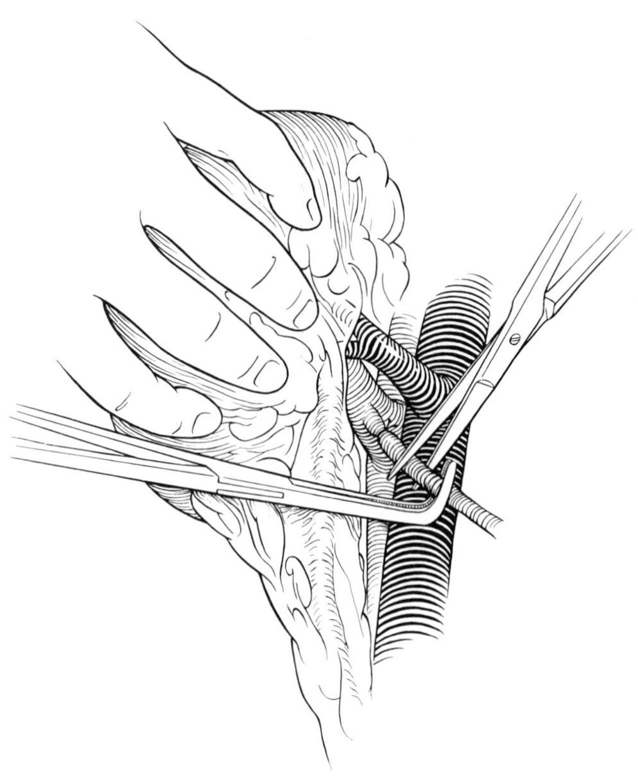

Figure 31.10. Gentle medial retraction of the kidney is continued to maintain exposure to the posterior hilar area. At this time, a careful search is made for the commonly occurring large lumbar vein that usually will be found entering the posterior aspect of the renal vein just lateral to the aorta, ascending form the paraspinous musculature dorsally. A 2–0 silk ligature is placed around it as it enters the renal vein while a right-angle hemostat is used to secure it proximally, well away from the first ligature. The vein is then transected with an adequate stump between the ligature and the right-angle hemostat, and a second silk tie is placed to secure the dorsal stump. Completion of this step results in the kidney being freed completely from all surrounding structures except the renal artery and vein.

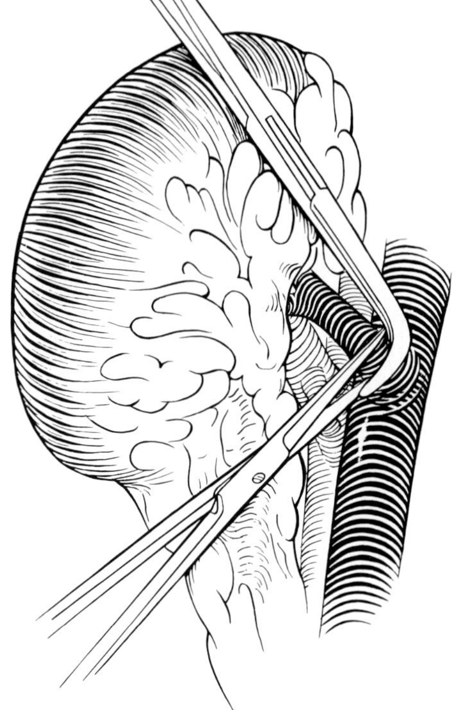

Figure 31.11. After ensuring an adequate diuresis from the donor kidney and ascertaining that the recipient is ready for transplantation, a right-angle hemostat is placed across the renal artery just distal to its aortic takeoff. The artery is then transected just distal to the hemostat.

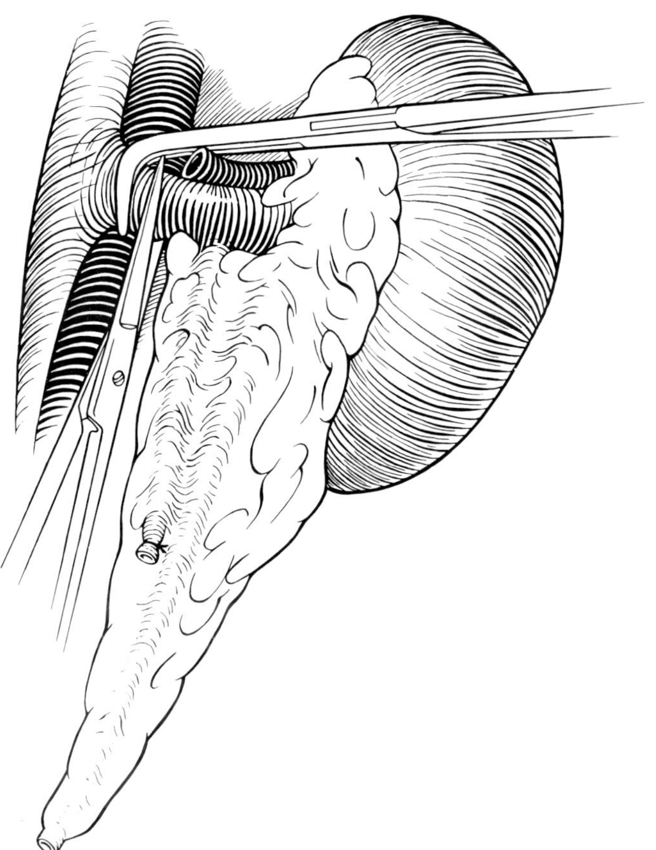

Figure 31.12. The kidney is retracted laterally while the renal vein is crossclamped distally with a right-angle clamp and transected. The kidney is then delivered to the perfusion table where it will be flushed with a chilled electrolyte solution. The renal vein is ligated with two separate 0 silk ligatures. The renal artery is secured in a similar fashion. Final hemostasis is accomplished by electrocoagulation, after which the renal bed is thoroughly irrigated with fresh, warm saline and the incision closed in a standard fashion. Drains are not used.

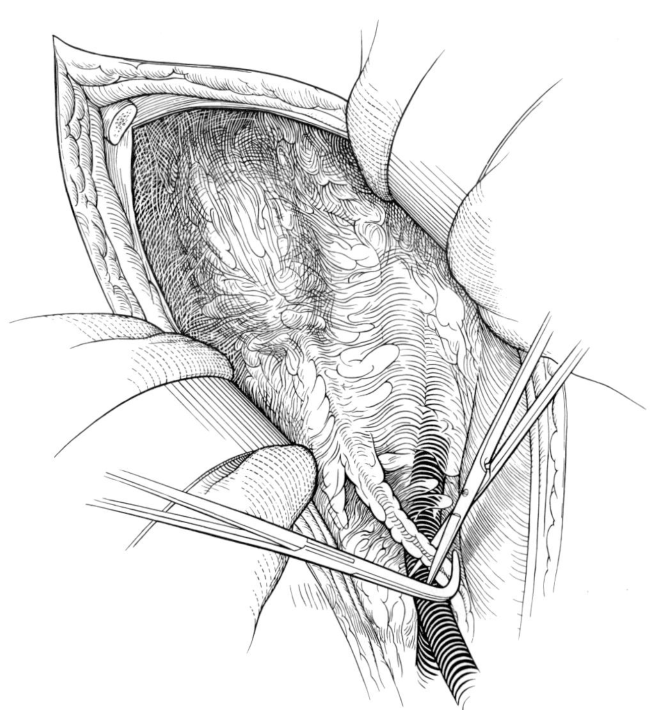

Figure 31.13. To perform a right donor nephrectomy, a 12th rib resection is generally performed. The peritoneum is reflected medially and the retroperitoneum entered. The right ureter is identified and transected as it crosses the iliac bifurcation in a fashion similar to that described for the left side.

Figure 31.14. The Forder retractor is positioned in place. On the right side, the gonadal vein is situated far enough medial to the ureter that it is not involved in preservation of ureteral blood supply. There are, however, many small venous tributaries coursing between the gonadal vein and periureteral tissue that must be spot fulgurated as close to the gonadal vein as possible so that ureteral vascularity is not compromised. The ureter is gently retracted laterally and the dissection is carried up along the lateral aspect of the gonadal vein and the anterolateral aspect of the vena cava, clearing the caval adventitia up to the entry of the renal vein.

Laterally, the ureteral dissection is carried up to the lower pole of the kidney, preserving a large amount of periureteral fat and adventitia. The perinephric fat covering the anterior, lateral, and posterior surfaces of the kidney is then dissected off, again staying at least 2–3 cm from the renal hilus both anteriorly and posteriorly. As with a left donor nephrectomy, a triange of perineprhic fat is retained between the lower pole and ureter to preserve ureteral blood supply

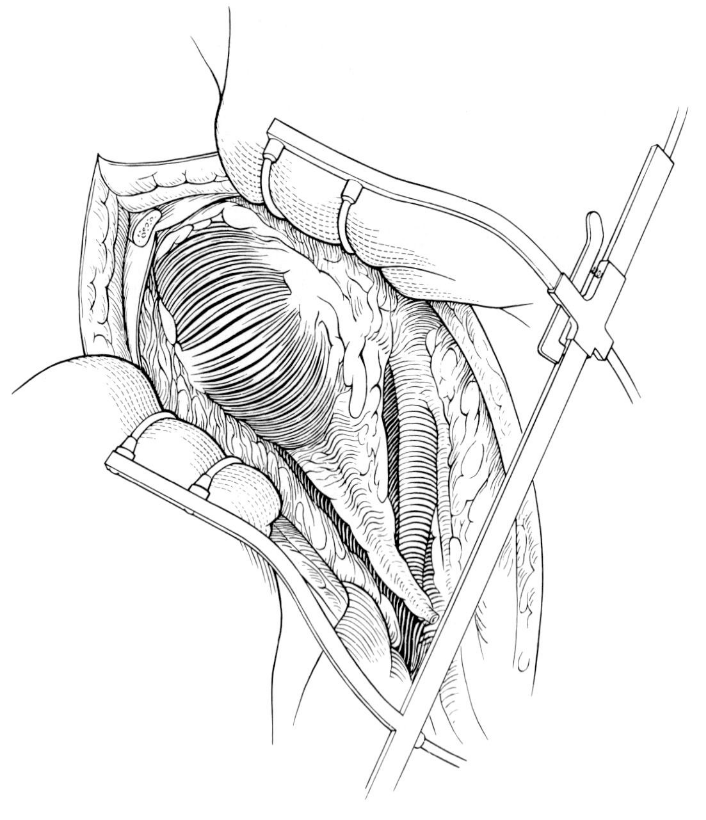

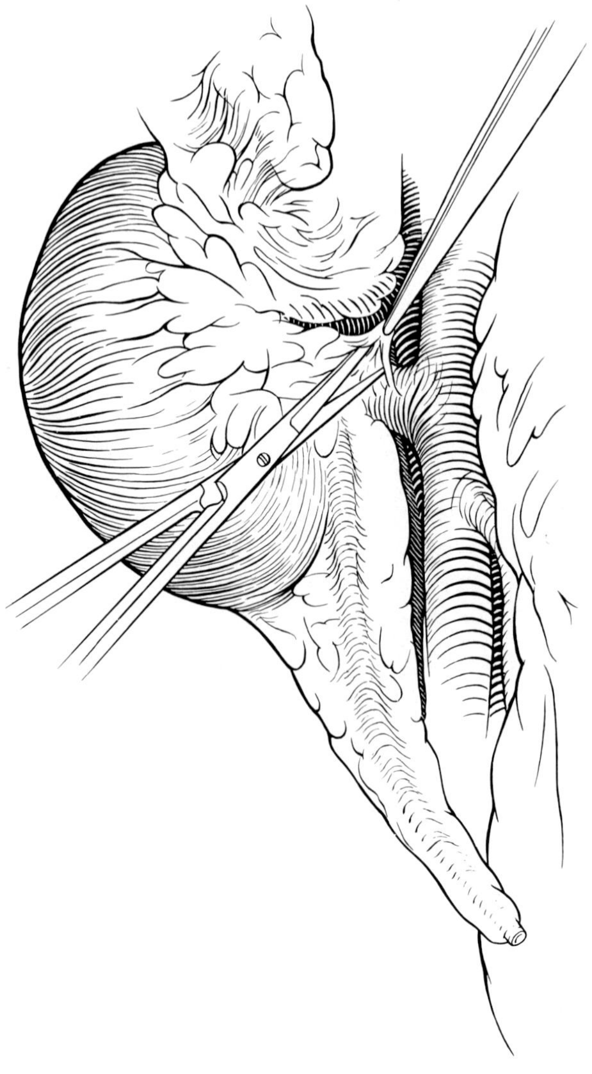

Figure 31.15. The kidney is gently retracted laterally and the dissection continued along the anterolateral aspect of the vena cava, transecting the small vascular, lymphatic, and nervous structures coursing from the aorta posterior to the vena cava and from the vena cava itself toward the kidney. Dissection and mobilization of the distal renal vein from surrounding structures should then be continued to clear completely the junction of the renal vein and vena cava anteriorly and inferiorly.

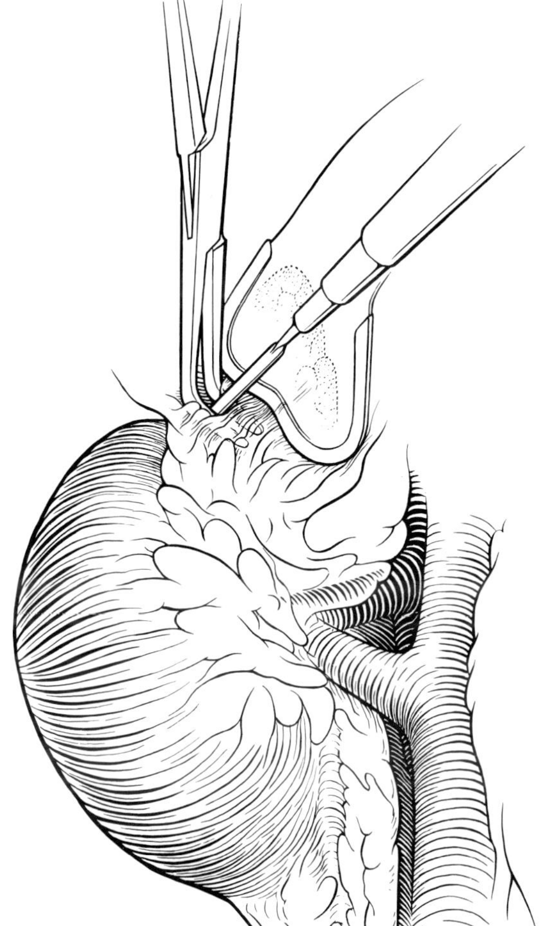

Figure 31.16. Attention is directed superiorly to the upper pole of the kidney where the lower margin of the adrenal gland is visualized. A Harrington Deaver is used to retract the adrenal gland gently medially. Staying midway between the capsule of the kidney and the lower pole of the adrenal gland, the dissection is carried laterally to medially with spot fulguration of the numerous small vessels in the web of tissue coursing between these two structures. Dissection of the superior aspect of the renal vein and lateral aspect of the vena cava can now be completed.

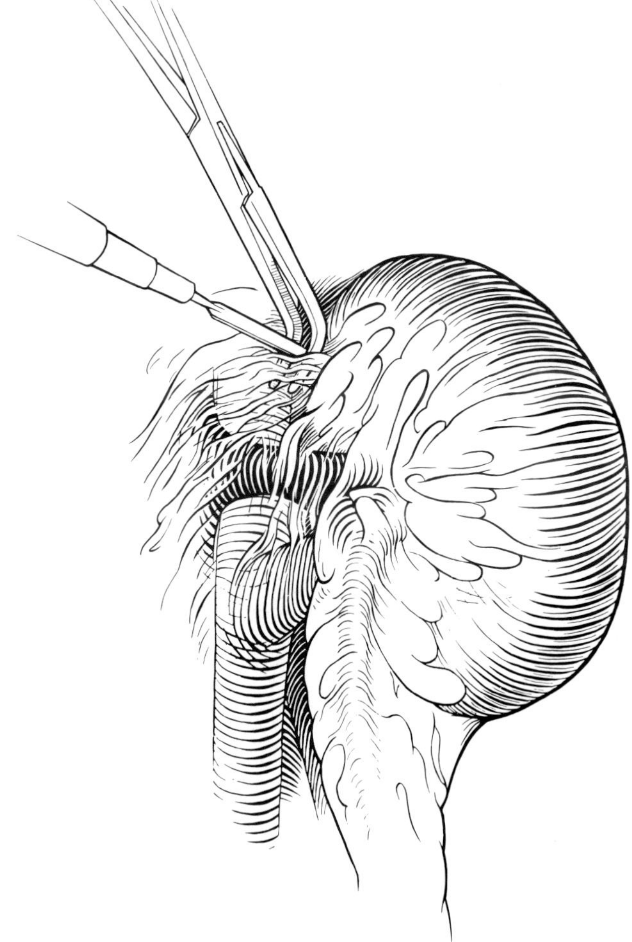

Figure 31.17. The kidney is reflected medially and the artery is identified visually and palpably coursing posterior to the vena cava. The remaining strands of connective tissue that lie between the superior pole of the kidney and the vena cava are now dissected off after spot coagulation.

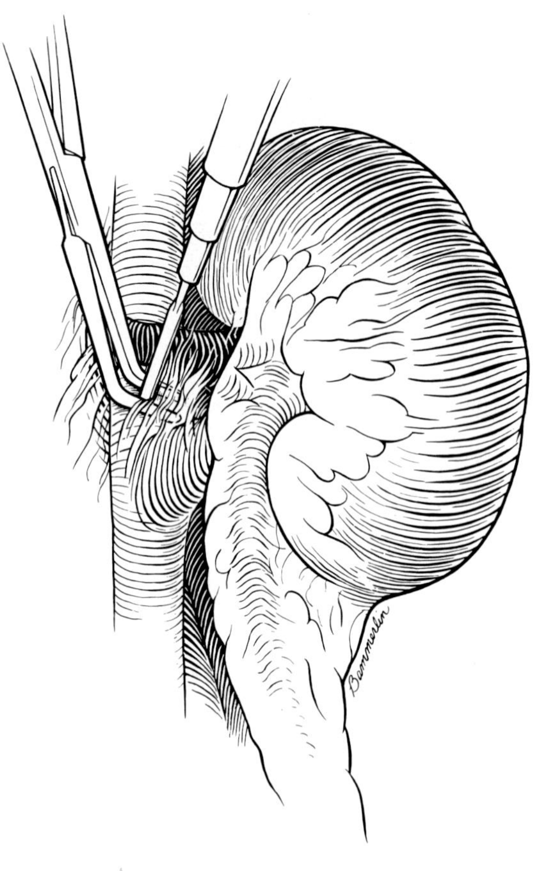

Figure 31.18. The renal artery is now freed from its periadventitial tissue at a level posterior to the vena cava. At this time, any pericaval adventitia remaining on the posterior aspect of its junction with the renal vein is cleared so that a Satisnsky clamp may be applied later for subsequent transection of the right renal vein with a cuff of vena cava.

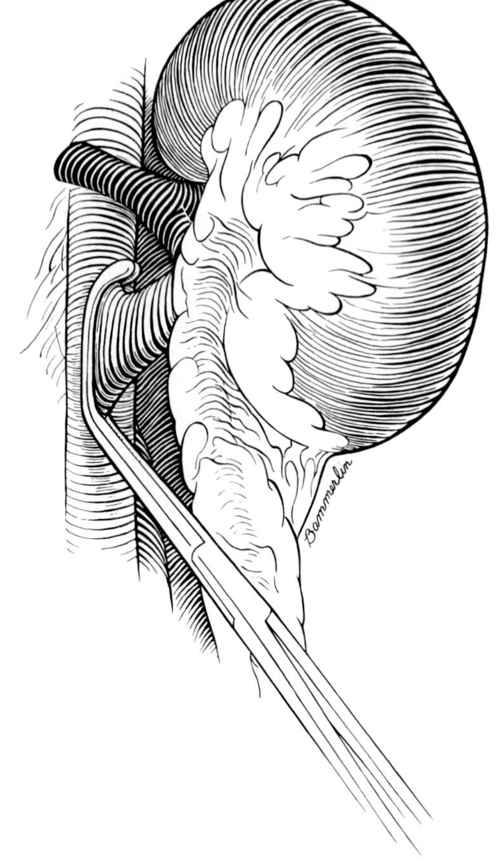

Figure 31.19. The kidney is now lying free, attached only by the artery and vein. After ensuring an adequate diuresis from the donor kidney and ascertaining that the recipient is ready for transplantation, the kidney is reflected medially to expose the proximal right renal artery. This is then clamped with a right-angle hemostat and transected just distal to the clamp. A medium-sized Satinsky clamp is then placed to occlude the vena cava partially at the entrance of the right renal vein, taking approximately 50% of the caval circumference. In that way, an adequate caval cuff will remain that will not subsequently slip out between the jaws of the clamp. The renal vein is then transected to include 2–3 mm of caval wall, thereby greatly aiding the implanting surgeon in performing the venous anastamosis in the recipient.

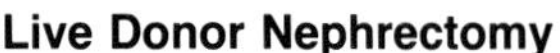

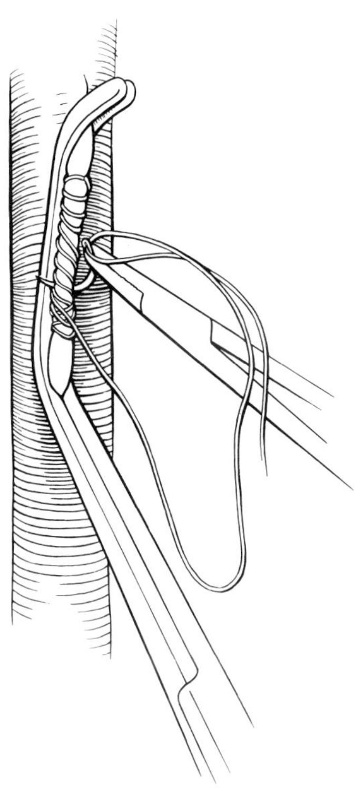

Figure 31.20. When the kidney is removed from the operative field, the artery is secured with two separate ligatures of 0 silk. The cavotomy is the closed with a running 5–0 vascular silk suture. This begins just above the superior aspect of the cavotomy and continues downward including bites of 1–2 into both the anterior and posterior caval walls until the lower aspect of the cavotomy is reached. The lowest suture should be placed 1–2 mm below the most caudad aspect of the cavotomy. It is then run back between previous bites up to the level of the highest suture where it is secured. The Satinsky clamp is then released and any residual oozing is controlled with gentle compression. Hemostasis is completed with electrofulguration, after which the area is irrigated with fresh, warm saline. The incision is again closed in a standard fashion without the use of drains.

POSTOPERATIVE CARE

A chest x-ray is routinely obtained in the recovery room to exclude the possibility of a pneumothorax. Nasal gastric suction is not routinely used. A ureteral catheter is left indwelling for 24 hr. All patients are assisted out of bed the first night, then ambulated at least three times daily because early ambulation appears important in preventing both pulmonary complications and the development of deep vein thrombosis. Intravenous fluids are continued at liberal rates until adequate oral alimentation is established. Postoperative antibiotics are not routinely used.

Suggested Readings

Bennett AH, Harrison JH: Experience with living familial renal donors. *Surg Gyneocol Obstet* 139:898, 1974.

Bergan JJ: Current risks to the kidney transplant donor. *Transplant Proc* 5:1131, 1973.

Conner WT, Van Buren CT, Floyd M, Kahan BD: Anterior extraperitoneal donor nephrectomy. *Urology* 126:443, 1981.

Dunn JF, Nylander WA, Richie RE, et al: Living related kidney donors. *Ann Surg* 203:637, 1986.

Kincaid OW: Techniques and hazards of renal angiography. *Renal Angiography*. Chicago, Year Book, 1976.

Levey AS, Hou S, Bush HL Jr: Kidney transplantation from unrelated living donors. *N Engl J Med* 314:914, 1986.

Penn I, Halgrimson CG, Ogden D, Starzl TE: Use of living donors in kidney transplantation in man. *Arch Surg* 101:226, 1970.

Ringden O, Friman L., Lundgren G, Magnusson G: Living related kidney donors: Complications and long-term renal function. *Transplantation* 25:221, 1978.

Ruiz R, Novick AC, Braun WE, Montague DK, Stewart BH: Transperitoneal live donor nephrectomy. *J Urol* 124:779, 1980.

Weinstein SH, Navarre RJ, Loening SA, Corry RJ: Experience with live donor nephrectomy. *J Urol* 124:321, 1980.

CHAPTER **32**

Technique of Renal Transplantation

ANDREW C. NOVICK

During the last 20 years, renal transplantation has become a safe and highly effective method for treating patients with end-stage renal failure. The 1-year patient survival rate after transplantation is 95%; 1-year graft survival rates for cadaver and live donor allograft recipients are 80% and 90%, respectively. In 1986, approximately 8000 patients with end-stage renal disease underwent renal transplantation and the pool of potential transplant recipients continues to increase in this country.

Renal transplant recipients are particularly susceptible to poor healing and infection because of the complications of uremia and the altered host responses induced by immunosuppressive therapy. These considerations demand meticulous attention to detail in performing transplantation surgery, with careful handling of tissues and strict adherence to basic operative principles of asepsis and hemostasis. Equally important in minimizing the morbidity associated with renal transplantation are anticipation of surgical complications and their prompt treatment when they occur.

In most cases, the renal allograft is implanted into one or the other iliac fossa. In determining which iliac fossa to employ for transplantation, one should consider both the anteroposterior relationships of the renal vessels and the anticipated method of arterial anastomosis. When end-to-end arterial anastomosis to the hypogastric artery seems likely, as in performing single artery transplantation in young patients, it is customary to place the right kidney in the left iliac fossa, and vice versa. When end-to-side arterial anastomosis to the external or common iliac artery is expected, as in older patients or when employing a Carrel aortic patch with multiple donor arteries, the right kidney will lie more comfortably in the right iliac fossa and the left kidney in the left iliac fossa. These are only relative considerations and, with proper positioning of the graft and renal vessels, either kidney may be inserted into either iliac fossa. A relative advantage of using the right iliac fossa is that the right iliac vein has a more horizontal course than the left and is more accessible for the venous anastomosis. This may assume clinical significance when transplanting a kidney with an unusually short renal vein.

In patients with a history of lower extremity thrombophlebitis, silent thrombosis of the iliac veins may have occurred and transplantation should be performed preferentially into the opposite iliac fossa. If ipsilateral transplantation is being considered, preoperative venography should be done to verify iliac venous patency. In patients with a prior failed renal transplant, the second graft is always placed in the unoperated contralateral iliac fossa.

When the recipient is anesthetized, a no. 18 French urethral catheter is inserted in the bladder. A urine specimen is sent for culture or, if the patient is anuric, the bladder is irrigated with saline and this fluid is cultured. The bladder is filled by gravity with 100–200 ml of 1% neomycin sulfate solution, and the catheter is clamped and connected to a closed drainage system. Shaving of the operative site is done in the operating room and the skin is prepared with an iodine solution for 10 min. Before commencing the operation, a single intravenous bolus of broad-sprectrum antibiotics is given. These include ampicillin, 2 gm; nafcillin, 2 gm; and tobramycin, 2 mg/kg. In patients allergic to pennicilin, clindamycin, 400 mg, is substituted for ampicillin and nafcillin.

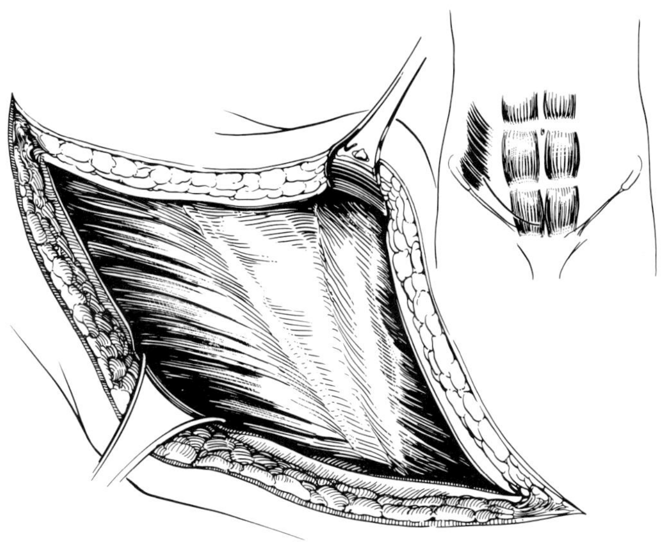

Figure 32.1. A lower quadrant transverse semilunar skin incision is made extending from the midline to just above the anterosuperior iliac spine. Throughout the operation, care is taken to achieve absolute hemostasis and to minimize blood loss.

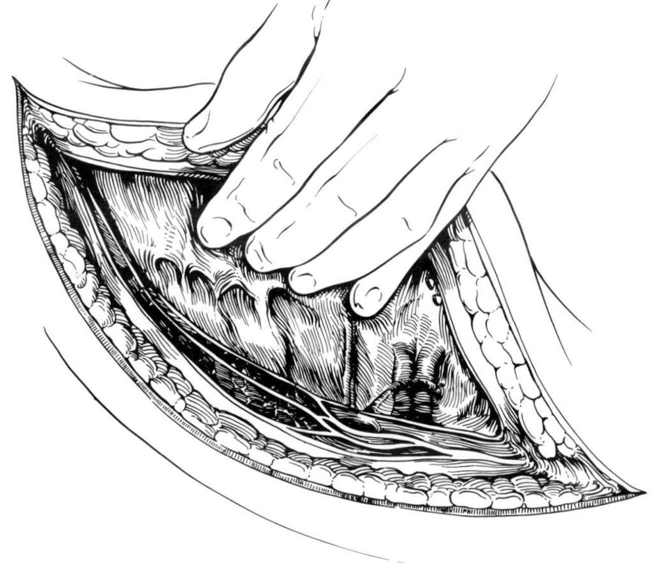

Figure 32.2. The external oblique, internal oblique, and transversus abdominis muscles are divided in line with the incision. The inferior epigastric vessels are identified lateral to the rectus muscle.

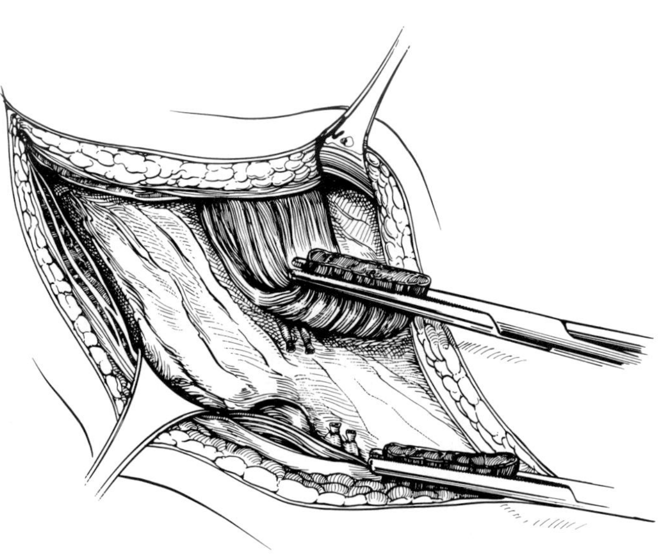

Figure 32.3. The inferior epigastric vessels are secured and divided. The rectus muscle is either retracted medially or, if exposure of the bladder is not adequate, this muscle is divided at its tendinous insertion to the symphysis pubus. In the female, the round ligament is ligated and divided. The spermatic cord in the male is mobilized and retracted medially to obviate post-operative hydrocele formation that commonly occurs after high cord ligation.

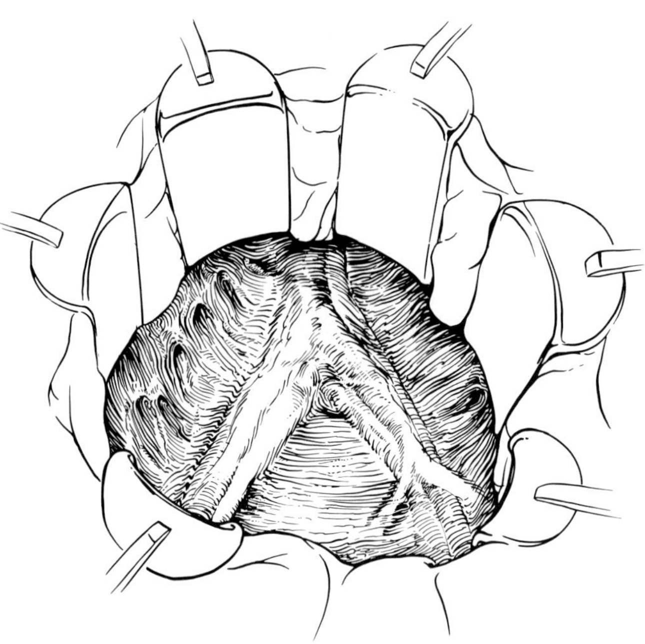

Figure 32.4. Extraperitoneal exposure of the iliac fossa is obtained by reflecting the peritoneum superiorly to the common iliac artery and medially to the bladder. A self-retaining ring retractor is inserted to maintain exposure of the operative field. The lateral blade of the retractor is doubly padded to avoid injury to the lateral femoral cutaneous nerve. The superior retractor blade is positioned to avoid compression of the common iliac artery, which may interfere with allograft perfusion after revascularization.

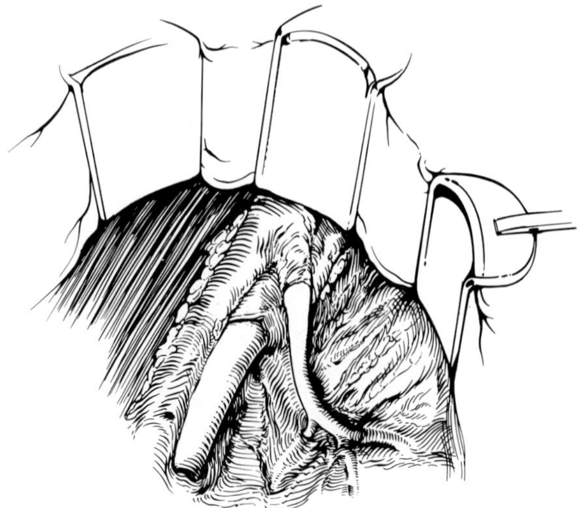

Figure 32.5. The external iliac vein is mobilized from the internal iliac origin to the femoral junction. To avoid postoperative lymphatic complications, all overlying lymphatic tissue is ligated and divided. If the donor kidney has a short renal vein, the internal iliac vein is divided to allow elevation of the external iliac vein and, thereby, to facilitate the venous anastomosis. End-to-end anastomosis of the renal artery to the hypogastric (internal iliac) artery is preferred, and the latter vessel is mobilized from its origin to the major anterior and posterior branches. Again, all overlying lymphatic vessels are ligated and divided. In such cases, it is unnecessary to mobilize the common and external iliac arteries.

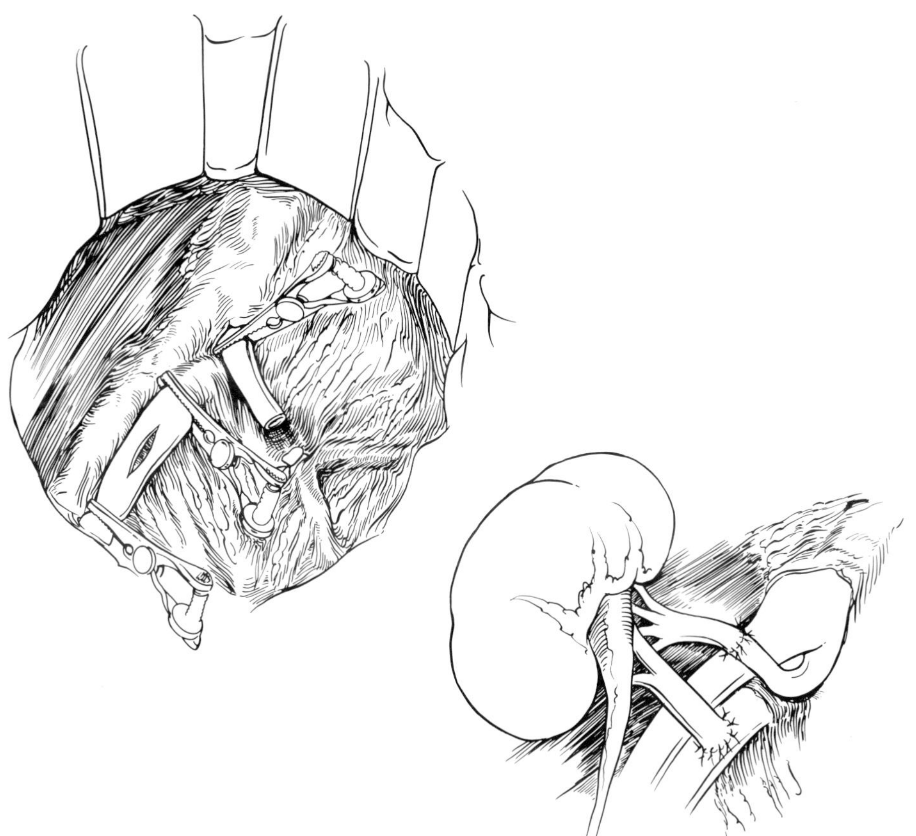

Figure 32.6. Vascular clamps are placed proximally and distally on the external iliac vein. A venotomy is performed by excising a narrow longitudinal ellipse from the anterolateral aspect of the vein. The hypogastric artery temporarily is occluded proximally, its major branches are ligated distally, and the artery is divided proximal to the ligatures. If mild atherosclerosis of the hypogastric artery is present, endarterectomy is performed to render this vessel suitable for anastomosis to the renal artery. Heparin solution is instilled into the lumen of the hypogastric artery and external iliac vein.

The kidney is then brought into the operative field and the artery and vein are examined. Any residual tissue surrounding the origin of these vessels is removed and, if the renal vein appears short, this is mobilized from the renal sinus to obtain greater length. The kidney is lowered into the incision and end-to-side anastomosis of the renal vein to the external iliac vein is performed with a continuous 5–0 vascular suture. End-to-end anastomosis of the renal artery to the hypogastric artery is performed with interrupted 6–0 vascular sutures, after aligning these vessels carefully to avoid angulation or kinking. After the arterial anastomosis is completed, all vascular clamps are removed and circulation to the kidney is restored.

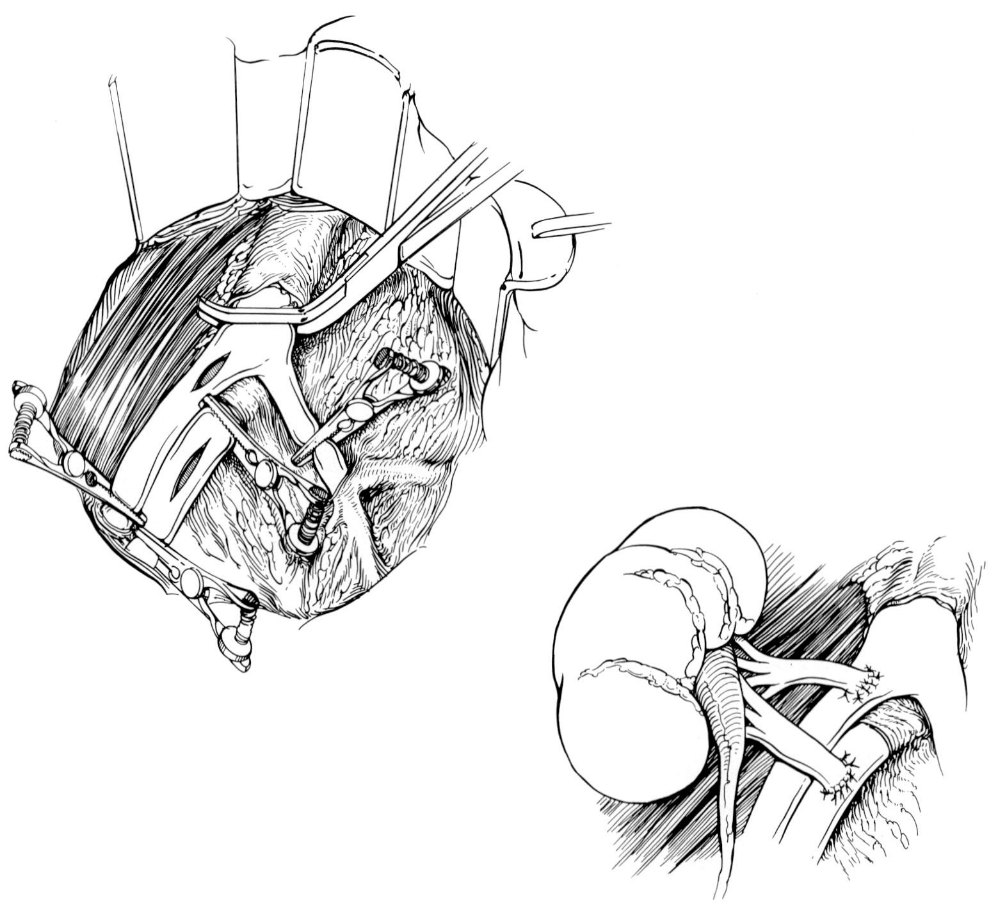

Figure 32.7. The indications for end-to-side arterial anastomosis to the common or external iliac artery are: extensive atherosclerosis of the hypogastric artery, significant discrepancy in size between the renal and hypogastric arteries, or multiple donor renal arteries encompassed by a Carrel aortic patch. In such cases, the external iliac artery and a contiguous segment of the common iliac artery are mobilized. Vascular clamps are placed across the common iliac, hypogastric, and external iliac arteries and an arteriotomy is performed in the recipient vessel. In general, our preference is to perform end-to-side arterial anastomosis to the common iliac artery because of its larger caliber. This may not be possible when renal arterial length is insufficient or when there is significant atherosclerosis of the common iliac artery. In such cases, arterial anastomosis is to the external iliac artery, which lies in closer proximity to the renal hilus and is less often diseased than the common iliac artery. The anastomosis is performed with interrupted 6–0 vascular suture unless anastomosis of a Carrel aortic patch is performed, in which case a continuous 5–0 vascular suture is used.

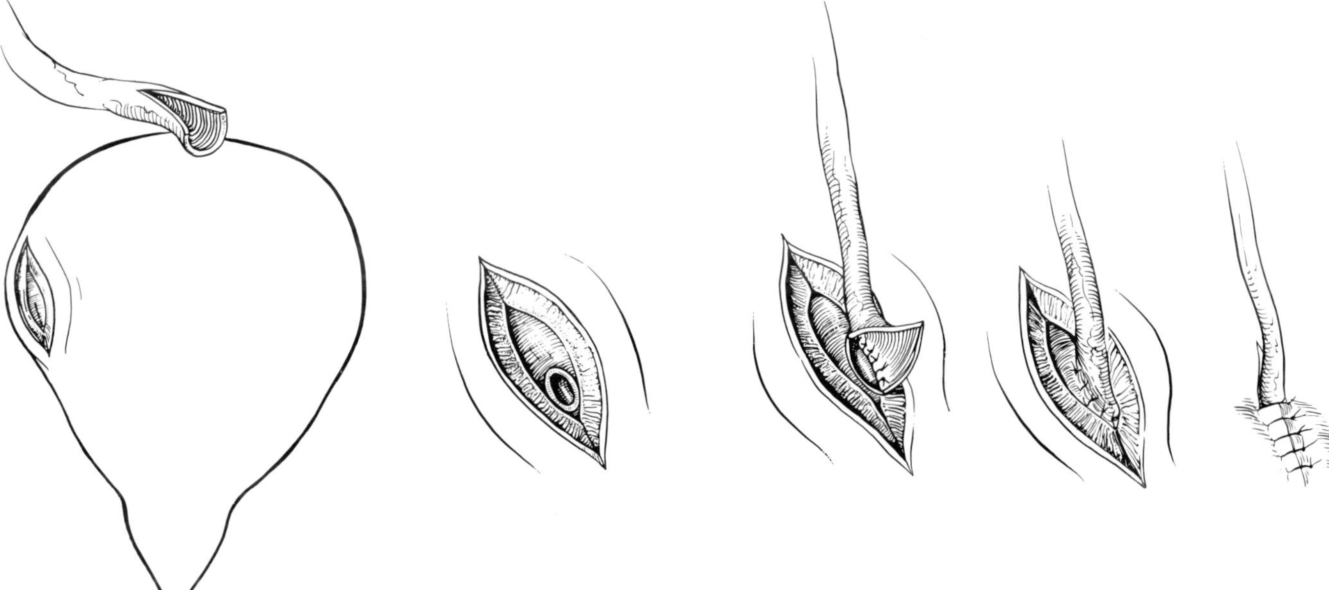

Figure 32.8. After completion of the vascular anastomoses, urinary tract reconstruction is achieved by ureteronecystostomy. This method is preferred over ureteroureterostomy or ureteropyelostomy because of a lower incidence of postoperative urinary fistulas. In performing ureteroneocystostomy, one should use the shortest length of ureter that will reach the bladder without tension because the allograft ureter receives its blood supply exclusively from branches of the renal artery. Since 1983, we have preferentially employed the extravesical ureteroneocystostomy technique originally described by Lich.

A 3-cm incision is made on the posterolateral aspect of the bladder. The perivesical fat, adventitia, and muscle of the bladder wall are incised to expose the mucosa over the entire length of the incision. The edges of the bladder muscle are undermined by pushing the mucosa away from the muscle. The distal end of the allograft ureter is spatulated for a short distance. A small opening is made in the bladder mucosa at the distal end of the incision and mucosa-to-mucosa anastomosis is done between the ureter and the bladder, using interrupted or continuous 4–0 chromic sutures. At the distal aspect of the suture line, one or two bites are inserted through the entire bladder wall to anchor the ureter and prevent it from pulling out of the tunnel. The bladder muscle then is reapproximated loosely over the ureter with interrupted 3–0 chromic sutures.

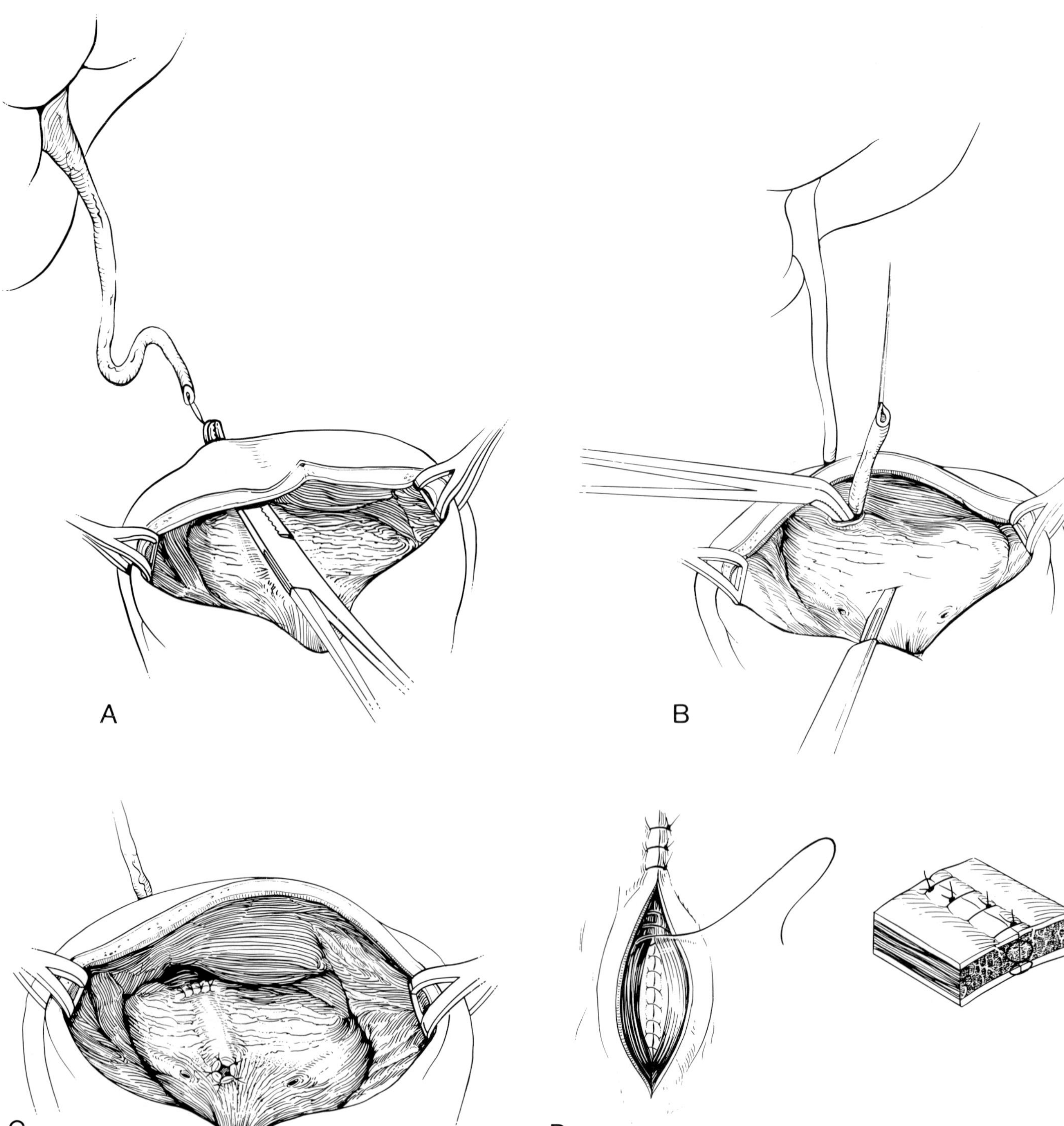

Figure 32.9. A-D, as an alternative to the method described above, a transvesical ureteroneocystostomy technique may be used. The bladder is opened through an anterior cystotomy and a stab incision is made in the posterolateral bladder wall. The donor ureter is brought through the stab incision and a 2- to 3-cm submucosal tunnel, directed toward the bladder neck, is fashioned. The ureter is then brought through the tunnel, taking care to avoid torsion on its longitudinal axis. The ureter is spatulated and anastomosed to the bladder with interrupted 4–0 or 5–0 chromic sutures. The sutures fixing the distal aspect of the ureter to the bladder are inserted deeply into the muscularis, while the remaining sutures are placed only through the bladder mucosa. The mucosa overlying the stab incision is closed with a continuous 5–0 chromic suture. The cystostomy incision is closed in three separate layers, with the second and third layers slightly overlapping the immediately underlying layer, to ensure a watertight repair.

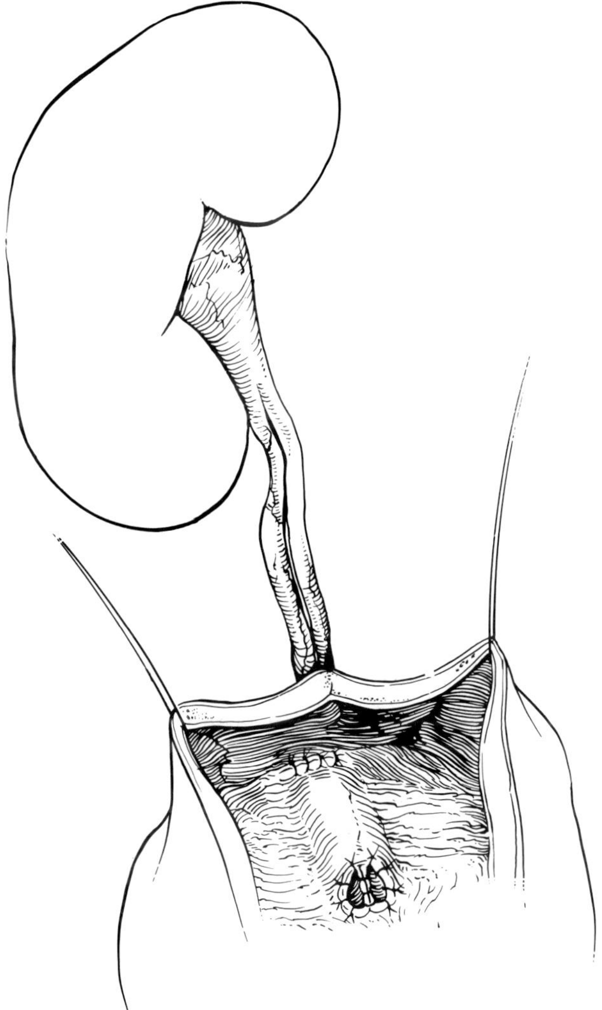

Figure 32.10. The transvesical ureteroneocystostomy technique is preferred for transplantation of kidneys with a double ureter. The two ureters are left in their common adventitial sheath and are brought through the posterior bladder wall and submucosal tunnel together, as with a single ureter. Both ureteral ends are spatulated, the medial ends are sutured together, and the lateral and distal aspects are anastomosed to the bladder as with a single ureter.

Multiple Renal Arteries

Multiple renal arteries occur unilaterally and bilaterally in 23% and 10% of the population, respectively. Important prerequisites to successful transplantation of kidneys with multiple arteries are: *(1)* proper techniques of organ procurement; *(2)* thorough arteriographic evaluation of potential living donors; and *(3)* selection of an appropriate method of arterial revascularization. When such kidneys are transplanted, failure to recognize and preserve an accessory renal artery may eventuate in ureteral necrosis, graft rupture, segmental renal infarction, postoperative hypertension, or calyceal fistula formation. A variety of techniques are available for performing multiple artery renal transplantation.

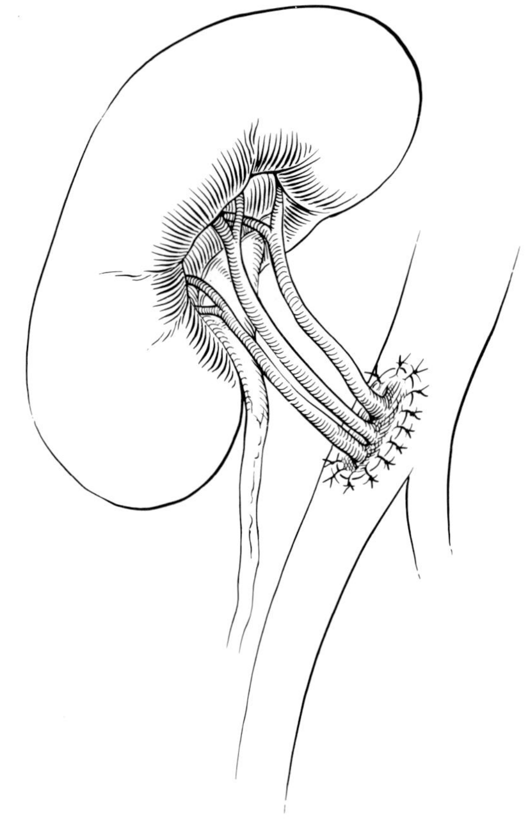

Figure 32.11. Anastomosis of a Carrel aortic patch encompassing all renal arteries to the recipient common or external iliac artery is the preferred method for arterial anastomosis of cadaver kidneys with multiple arteries. This requires that cadaver donor nephrectomy be performed en bloc with the aorta and vena cava. Use of such an aortic patch is not possible when kidneys are harvested separately, when polar vessels are injured inadvertently during removal, when there is significant atherosclerosis of the perirenal aorta, or when the renal arteries are widely separated on the aorta. Likewise, in live donor renal transplantation, a cuff of aorta should never be taken because of the increased risk to the donor.

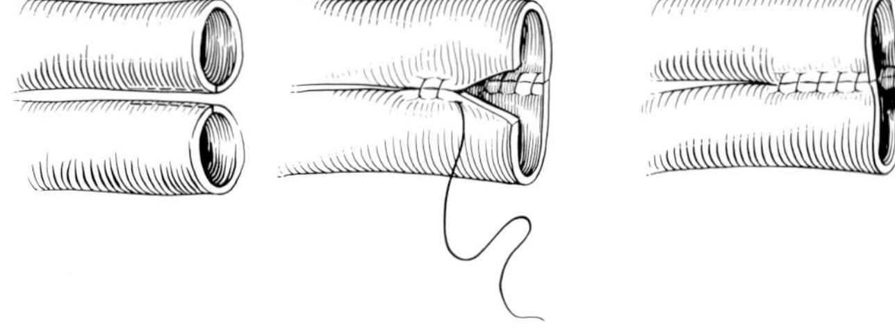

Figure 32.12. When two adjacent renal arteries of comparable size are present, our preferred method is extracorporeal side-to-side anastomosis of the two vessels to create a common ostium. This is done just before implantation, with the kidney cooled in ice saline solution. Continuous 6–0 or 7–0 vascular sutures are employed for the repair, with optimal magnification provided by 3.5 × loupes. Revascularization in the recipient involves only a single arterial anastomosis, preferably end-to-end to the hypogastric artery, with no increase in the warm renal ischemia time. This method is technically simple and, hemodynamically, yields less resistance to flow than do separate vascular anastomoses because of the greater cross-sectional area of the coapted vessels.

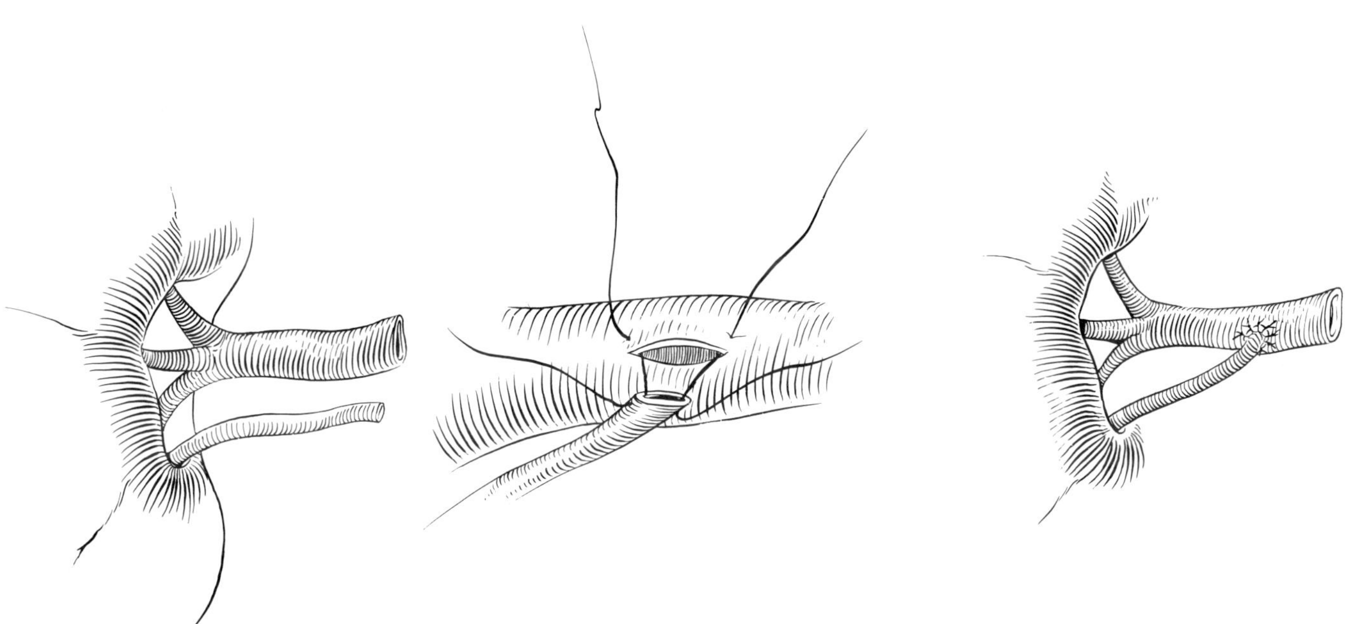

Figure 32.13. When two renal arteries of disparate caliber are present, our preferred technique is end-to-side reimplantation of the smaller artery into the larger one. A short linear arteriotomy is made in the side of the larger artery, without removing any of the vessel wall, to obviate narrowing of the arterial lumen. The smaller artery is spatulated and end-to-side anastomosis to the larger vessel is done with interrupted 7–0 vascular sutures, using microvascular instruments and 3.5 × loupes for magnification. A small catheter or probe may be placed through the suture line during its construction to prevent accidental entrapment of the back wall. The completed anastomosis is tested for patency and integrity by gentle perfusion of the main renal artery. The transplant operation is then done as with a single renal artery. The advantages of this method are that *(1)* it is technically simple, *(2)* it involves anastomosis of vessels that are similar in thickness, *(3)* only one arterial anastomosis is required in the recipient, and *(4)* warn renal ischemia time is not prolonged. This technique can also be used for transplant kidneys supplied by more than two renal arteries of varying caliber.

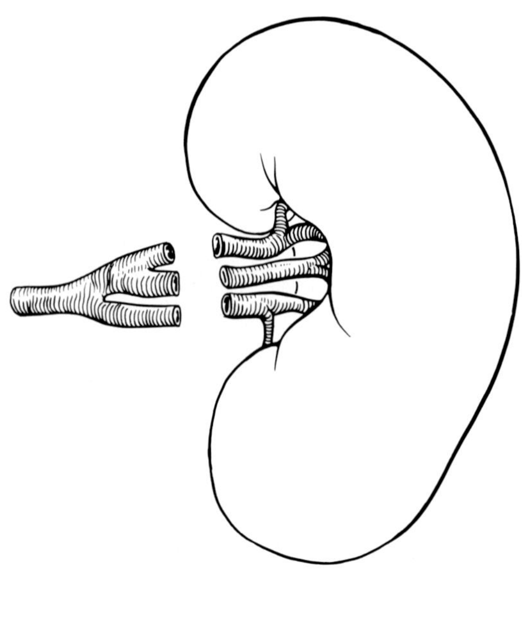

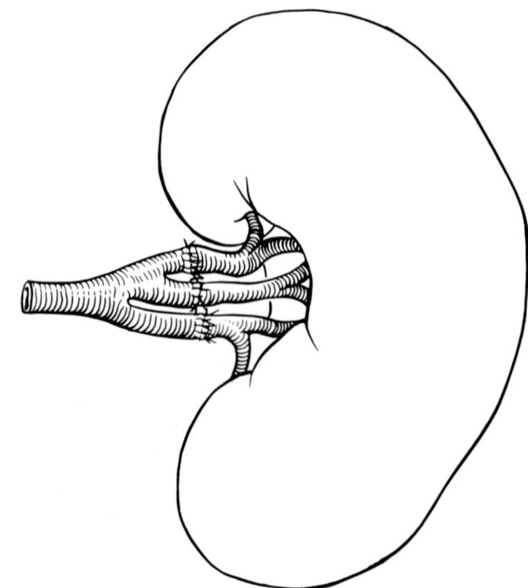

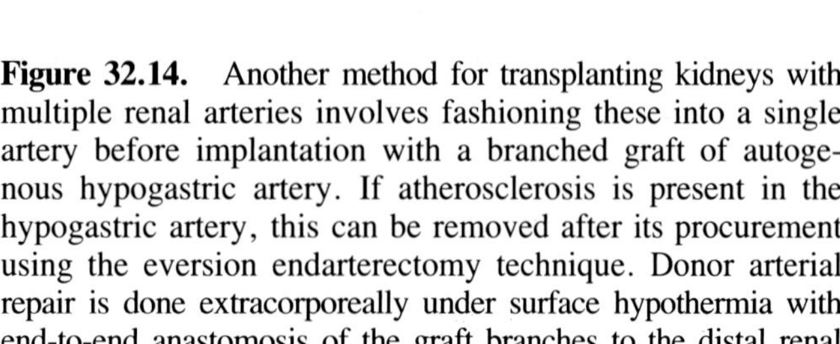

Figure 32.14. Another method for transplanting kidneys with multiple renal arteries involves fashioning these into a single artery before implantation with a branched graft of autogenous hypogastric artery. If atherosclerosis is present in the hypogastric artery, this can be removed after its procurement using the eversion endarterectomy technique. Donor arterial repair is done extracorporeally under surface hypothermia with end-to-end anastomosis of the graft branches to the distal renal arteries. The kidney is then transplanted as with a single renal artery, with no added warm ischemia time. This technique is particularly useful to transplant kidneys with more than two renal arteries or when insufficient arterial length is present to permit use of the previous two methods described. Should extensive calcification of the hypogastric artery render it unsuitable as a reconstructive graft, a branched saphenous vein graft can be used alternatively in the same fashion.

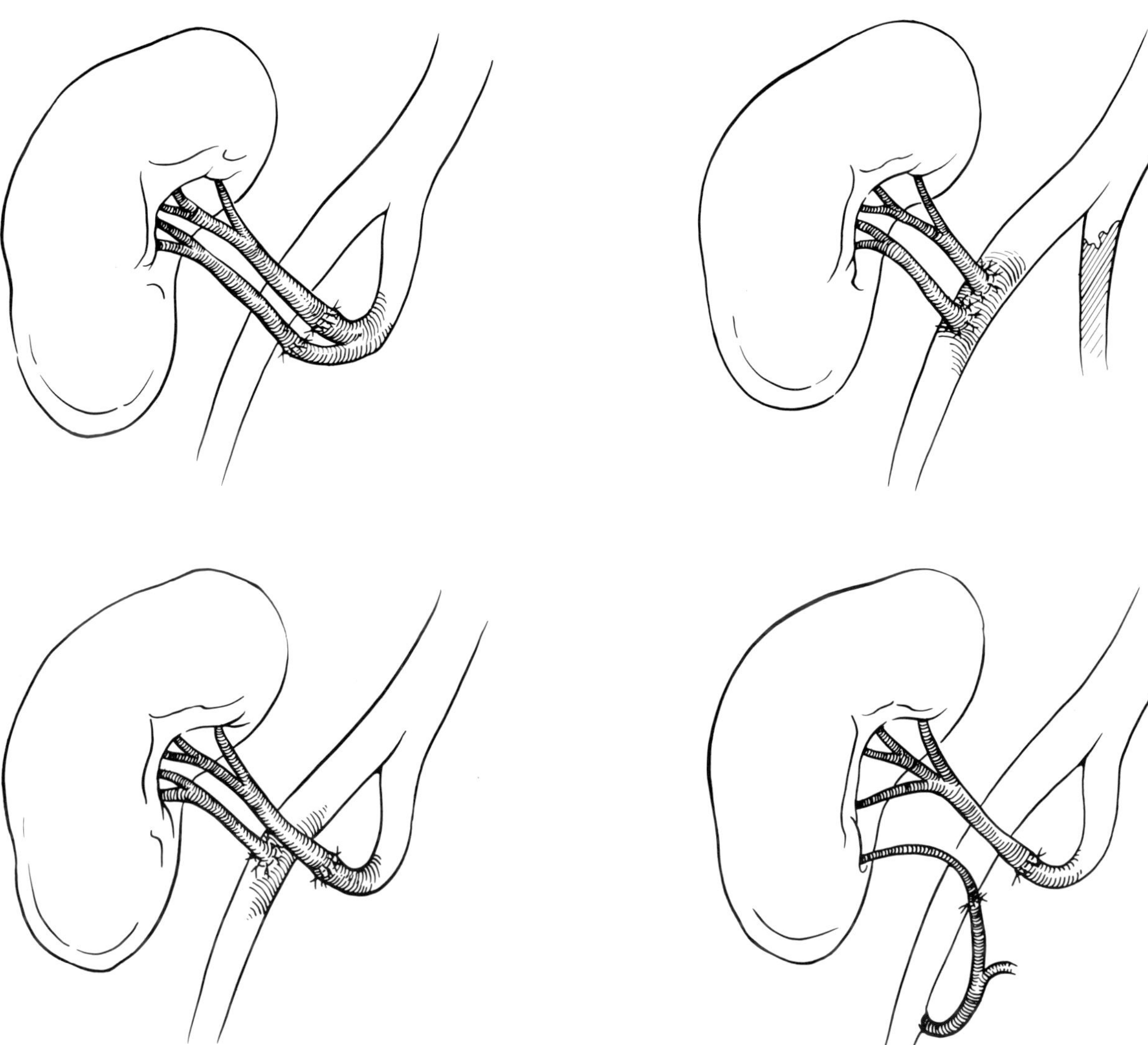

Figure 32.15. Additional techniques for performing multiple artery transplantation include arterial anastomoses to the branches of the hypograstric artery *(top left),* separate arterial anastomoses to the external and/or common iliac arteries *(top right),* separate arterial anastomoses to the hypogastric and external iliac arteries *(bottom left),* and polar artery anastomosis to the inferior epigastric artery *(bottom right).* These techniques all require performance of multiple arterial anastomoses in situ that result in a prolonged warm ischemia time. Therefore, when a Carrel aortic patch is not available, we prefer extracorporeal arterial reconstruction employing one of the three methods described above. These latter techniques have proven to be readily applicable, either individually or in combination, to most anatomic variants presented by kidneys with multiple arteries.

Multiple Renal Veins

Multiple renal veins are less common than multiple arteries and more frequently involve the right kidney. Small renal veins simply can be ligated without risk. When double renal veins of equal size are present, both of these must be preserved to avoid increased intrarenal venous pressure after revascularization. The optimum method involves implanting these together with a cuff of vena cava obtained at the time of nephrectomy. When this is not available, extracorporeal venous reconstruction is performed as described for multiple arteries with either conjoined or end-to-side anastomosis of the two veins.

Transplantation in Children

There are special surgical considerations when renal transplantation is performed in young pediatric patients. In children weighing less than 20 kg, the iliac fossa is too small to accommodate a kidney from an adult donor. In this event, the graft must be inserted in a more cephalad location.

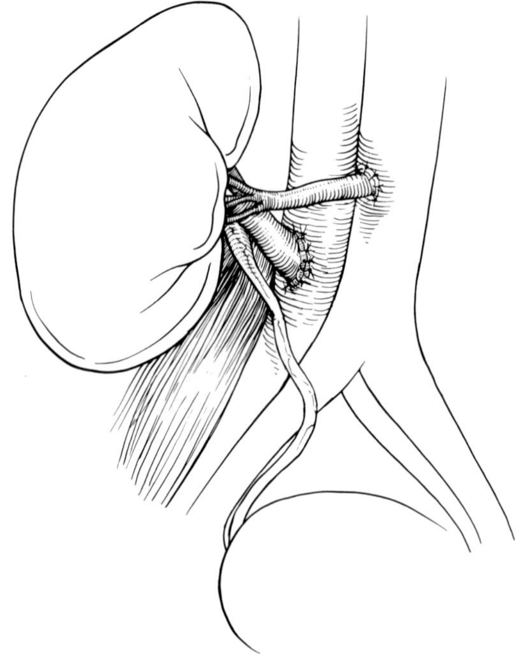

Figure 32.16. A midline transperitoneal incision is made and the cecum and ascending colon are reflected medially to expose the aorta, the vena cava, and the common iliac vessels. The graft is placed retrocecally with end-to-side anastomosis of the renal vein either to the vena cava or to the right common iliac vein. The renal artery is anastomosed end-to-side to either the aorta or the right common iliac artery. Immediately after revascularization of the allograft, 300 ml of albumin are administered as an intravenous bolus to replenish the suddenly depleted intravascular volume and to ensure adequate renal perfusion. The ureter generally reaches the bladder easily, remaining retroperitoneal throughout its course, and a ureteronecystostomy is performed. An alternate surgical approach for performing transplantation in children involves the use of extraperitoneal incision extending from the tip of the 12th rib to the symphysis pubis. This method is particularly helpful in children who have been managed with peritoneal dialysis. Very small children, weighing less than 8 kg, will require transplantation of a pediatric cadver graft.

Transplantation with Urinary Diversion

In some patients, the bladder may be unsuitable for transplantation due either to severe neurogenic disease or postinflammatory contracture. In such cases, renal transplantation must be performed in conjunction with supravesical urinary diversion. The most common technique involves the creation of an intestinal (generally ileal) conduit with a lower quadrant stoma at a separate operation before transplantation; 4–6 weeks later, the transplant operation is performed.

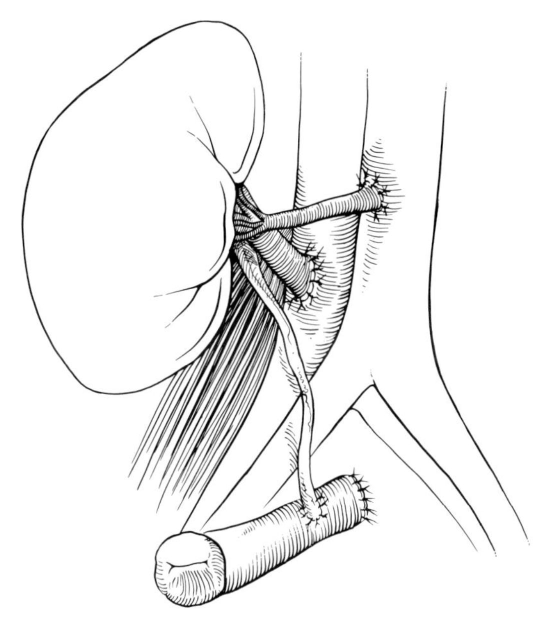

Figure 32.17. The preferred method for performing transplantation into an ileal conduit is to place the allograft retrocecally, as in pediatric transplantation, with anastomosis of the renal vessels either to the aorta and vena cava or to the common iliac vessels. This allows gravity-dependent urinary drainage and a more direct ureteroenteric anastomosis than when transplantation into the iliac fossa is done.

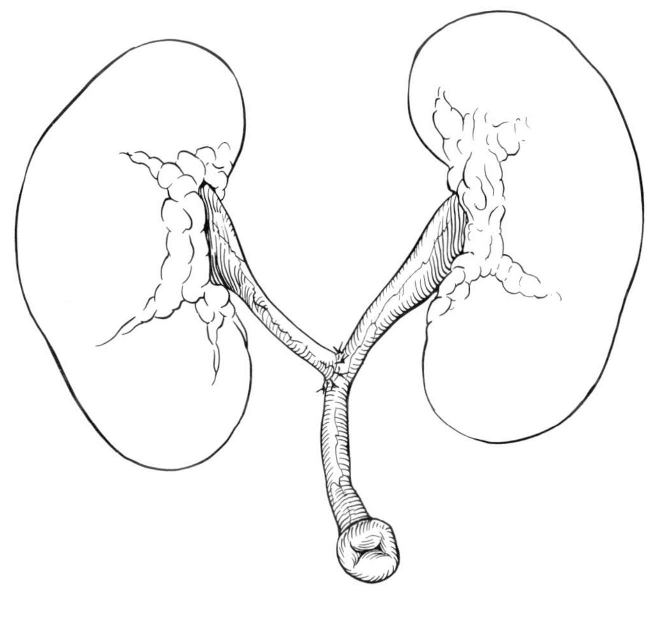

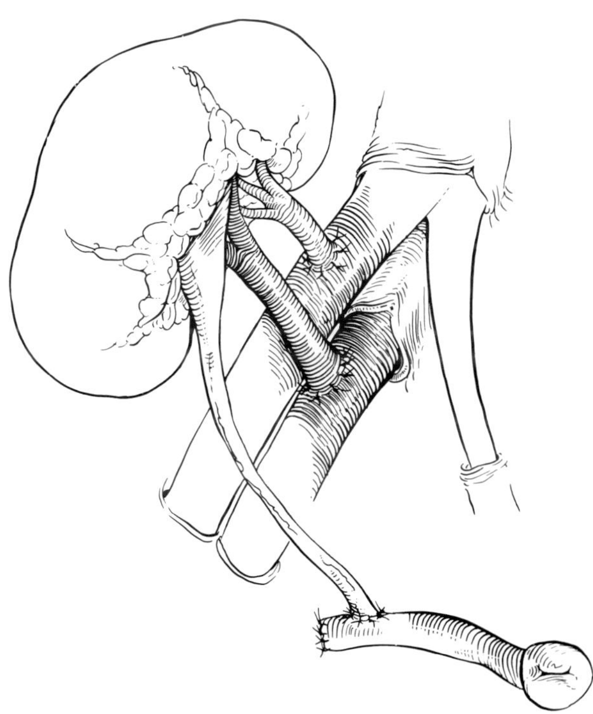

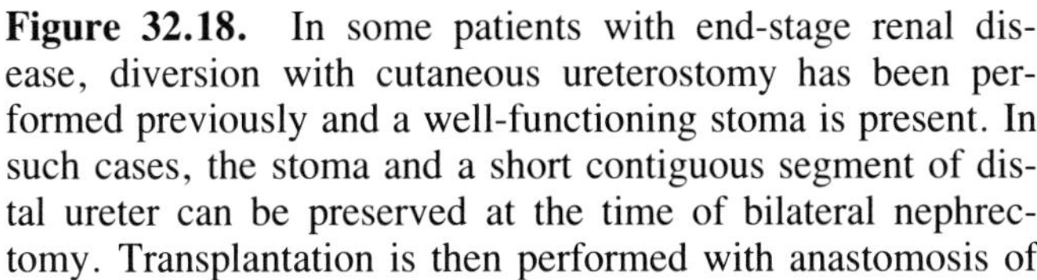

Figure 32.18. In some patients with end-stage renal disease, diversion with cutaneous ureterostomy has been performed previously and a well-functioning stoma is present. In such cases, the stoma and a short contiguous segment of distal ureter can be preserved at the time of bilateral nephrectomy. Transplantation is then performed with anastomosis of the allograft ureter to the retained native ureter just below the abdominal wall, thus, obviating the need for an intestinal segment. Using this method, satisfactory urinary drainage is achieved through the normal peristaltic ability of the allograft ureter, and the retained dilated ureter functions solely as a short conduit and stoma.

RENAL AUTOTRANSPLANTATION

Transfer of a kidney from one site to another in the same patient evolved as a logical extension of the field of renal allotransplantation. The first successful autotransplant was performed in 1962 by Hardy in a patient whose ureter had been severely damaged by previous aortic surgery. In 1963, Woodruff achieved the first successful autotransplant for renovascular hypertension. Effective methods of renal preservation and microvascular surgical techniques subsequently resulted in the advent of extracorporeal (bench) renal surgery for selected patients with complicated upper urinary tract disorders.

The current indications for renal autotransplantation with or without bench surgery include complicated renovascular disorders, extensive ureteral damage, and occasional patients with large renal neoplasms. The indications and techniques for performing extracorporeal renal surgery in patients with renovascular disease (chapter 28) and renal carcinoma (chapter 11) are reviewed elsewhere in this book.

In patients undergoing renal autotransplantation, preoperative renal and pelvic arteriography should be done to define renal arterial anatomy and to ensure relatively disease-free iliac vessels. Autotransplantation of kidneys involved with severe renal parenchymal and/or small vessel disease should be avoided. Such kidneys generally flush poorly after their removal, often leading to irreversible ischemic damage and nonfunction postoperatively. In patients with bacteriuria, organism-specific parenteral antibiotic therapy is initiated 48 hours preoperatively.

Renal autotransplantation is generally performed through an anterior subcostal transperitoneal incision combined with a separate lower-quadrant transverse semilunar incision. For nonobese patients, a single midline incision extending from the xyphoid process to the symphysis pubis may be used alternatively. Immediately after its removal, the kidney is flushed with 500 ml of chilled Collins intracellular electrolyte solution. If an extracorporeal operation is to be done, the flushed kidney is then placed in a basin of ice slush saline for hypothermic preservation outside the body. When the kidney is ready for autotransplantation, this is always done into the prepared iliac fossa using the same vascular techniques as described earlier in this chapter for renal allotransplantation.

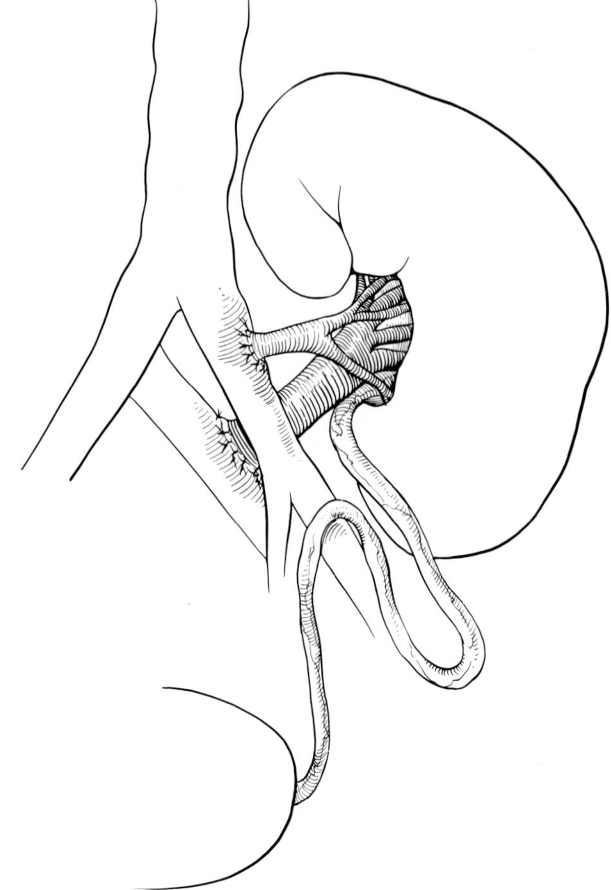

Figure 32.19. Occasionally, renal autotransplantation is performed without an extra-corporeal operation, as in patients with main renal artery stenosis and a diseased but patent aorta. In the latter circumstance, autotransplantation into the iliac fossa is done with the ureter left intact. Although it may follow a redundant course to the bladder after autotransplantation, normal ureteral peristalsis provides effective drainage of urine from the kidney. In such cases, care must be taken not to rotate the kidney in moving it so as to produce an obstructive torsion of the ureter.

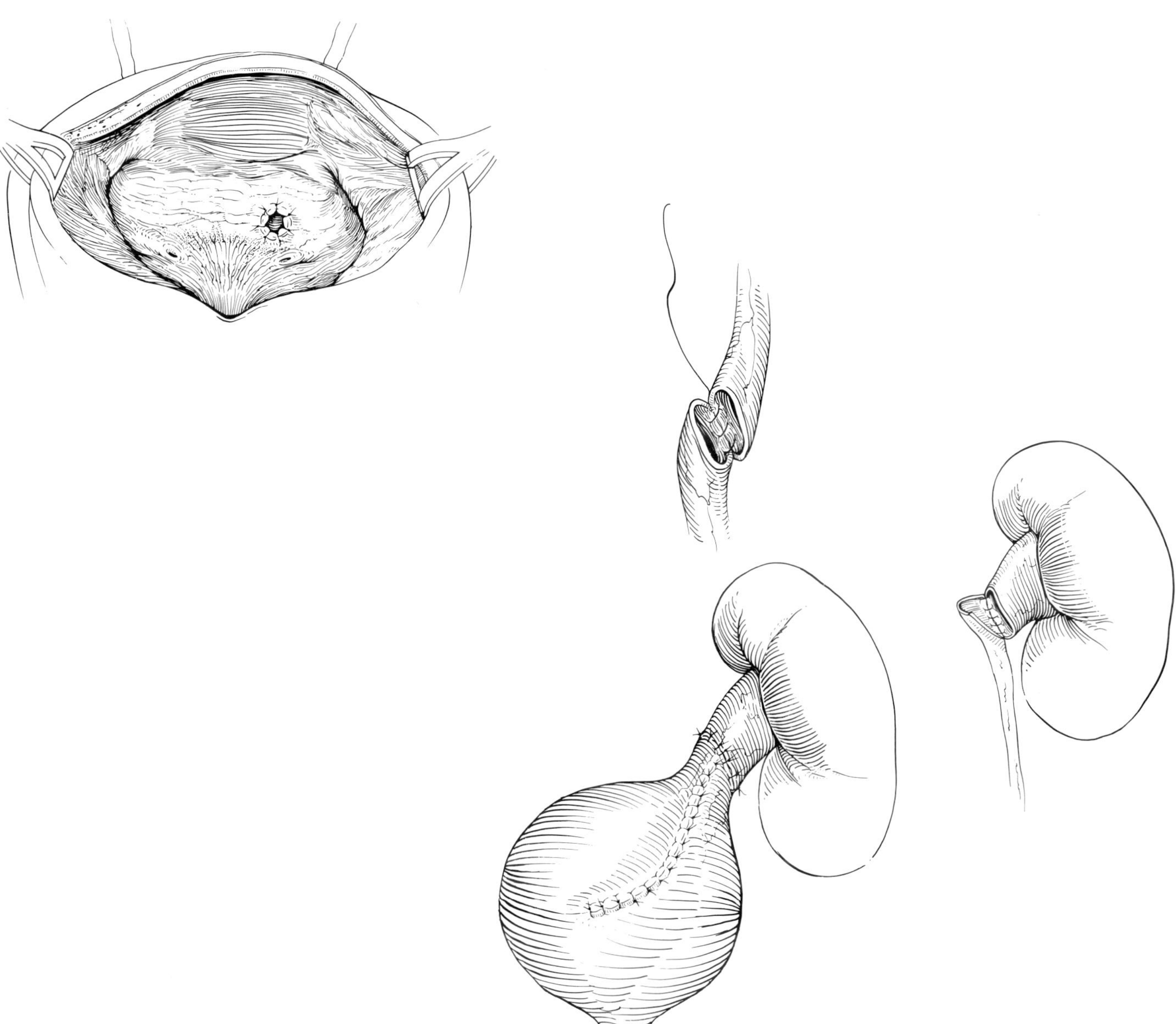

Figure 32.20. Another indication for renal autotransplantation without an extracorporeal operation is in patients with extensive ureteral loss. Various methods are available for restoring urinary continuity after autotransplantation in such cases. Ureteroneocystostomy is the preferred technique when there is an adequate length of unobstructed proximal ureter. In some cases where extensive fibrotic obstruction of the upper ureter is present, the strictured areas are resected and the proximal ureter or renal pelvis is anastomosed to the lower, disease-free ureter. When it is necessary to resect the entire ureter, direct pyelovesicostomy with or without a Boari bladder flap is done. The latter technique is specifically indicated in patients with a history of recurrent colic from renal calculi.

Suggested Readings

Bodie B, Novick AC, Rose M, Straffon RA: Long-term results of renal autotransplantation for ureteral replacement. *J Urol* 136:383, 1986.

Hardy JD: High ureteral injuries: Management by autotransplantation of the kidney. *JAMA* 184:97, 1963.

MacGregor P, Novick AC, et al: Renal transplantation in end-stage renal disease patients with existing urinary diversion. *J Urol* 135: 686, 1986.

Novick AC: Surgery of renal transplantation and complications. In: Novick AC, Straffon RA (eds): *Vascular Problems in Urologic Surgery*. Philadelphia, WB Saunders, 1982.

Novick AC: The value of intraoperative antibiotics in preventing renal transplant wound infections. *J Urol* 125:151, 1981.

Novick AC, Magnusson M, Braun WE: Multiple-artery renal transplantation: emphasis on extracorporeal methods of donor arterial reconstruction. *J Urol* 122:731, 1979.

Novick AC, Stewart BH, Straffon RA: Extracorporeal renal surgery and autotransplantation: Indications, techniques and results. *J Urol* 123:806, 1980.

Palleschi J, Novick AC, et al: Vascular complications of renal transplantation. *Urology* 16:61, 1980.

Salvatierra O, Olcott C, Amend WJ, Cochrum KC, Feduska NJ: Urological complications of renal transplantation can be prevented or controlled. *J Urol* 117:421, 1977.

Starzl TE, Marchioro TL, Morgan WW, Waddell WR: A technique for use of adult renal homografts in children. *Surg Gynecol Obstet* 119:106, 1964.

Woodruff MFA, Doig A, Donald KW, Nolan B: Renal autotransplantation. *Lancet* 1:433, 1966.

CHAPTER **33**

Transplant Nephrectomy

RICHARD M. LEWIS

Indications for surgical removal of renal allografts include acute, catastrophic events (fortunately rare), such as intractable hemorrhage secondary to graft rupture or loss of integrity of vascular anastomoses, fulminant necrosis resulting from vascular thrombosis or hyperacute rejection, irreparable urinary fistulae, or severe perinephric infection (1–8). More commonly, transplant nephrectomy is performed when loss of graft function is accompanied by fever, malaise, hyptertension, graft pain and/or tenderness associated with accelerated or acute rejection, marked hypertension, and/or severe nephrosis resulting from glomerulopathic process such as recurrent focal sclerosing glomerulonephritis (1–7, 9–11). In the absence of such overt clinical stigmata, nonfunctioning renal allografts may remain in situ without impacting adversely on long-term morbidity (1–6, 12).

Optimum timing and execution of transplant nephrectomy require knowledge of the time elapsed since initial implantation, the original operative approach (extraperitoneal or transperitoneal), the number and anatomy of vascular and ureterovesical anastomoses, and pertinent complications such as disseminated or localized infection, graft rupture, disruption of vascular anastomoses, lymphocele, or urinary fistula. In addition, the anteroposterior orientation of the hilar structures is derived from knowledge of whether a right or left donor kidney was utilized.

Preoperative preparation of the patient requires adequate dialysis and either complete discontinuation of immunosuppressive therapy or reduction of same to the lowest corticosteroid dose required to prevent acute adrenal insufficiency (5, 13). Circumstances permitting, infectious, cardiopulmonary, coagulopathic, and other medical problems are definitively treated before surgery. In the absence of localized infection, limited, broad spectrum perioperative antibicrobial therapy is sufficient for wound prophylaxis (14, 15).

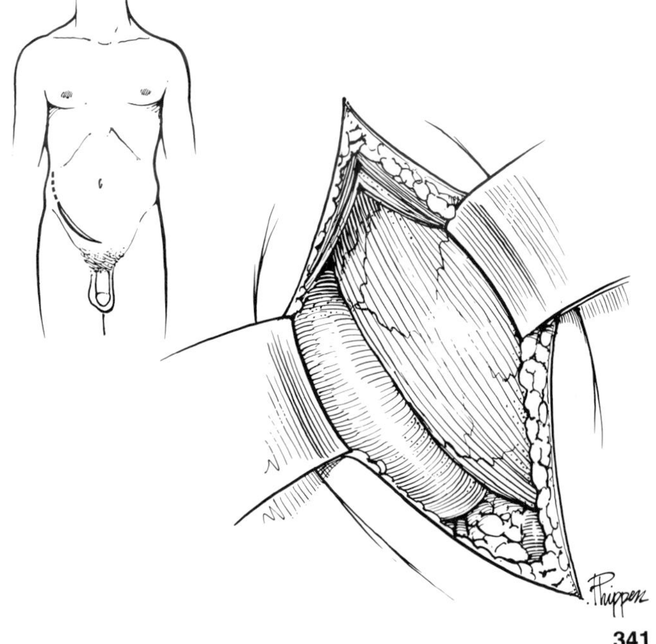

Figure 33.1. The patient is supine and placed on the operating table in the slight Trendelenburg position to facilitate superomedial retraction of the peritoneum and its contents. If the patient is producing urine, a Foley catheter is placed transurethrally to ensure that the bladder remains empty and thereby optimizes subsequent exposure of the paravesical space. The previous transplant incision is opened or excised over its entire length and extended cephalad as needed to facilitate exposure. The superficial fascia is divided along the line of the incision exposing an underlying suture line that usually encompasses the external oblique aponeurosis superolaterally and the anterior rectus sheath inferomedially. Old sutures are removed and the line of closure divided. The inner line of closure, consisting of the internal oblique muscle and its investing fascia as well as the subjacent transversalis fascia, is identified and opened in similar fashion. These musculofascial layers may be either well defined or nearly obliterated by scar tissue making it difficult to establish normal anatomic planes of dissection. Once the deep line of exposure is developed as described, the surface of the allograft usually can be visualized within the operative field.

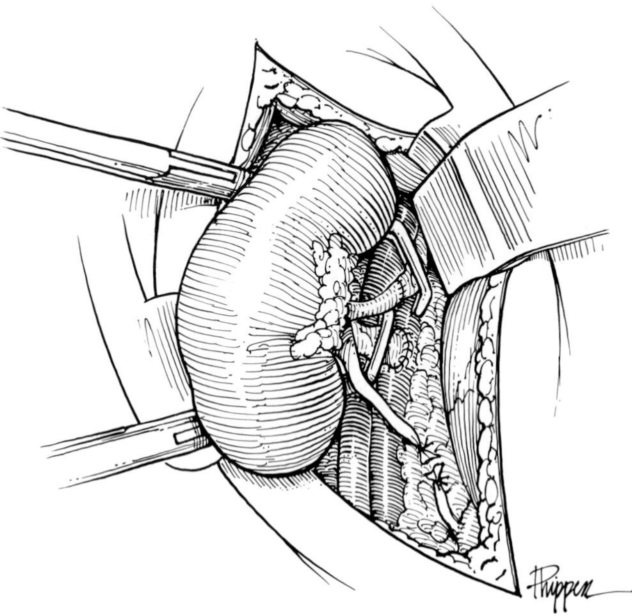

Figure 33.2. When anatomic planes can be defined readily, the plane between the anteromedial surface of the allograft and the peritoneum is developed by an extracapsular dissection that may be approached caudally from the previously defined paravesical space, cephalad from an area free of cicatrization above the upper pole, and/or directly over the midportion of the allograft. The posterolateral surface is dissected away from the floor of the iliac fossa in similar fashion. Dissection of the right paravesical space is undertaken with particular attention paid to rapid identification and averting injury to the distal aspects of the external iliac vessels. The transplant ureter is identified, mobilized, ligated with a 0-chromic ties, and sharply divided.

A self-retaining retractor may then be placed to facilitate exposure of the hilar structures. The approach to the allograft vessels in this situation is individualized and governed by their anteroposterior orientation (determined on the basis of whether the allograft was the donor's right or left kidney) and the distribution of local scarring. Mobilization of the allograft vessels is carefully undertaken from alternating cephalad, caudad, medial, and lateral directions to allow for rapid placement of a hilar clamp if needed to control inadvertent hemorrhage. Once mobilized, the renal artery or arteries and, subsequently, the vein(s) may be divided individually, or together, above one or two occlusive vascular clamps. The allograft is removed from the operative field and individual vessels are suture ligated.

After removal of the allograft, hemostasis is achieved and the wound is irrigated with saline and neomycin-bacitracin solution. When the wound is closed primarily, the fascial closure is performed in two layers using interrupted, 0-ethibond suture placed in a figure-eight or Tom Jones fashion. Either skin staples or 3–0 dermalon, interrupted vertical mattress sutures are used for skin closure. Drains are not introduced unless there is difficulty with hemostasis or localized infection is present (16). Construction of a peritoneal window is not performed routinely.

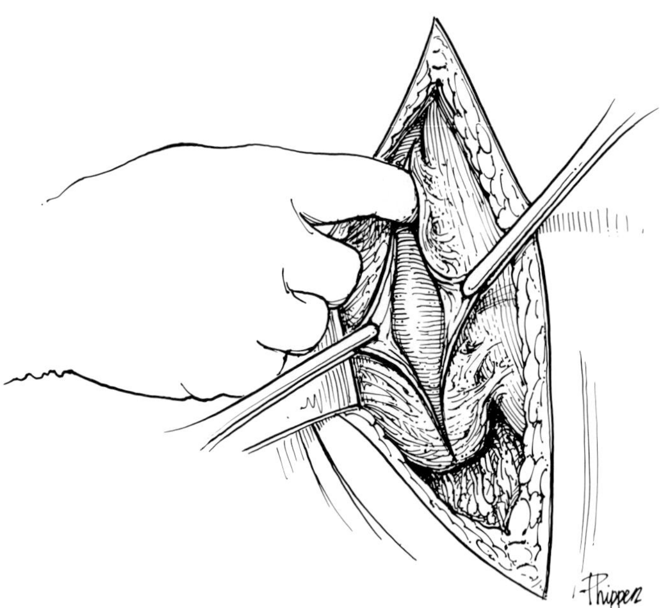

Figure 33.3. Definition of the planes of dissection as described above may be undertaken with relative ease in the early posttransplant period but is frequently precluded by the presence of a thick pseudocapsule combined with dense perinephric scarring and adhesion formation that develops over more extended periods of time. Mobilization of the allograft in the latter instance may be most optimally carried out via an intracapsular dissection (13, 17). The renal capsule is incised over the long axis of the allograft and then separated from subjacent parenchyma by blunt dissection (12, 13, 17) in which the capsule is then retracted away from the parenchyma and may be divided circumferentially to optimize access to the hilar structures.

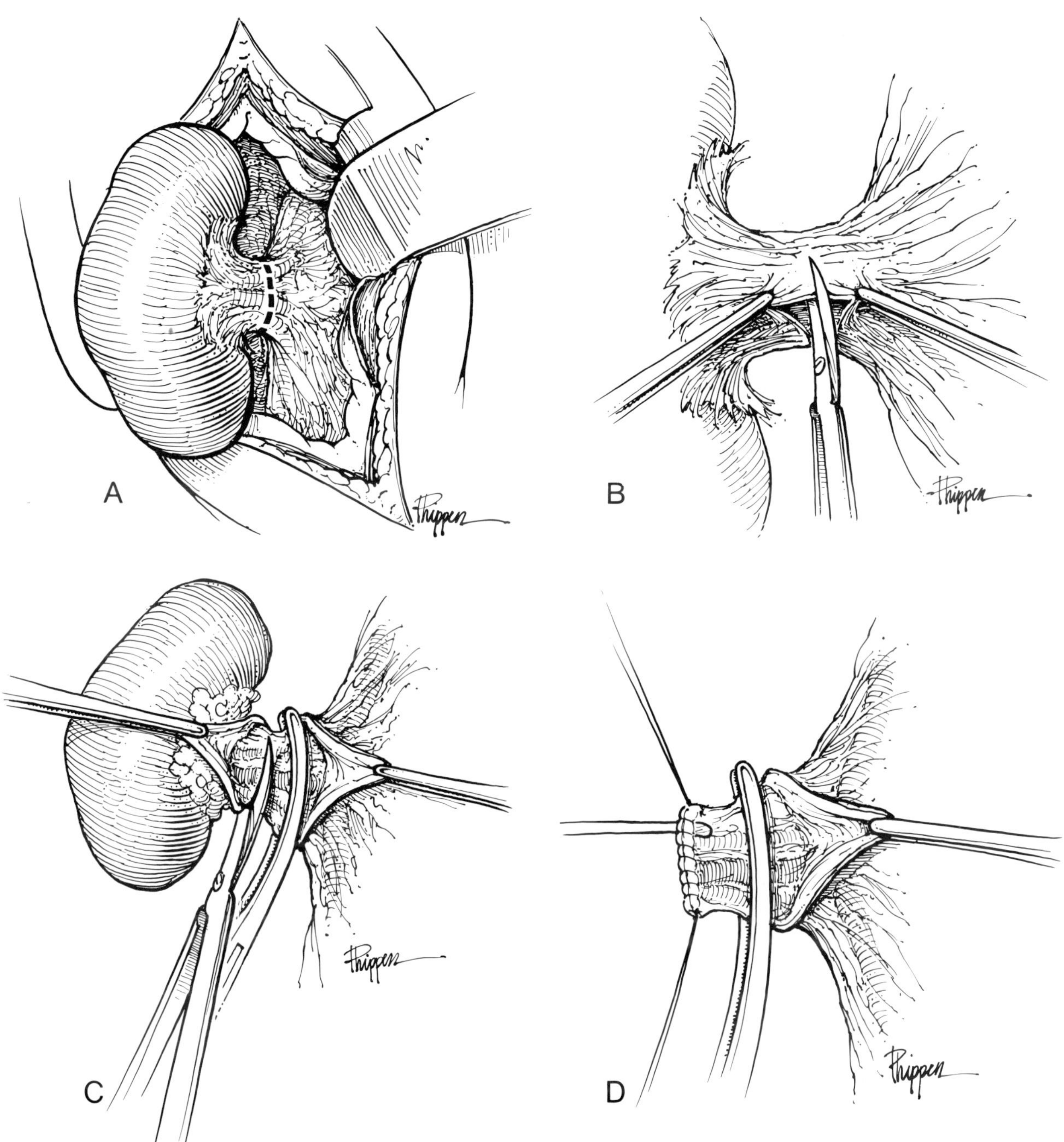

Figure 33.4. A-D, one may then encounter an umbrella of dense scar tissue enveloping the hilar structures and extending outward over the perihilar region, proximal and distal iliac vessels, and the paravesical space. This layer of scar tissue may be incised circumferentially about the hilar area to allow access to the underlying renal artery(ies), veins(s), proximal ureter, and interdigitating fatty and lymphatic tissue. With care taken to avoid injury to the subjacent external iliac vessels that are commonly tented upward by perihilar cicatrization, these structures may then be dissected separately or occluded together between one or two vascular clamps. When the hilar structures are divided together, sufficient tissue must be left above the vascular clamp(s) to allow for adequate hemostasis to be obtained by suture ligation of the hilar remnant using a running Prolene suture reinforced with interrupted, horizontal mattress sutures (17).

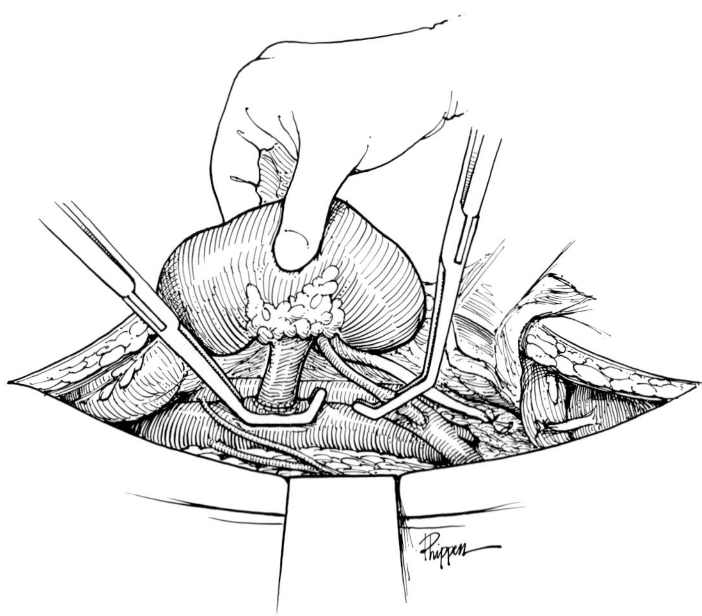

Figure 33.5. If the allograft was placed transperitoneally, nephrectomy is also performed through the initial operative incision. The bowel is mobilized and retracted away from the allograft. Particular care must be taken to avoid tearing the fragile vena cava during the course of the dissection. Depending on it's length and how readily it can be mobilized, the renal vein may be ligated distal to the caval anastomosis or resected above an atraumatic (e.g., Satinsky) vascular clamp partially occluding the subjacent inferior vena cava, which is then closed with a running, cross-stitched 5–0 or 6–0 Prolene suture. Once the allograft has been removed, hemostasis achieved, and the wound adequately irrigated, the peritoneum is separately closed with running, chromic suture. This is followed by a single layer fascial closure using interrupted, ethibond sutures placed in a figure-eight or Tom Jones fashion.

COMPLICATIONS AND POSTOPERATIVE MANAGEMENT

The major complications associated with transplant nephrectomy are wound infection, hemorrhage, and vascular injury (3, 5, 14, 16). When local infection is present at the time of surgery, prevention of subsequent sepsis is achieved best by leaving the wound open to closure by secondary intention and appropriate use of antibicrobial therapy (13, 15, 17). Wound infection after primary closure also can be prevented effectively by appropriate use of prophylactic antibicrobial therapy as noted above (14, 15). Extended postoperative antimicrobial therapy is not administered unless hematoma, perinephric, urinary tract, or other overt clinical infections are present at the time of surgery (8, 15).

A 6% incidence of significant intraoperative hemorhage has been reported (12). Postoperative hemorrhage may occur acutely or be delayed (3, 5, 12) and has been reported to develop more often in association with removal of allografts with arteries anastomosed end-to-side to the recipient external iliac artery vs. end-to-end to the recipient hypogastric artery (18). Heparinzation during hemodialysis has also been implicated as a significant risk factor for delayed hemorrhage (5). Injury to the iliac vessels is managed by primary repair or ligation with concomitant bypass grafting if necessary to maintain viability of the lower extremity (3, 5). Iliofemoral bypass is contraindicated in the presence of overt wound infection and, if grafting is necessary in such situations, femoral-femoral or axillofemoral approaches have been recommended (5).

In the absence of local infection, a permanent, chronic peritoneal dialysis catheter may be placed after closure of the transplant nephrectomy operative wound. Frequent, small volume exchanges may be attempted within 24–48 hours postoperatively and often suffice for adequate renal replacement therapy regardless of whether the peritoneum remained intact or was entered and subsequently repaired during the transplant nephrectomy (19).

References

1. Gustafsson A, Groth CG, Halgrimson CG, Penn I, Starzl TE: The fate of failed renal homografts retained after retransplantation. *Surg Gynecol Obstet* 137:42, 1973.
2. DiSesa VJ, Tilney NL: Conservative management of the failed renal allograft: Indications for transplant nephrectomy. *Curr Surg* 418, 1982.
3. Sinha SN, Castro JE: Allograft nephrectomy. *Br J Urol* 48:413, 1976.
4. Marshall V: Renal transplantation—15 years experience. *Br J Urol* 68:1, 1981.
5. Smith RB, Ehrlich RM: Complications of transplant nephrectomy. *Urol Clin North Am* 3:643, 1976.
6. Silberman H, Fitzgibbons TJ, Butler J, Berne TV: Renal allografts retained in situ after failure. *Arch Surg* 115:42, 1980.
7. Smolev JK, Mcloughlin MG, Rolley R, Sterioff S, Williams GM: The surgical approach to urological complications in renal allotransplant recipients. *J Urol* 117:10, 1977.
8. Kyriakides GK, Simmons RL, Najarian JS: Wound infections in renal transplant wounds: Pathogenetic and prognostic factors. *Ann Surg* 182:772, 1975.
9. Zimmerman CE: Renal transplantation for focal segmental glomerulosclerosis. *Transplantation* 29:172, 1980.
10. Pinto J, Lacerda G, Camerson JS, Turner DR, Bewick M, Ogg CS, et al: Recurrence of focal segmental glomerulosclerosis in renal allografts. *Transplantation* 32:83, 1981.
11. Hoyer JR, Vernier RL, Najarian JS, Raij L, Simmons RL, Michael AF: Recurrence of idiopathic nephrotic syndrome after renal transplantation. *Lancet* 1:7773, 1972.
12. Chiverton SG, Murie JA, Allen RD, Morris PJ: Renal transplant nephrectomy. *Surg Gynecol Obstet* 164:324, 1987.
13. Voesten HGJ, Slooff MJH, Hooykaas JAP, Tegzess AM, Kootstra G: Safe removal of failed transplanted kidneys. *Br J Surg* 69:480, 1982.
14. Novick AC: The value of intraoperative antibiotics in preventing renal transplant wound infections. *J Urol* 125:151, 1981.
15. Kohlberg WI, Tellis VA, Bhat DJ, Driscoll B, Veith FJ: Wound infections after transplant nephrectomy. *Arch Surg* 115:645, 1980.
16. Banowsky LH, Montie JE, Braun WE, Magnusson NO: Renal transplantation III: Prevention of wound infections. *Urology* 4:656, 1974.
17. Sutherland DER, Simmons RL, Howard RJ, Najarian JS: Intracapsular technique of transplant nephrectomy. *Surg Gynecol Obstet* 146:952, 1978.
18. Mosley JG, Castro JE: Arterial anastomoses in renal transplantation. *Br J Surg* 65:60, 1978.
19. McDonald MW, Serioff S, Engen DE, Zincke H, Kurtz SB: Renal transplantation in patients with indwelling continuous ambulatory peritoneal dialysis catheters. *J Urol* 137:849, 1987.

CHAPTER 34

Dialysis Access Surgery

THOMAS R. HEFTY
THOMAS R. HATCH
JOHN M. BARRY

Hemodialysis and peritoneal dialysis have become routine procedures in supporting patients with renal failure. Because prolonged dialysis may be required, a conservative approach in providing access for dialysis that will preserve future access sites is preferred. The introduction of the external arteriovenous (AV) shunt for hemodialysis marked the beginning of our ability to offer repeated vascular access for dialysis. Subsequently, Brescia and associates described a surgically created AV fistula to arterialize a vein that could be repeatedly punctured for vascular access. In the past two decades, several other options have been developed including graft AV fistulas, central venous catheters for hemodialysis, and surgically placed catheters for peritoneal dialysis. Although a great deal of surgical ingenuity has led to many technical variations, only the more commonly used procedures will be described here.

An algorithm that reflects our decision-making process for dialysis access surgery is shown in Figure 34.1. In centers where renal transplantation is performed by urologists, the capability for access surgery contributes significantly to continuity of care.

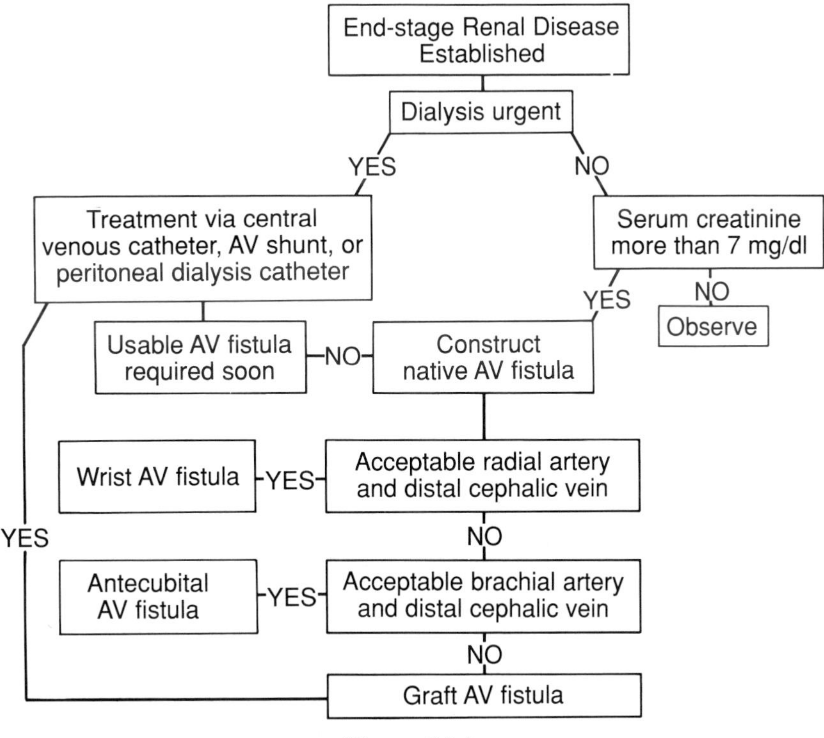

Figure 34.1.

PREOPERATIVE ASSESSMENT AND ANATOMY

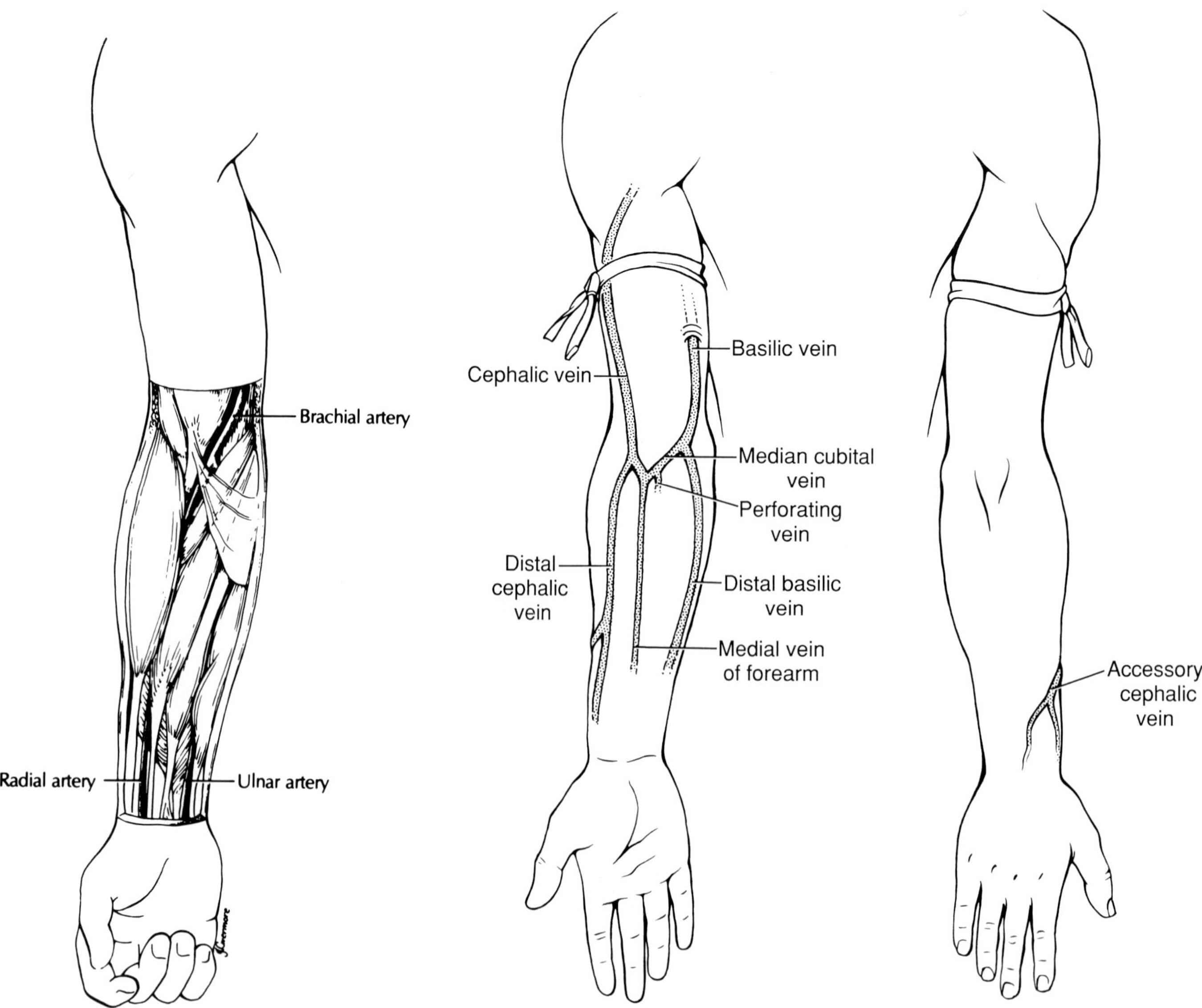

Figure 34.2. The patient's extremities are examined in a warm room using a venous tourniquet. Attention is paid to the size and patency of the distal cephalic, accessory cephalic, and proximal cephalic veins. The cephalic, medial cubital, and basilic veins make a variable "M" in the antecubital fossa.

Figure 34.3. The radial, ulnar, and brachial arteries are palpated. An Allen's test is done by compressing the radial artery while the patient clenches his fist. Return of color to the relaxed hand within 3 sec indicates patency of the ulnar artery and palmar arches. The converse can be done to assess the radial artery. The radial artery is below the antebrachial fascia at the wrist and the brachial artery is below the tough bicipital aponeurosis.

Examination of the ankle includes palpating the greater saphenous vein for patency and palpating the dorsalis pedis and posterior tibial arteries.

The selected extremity is scrubbed and the nails are clipped before surgery. The patient receives a prophylactic dose of antibiotic to cover skin organisms before surgery and for 24 hours postoperatively. Sedation is a useful adjunct to local anesthesia during the procedure.

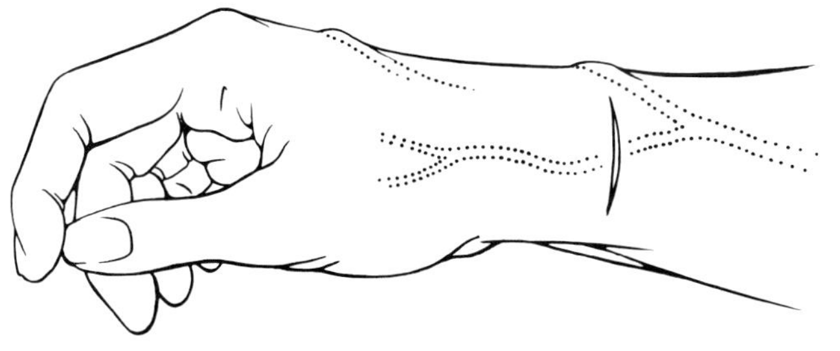

ARTERIOVENOUS SHUNT

Figure 34.4. The incision is planned 4 cm above the styloid process of the radius to allow for wrist motion without shunt kinking or erosion. The skin overlying the radial artery and cephalic vein is infiltrated with plain 1% lidocaine (epinephrine is omitted to reduce vasospasm).

A longitudinal incision through the antebrachial fascia is made to expose the radial artery with its two venae comitantes. Each vessel is isolated by gentle dissection and a 2–0 silk strand is placed around it for traction. The vein is addressed first because adequate venous return is ncessary for success. It is usually unnecessary to divide branches.

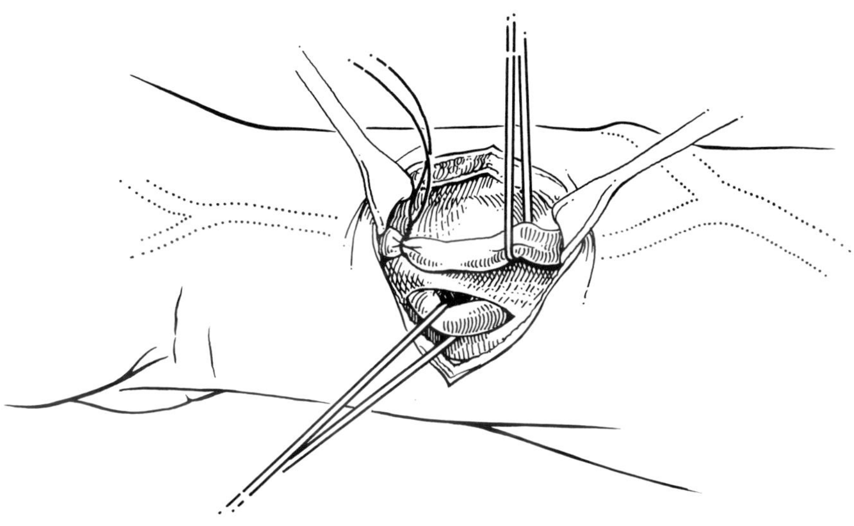

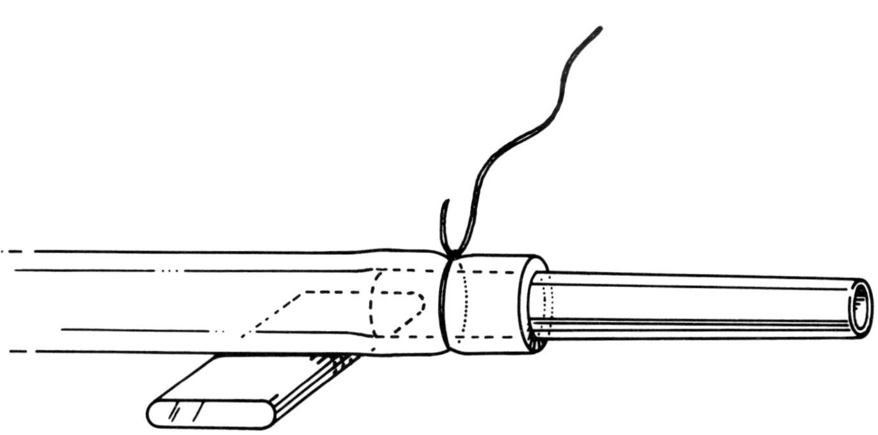

Figure 34.5. Depending on vessel size, small, medium, or large vessel tips are secured to the winged Ramirez Silastic cannula with a 2–0 silk tie leaving one strand long.

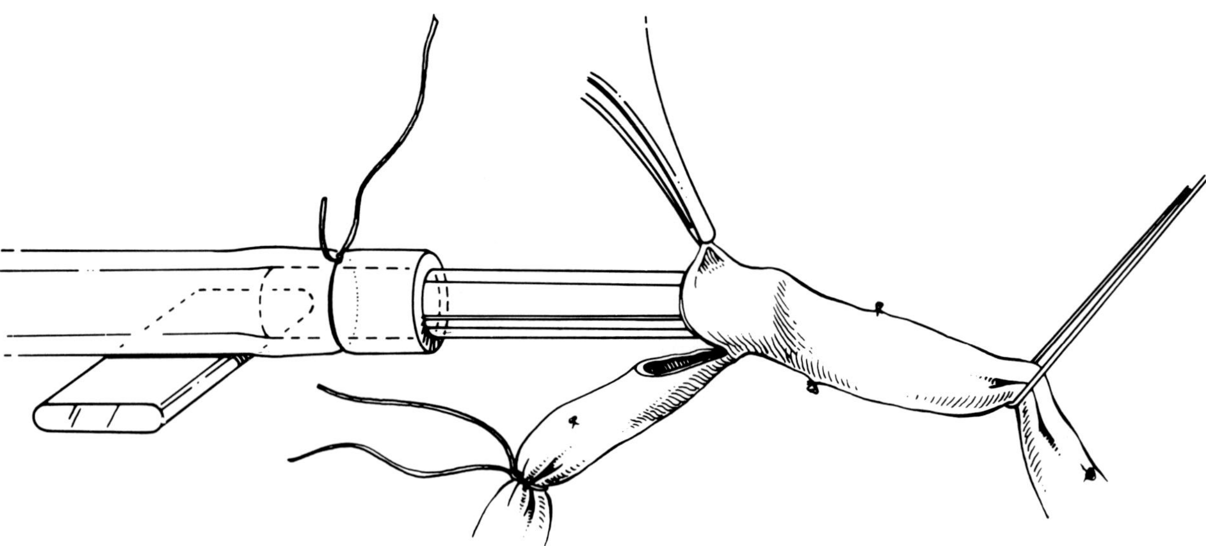

Figure 34.6. The vein is ligated distally with a 2–0 silk ligature that is clamped to the surgical drapes for counter traction. A proximal 2–0 silk is passed around the vessel and left untied to be used for traction and hemostasis. An 11 blade is used to open the vein obliquely for half of its diameter. The overhanging edge of the vessel is grasped with fine serrated forceps and gentle dilatation is done with vessel dilators or with a small closed hemostat. The cannula tubing with vessel tip has been filled with heparinized saline and clamped.

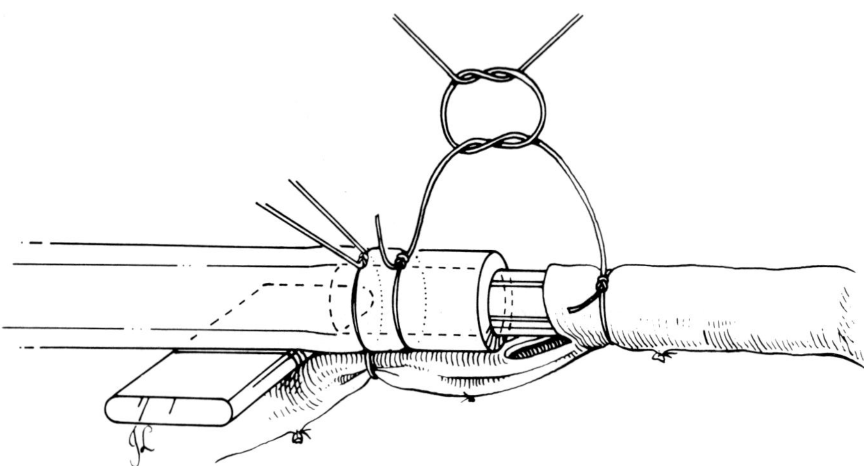

Figure 34.7. The vessel tip is gently advanced into the vein and the proximal 2–0 silk ligature is tied on the vein and indwelling vessel tip. One limb of the suture is trimmed. The limbs of 2–0 silk left long on the shunt tubing and proximal vein are tied together and the distal silk ligature is tied around the cannula for added stability.

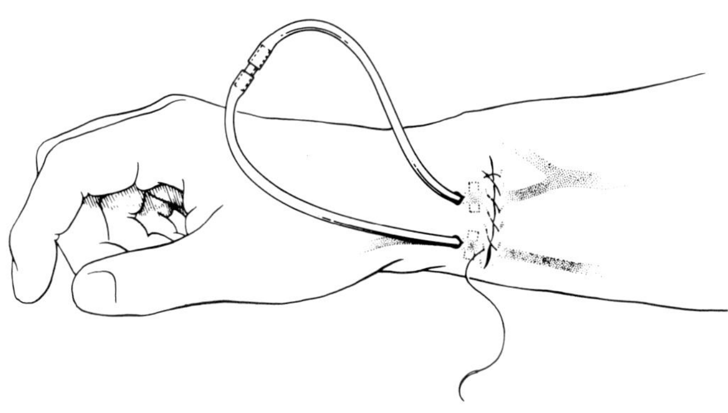

Figure 34.8. A small space is dissected with a hemostat for the wings of the shunt tubing and the tubing is brought out through a small stab incision 1–2 cm distal to the skin incision. Heparinized saline is flushed through the venous limb to confirm patency. The artery is handled in a similar fashion with special attention to gentle dilatation. Traction on the proximal silk tie by the assistant will provide hemostasis. Avoid damaging or "bunching up" the intima by forcing in too large a vessel tip into the artery. The arterial and venous limbs of the shunt are joined by a straight connector and taped securely.

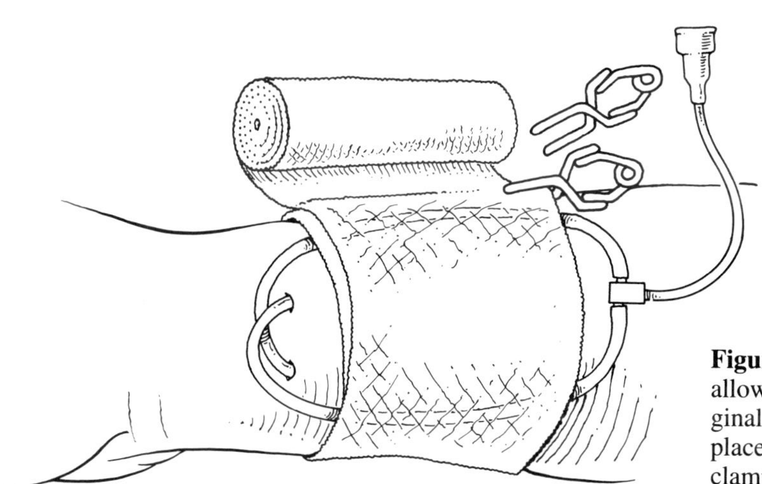

Figure 34.9. An optional "T" connector may be used that allows easy access for drawing blood and for flushing a marginal shunt with heparinized saline. A soft gauze wrapping is placed around the incision and shunt tubing and two shunt clamps are attached to the dressing for emergency occlusion.

When suitable vessels for an arteriovenous shunt are not available in the upper extremity, an ankle shunt may be performed. This operation is most suitable for an individual who is not expected to be ambulatory soon. Arterial supply to the toes can be assessed by compressing the posterior tibial and dorsalis pedis arteries and squeezing the foot from toe to heel. Capillary refill is observed on releasing one artery or the other. The great saphenous vein is isolated just anterior to the medial malleous and it is cannulated as described for the wrist AV shunt.

The posterior tibial artery is exposed posterior to the median malleolus deep to the flexor retinaculum. Alternatively, the dorsalis pedis artery may be used below the ankle and is deep to the inferior extensor retinaculum and medial to the extensor hallucis brevis muscle. Once the vessels are exposed, the procedure is identical to that described for a wrist AV shunt.

The availability of subclavian central venous catheters for acute dialysis has largely eliminated the need for ankle AV shunts.

CENTRAL VENOUS CATHETER

The uremic patient in need of acute hemodialysis can be managed by placing a subclavian vein catheter. In contrast to femoral vein catheters, the patient is free to walk and can be managed as an outpatient while an AV fistula matures. The physician placing the subclavian catheter should be familiar with the procedure of subclavian central venous catheter placement.

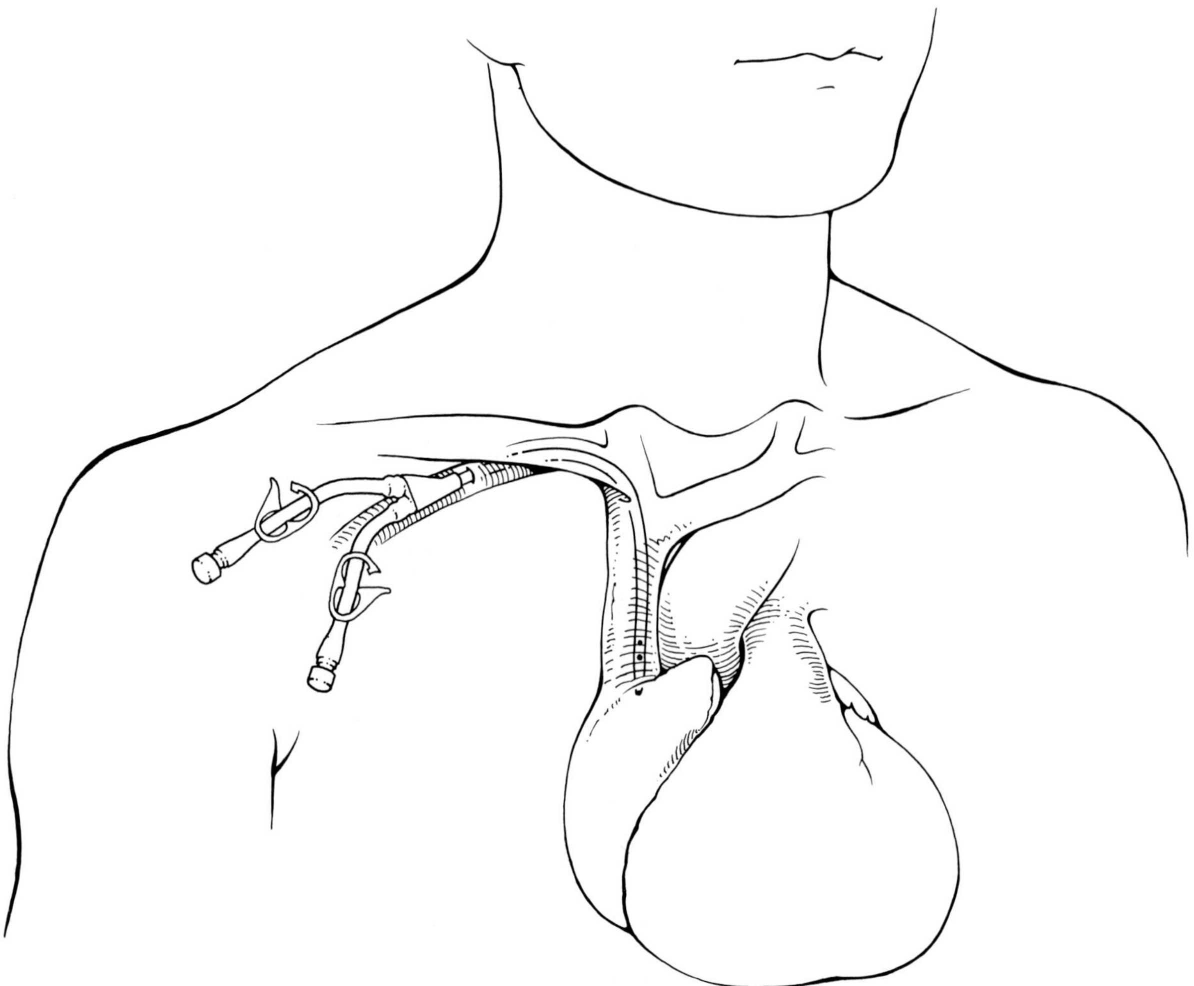

Figure 34.10. Aseptic technique is used and once the vein is located, a .038-inch guidewire is advanced approximately 8 inches. With the guidewire in place, the tract through the subcutaneous tissue is dilated. A double-lumen catheter is preferred to minimize the need for heparinization during dialysis. It is advanced with gentle rotation through the subcutaneous tissue into the subclavian vein.

A final position with the tip of the catheter near junction of the superior vena cava and right atrium is desired. The catheter is then flushed and heparinized saline is left indwelling. The catheter is sutured to the skin, and a sterile dressing is applied. A portable chest x-ray is then done to examine the position of the catheter and to check for the possible complication of pneumothorax. Dressing changes are done with each dialysis treatment and the subclavian catheter is removed if there is any sign of infection.

ARTERIOVENOUS FISTULA

Anastomosis of the end of the distal cephalic vein to the side of the radial artery prevents venous engorgement and disfigurement of the hand that can result from a side-to-side anastomosis. Five vascular instruments are required for this procedure including a Castroviejo needle holder, two fine serrated forceps, a Heifitz clip, and angled Westcott scissors. Vessel loops, a no. 3 Fogarty embolectomy catheter, two 7–0 polypropylene sutures on a cardiovascular needle, sewing towels, warmed heparinized saline, and GU irrigation are also used.

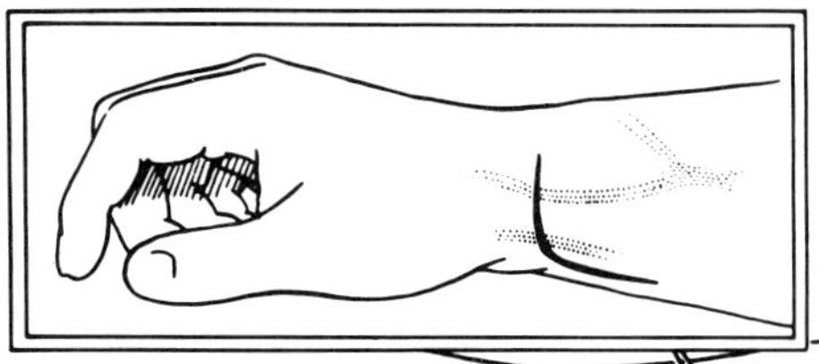

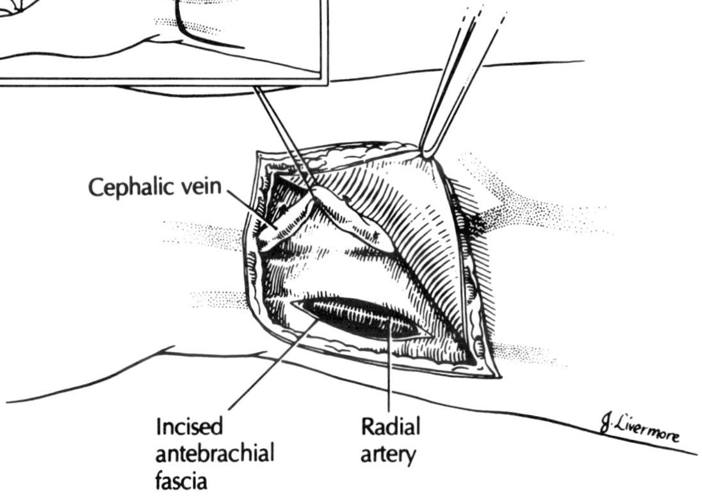

Figure 34.11. A transverse incision over the distal cephalic vein is curved proximally over the axis of the radial artery. A triangular flap of skin and subcutaneous tissue is raised. The veins are mainly above the superficial branches of the radial nerve that are spared wherever possible. A hemostat on the subcutaneous tissue at the corner of the flap will serve as a self-retaining retractor. Branches of the cephalic vein are divided between 4–0 silk ligatures. If the cephalic vein overlying the radius is thrombosed or inadequate, a small extension of the incision toward the ulna will allow dissection of the accessory cephalic vein draining the superficial dorsal veins of the hand.

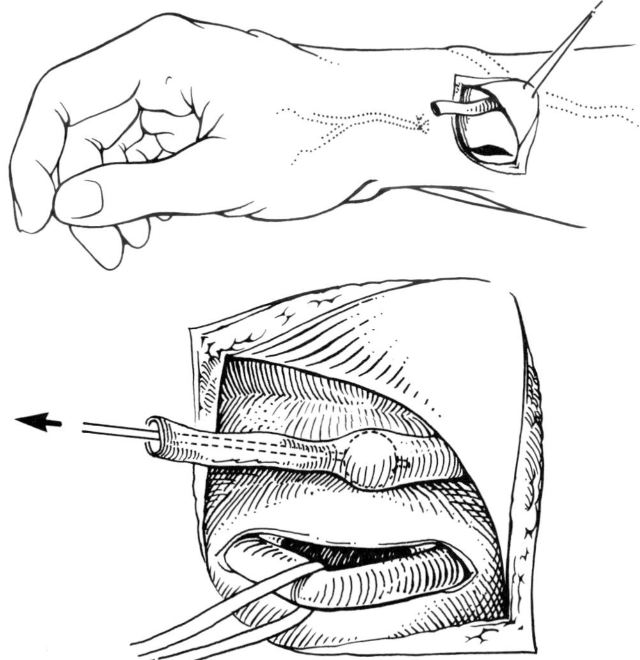

Figure 34.12. After proximal mobilization, the vein is dissected as far distally as possible, ligated with a 2–0 silk, and divided. A no. 3 Fogarty catheter is passed about 30 cm up the vein, the balloon is inflated, and the catheter is withdrawn gently to dilate the vein. The vein is then flushed with heparinized saline. A Heifitz clip is applied if back bleeding occurs.

The antebrachial fascia is incised and the radial artery is mobilized for about 3 cm dividing small branches between 4–0 silk ligatures.

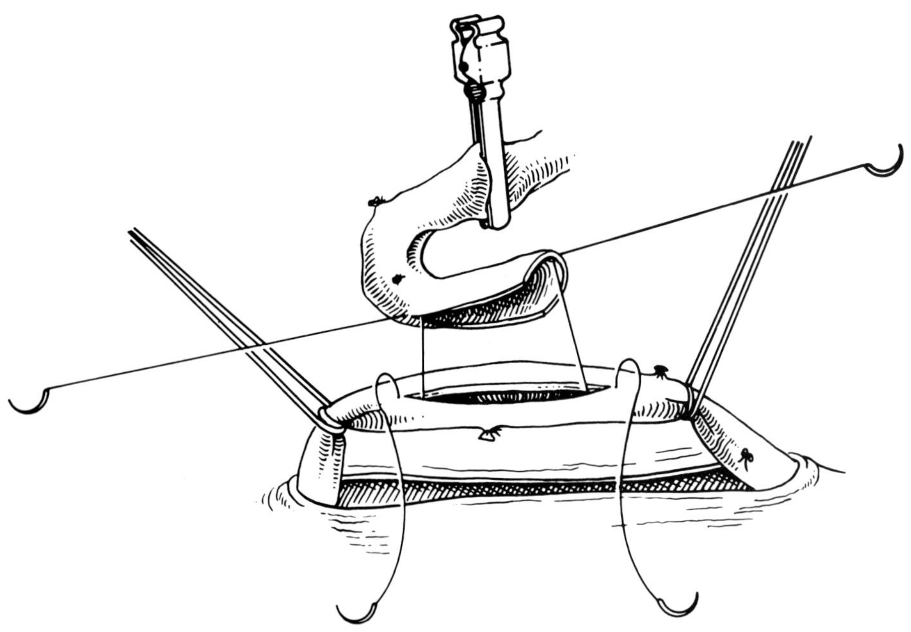

Figure 34.13. Thin vessel loops are doubly passed around the artery distally and proximally, and clamped to the drapes to occlude and elevate the artery. A 5 to 10-mm longitudinal arteriotomy is made with a no. 11 blade and Westcott scissors and flushed with heparinized saline. The distal vein is spatulated approximately 5 mm on its ulnar aspect and swung to the artery in a smooth curve. Sewing towels are placed and double-armed 7–0 cardiovascular polypropylene sutures are passed from inside out at the heel and toe of the anastomosis.

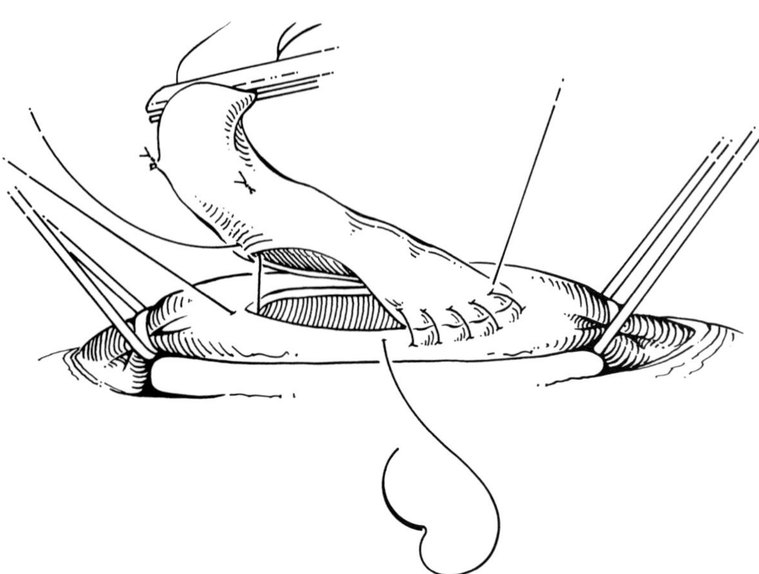

Figure 34.14. One limb of the suture at the toe of the anastomosis is run past the heel by two or three stitches and tagged. The remaining limb of the toe suture is then run for approximately three stitches and tagged. The artery may be dilated through the uncompleted portion of the anastomosis at this time.

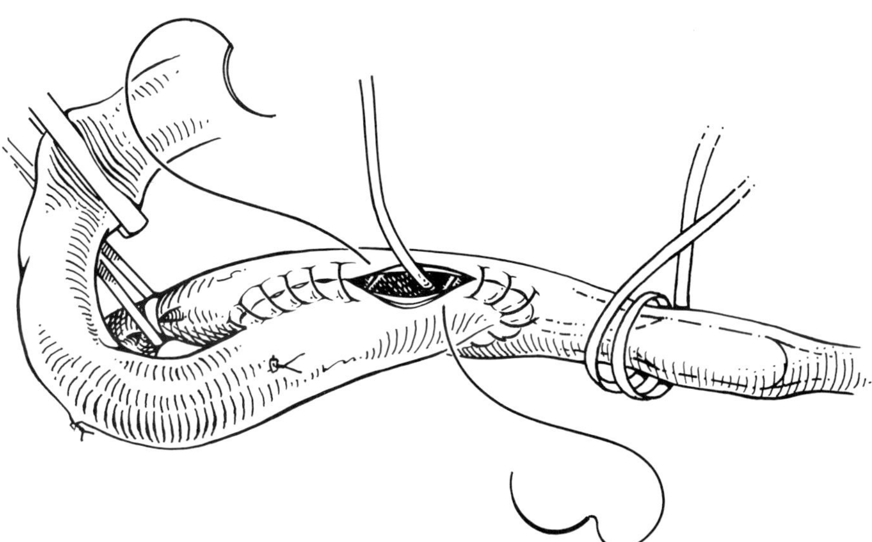

Figure 34.15. Vessel dilators are passed a short distance in the proximal radial artery by relaxing tension on the proximal vessel loop. The anastomosis is then completed and the sutures tied. The vessel loops are loosened to allow flow through the fistula. Minor bleeding can be controlled with sponge pressure for a few minutes. Occasionally, additional 7–0 or 6–0 sutures will be needed.

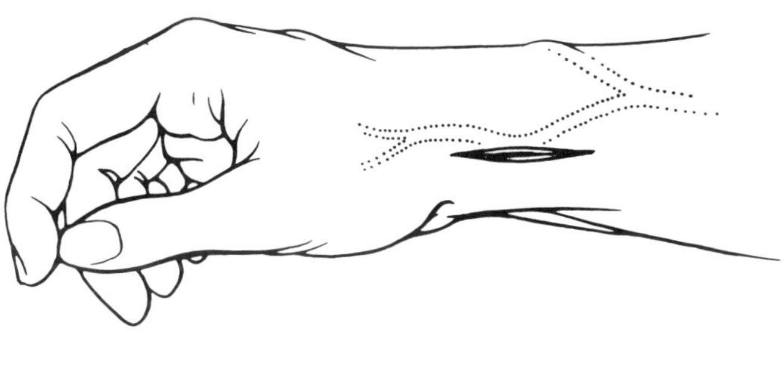

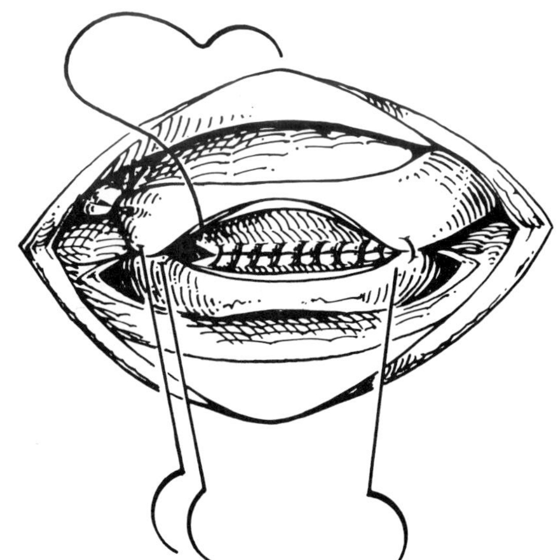

Figure 34.16. An alternative technique utilizing a side-to-side anastomosis is illustrated. This is useful when the vein closely overlies the artery and is done by sewing the back wall from the inside of the anastomosis. After completion of the anastomosis, the fistula can be converted to a functional end-to-side anastomosis by ligation of the vein distally.

The wound is irrigated with antibiotic solution and closed with interrupted 4–0 polyglycolic acid suture in the subcutaneous tissue and running subcuticular 4–0 polyglycolic acid on the skin. Care is taken not to compress the vein with closure. Postoperative care includes a warm pad on the arm to promote vasodilatation and 24 hr of antibiotic coverage. Early thrombosis is treated with exploration and thrombectomy with revision of the fistula if needed. Anticoagulation should be considered if no technical problems are detected at exploration.

ANTECUBITAL AV FISTULA

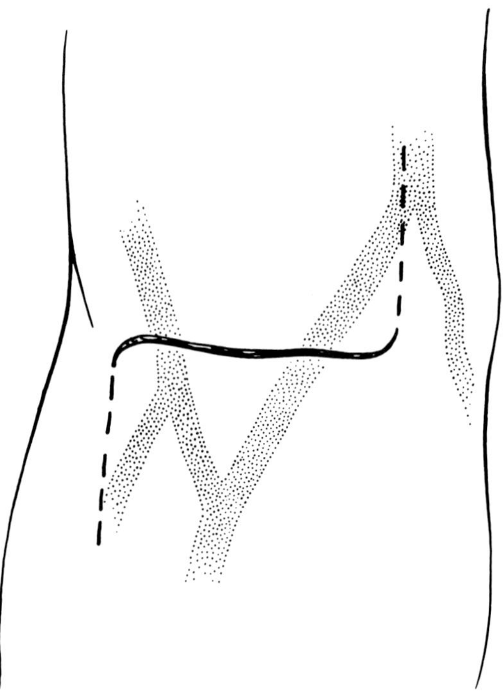

Figure 34.17. When the vessels at the wrist are small or occluded, an antecubital AV fistula may be created using the same set of instruments. The skin is infiltrated with 1% lidocaine and a transverse incision is made. It will rarely be necessary to extend the transverse incision as shown.

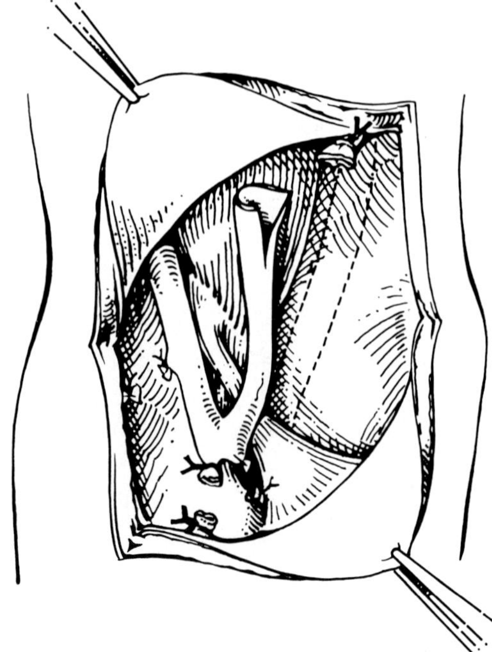

Figure 34.18. Below the superficial fascia, the medial cubital and cephalic veins can be dissected distally to their juncture with the median vein of the forearm and the perforating vein. If the valvular anatomy allows retrograde flow down the medial cubital vein to the cephalic vein, the median vein of the forearm and perforating vein may then be divided between 2–0 silk ligatures. The medial cubital vein is ligated proximally, divided, and spatulated on its posteromedial aspect for approximately 5 mm. The vein is gently dilated with a no. 1 Fogarty catheter, flushed with heparinized saline, and any back bleeding is controlled with a Heifetz clip.

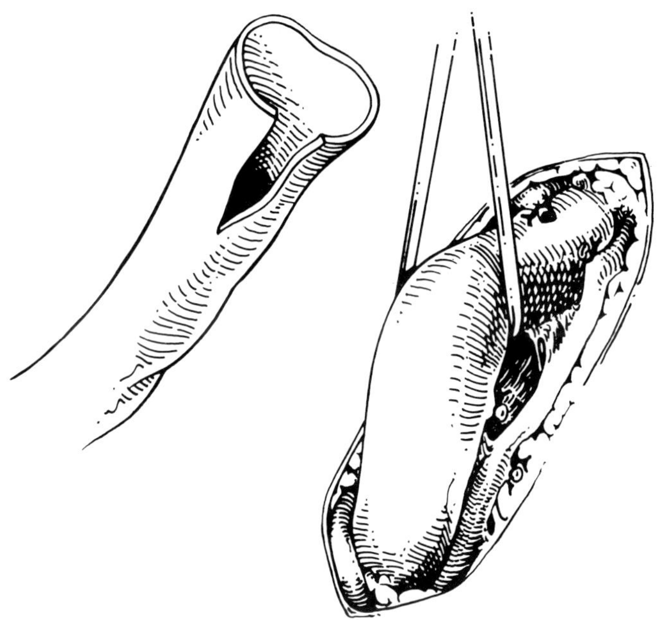

Figure 34.19. The brachial artery is approached by exposing the fibrous bicipital aponeurosis over the palpable pulsation. This layer and the space below it is infiltrated with 1% lidocaine taking care not to puncture the artery and, thereby, cause a hematoma. A 2- to 3-cm opening in the direction of the artery is made through the deep fascia exposing the brachial artery surrounded by fat and its two venae comitantes. With hemostat dissection, a vessel loop is placed around the artery for traction. The venae comitantes can usually be rolled off the artery either medially or laterally but, occasionally, a vein crossing anteriorly will need to be divided between two 4–0 silk ligatures. Small branches of the artery are divided between 4–0 silk ligatures. Small branches of the artery are divided between 4–0 silk ties, and 2 cm of artery is isolated between double wrapped vessel loops.

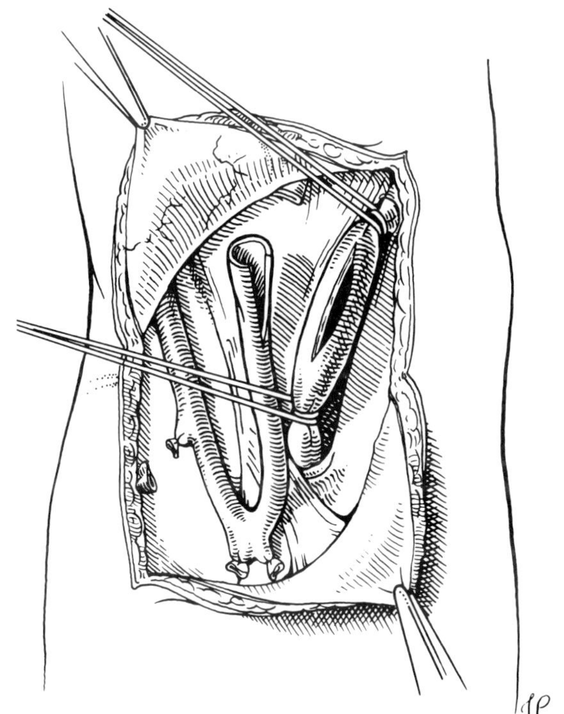

Figure 34.20. After securing the vessel loops to the drapes, a 1-cm longitudinal arteriotomy is made with a no. 11 blade and the Wescott scissors. Blood is flushed out with heparinized saline. The anastomosis is then done as described for a wrist fistula.

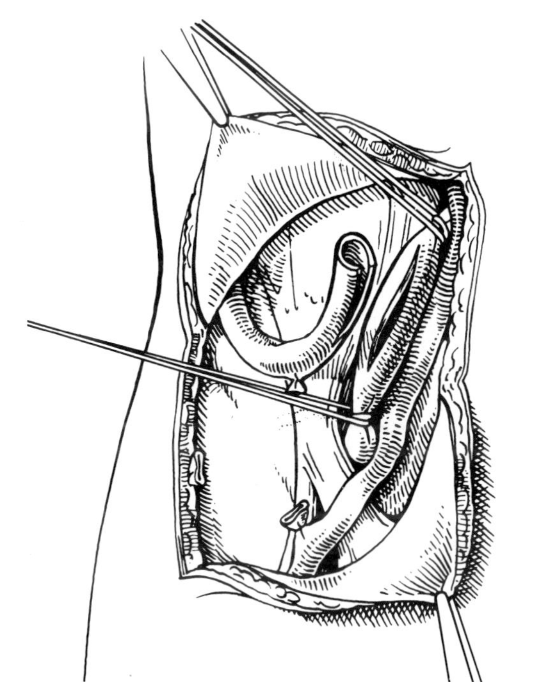

Figure 34.21. When the medial cubital vein is not usable, the cephalic vein is dissected distally as far as possible, extending onto the median vein of the forearm if added length is needed. The vein is ligated and divided as far distally as possible after the perforating vein is divided. The vein is spatulated on its posterolateral aspect. Undermining the superior wound edge and ligating and dividing any lateral tributaries to the cephalic vein will allow increased medial mobility without venous compression. The anastomosis is done as previously described.

FOREARM GRAFT ARTERIOVENOUS FISTULA

Loop forearm grafts are indicated when the vessels are inadequate for creation of a native fistula. A graft AV fistula is also useful when obesity makes access of the native vein difficult or when there is insufficient time for a native fistula to mature. Vascular graft materials used at our institution for this purpose have included chemically prepared bovine carotid arteries (Artegraft, Johnson & Johnson) and expanded polytetrafluoroethylene (PTFE, GORE-Tex, Impragraft). Various sizes of each type are available.

The preoperative assessment and anatomy is the same as described previously. Perioperative intravenous antibiotics are important to cover the patient for skin organisms when placing a loop forearm graft.

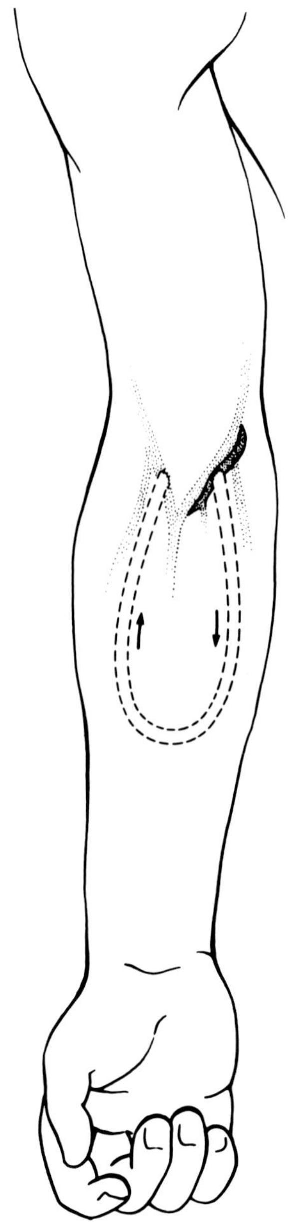

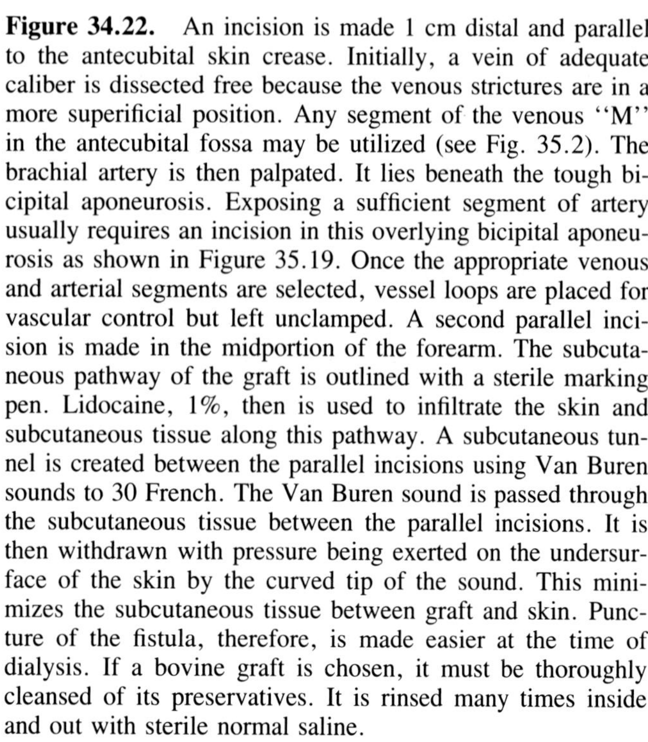

Figure 34.22. An incision is made 1 cm distal and parallel to the antecubital skin crease. Initially, a vein of adequate caliber is dissected free because the venous strictures are in a more superficial position. Any segment of the venous "M" in the antecubital fossa may be utilized (see Fig. 35.2). The brachial artery is then palpated. It lies beneath the tough bicipital aponeurosis. Exposing a sufficient segment of artery usually requires an incision in this overlying bicipital aponeurosis as shown in Figure 35.19. Once the appropriate venous and arterial segments are selected, vessel loops are placed for vascular control but left unclamped. A second parallel incision is made in the midportion of the forearm. The subcutaneous pathway of the graft is outlined with a sterile marking pen. Lidocaine, 1%, then is used to infiltrate the skin and subcutaneous tissue along this pathway. A subcutaneous tunnel is created between the parallel incisions using Van Buren sounds to 30 French. The Van Buren sound is passed through the subcutaneous tissue between the parallel incisions. It is then withdrawn with pressure being exerted on the undersurface of the skin by the curved tip of the sound. This minimizes the subcutaneous tissue between graft and skin. Puncture of the fistula, therefore, is made easier at the time of dialysis. If a bovine graft is chosen, it must be thoroughly cleansed of its preservatives. It is rinsed many times inside and out with sterile normal saline.

Figure 34.23. The graft is then pulled through the subcutaneous tissue with uterine packing forceps. With a bulb syringe, the graft is distended with heparinized saline to ensure that there are no kinks. The ends of the graft are then tailored in an angled fashion. The venous anastomosis is performed initially after the vessel loops are placed under tension and clamped to the drapes. Performing the venous anastomosis first decreases the ischemic time of the forearm. To perform a running anastomosis, 6–0 polypropylene is used. The arterial anastomosis is then done in a similar fashion.

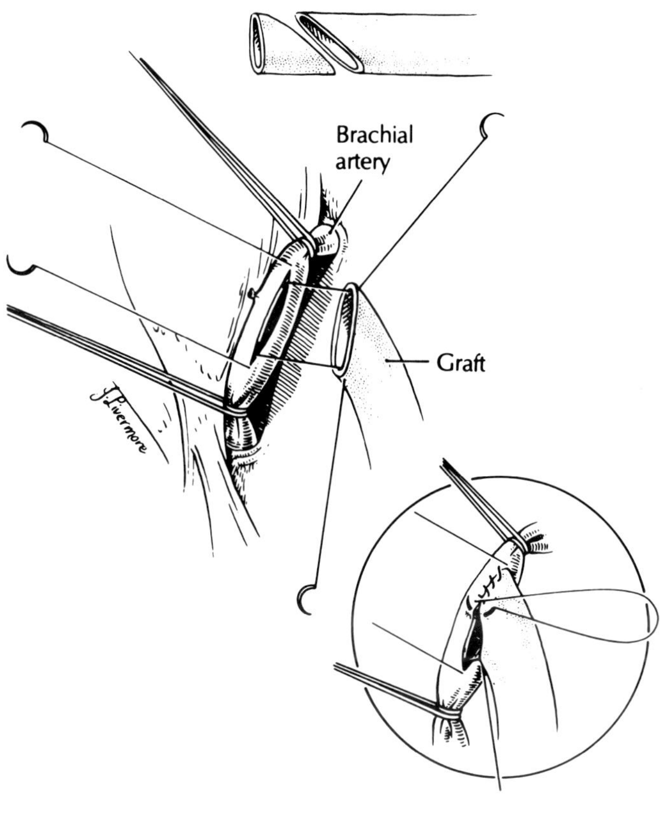

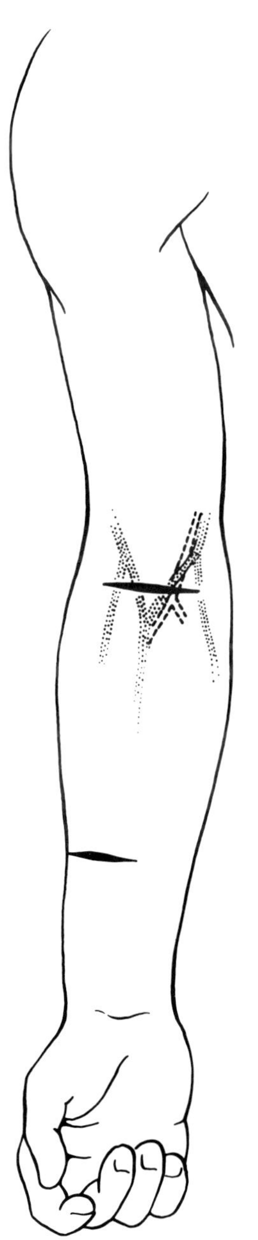

Figure 34.24. The final position of the graft is illustrated. Although these grafts may be used on an emergent basis, it is optimal to wait 2–3 weeks. This allows the edema to subside and decreases the potential for hematoma formation around the graft after needle puncture.

THIGH GRAFT ARTERIOVENOUS FISTULA

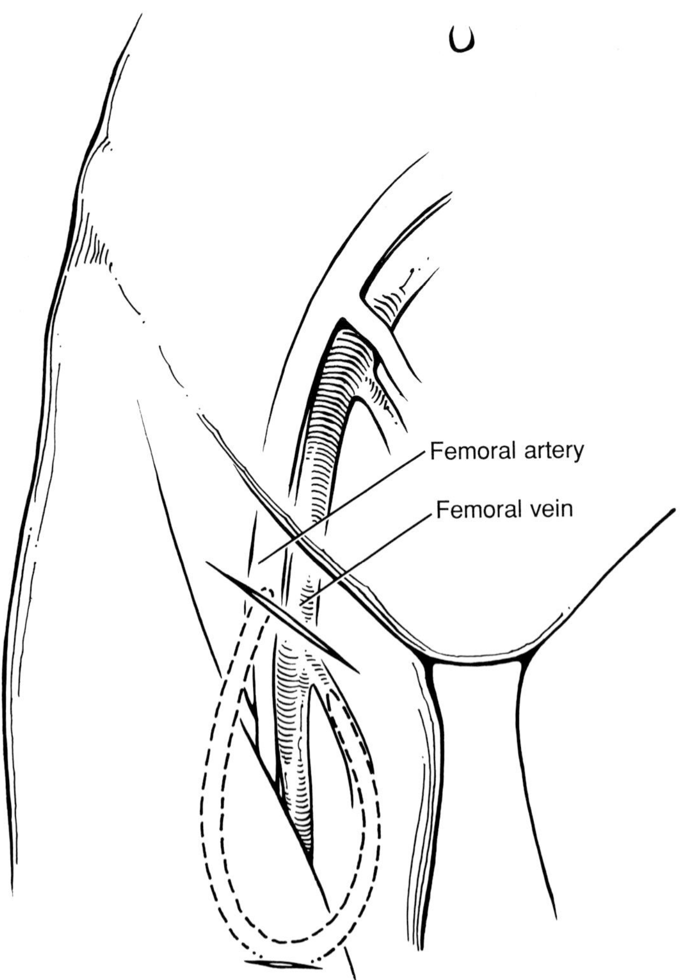

Figure 34.25. When suitable vessels are not available for placement of a loop graft in the upper extremities, we have utilized the inguinal region. Grafts in this region have not hindered the daily activities of our patients and provide excellent vascular access for the dialysis nurse.

The proximal femoral artery and proximal saphenous vein are used most frequently to create a loop graft in this region. This technique is the same as described previously except that the surgeon generally stands when operating in this region.

Chronic Ambulatory Peritoneal Dialysis Access

Certain patients in chronic renal failure may choose chronic ambulatory peritoneal dialysis (CAPD) as an alternative to hemodialysis. This method allows the patient freedom from regular visits to a hemodialysis unit. Before a peritoneal catheter is placed, the patient must demonstrate an understanding of this dialysis technique, be able to perform dialysate exchanges in a sterile fashion, and have adequate eyesight and finger dexterity to carry out this routine on a daily basis.

This method of dialysis is frequently used in children. Parents of these children generally assume responsibility for the daily exchanges. It has been suggested that children on CAPD have better growth compared to children on hemodialysis.

We commonly use a Toronto-Western or coiled Tenckhoff catheter. The Toronto-Western catheter has two Silastic discs at its distal tip to prevent catheter entanglement with the omentum and intestines. With the coiled Tenckhoff CAPD catheter, the distal tip is coiled several times to prevent omental obstruction of the catheter.

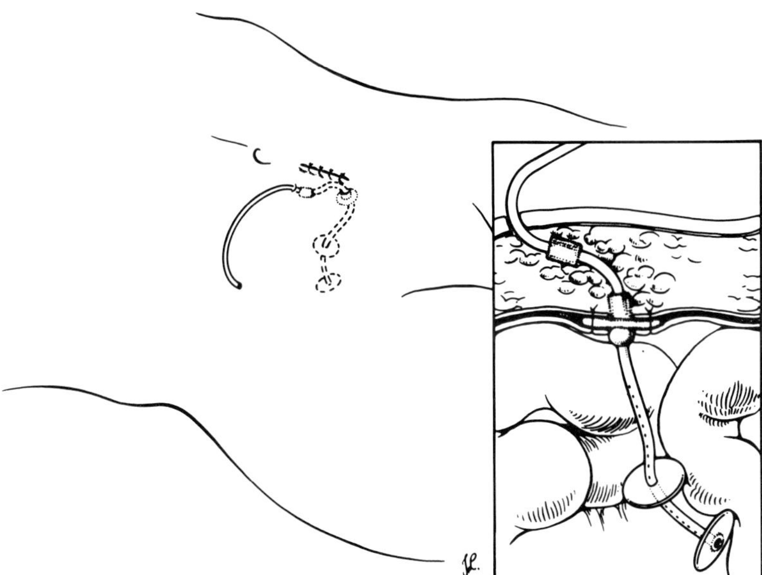

Figure 34.26. The catheter exit site is marked on the patient's abdomen carefully avoiding the beltline. We give perioperative intravenous antibiotics to cover the patient for skin organisms. The patient is placed in the supine position on the operating room table. An area 4 cm inferior and 4 cm lateral to the umbilicus directly over the rectus muscle is infiltrated with 1% lidocaine without epinephrine. A 5-cm horizontal incision is then made directly over the anterior rectus sheath. The rectus muscle is split to expose the posterior rectus fascia. A small incision no longer than 1 cm is made in the posterior fascia and peritoneum. The edges are then grasped with a hemostat. If any portion of the omentum comes through this incision, it is grasped and delivered through the wound. A partial omentectomy is then performed to reduce the incidence of catheter entanglement.

The CAPD catheter is then passed through this small incision. Using 2–0 polypropylene, a purse-string suture is placed in the posterior fascia and peritoneum that also incorporates the fibers of the cuff of the peritoneal dialysis catheter. The purse-string is then tied down and 500 ml of dialysate is infused through the catheter. If inflow and outflow of this dialysate is rapid and there is no evidence of obstruction, a subcutaneous tunnel is then made and the catheter is brought through the previously chosen exit site on the abdomen. The anterior fascia is closed with a running 2–0 polyglycolic acid.

When the need for dialysis is urgent, peritoneal dialysis may be initiated immediately after surgery. However, leakage of dialysate through the incision will be more likely in this situation.

Suggested Readings

Brescia MJ, Cimino JE, Appel K, Hurwich BJ: Chronic hemodialysis using venipuncture and a surgically created arteriovenous fistula. *N Engl J Med* 275:1089, 1966.

Chinitz JL, Yokoyama T, Bower R, Swartz C: Self-sealing prosthesis for arteriovenous fistula in man. *Trans Am Soc Artif Intern Organs* 18:452, 1972.

Potter DE, San Luis E, Wipfler JE, Portale AA: Comparison of continuous ambulatory peritoneal dialysis and hemodialysis in children. *Kidney Int* 30:S-11, 1986.

Quinton WE, Dillard D, Scribner BH: Cannulation of blood vessels for prolonged hemodialysis. *Trans Am Soc Artif Int Organs* 6:104, 1960.

Schwarzbeck A, Brittinger WD, Strauch M: Percutaneous cannulation of subclavian vein for acute haemodialysis. *Proc Eur Dial Transplant Assoc Eur Ren Assoc* 15:575, 1978.

Tenckhoff H, Schecter H: A bacteriologically safe peritoneal access device. *Trans Am Soc Artif Intern Organs* 14:181, 1968.

Wedgwood KR, Wiggins PA, Guillou PJ: A prospective study of end-to-side vs. side-to-side arteriovenous fistulas for haemodialysis. *Br J Surg* 71:640, 1984.

SECTION 8

Operative Procedures in the Retroperitoneum

CHAPTER 35

Retroperitoneal Lymphadenectomy

JOHN P. DONOHUE

Significant changes are under way in the evolution of the technique of retroperitoneal lymphadenectomy. For low stage disease, a number of workers both here and abroad have described techniques that permit ejaculation postoperatively in up to 90% of the cases (1–3). The postganglionic fibers of the lumbar sympathetic chain can be identified and preserved, particularly when there is no clinical evidence of disease in cases that appear to be of stage I classification. Also, in clinically advanced disease, the distribution of nodes has been well described (4) and a template for dissection that will include these is achieved readily by experienced groups. Finally, the role of surgery in still further advanced disease is now well established as "postchemotherapy," and the nature and extent of this surgery has also been thoroughly described (5, 6). Briefly, it involves an extended bilateral (as opposed to a modified unilateral) dissection, which has become feasible in low stage disease as noted above.

SURGERY FOR LOW STAGE DISEASE

Quite understandably, surgery itself for low stage disease has been questioned. This is appropriate in view of the fact that, in our series and in the experience of many others, about 70% of our clinically negative patients will indeed have negative lymph nodes. Assuming only a slight pathologic sampling error, this implies that there was no therapeutic effect to the retroperitoneal lymph node dissection (RPLND) surgery. The arguments (pro and con) for surgery for low stage disease have been well developed and discussed elsewhere. Patients who relapse in surveillance studies do so most often in the retriperitoneum as one would expect. Unfortunately, this area is difficult to monitor and will require even more aggressive and frequent study in the future (e.g., examining the abdominal computed axial tomography (CAT) scans every 6 weeks as opposed to every 3 months, as had been suggested. If the patients are selected carefully on the basis of primary testicular pathologic characteristics and if all patients who show suspicious results on any clinical parameter (e.g., lymphangiogram) are excluded, there is no question that satisfactory data can be obtained. In fact, most (but not all) patients can be salvaged at clinical relapse, with the salvage rate now estimated to be in the 95th percentile (7). Unfortunately, this is not an improvement in survival statistics, but, in fact, is lower in terms of absolute survival, which was in excess of 99% if one accepts the data from the largest American series. The only positive thing that can be said for surveillance is that patients who were truly negative were spared an operation that offered no therapeutic benefit.

Improvements in technique of staging RPLND now render moot the primary argument against the procedure. This argument is that young men become sterile from ejaculatory impotence after surgery at a time of life before marriage when this is most threatening. It is of great interest that worldwide data are being generated regarding preservation of ejaculation, and thus, of fertility, after RPLND surgery. Therefore, the main emotional and social argument against RPLND in low stage disease has been defused by the nerve-sparing modifications emerging on both sides of the Atlantic (1–3).

SURGICAL TECHNIQUE

The technique of the surgery has been thoroughly described in earlier publications cited (8). The exposure is obtained by making a midline incision from xyphoid to pubis. Drapes and a circular plastic wound protector are placed and, currently, we are using a self-retaining ring retractor that is affixed to the table. After careful exploration of the abdomen, the root of the small bowel is divided. For low stage disease, it is not necessary to divide the right posterior colonic mesentery and to mobilize the bowel completely, placing it in a bowel bag on the patient's chest. Rather, the viscera can be retracted in wet laparotomy pads, exposing the interaortocaval and the periaortic groups of nodes. We also divide the inferior mesenteric vein between suture ligatures to mobilize better the left colonic mesentery and to permit improved elevation and mobilization of the pancreas. This is not necessary in staging RPLND for clinically negative patients, particularly those with right-sided primary tumors. In those with left-sided primary tumors, this vein should be divided and the colonic mesentery mobilized to facilitate retraction and exposure in this area.

The basic principle of dividing the nodal and adventitial packages as they surround the great vessels in a longitudinal manner is indicated in Figure 35.1. This is accomplished most easily at the 12 o'clock position over both the cava and the aorta. It is also done over the renal vein in order to begin the dissection with a transverse unfurling of the nodal package, establishing the superior margin of the dissection.

For low stage disease, care must be taken when dividing the nodal package at the 12 o'clock position to avoid the preaortic tissues below the inferior mesenteric arterry, providing all tissue appears completely negative for tumor. This will permit the patient to ejaculate postoperatively. Therefore, the preaortic "split" is confined to the level of the inferior mesenteric artery takeoff and then the tissue is rotated laterally off the great vessels. The lumbar vessels are ligated between 2–0 silk sutures in continuity, then divided. We also place a small vascular clip proximal to the ligatures for added security before dividing them, allowing mobilization of the great vessels off the posterior body wall. It also permits better exposure, ensures better vascular control, and lowers inadvertent blood loss that may occur in the absence of this prospective exposure approach. Of course, it is not necessary to divide the lumbar vessels when doing a node dissection for low stage disease; however, in our experience, this facilitates exposure and completeness of lymphatic clearance (see Fig. 35.2 and 35.3 for dissection boundaries in low stage disease).

HIGH STAGE DISEASE

Normally, platinum-based consolidation chemotherapy is given to reduce or eliminate the tumor burden and then the patient is reevaluated. If the tumor has been eliminated to the extent that a complete remission (CR) is obtained, we simply follow the patient, secure in the knowledge that 10% or fewer will relapse. Furthermore, they tend to relapse by metastasizing into the chest and, therefore, retroperitoneal lymphadenectomy is unnecessary in someone who has truly negative results on computed tomography (CT) scan of the abdomen *after* completion of chemotherapy. When analyzing recurrence in this group, we have found that only one in four patients who does relapse actually will have recurrence in the belly. Therefore, retroperitoneal lymphadenectomy in this group is unwarranted *if* they have a solid CR after chemotherapy.

Unfortunately, about 30% of the patients do not obtain a CR but eventually require postchemotherapy surgery. Any residual mass lesion after chemotherapy should be excised for both histologic assessment and assignment of further therapy in the event of persistent malignant elements. The approach to patients with advanced disease after chemotherapy has been extensively described (9).

Patients with bulky, teratomatous tumors present difficult problems, particularly if the tumor is massive, and even more so if it contains abundant immature elements. The significance of a resected teratoma and its relapse potential is the subject of much interest and current study (10). Regression analysis studies reveal that primary factors in postchemotherapy relapse in teratoma patients are: *(a)* site, *(b)* tumor burden, and *(c)* histologic features of the surgical specimen.

There is a highly significant difference between primary mediastinal tumor relapse and that of lung or abdomen, or lung and abdomen. There is also a significant difference between small versus moderate versus massive disease resected after chemotherapy. Those with the most bulky disease relapse most commonly. Usually, relapse is outside the field of resection, but it also is not uncommon to have relapse occur within the field of dissection, particulary related to posterior body wall foramena, gastrointestinal viscera, or deep pelvic or mediastinal nodes. This has been described in earlier communications (10, 11).

Finally, those patients with cancer in the histologic surgical specimen represent a more difficult group because they do not

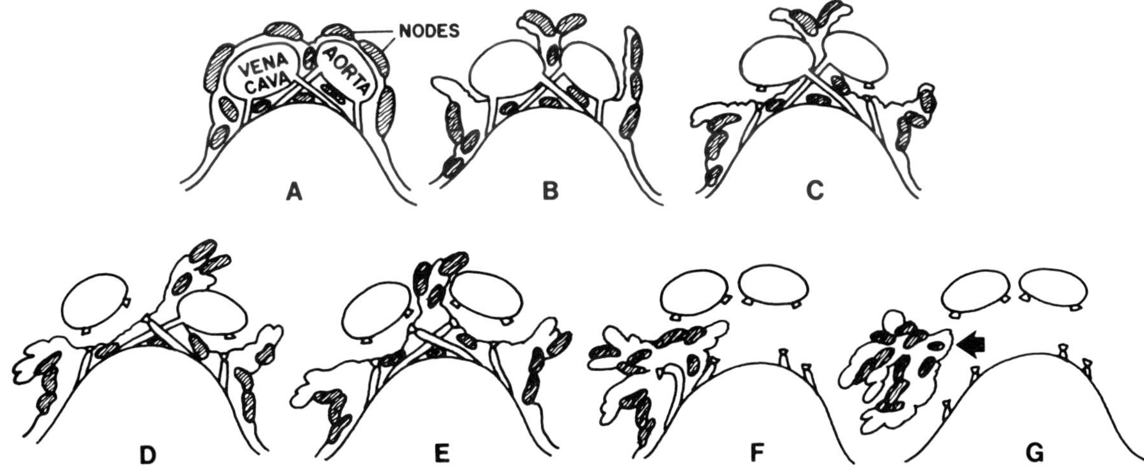

Figure 35.1. Axial view of the great vessels relative to the lymphadic package surrounding them. If one wishes to do a complete bilateral lymphadenectomy, it is useful to divide the lumbar vessels (as pictured in **C, D, E**) and elevate these vessels away from the lymphatic package that has been divided on the anterior surface of the great vessel and then rotated lateral to these. This permits removal of the lymphatic package from the posterior body wall (as pictured in **F** and **G**).

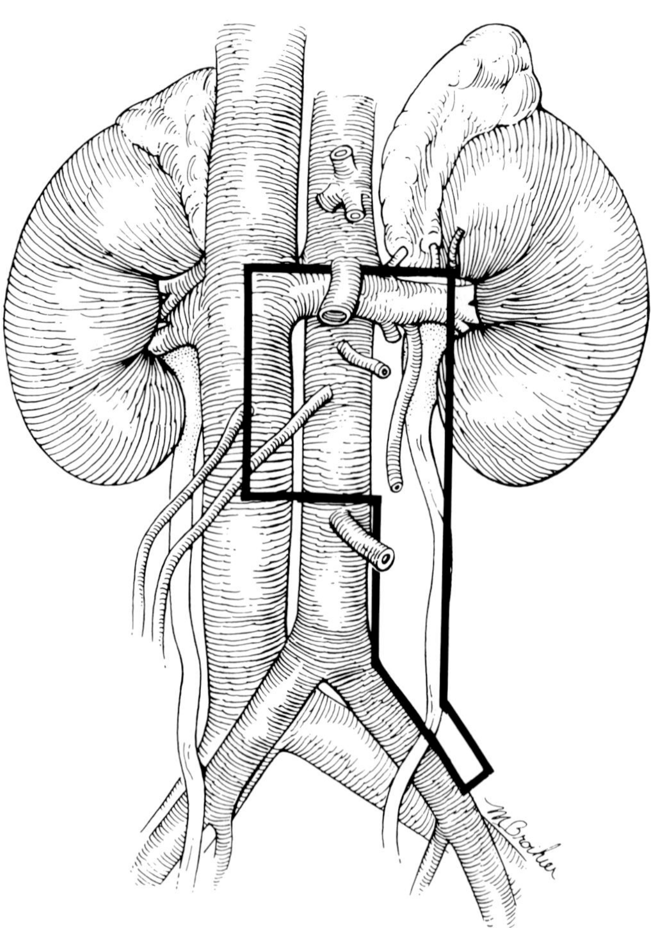

Figure 35.2. Template or boundary of dissection margins for low-stage left-sided testis tumor. The primary zone of spread is left paraaortic. Selection of interaortacaval nodes (right paraaortic) should be limited to a sampling of nodes in this area if one wishes to do a more limited dissection that would permit nerve-sparing of postganglionic sympathetic fibers, especially from the right sympathetic chain. It is critical to avoid preaoritc dissection below the level of the inferior mesenteric artery where many of the sympathetic fibers converge into what may be called the hypogastric plexis.

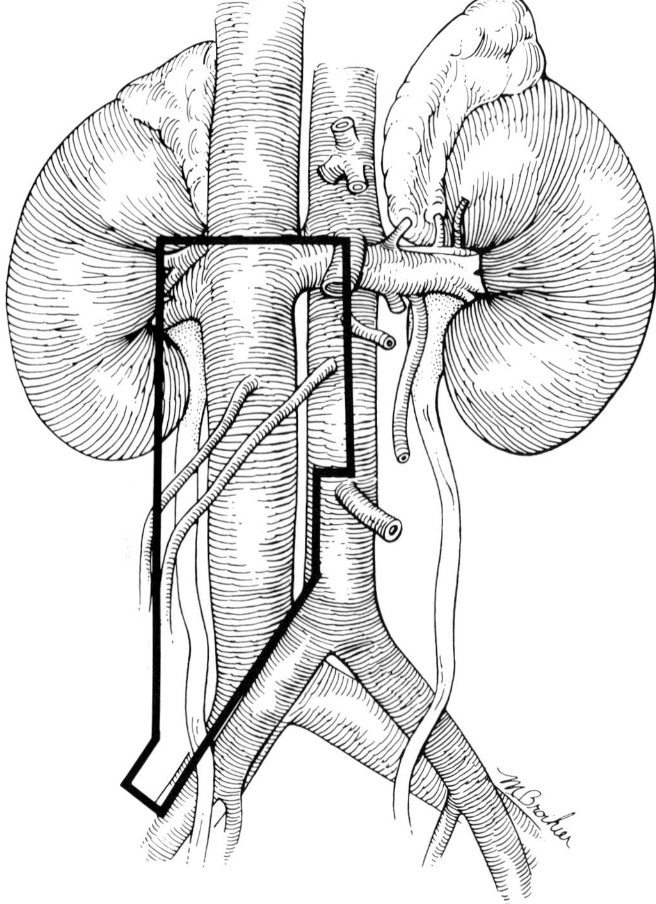

Figure 35.3. Outline or boundaries of dissection for right-sided primary testis tumor. Primary zone of spread from the right side is the interaortacaval zone, i.e., right paraaortic nodes. Again, care must be taken to avoid preaortic dissection below the level of the inferior mesenteric artery. Also, in the nerve-sparing technique, it is possible to identify the postganglionic fibers of the sympathetic nervous system arising from the right sympathetic chain and passing on the medial surface of the vena cava as they decussate in the preaortic zone and continue caudad into the pelvis.

respond as well to chemotherapy. If the resection is complete, they still have a fair chance of cure with the addition of salvage chemotherapy. One of the most difficult subsets in this histologic analysis are those with sarcomatous elements in the resected surgical specimen. Analysis reveals these patients to be at particularly high risk for relapse.

Of considerable interest also, when reviewing histologic findings is the occasional patient with nongerm cell elements in resected tumor. Ulbright and associates (10) have described such elements as adenocarcinoma, embryonal rhabdomyosarcoma, etc. in these tumors. Of interest is the fact that, in most cases, these nongerm cell elements were found in the primary tumors.

In three of 11 patients, primary mediastinal tumor was found to have these elements initially. Another primary retroperitoneal tumor was found to have nongerm cell elements and the remaining cases were found to have primary nongerm cell elements coexistent with the primary testicular tumor. The heterogeneity among germ cell tumors in the testis is becoming well recognized.

New insights are provided by study of tumors resected after chemotherapy. In reviewing 269 cases of teratoma seen at Indiana University Medical Center from 1974–1982, 11 patients with nonseminomatous germ cell tumors (NSGCT) were found to have elements of nongerm cell malignancies as noted above. Apparently, platinum-based combination chemotherapy eliminated the more sensitive germ cell elements, unmasking the remaining nongerm cell elements that persisted after chemotherapy.

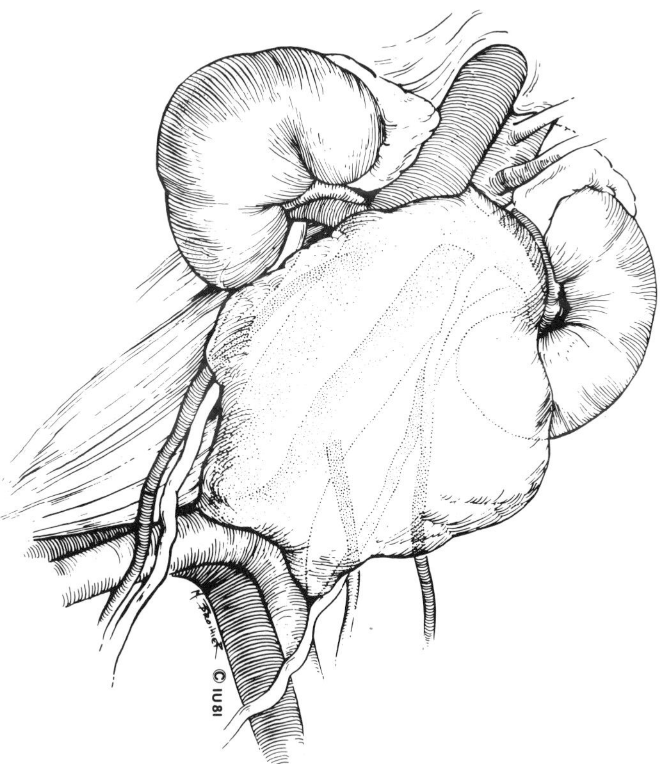

Figure 35.4. Anterior aspect of typical postchemotherapy tumor. Often, this is wrapped around the great vessels.

The technique of resecting the retroperitoneum after chemotherapy is also well described in earlier publications (12). The basic strategy of postchemotherapy RPLND for residual bulk disease is shown in Figures 35.4–35.7. Not only should the tumor itself be excised, but tissues within the original retroperitoneal template of nodal drainage from the testis should be removed as well. Therefore, with few exceptions, a full bilateral RPLND is indicated in postchemotherapy dissections. Normally, the exposure is the same as described for low stage disease.

In most cases, not only is the root of the small bowel mesentery incised but also the posterior attachments to the cecum and the mesocolon of the right side are divided, and bowel is mobilized up and away from the anterior aspect of Gerota's fascia and placed in the chest in a bowel bag. Such cases commonly require additional exposure, therefore, we usually divide the inferior mesenteric vein between silk ligatures and then mobilize the left colonic mesentery. The inferior mesenteric artery is usually divided to complete mobilization of the left colonic mesentery and retract this away from the tumor and the retroperitoneal nodes. Of course, the lumbar postganglionic fibers will be dissected during the preaortic dissection, and most of these patients will not be able to ejaculate if a complete dissection has been accomplished in the lower periaortic zone.

A basic strategy is to begin anterior to the great vessels again either in the iliac or left renal venous area. The longi-

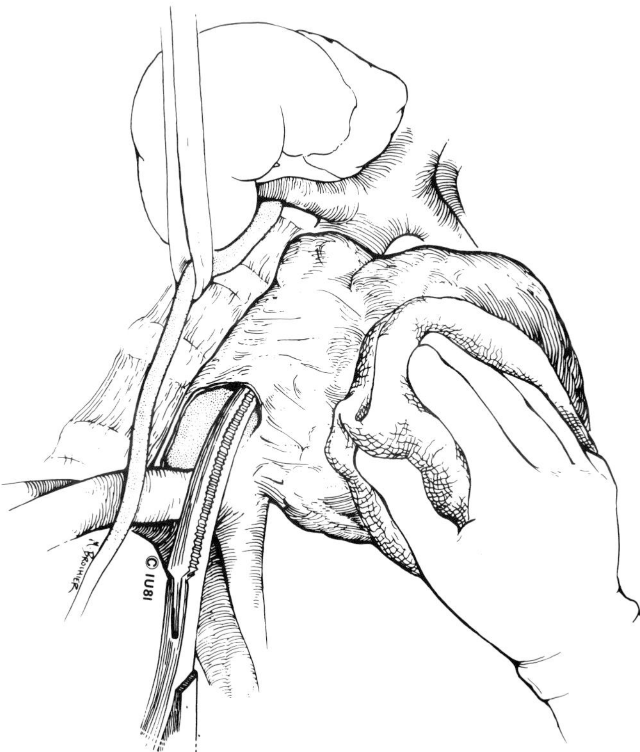

Figure 35.5. Dissection in the subadvanticial plane of the vena cava. This is often required to develop a plane of clevage and to mobilize the tumor off the great vessel. Dividing the lumbar vascular attachments greatly facilitates this.

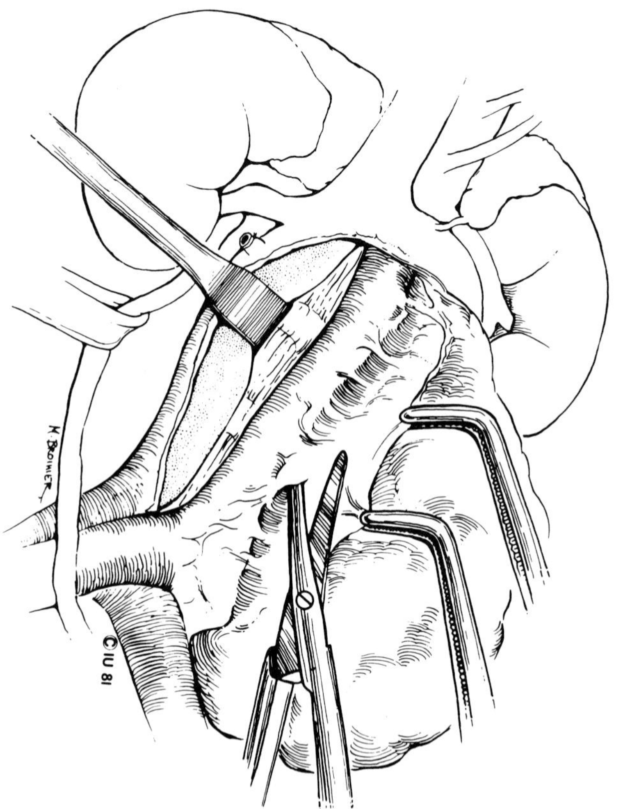

Figure 35.6. Extra or preadventitial dissection of the tumor off the aorta. If possible, the adventitia on the aorta should be preserved so as to give it the necessary strength for suture repair of arteriotomies, etc. Occasionally, subadventitial dissection is necessary but it is also hazardous as noted in text.

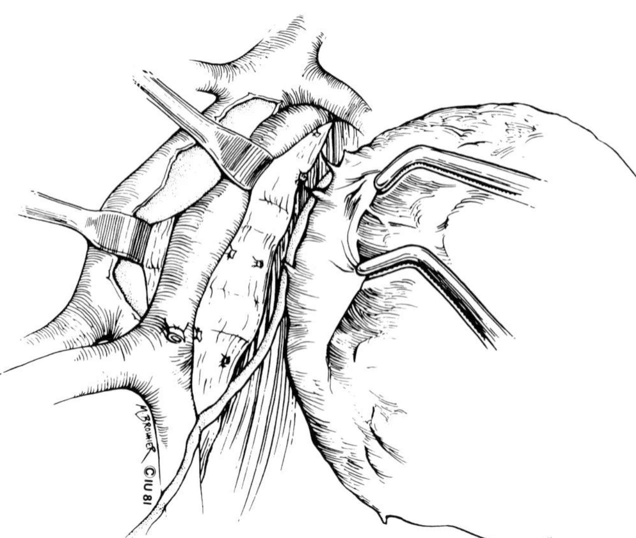

Figure 35.7. Completion of the dissection of the tumor off the great vessels and posterior spinous ligaments and ureter. Placement of right-angle clamps on the specimen assist in the rotation and elevation of the specimen.

tudinal split is made over the great vessels, sometimes with the need to retract tumor laterally as one does so. Dividing the lumbar vessels allows retraction of the great vessels off and away from the tumor and when this is accomplished, the tumor then can be resected from the posterior body wall. At this point, the lumbar vessels are controlled at the foramena with clips, suture ligatures, or both. Bovie cautery, using an extender if necessary, is usually quite helpful in postchemotherapy dissections. This strategy is depicted graphically in Figures 35.4–35.7.

One should note particularly the need for specialized vascular techniques in some patients. We have resected the vena cava in 18 patients in our series, usually because of involvement with tumor. In a number of cases, the tumor extended inside the cava and was found to be inseparable from it. Of interest is the fact that, in postchemotherapy patients, the intracaval tumor may well be cystic and teratomatous, reflecting changes wrought by chemotherapy. The patients with caval resection are at high risk for postoperative ascites and leg lymphedema, both of which are reversible in time.

Care should be taken to avoid a subadventitial plane of cleavage on the aorta, particularly any extended dissection on this plane. The vascularity of the wall of the aorta is much impaired in patients who are left with an extensive subadventitial dissection. We have noted difficulty in repairing arteriotomies and there is a tendency for a vessel to leak or rupture postoperatively if hypertension develops. In five patients, it has been necessary for us to replace such damaged aortas with knitted Dacron graft material (five of over 200 postchemotherapy patients). In each case, the graft was well tolerated and the immediate outcome was favorable.

Another word of caution relates to suprahilar disease, which can take two forms. Direct extension from a massive infrahilar tumor may project into the suprahilar zone. In this case, it is usually precrural and can be rolled down and away from the great vessels. Occasionally, it needs to be removed en bloc, with one kidney or the other being inseparable form the renal hilum. The usual path of lymph flow into the chest from the retroperitoneum is periaortic and posterior. CAT scans have taught us that most suprahilar positive nodal disease is in the retrocrural zone. If this enlarges, it becomes expedient to use a thoracoabdominal approach, reflecting the essential nature of a posterior mediastinal fixed tumor. With early and low bulk involvement, this part of the dissection can be done through the anterior approach, even if it requires splitting the crus for a few centimeters. This can always be repaired by direct suture reapproximation of the crura and the posterior ligamentous attachments of the spine. The cysterna chyli is based anywhere from L-1 to T-10 in the posterior periaortic retrocrural space together with the azygos and hemiazygos venous systems, and it can usually be recognized as such. This must be handled with great care and then suture-ligated or clipped at its base so as to avoid leakage and subsequent ascites. About 1% of our advanced cases will develop postoperative ascites; they usually can be managed conservatively with hyperalimentation and then oral feedings with medium- and short-chain lipoprotein diet. Surgical intervention with peritoneal venous shunting, for example, is a rarely needed alternative to conservative management

Concerning high stage disease, RPLND remains a great challenge. The selection of cases for surgery depends on clinical studies. One could argue that CT scan is must too insensitive in these postchemotherapy patients, but it is reasonably accurate. Our retrospective analysis suggests that of those who achieve a complete remission with chemotherapy alone, less than 5% will ever relapse in the retroperitoneum after chemotherapy. With close follow-up and repeat CT scans, these patients will be detected. This is quite different from the clinical stage I model patient who has not had chemotherapy, for in the best of hands, 20% or more of this clinical stage I group will have positive nodes and relapse clinically. Furthermore, without prior chemotherapy, the relapse in this same group tends to be rapid and fulminating. If relapse occurs in the retroperitoneum in the postchemotherapy group, it usually is delayed in its presentation. Therefore, our own practice is to permit clinical staging in the postchemotherapy patients in order to direct selection of patients for surgery. Those with a radiographic lesion in the retroperitoneum undergo a complete bilateral retroperitoneal lymphadenectomy. Patients in stage II or stage III who achieve completely negative results are followed with interval CT scans (about very 3 months in the first year postchemotherapy, every 4–6 months in the second year, and yearly thereafter for those enjoying a continuing CR).

The same is true for chest disease. We resect persistent radiographic lesions and give salvage chemotherapy for those with any residual malignancy in the resected specimen. If there is scar necrosis or simple teratoma in the resected specimen, we withhold salvage chemotherapy.

At the present time, we are undecided as to whether those with abundant immature elements in a resected teratoma should have further or salvage chemotherapy. So far, we have chosen to withhold further chemotherapy and later, if patients relapse, we treat them with chemotherapy or surgery.

RPLND for low stage disease has been scaled down (Figs. 35.2 and 35.3), modified downward with coincident increase in preservation of ejaculation. At this time, it seems the safest and least risky approach for stage I clinical disease. RPLND for high stage disease is usually extended bilaterally and, at times, requires extensive combined chest and pelvic procedures. Therefore, there is a wide spectrum in the technical demands of RPLND surgery depending on the clinical presentation.

References

1. Lange PH, Narayian P, Fraley EE: Fertility issues following therapy for testicular cancer. *Semin Urol* 11:264, 1984.
2. Loehrer PJ, et al: Teratoma following cis-platinum based combination chemotherapy for non-seminomatous germ cell tumors: a clinicopathologic correlation. *J Urol* 135:1183, 1986.
3. Loehrer PJ, Sledge GW, Einhorn LH: Heterogeneity among germ cell tumors of the testis. *Semin Oncol* 12:304, 1985.
4. Patton JF, Mallis N: Tumors of the testis. *J Urol* 81:457, 1959.
5. Richie J, Garnick M: Modified lymph node dissection in clinical stage I testis cancer (Abstr 179). Societe Int. d'Urologie, Vienna, June 23–28, 1985.
6. Skinner DG, Fraley EE, Donohue JP, Staubitz W: VIII. Surgical standing of testicular tumors. IX. Historical perspectives on node dissection. XI. Transabdominal lymphadenectomy. In Donohue JP (ed): *Testis Tumors,* Vol. 7. International Perspectives in Urology. Baltimore, Williams & Wilkins, 1983, pp. 145–206.
7. Young JD Jr: Retroperitoneal surgery. In Glenn JF, Boyce WH (eds): *Urologic Surgery*. New York, Harper & Row, 1975, p. 848.
8. Fraley EE: Transthoracic retroperitoneal lymphadenectomy for testicular cancer. In Donohue JP (ed): *Testis Tumors,* Vol. 7. International Perspectives in Urology. Baltimore, Williams & Wilkins, 1983, p. 169.
9. Skinner DG: Management of non-seminomatous tumors of the testis. In Skinner DG, deKernion JB (eds): *Genitourinary Cancer*. Philadephia, WB Saunders, 1978, pp. 470–493.
10. Ulbright TM, Loehrer PJ, Roth LM, et al: The development of non-germ cell malignancies within germ cell tumors: A clinicopathologic study of 11 cases. *Cancer* 54:1824, 1984.
11. Van Buskirk KE, Young JG: Evolution of the bilateral antegrade retroperitoneal lmph node dissection in the treatment of testicular tumors. *Milit Med* 133:575, 1968.
12. Whitmore WF Jr: Treating germinal tumors of the testis. *Cont Surg* 6:17, 1975.

Suggested Readings

Chevassu M: Tumeurs du testicule (Thesis). Paris, 1906.

Chevassu M, Prique: Teratoma du testicule. *Bull Soc d Chir* (Paris) 14–60, 1898.

Cooper JF, Leadbetter WF, Chute R: Thoracoabdominal approach for retroperitoneal gland dissection: Its application to testis tumors. *Surg Gynecol Obstet* 90:486, 1950.

Donohue JP: Retroperitoneal lymphadenectomy: The anterior approach including bilateral suprarenal-hilar dissection. *Urol Clin North Am* 4:509, 1977.

Donohue JP, Einhorn LH, Williams SD: Cytoreductive surgery for metastatic testis cancer: Considerations of timing and extent. *J Urol* 123:876, 1980.

Donohue JP, Zachary JM, Maynard BR: Distribution of nodal metastases in nonseminomatous testis cancer. *J Urol* 128:315, 1982.

Donohue JP, Rowland RG: The role of surgery in advanced testicular cancer. *Cancer* 54:2716, 1984.

Fossa SD, Klepp O, Ous J, et al: Unilateral retroperitoneal lymph node dissection in patients with non-seminomatous testicular cancer in clinical state. *J Eur Urol* (in press).

Herr H, Segani P, Whitmore W, et al: Non-operative management of selected clinical stage I patients with non-seminomatous testicular cancer. *J Urol* 135:500, 1986.

Hinman F: Operative treatment of tumors of the testicle. *JAMA* 63:2009, 1914.

Weisbach L, Boedefeld E: Modified lymph node dissection to preserve fertility. (Abstr 180) Societe Int. d'Urologie, Vienna, June 23–28, 1985.

CHAPTER **36**

Operations on the Ureter

ERNEST E. HODGE

Operative procedures on the ureter are aimed primarily at alleviating intrinsic or extrinsic obstruction or repairing urine fistulae resulting as a complication of either primary disease (lithiasis, infection, tumor, etc.) or ureteral injury. In addition to correcting these processes, the proposed intervention should provide for the maintenance or restoration of urinary continuity with allowance for optimal preservation of renal function and the least opportunity for recurrence. Historically, ureteral operations were embarked upon with trepidation due to a high incidence of complications that often resulted in loss of the ipsilateral renal unit. Although by no means totally eliminating such complications, surgical advances during the past few decades have allowed for the successful accomplishment of the above goals with regularity.

An appreciation of the anatomic relationships of the ureter and identification of the "normal" ureter both proximally and distally to the disease process is required to avoid unnecessary mobilization of the ureter and to minimize the risk of inadvertent ureteral injury. Prevention of devascularization of the ureter requires an understanding of its blood supply and preservation of its adventitial sheath, especially in the midureter where the blood supply is most tenuous. Longitudinal ureterotomies are usually preferred as they are the least disruptive of the vascular supply to the ureter.

Before arrival in the operative theater, every effort should be undertaken to assure optimization of the patient as a surgical candidate. Many situations considered surgical emergencies in the past now can be evaluated safely preoperatively, with open intervention occurring in a more elective fashion. Thorough radiographic study will not only delineate the site of pathology, but also will uncover alteration of normal anatomy. Temporary urinary diversion, either via retrograde ureteral catheterization or percutaneous nephrostomy, will often assist in correction of azotemia and other metabolic abnormalities and enhance efforts to treat infection. Currently available broad spectrum antimicrobial therapy allows eradication of even the most resistant organisms, which thereby reduces the chance of surgical contamination from infected urine. In selected cases, the placement of intraureteral stents before surgery is also helpful for localization of the ureter intraoperatively.

Reconstruction of the ureter should be performed with specific objectives in mind. Adequate intraluminal capacity can be assured by incorporating only small amounts of tissue in ureterotomy closure, while the preparation of transected ureteral segments should utilize either oblique incisions or spatulation so that a wide elliptical anastomosis may be done. Ideally, ureteral repairs should be watertight, although the avoidance of vascular compromise is also essential. Tension-free anastomoses are created by sufficient proximal and distal ureteral mobilization. Finally, surrounding the anastomosis with fat, peritoneum, or omentum will help prevent fixation and angulation of the ureter during the healing process.

The appropriate suture material for use in ureteral surgery also should be considered carefully. As a basic principle, small (4–0 or less) absorbable suture material is indicated. Traditionally, chromic catgut has been widely employed in ureteral surgery. Polydioxanone (PDS) is a newer absorbable monofilament synthetic suture that has several appealing characteristics; including longer absorption time, longer retainment of suture strength, minimal local tissue reaction and no increased risk of calculus formation. Controversy concerning postoperative ureteral stenting has generally centered around the attendant complications, such as migration, chemical irritation, infection and calculus formation. However, recent refinements have allowed for liberalization in the use of such stents when appropriate sizes are chosen and they are positioned properly. The commonly used double J stent should be small enough to prevent impingement upon the ureteral mucosa and positioned such that the proximal coil is in the renal pelvis, rather than the upper ureter or infundibulocalyceal system, and the length of the stent should place the distal coil well within the bladder. The surgical site should be drained, especially if there is concern regarding postoperative urine leakage, and the development of closed suction drainage systems has dramatically diminished difficulties historically encountered with wound drainage. Optical magnification and improved illumination obtained with the use of opthalmologic loupes and headlamps has significantly enhanced the accuracy of surgical procedures on the ureter, especially those in the pelvis.

Over the past few years, the indications for open operative intervention on the ureter have diminished, due to the advent and efficacy of endourologic techniques. Nonetheless, it is appropriate for practicing urologists to remain familiar with the surgical principles involved in ureteral surgery. This chapter will focus on ureterolysis for retroperitoneal fibrosis, ureterolithotomy, ureteroureterostomy, and transureteroureterostomy. Operations directed at disorders of the ureteropelvic junction and the ureterovesical junction as well as endourologic and ureteral replacement procedures (autotransplantation, etc.) are discussed elsewhere.

URETEROLYSIS FOR RETROPERITONEAL FIBROSIS

Despite being described by Albarran in 1905, retroperitoneal fibrosis did not gain acceptance as a primary disease process until Ormond reported two cases in 1948. Subsequently, numerous reports of this pathology have appeared in the literature. Whereas idiopathic retroperitoneal fibrosis occurs infrequently, increasing accounts of fibrosis thought to be secondary to suspected causes are being noted. Due to the insidious nature of the disease, accurate diagnosis and appropriate therapy are often delayed.

The exact etiology of idiopathic retroperitoneal fibrosis is not known, although it has been suggested that it may be a form of connective tissue disease and possibly a hypersensitive angitis due to its intimacy with the vascular tree. Methysergide, used in the treatment of migraine headaches has been proven to cause fibrosis in the retroperitoneum and other organs. While lacking the evidence existing for methysergide, association has been described with numerous other drugs. These include amphetamines, lysergic acid diethylamide (LSD), phenacetin, haloperidol, and the antihypertensive agents hydralazine, reserpine, methyldopa, and propranalol. The cause of drug-induced retroperitoneal fibrosis is thought to be due to elevated serotonin levels, although definitive support for this is lacking. Other etiologies of secondary fibrosis include cancer, retroperitoneal trauma and hemorrhage, vascular disorders such as aneurysms, and prior retroperitoneal surgery with the latter two being reported much more commonly recently.

Although approximately 90% of patients will complain of pain, usually a dull backache, there are no pathognomonic signs or symptoms that will expose the disease. The suspicion of retroperitoneal fibrosis is usually raised by radiographic evaluation for unexplained renal insufficiency. The typical radiographic triad upon intravenous or retrograde pyelography comprises proximal hydronephrosis, medial deviation of the ureters in the L-5 to S-1 area, and evidence of extrinsic ureteral compression. If the degree of azotemia precludes pyelography, ultrasound, computed tomography (CT), or magnetic resonance imaging will demonstrate the retroperitoneal mass. It should be noted that radiographic findings suggest the diagnosis of idiopathic retroperitoneal fibrosis, but this can only be confirmed by tissue examination as other processes, especially malignancy, can be indistinguishable.

Treatment is invariably directed at correction of the obstructive uropathy with the intent to normalize renal function. Medical management consists of the immediate cessation of implicated drugs, especially methysergide, as this alone has resulted in complete reversal of the process in some patients. The role of corticosteroids appears to be limited to the unusual patient who presents early with only minimal changes of obstruction and renal function. Nonoperative management of patients with more advanced disease, including severe azotemia, should include ureteral catheterization, which usually can be done with surprising ease despite the degree of obstruction present. The inability to pass ureteral catheters would necessitate placement of percutaneous nephrostomies. However, if one is to consider this form of management for any length of time, a retroperitoenal biopsy should be performed so as not to fail to treat an underlying malignancy.

The overwhelming majority of patients will require surgical correction. Owing to the propensity for bilaterality of the disease, nephrectomy should be entertained only if complete functional loss of the kidney has been documented. Segmental ureteral resection is rarely, if ever, effective and is contraindicated in this disease. Ureterolysis with simultaneous deep tissue biopsy and separation of the ureter from the fibrotic process has become the procedure of choice. The surgical approach is via a midline transperitoneal incision that allows for simultaneous exposure of both ureters. Commonly, even when radiographic evaluation suggests minimal or no obstruction of one ureter, there is still significant periureteral fibrosis found at the time of surgical exploration. Prophylactic ureterolysis is advocated in this setting to avoid the necessity of a subsequent operative procedure. The technique of ureterolysis is described in Figures 36.1–36.7.

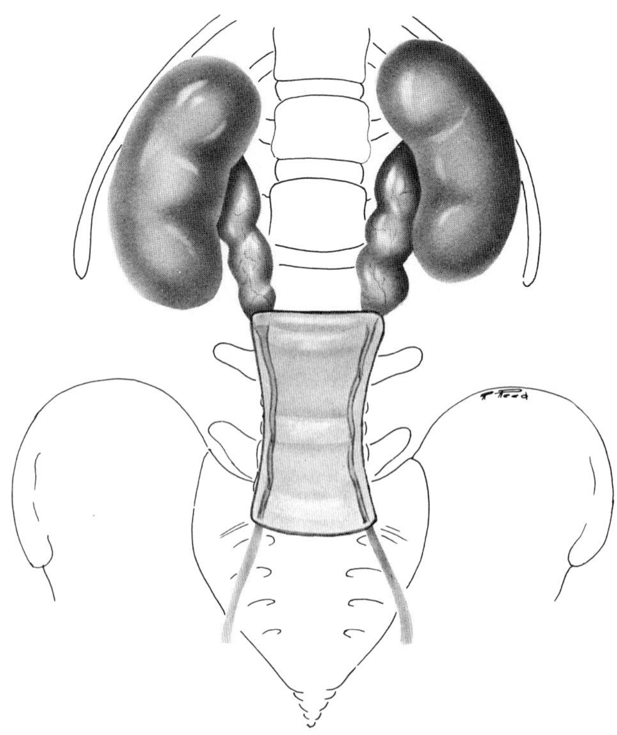

Figure 36.1. *Pathology*. Grossly, retroperitoneal fibrosis is a flat, firm gray-white fibrous mass of varying thickness that may envelop the great vessels and affect one or both ureters. Bilateral ureteral encasement usually develops. At times, the lesion may appear almost cartilaginous or porcelain-like. Although the lesion may extend upward to the level of the kidneys or downward into the bony pelvis, it is found most often over the sacral promontory and is well demarcated. Significant obstruction is usually confined to the middle one-third of the ureters.

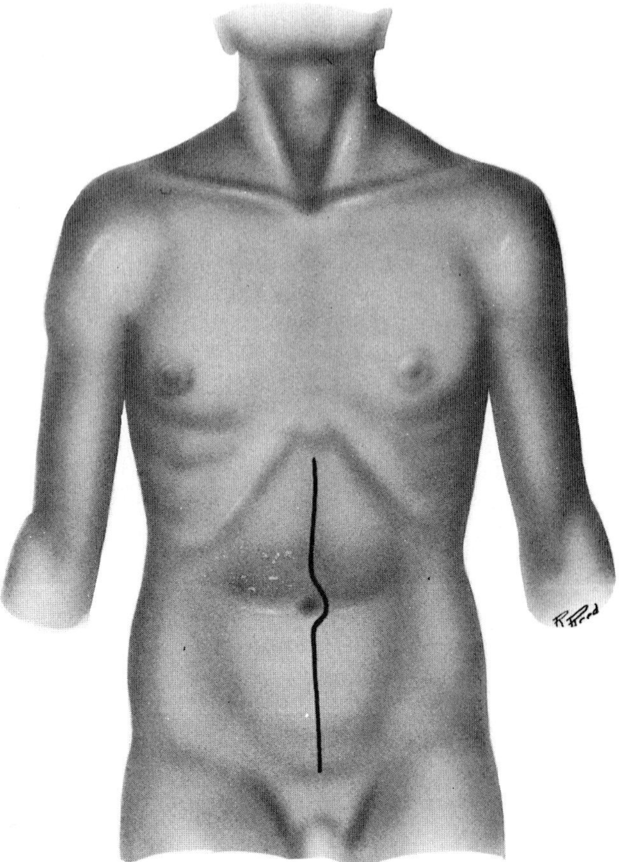

Figure 36.2. With the patient supine, under general endotracheal anesthesia, a midline incision is made from the xiphoid process to just above the pubis, circumventing the umbilicus.

Figure 36.3. After opening the peritoneal cavity, a systematic inspection of viscera should be made to determine the presence or absence of unsuspected malignant disease. The retroperitoneal region is exposed by retraction of the descending colon to the left, the transverse colon superiorly, and the right colon and the entire small bowel to the right. In some instances, the limited size of the peritoneal cavity prevents adequate exposure of the retroperitoneal region by retraction of the viscera; in this event, the transverse colon should be exteriorized to the anterior chest wall, and the entire small bowel should be exteriorized to the right. The intestines should be protected by moistened, folded hand towels or packs. Individual retractors or a self-retaining retractor of the Smith ring type, as illustrated, are appropriately placed to expose the posterior peritoneum. Usually, the posterior peritoneum overlying the sacral promontory and the great vessels is scarred and densely adherent to the fibrosis. In cases where central involvement of the great vessels is massive, with dense fibrosis of the entire posterior peritoneum, it may be easier to reflect the colon medially and expose each ureter laterally from the more normal margins of the retroperitoneal space.

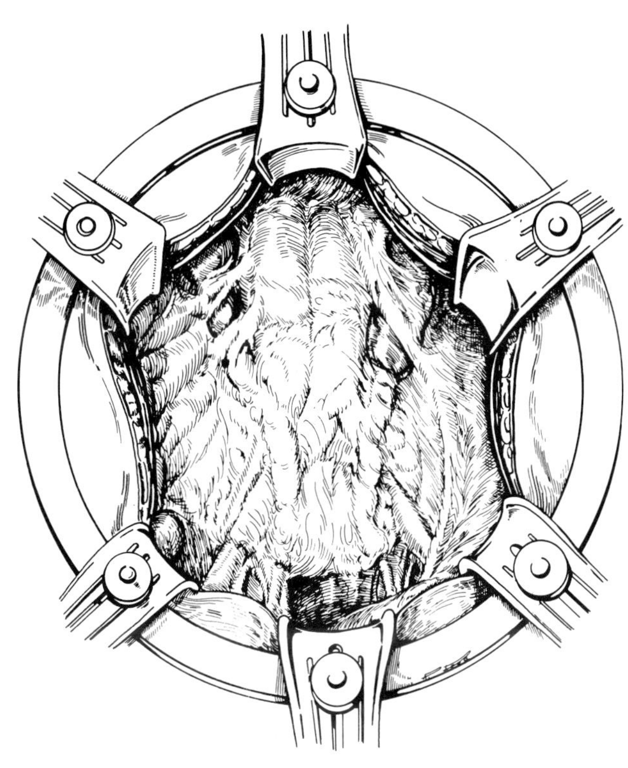

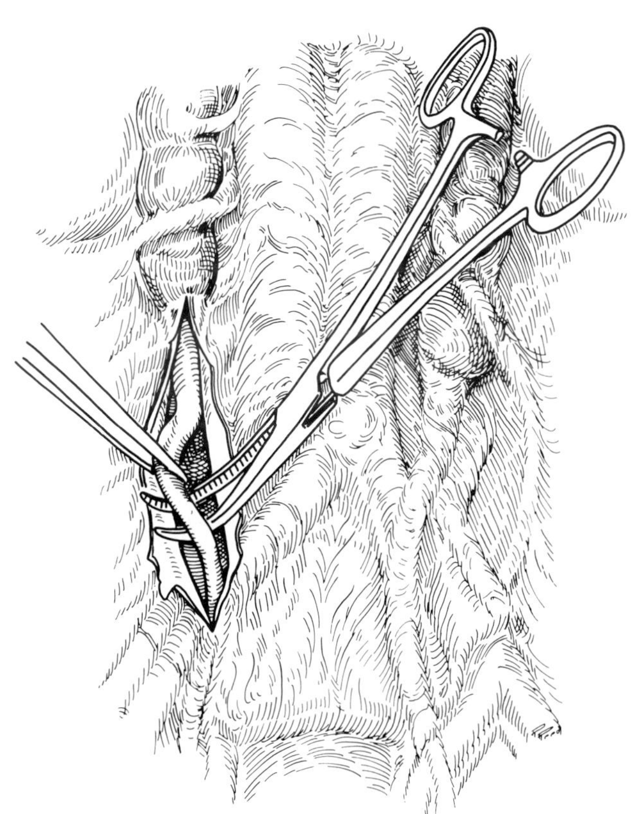

Figure 36.4. The posterior peritoneum is incised in the midline between the duodenum and the inferior mesenteric vein, and this incision is carried inferiorly over the sacral promontory. The duodenum is mobilized and retracted to the right. Flaps of posterior peritoneum are developed and the retractors are placed under these flaps, exposing the entire retroperitoneal region and both ureters. The extent of fibrosis should be determined and a deep and generous biopsy specimen taken from the lesion for frozen section. The dilated and tortuous upper ureters are easily identified. Ureterolysis can usually be accomplished with ease. Mobilization of the ureters is done best by blunt dissection using a right-angled hemostat. The dissection of the right ureter is begun where the proximal dilated and tortuous ureter enters the fibrotic mass. The blunt tip of the right-angled hemostat is placed immediately adjacent to the adventitia of the ureter and inserted into the layer of fibrosis. The jaws of the instrument are gently spread, separating the ureter from the fibrotic tissue. Once an appropriate plane is established, the ureters usually separate easily. However, on occasion, sharp dissection will be required. As the ureter is freed, it will promptly fill with urine; if not, this signifies incomplete removal of fibrotic tissue. While injury to the major blood vessel is usually not a great hazard, as the vessels are well protected by the fibrosis, one would be wise to have adequate amounts of blood prepared preoperatively. The ureter must be lysed completely.

Figure 36.5. The right ureter has been completely lysed and an identical procedure is then performed on the left ureter. Again, the dissection of the left ureter is begun where the proximal dilated and tortuous segment enters the fibrotic mass. If the proximal dilated ureter is tortuous, ureteral adhesive bands should be divided by sharp dissection to ensure ureteral straightening up to the renal pelvis on both sides. The gonadal vessels, although not readily apparent, will be encountered and must be sacrificed on each side.

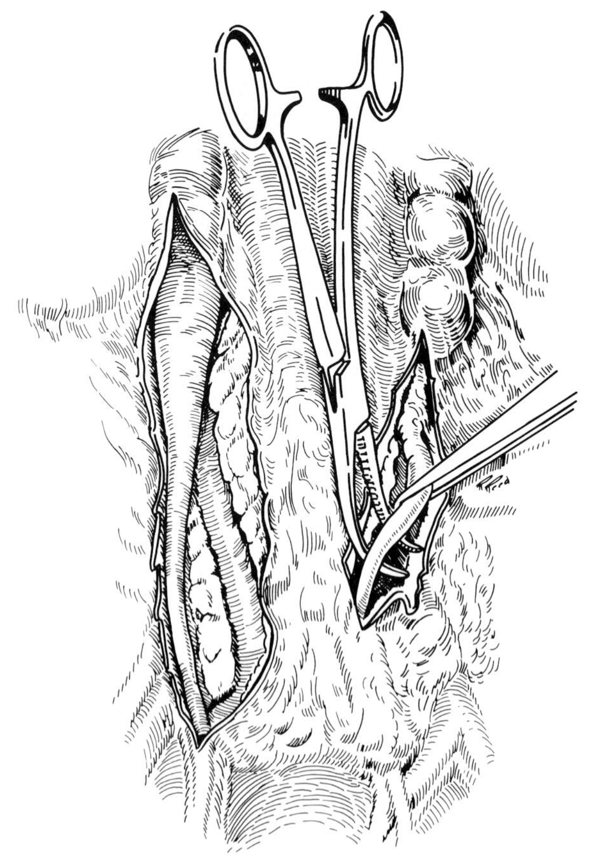

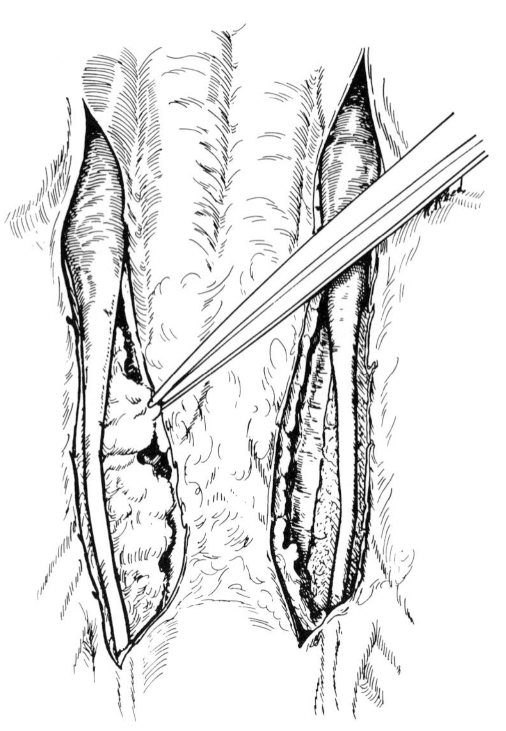

Figure 36.6. When both ureters have been lysed, they may be managed in either one of two ways. The ureters may be transplanted to an intraperitoneal position, or transposed laterally and anteriorly, interposing retroperitoneal fat between the ureters and the fibrosis. We prefer the latter procedure, as shown here, because it avoids the possibility of obstruction where the ureter passes through the peritoneum. Retroperitoneal fat is grasped with straight forceps and placed between the ureter and the pathologic process. Alternatively, omental flaps can be used to isolate the ureters in the lateral and anterior positions.

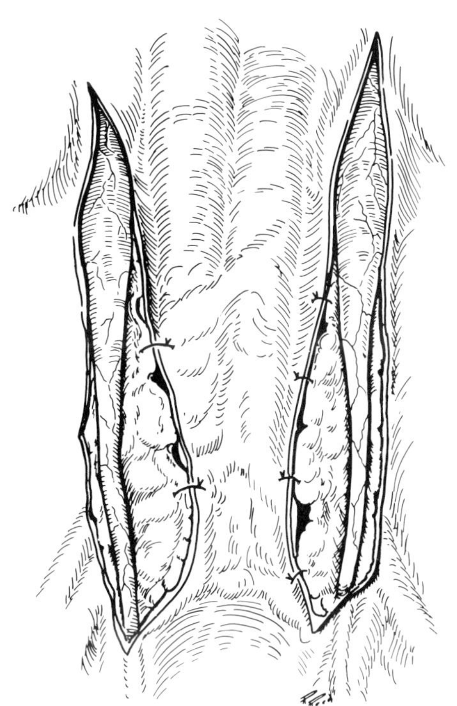

Figure 36.7. The retroperitoneal fat interposed between both ureters and the fibrosis is fixed in place by fine, interrupted sutures. The posterior peritoneum is then closed with a continuous 00 chromic suture and the anterior abdominal wall is closed. Retention sutures are recommended because of delayed wound healing, which can be anticipated in patients with renal insufficiency.

Postoperative Care

Long-term corticosteroid therapy is recommended as it has been demonstrated to be of benefit in preventing restenosis. While many patients will be able to resume oral intake soon after surgery, their nutritional status should be evaluated and early insitution of parenteral hyperalimentation is encouraged, especially if a patient appears destined for several days of ileus superimposed upon previous inadequate nutrition during the state of azotemia. Ureteral catheters, if present, may be left until the patient has recuperated adequately. The patient may even be discharged and the stents removed in the outpatient setting. If nephrostomy tubes were placed, these should be clamped several days postoperatively and remain clamped for approximately 24 hours. If the patient tolerates clamping of the tubes without incident, they may be removed. If difficulties are encountered after clamping, conversion to internal stents via the already established percutaneous access may be indicated. Periodic serum creatinine and blood urea nitrogen determinations should reflect continued regression of azotemia. If this does not occur, it signifies inadequate ureterolysis or irreversible renal damage. Many patients have taken as long as 3–4 months to demonstrate normalization of their renal function. Patient monitoring should be continued on a long-term basis and subsequent radiographic evaluation, usually at 3–6 months, should be performed.

UTRETEROLITHOTOMY

The introduction of extracorporeal shock wave lithotripsy and refinement of various endourologic procedures for stone destruction and removal has relegated ureterolithotomy, once the mainstay of interventional therapy for ureteral calculi, to little more than historical interest. It should be remembered that the majority of renal calculi, including virtually all those that are smaller than 0.5 cm, will pass spontaneously. The practicing urologist should be cautioned to respect the time-honored indications for intervention in patients with ureterolithiasis, such as significant pain, marked obstruction, or infection and avoid the temptation of utilizing newer methods for less compelling indications as the potential for complications is always present. Despite recent advances, there are still occasions (usually because of the inability to otherwise remove a stone with alternative procedures) when an open ureterolithotomy is warranted.

The surgical approach for ureterolithotomy is dependent upon the location of the stone. Stones usually will become lodged in areas where the ureter is most narrow, namely, the ureteropelvic junction, the point where the ureter crosses anterior to the iliac vessels and the ureterovesical junction. Historically, approximately 65% of ureterolithotomies have been performed for stones in the upper ureter while 15% have occurred in the midureter and 20% in the lower ureter. The upper ureter is most commonly approached via a flank incision, either through the bed of the 12th rib or subcostally. Alternatively, there are also many advantages associated with use of a posterior lumbotomy incision for upper ureterolithotomy. Access to the midureter can readily be obtained through an anterior extraperitoneal muscle-splitting (Foley) incision. The lower ureter can be exposed through a midline suprapubic or Pfannenstiel incision. However, our preference is the use of a modified curvilinear lower abdominal incision (Gibson) such as is commonly used for pelvic exposure in renal transplant operations. In selected females, ureterolithotomy in the distal ureter may be performed via a vaginal approach. Stones impacted in the most distal intramural ureter often require transvesical exposure for removal.

Immediately before performing ureterolithotomy, several items deserve the urologist's consideration. The patient should be adequately hydrated with correction of any fluid and electrolyte imbalances that may have developed as a result of nausea and vomiting commonly associated with renal colic. A urine culture should have been obtained and organism-specific antimicrobial therapy should be instituted preoperatively. It is of utmost importance that appropriate radiographs be taken immediately before surgery to assure that there has been no migration of the stone. Figure 36.8–36.15 depict the removal of a calculus from the right upper ureter and the left lower ureter.

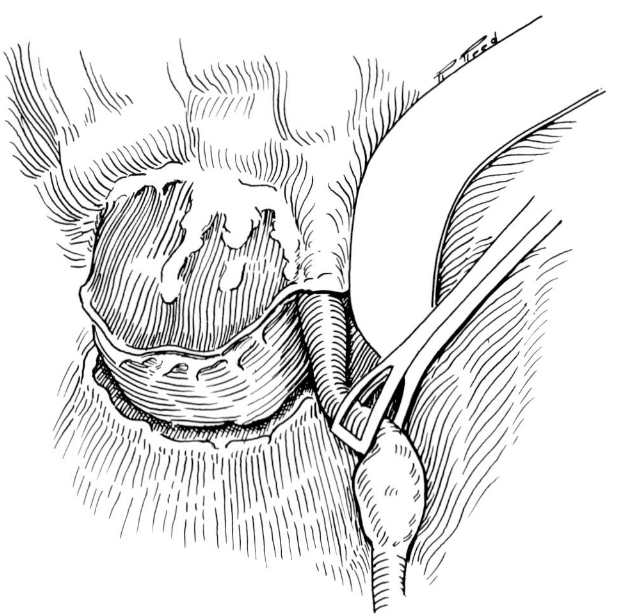

Figure 36.8. After an appropriate extraperitoneal surgical incision, Gerota's fascia is opened and the upper ureter is palpated by blunt dissection above the suspected location of the stone. As soon as the ureter is identified, a Babcock forceps is gently placed across the ureter to provide both gentle traction and to prevent the calculus from migrating back into the renal pelvis, where retrieval may be extremely difficult.

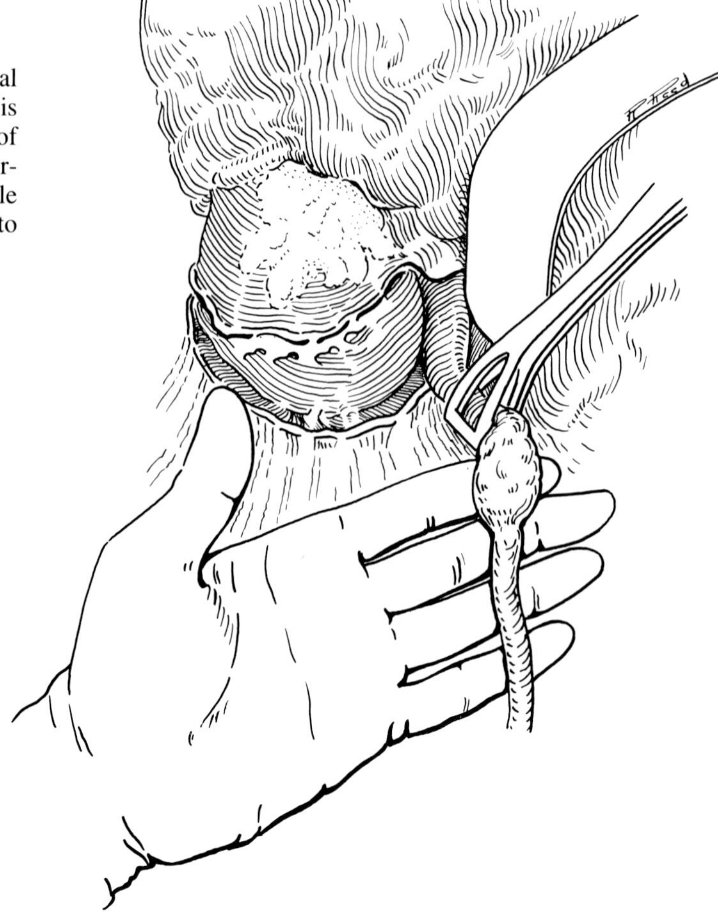

Figure 36.9. The ureter is then dissected bluntly downward to a point where the calculus can be palpated within its lumen. Care should be taken not to damage the muscularis of the ureter during this dissection, nor to devascularize the ureter. The ureter is then gently mobilized and the stone exposed by placing the fingers behind the ureter and pressing the stone forward with the index finger of the operator's hand.

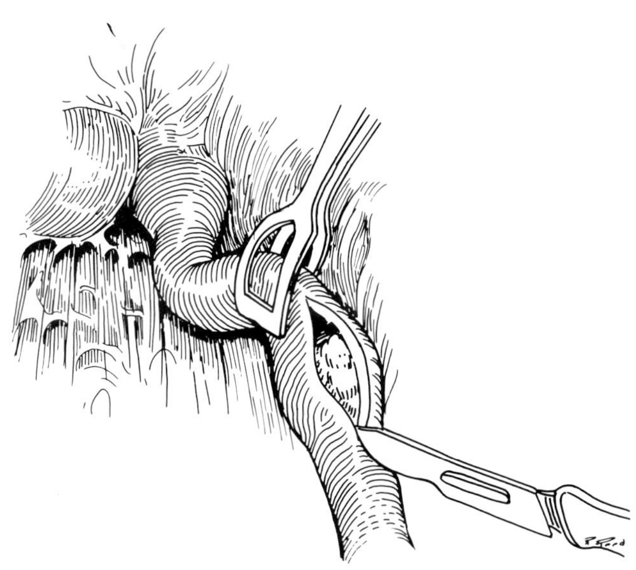

Figure 36.10. A short vertical ureterotomy is then made with the scalpel blade, cutting down upon the stone and taking care not to injure the posterior wall of the ureter.

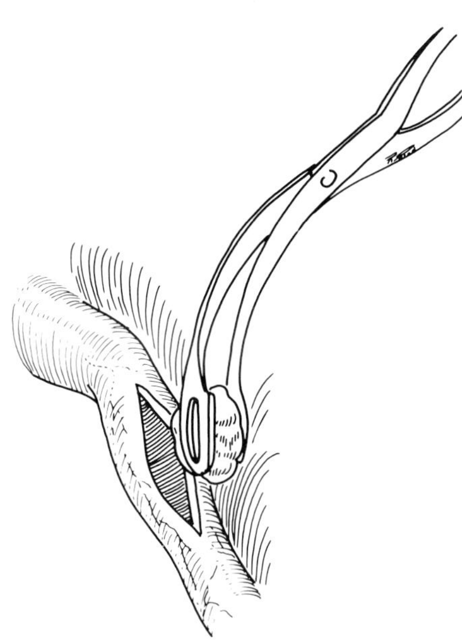

Figure 36.11. The stone is gently extracted with forceps, care being taken not to fragment the stone or to allow calcareous particles to pass down the ureteral lumen.

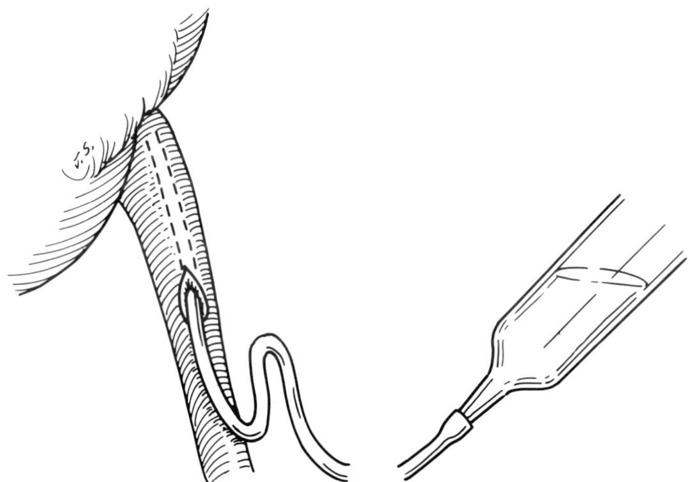

Figure 36.12. The patency of the ureteral lumen is then tested by passing ureteral catheters of appropriate size both upward into the renal pelvis and downward into the bladder, irrigating vigorously with an antiseptic solution as the catheter is withdrawn. If significant edema or inflammation exists, a double J ureteral stent may be placed at this time.

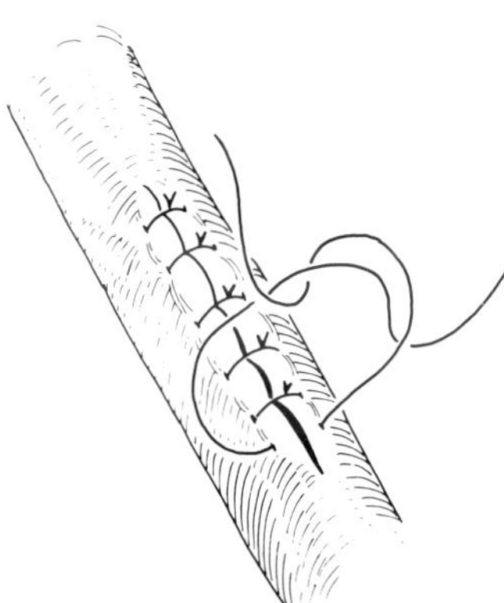

Figure 36.13. The ureterotomy incision is then closed with 5–0 chromic catgut, vicryl, or PDS sutures placed 1–2 mm apart, including only adventitia and a small bit of ureteral musculature. The ureter is observed briefly to be sure that a watertight closure has been achieved, after which a Penrose or closed suction drain is placed down to the site of the ureterotomy and brought out through a separate stab incision in the flank.

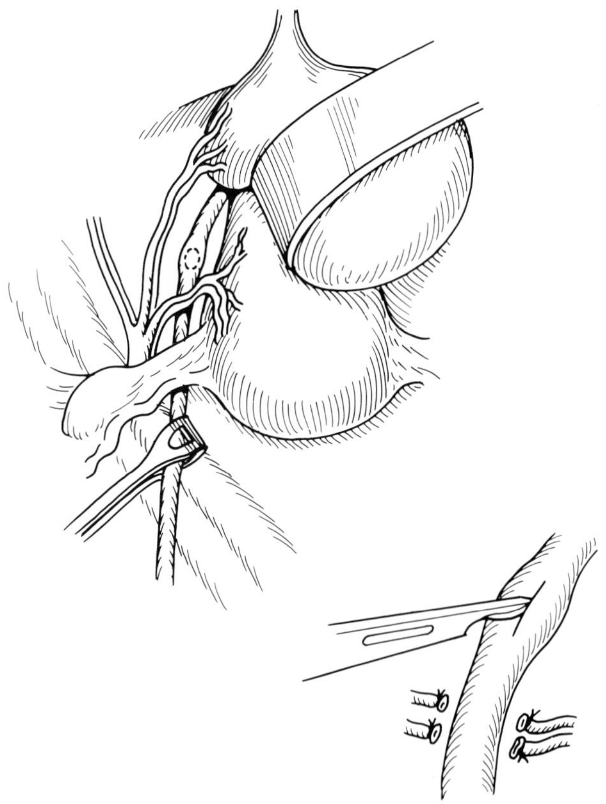

Figure 36.14. During a distal ureterolithotomy, the operation is kept retroperitoneal and the lower ureter is exposed as it courses downward across the iliac vessels. The division of the obliterated umbilical vessels often assist in the identification of the ureter at this level. In this illustration, the procedure is viewed from the head of the table as seen by the operating surgeon. When the stone is known to be located in the lower ureter below the iliac bifurcation, it is prudent to identify the ureter first at the level of the iliac vessels and, again, to immediately place a Babcock forceps around the ureter to prevent the stone from becoming dislodged and migrating upward out of the operative field.

The ureter is then gently dissected away from surrounding structures in a downward fashion while, at the same time, the bladder is reflected medially. The bladder is to be maintained in an empty state with an indwelling Foley ureteral catheter. A fixed ring retractor, such as the Smith ring or Bookwalter retractor, can be of great help in maintaining exposure during this operation. In the female, if the stone is lodged below the level of the uterine vessels, it is essential to secure and transect the uterine vessels before proceeding downward with additional ureteral dissection. This allows for better exposure of the lower ureter and also diminishes operative bleeding.

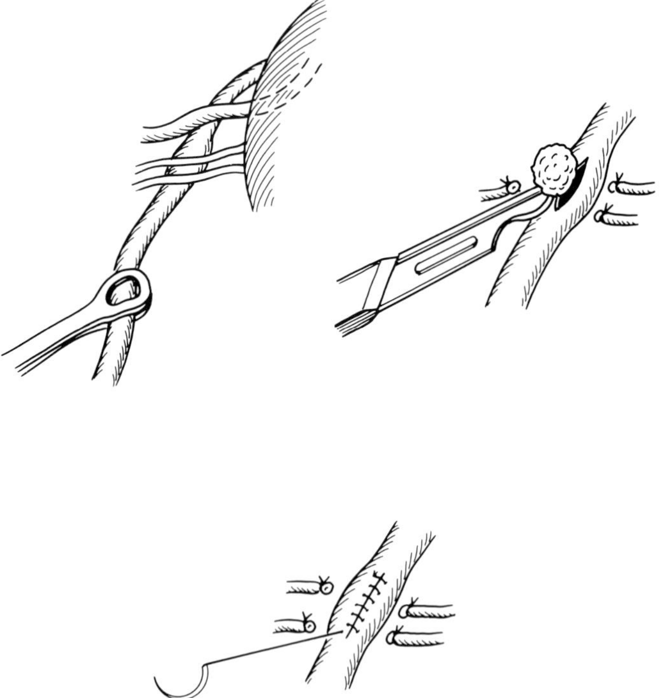

Figure 36.15. Care should be taken not to strip the ureter of its blood supply during downward dissection but to elevate it gently into the operative field with a series of Babcock clamps, maintaining posterior and medial vascular attachments whenever possible. In the male, branches of the vesical arteries must be divided and ligated to gain optimal exposure of low-lying stones, with care also being taken to avoid injury to the vas deferens. At this point, the stone usually can be palpated readily in the lower ureter, and by retracting the bladder medially, the ureter containing the stone can be brought readily into the operative field. An incision is then made sharply over the stone itself with the scalpel, with care being taken not to extend the incision too far beyond the extent of the stone. The incision should be just large enough to tease the stone gently from the ureteral lumen, usually by utilizing the tip of the knife blade with the assistance of smooth forceps.

After removal of the stone, the upper Babcock forceps is released and there should be a copious flow of urine from the upper ureter if significant obstruction was present due to the stone. Again, catheters of appropriate size are then passed upward to the level of the renal pelvis and downward into the bladder to be sure that any residual tiny calcareous debris is irrigated from the collecting system, and also to ensure that there is no evidence of obstruction below the site of the ureterotomy. An internal ureteral stent is placed if indicated, the ureterotomy is closed, and appropriate drains are placed.

Postoperative Care

Utilizing the operative technique described above, and in the absence of massive inflammatory changes or abscess formation around the ureter, healing usually takes place promptly and postoperative drainage is minimal. The patient should remain on culture-specific antimicrobial medications for several days after surgery and a follow-up intravenous pyelogram should be obtained 1–2 months later. The stones should be analyzed, appropriate metabolic studies obtained, and whenever possible, a medical regimen (including maintenance of adequate hydration) should be advised to prevent the future formation of stones.

URETEROURETEROSTOMY

The ability to join ureters or ureteral segments safely to each other has provided the urologist with an appropriate therapeutic option for a variety of situations. Partial ureteral resection and direct end-to-end anastomosis may be utilized for correction of focal ureteral obstruction, for the removal of localized ureteral tumors either in solitary kidneys or other situations where nephroureterectomy may be contraindicated, or for the repair of ureteral trauma. Ipsilateral ureters of a duplicated system may be joined to each other to alleviate obstruction of the upper pole moiety, or to allow for a simpler reimplantation of only a single ureter in conditions where reflux exists in both ureters. We have recently utilized ureteroureterostomy for the joining of duplicated ureters before reimplantation at the time of renal transplantation. In the latter situations, when joining ureters of duplicated systems, extreme caution is indicated during the dissection of the recipient ureter in order to minimize disruption of the ureteral blood supply.

Although ureteroureterostomy has proven to be of significant benefit, it should not be attempted if circumstances do not allow for sufficient mobilization of the ureters or ureteral segments to perform a tension-free anastomosis. Nor should it be performed if the surgical field is involved with active infection, previous exposure to irradiation, or severe inflammatory reaction from any process. As previously mentioned, ureteroureterostomy would not be appropriate in the treatment of ureters mobilized from retroperitoneal fibrosis. Figure 36.16–36.21 describe the technique of ureteroureterostomy after removal of a short segment of right ureter containing a solitary tumor.

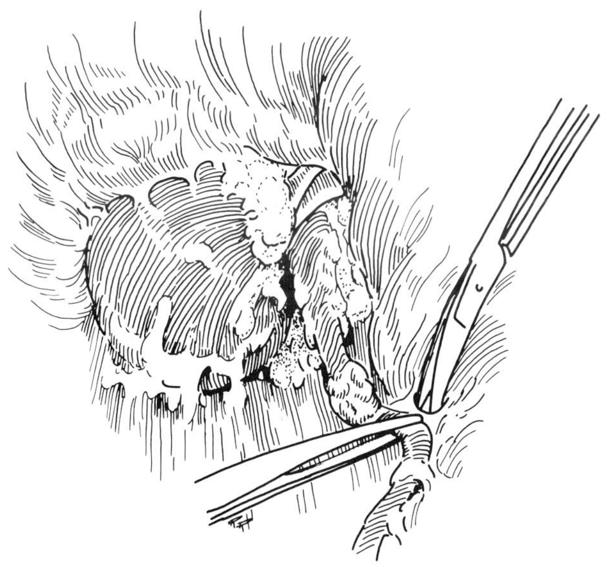

Figure 36.16. The ureter has been isolated by sharp and blunt dissection above and below the tumor, care being taken not to disturb the paraureteral tissues around the tumor itself.

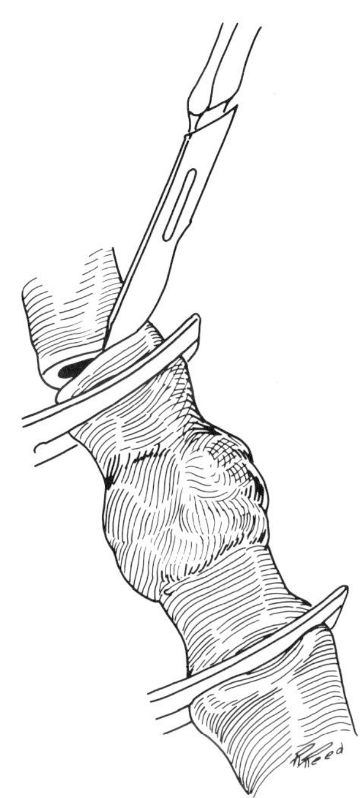

Figure 36.17. The ureter is cross-clamped just above and below the tumor, and the ureter transected with a scalpel as shown.

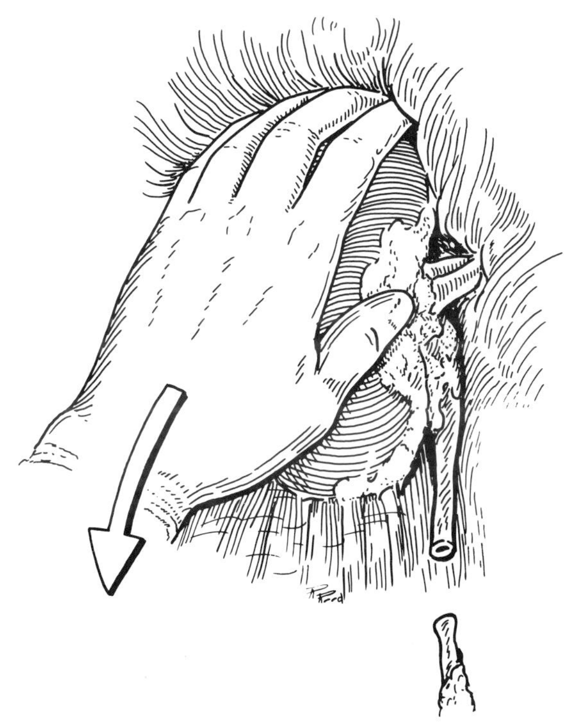

Figure 36.18. The ureter must be mobilized sufficiently to allow end-to-end anastomosis without tension. In some cases, the entire kidney also must be mobilized and brought downward to accomplish this. If the renal pedicle is sufficiently long, additional ureteral length of up to 3.5 cm can be gained by this simple maneuver.

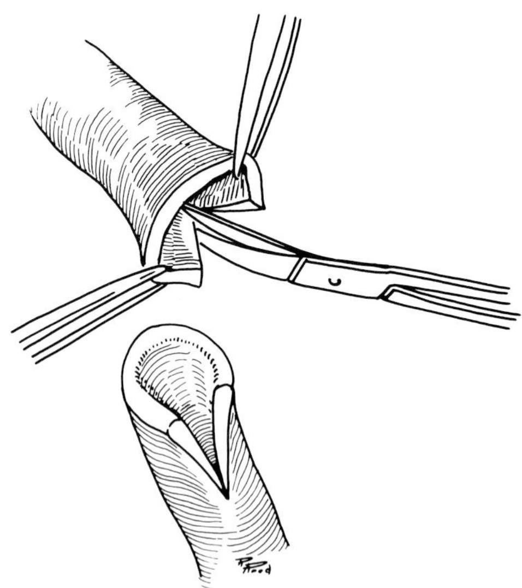

Figure 36.19. Each end of the transected ureter is then spatulated for a distance of 1–2 cm. If an internal ureteral stent is to be left, it should be placed at this time.

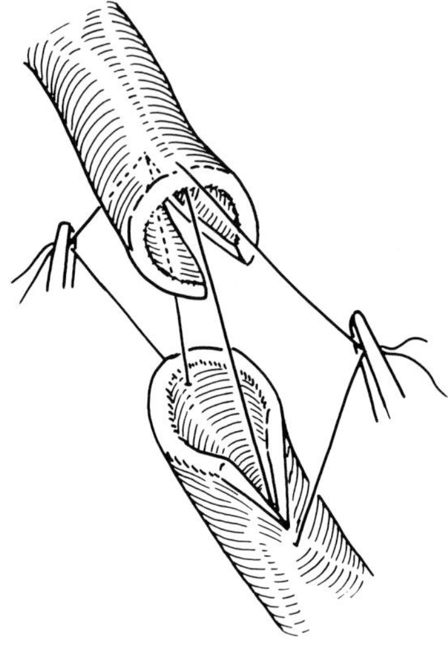

Figure 36.20. Stay sutures of 5–0 chromic, vicryl, or PDS are placed into the apex of each ureteral segment and brought through the midportion of the opposite ureteral wall as shown.

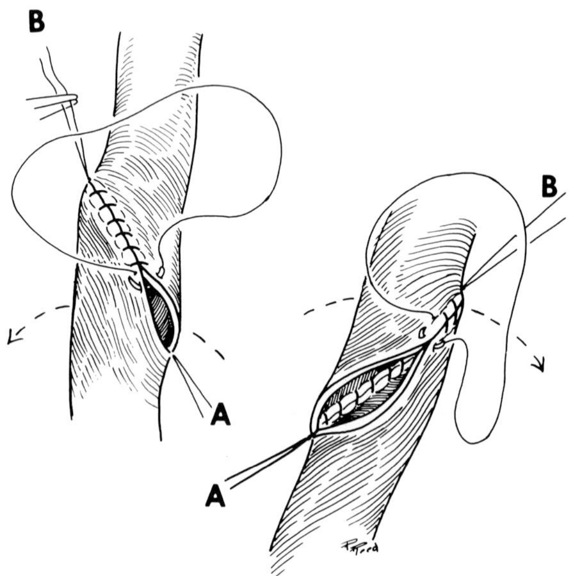

Figure 36.21. The ureteral walls are then anastomosed carefully by either running or interrupting the 5–0 sutures, with each bite being taken approximately 1 mm apart and 1–2 mm from the ureteral edge, and care being taken to approximate the ureteral edges accurately. Ureteral patency and watertightness can be tested by giving intravenous indigo carmine and observing the suture line for several minutes after intravenous diuresis has been instituted. Appropriate drains should be placed and the wounds closed.

Postoperative Care

The surgical drains are removed once drainage from the wound has ceased. An ultrasound can easily assure the absence of any undrained fluid collection or assess the development of hydronephrosis. If placed, ureteral stents may be left for 4–8 weeks with an intravenous pyelogram or retrograde ureteropyelogram being performed before removal. The patient should be followed carefully for the possible development of obstruction or leakage at the site of repair with either ultrasound, nuclear scan, or intravenous pyelogram being performed 2–3 months later.

TRANSURETEROURETEROSTOMY

Despite the description of its clinical applicability in 1934, transureteroureterostomy has been slow to gain wide acceptance due to the concern of potentially placing the normal recipient renal unit at unnecessary risk. Although complications with transureteroureterostomy have been reported, these have generally been in ill-advised settings; and several large reports have documented that, with meticulous attention to the principles described in this chapter, the procedure can be performed with minimal risk. Transureteroureterostomy should be used for correcting problems associated with the lower ureter (as there will usually be insufficient length if one attempts to address problems with the upper ureter) or if there is need to avoid operating in the pelvis. Recently, transureteroureterostomy has been employed in undiversion operations where ureteral length has already been compromised and, again, the procedure can be simplified with the reimplantation of only a single ureter.

Transureteroureterostomy is to be condemned in the same situations that were described as prohibitive for ureteroureterostomy. Additionally, transureteroureterostomy should not be considered in patients with stone disease, upper tract urothelial tumors, or abnormalities of the distal recipient ureter, such as obstruction or reflux. A transureteroureterostomy is best performed through a midline transabdominal incision with exposure of the entire retroperitoneum as previously described (see section on ureterolysis for retroperitoneal fibrosis). The procedure is described below and in Figure 36.22.

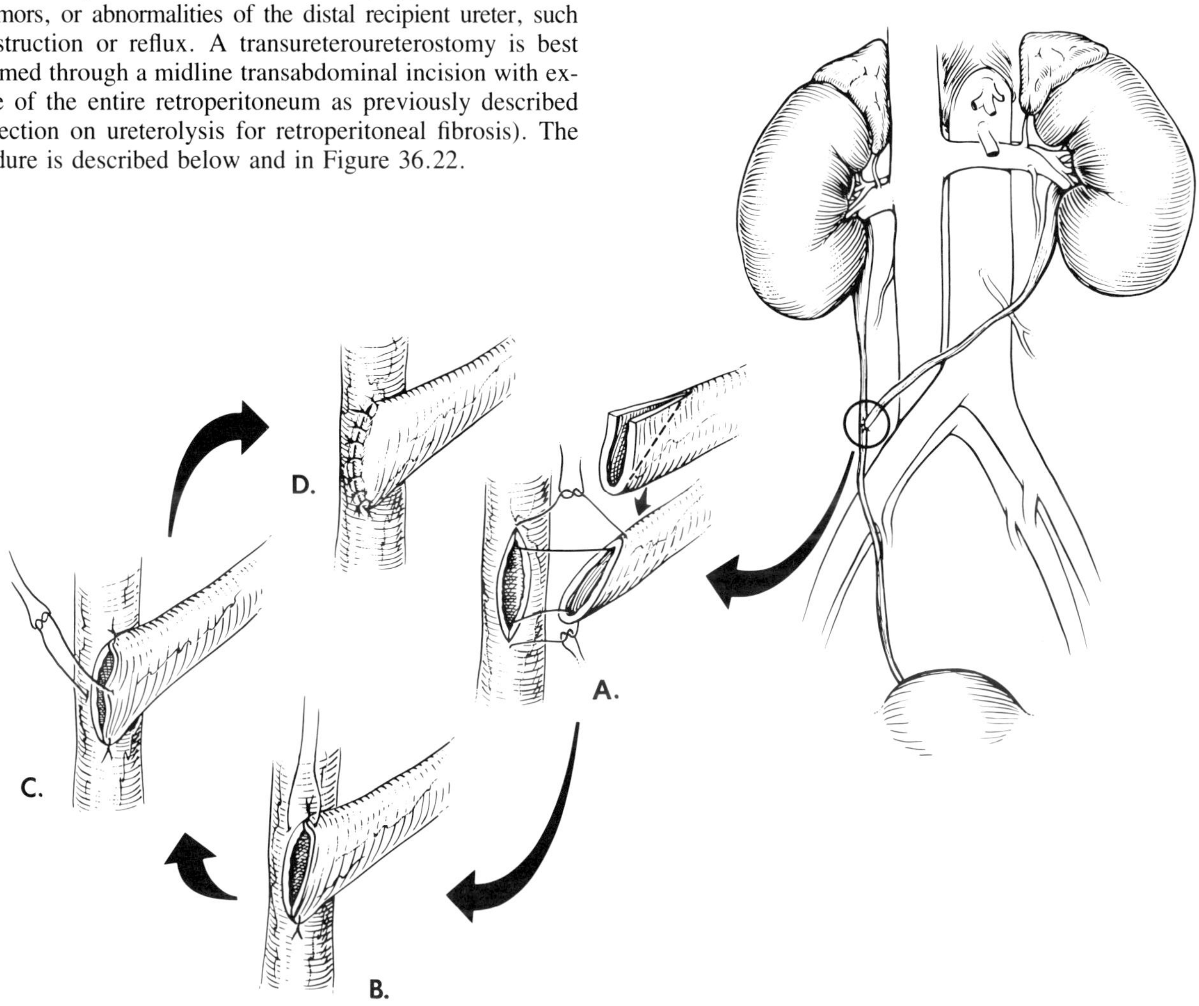

A.
B.
C.
D.

Figure 36.22. After exposure of the retroperitoneum, the colon on the side of the donor ureter is reflected. The ureter is then widely mobilized with all paraureteral tissue, including the gonadal vessels, being incorporated into the dissection, The dissection is carried as far proximally as necessary to obtain sufficient length of ureter for it to be anastomosed to the recipient ureter without tension or angulation. The donor ureter is then passed posterior to the peritoneum and anterior to the great vessels. It is occasionally necessary, especially in left-to-right procedures, to pass the ureter above the inferior mesenteric artery as illustrated to prevent acute angulation at that level. The posterior peritoneum is then incised over the recipient ureter with extreme care to avoid excessive paraureteral dissection. The anastomosis should be designed to create a slight angle at the junction of the ureters rather than the ureters ending up perpendicular to each other.

The donor ureter is then either spatulated or obliquely transected in preparation for anastomosis. Some dilated ureters may already possess sufficient intraluminal caliber without modification before anastomosis. A ureterotomy is then created in the recipient ureter exactly parallel to its long axis with an appropriate length to accomidate the donor ureter. Stay sutures of 5–0 chromic, vicryl, or PDS sutures are placed in the apex of the recipient ureterotomy and in a corresponding position in the end of the donor ureter. If indicated, an intraureteral stent is inserted at this time with the proximal end being placed into the renal pelvis of the donor ureter and the distal end passed through the recipient ureter into the bladder.

The 5–0 chromic, vicryl, or PDS sutures are then used to complete the anastomosis, usually in an interrupted fashion, although the posterior wall of the anastomosis is often easier completed with a running suture. Once the anastomosis has been completed, appropriate drains are positioned. The opening in the posterior peritoneum is then closed with a running 3–0 chromic suture, the reflected colon repositioned and tacked into place with several interrupted 3–0 chromic sutures, and the wound closed in a usual fashion.

Postoperative Care

The postoperative care is the same as described for uretero-ureterostomy.

Suggested Readings

Albarran J: Retention renal par periureterite; liberation externe de l'uretere. *Ass Fr Urol* 9:511, 1905.

Bergman H: *The Ureter,* 2nd ed. New York, Springer-Verlag, 1981.

Bickerton MW, Duckett JW: Suture Materials and Wound Healing, Lesson 15, Vol. 111, AUA Update Series, 1984.

Cass AS, Schmaelzle JF, Hinman F: Ureteral anastomosis in the dog: Comparing continuous with interrupted sutures. *Invest Urol* 6:94, 1968.

Ehrlich RM, Skinner DG: Complications of transureteroureterostomy. *J Urol* 113:467, 1975.

Graham JR, Suby HI, LeCompte PR, Sadowsky NL: Fibrotic disorders associated with Methysergide therapy for headache. *N Engl J Med* 274:359, 1966.

Hache, L, Utz DC, Wooner LB: Idiopathic fibrous retroperitonitis. *Surg Gynecol Obstet* 115:737, 1962.

Hamm FC, Weinbert SR, Waterhouse K: End-to-end ureteral anastomosis: Simple original technique. *J Urol* 87:43, 1962.

Hendren WH, Hensle TW: Transureteroureterostomy experience with 75 cases. *J Urol* 123:826, 1980.

Hewitt CB, Nitz GL, Kiser WS, Straffon RA, Stewart BH: Surgical treatment of retroperitoneal fibrosis. *Ann Surg* 169:610, 1969.

Higgins CC: Transureteroureteral anastomosis: Report of a clinical case. *J Urol* 34:349, 1935.

Hodges CB, Barry JM, Fuchs EF, Pearse HD, and Tank ES: Transureteroureterostomy: Twenty-five year experience with 100 patients. *J Urol* 123:834, 1980.

Koontz WW Jr, Klein FA, Vernon Smith MJ: Surgery of the Ureter. In Walsh PC, Gittes RF, Perlnutter AD, Stoney TA (eds): *Campbell's Urology,* 5th ed. Vol. 3, Chapter G4. Philadelphia, WB Saunders, 1986.

Lapides J, Caffny EL: Observations on healing of ureteral muscle: Relationships to intubated uretertomy. *J Urol* 76:47, 1955.

Nesbit RM: Elliptical anastomosis and urologic surgery. *Ann Surg* 130:796, 1949.

Nitz GL, Hewitt CB, Straffon RA, Kiser WS, Stewart BH: Retroperitoneal malignancy masquerading as benign retroperitoneal fibrosis. *J Urol* 103:46, 1970.

Novick AC: Posterior surgical approach to the kidney and ureter. *J Urol* 124:192, 1980.

Ormond JK: Bilateral ureteral obstruction due to envelopment and compression by an inflammatory retroperitoneal process. *J Urol* 59:1072, 1948.

Straffon RA: Surgery for calculus disease of the urinary tract. In Walsh PC, Gittes RF, Perlnutter AD, Stoney TA (eds): *Campbell's Urology,* 5th ed. Vol. 3, Chapter G4. Philadelphia, WB Saunders, 1986.

Weiss RM, Coolsaet BLRA: The ureter. In Gilenwater JV, Graphack JT, Hawards SS, Duckett JW (eds): *Adult and Pediatric Urology,* Vol. 1, Chapter 26. Chicago, Year Book, 1987.

Utz DC, Moghaddam A: The clinical guise of retroperitoneal fibrosis. *Clin Obstet Gynecol* 10:238, 1967.

CHAPTER 37

Intestinal Ureteral Replacement

ANDREW C. NOVICK

Replacement of the ureter with a segment of ileum was first performed clinically by Schoemaker in 1906 and was extensively evaluated by Moore and Goodwin in the 1950s. The primary indication for this operation is in patients with extensive ureteral damage where urinary continuity cannot be restored by conventional techniques such as ureteroneocystostomy with a psoas hitch and/or Boari flap, ureteroureterostomy, or transureteroureterostomy. This operation may also be indicated in patients with multiple recurrent renal calculi and repeated episodes of ureteral obstruction, to prevent recurrent colic by enabling spontaneous stone passage directly to the bladder.

The ileum possesses several properties that render it suitable for ureteral replacement in properly selected patients: *(a)* it is readily accessible and mobile; *(b)* it can be obtained on a broad mesenteric pedicle that provides good blood supply; *(c)* it has peristaltic activity; *(d)* fluid and electrolyte disorders are rarely observed in patients with normal renal function; and *(e)* complications at the donor site are uncommon.

All patient candidates for this operation must undergo a thorough lower urinary tract evaluation including a voiding cystourethrogram, cystometrogram, and cystoscopy. Any existing bladder outlet or urethral obstruction should be relieved before intestinal ureteral replacement, both to avoid dilatation and stasis in the intestinal segment and to ensure free passage of mucus from the bladder postoperatively.

Intestinal ureteral placement is contraindicated in patients with uncorrected bladder outlet obstruction, urinary incontinence, a neurogenic bladder, inflammatory small bowel disease, poor general medical condition, or a serum creatinine level >2.0 mg/dl. In patients with azotemia, use of the ileum in a closed urinary system has led to hyperchloremic acidosis from electrolyte reabsorption; in such cases, ileal ureteral replacement should be done in conjunction with cutaneous pyelo- or ureteroileostomy.

The ileum is the most commonly employed intestinal segment for ureteral replacement and its use, therefore, is described in this chapter. It is appropriate to state, however, that the large bowel is endowed with similar favorable properties and also may be used successfully in this fashion.

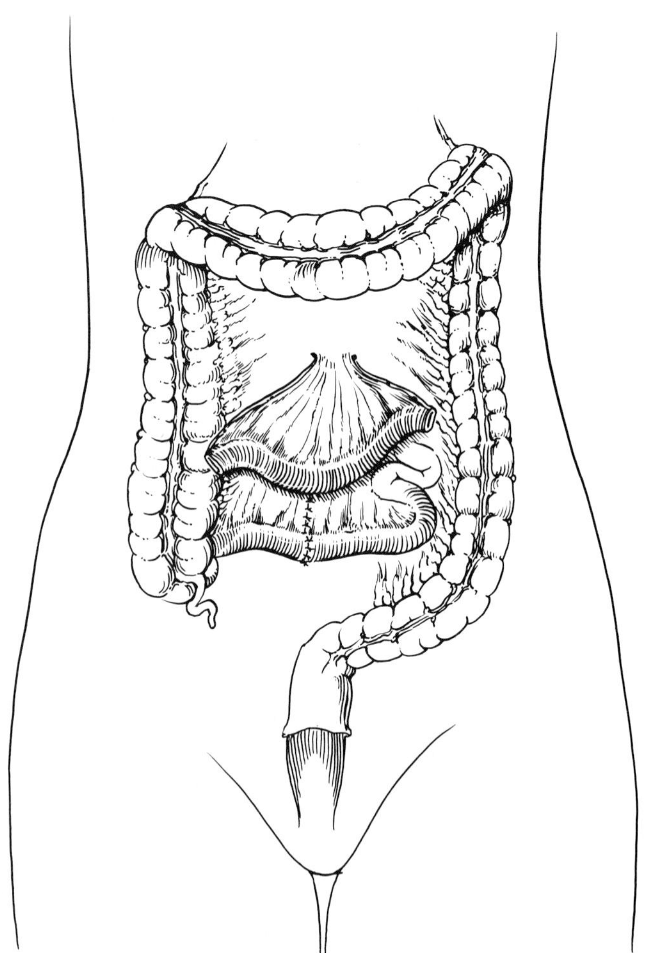

Figure 37.1. The patient is placed on a mechanical and antibiotic bowel prep for 24 hr before surgery. The operation is perrformed through either a midline or paramedian transperitoneal abdominal incision. The ileocecal valve is identified and an appendectomy is done. A segment of ileum is isolated approximately 20 cm from the ileocecal valve to allow the distal end to reach the bladder without tension. The ileal segment should be as short as possible, preferably less than 25 cm, because an excessively long segment may predispose to poor drainage, infection, and electrolyte disorders postoperatively. The mesentery is divided proximally and distally taking care to preserve blood supply to the ileal segment from the last intestinal branch of the superior mesenteric artery. A two-layer enteroenterostomy is done posterior to the ileal segment using an inner layer of continuous 3–0 chromic suture and an outer layer of interrupted 4–0 silk seromuscular sutures. The isolated ileal segment is then irrigated thoroughly with 1% neomycin solution.

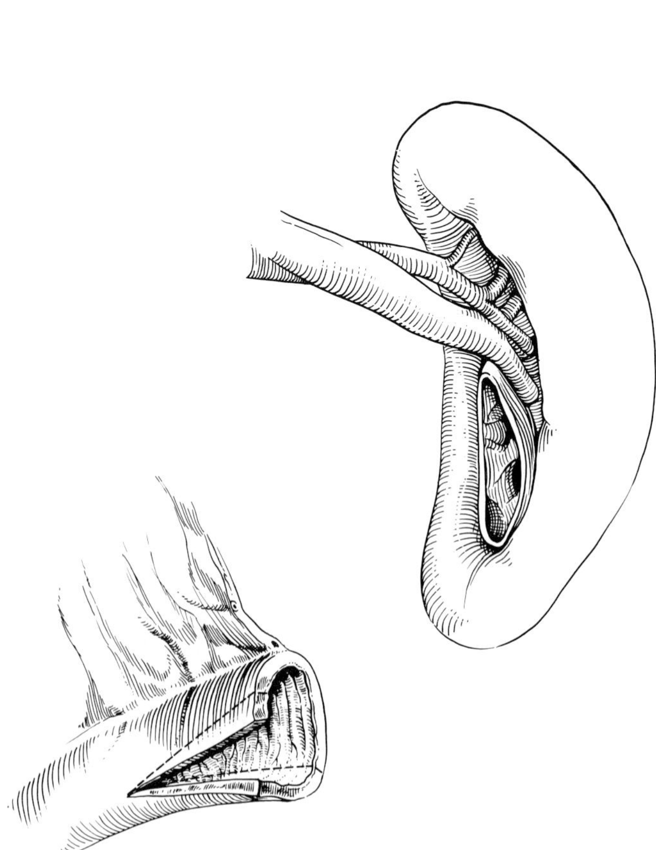

Figure 37.2. The renal pelvis and upper ureter are identified by incising the posterior peritoneum lateral to the large bowel, which is then reflected medially on either side. In most cases, the entire ileal segment is passed through a window in the colonic mesentery to lie completely in the retroperitoneum. Alternatively, only the proximal end of the ileum may be brought through an opening in the mesentery of the colon for anastomosis to the upper urinary tract. In all cases, the ileal segment is used in an isoperistaltic direction. The site of anastomosis of the proximal ileum to the upper urinary tract is determined by the existing anatomy and the specific indication for which ileal ureteral replacement is being done. In patients with multiple recurrent renal colic, the proximal ileum is usually sutured to the renal pelvis, lower infundibulum, and calix to facilitate stone passage through as wide an anastomosis as possible. In such cases, the renal pelvis is opened and any existing calculi are removed from the kidney. A nephrostomy tube is then inserted. The proximal ileum is spatulated in preparation for pyeloileal anastomosis.

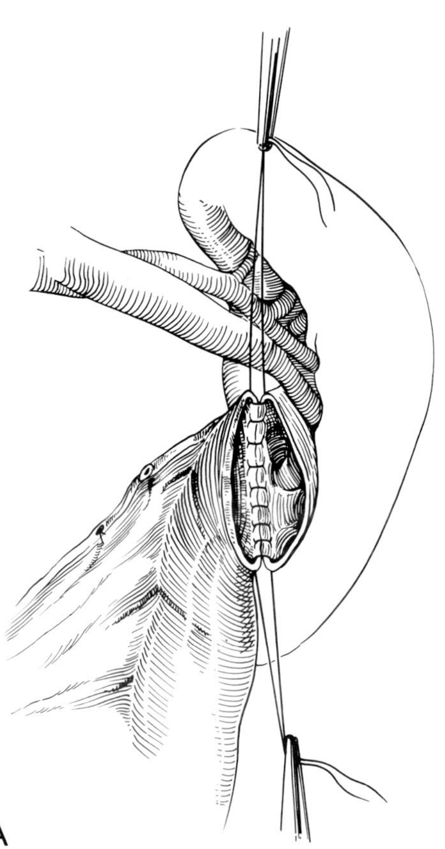

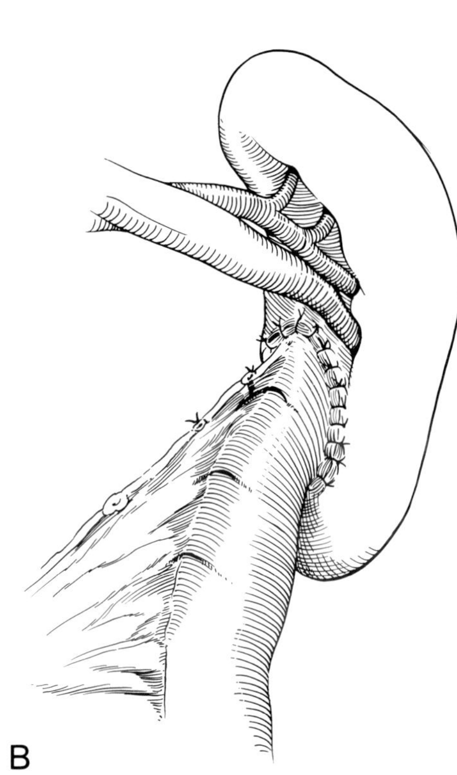

Figure 37.3. A and B, the proximal ileum is anastomosed to the renal pelvis, lower pole infundibulum, and calix with interrupted 3–0 chromic sutures taking care to avoid eversion of intestinal mucosa through the suture line. The ureter may be left in situ to facilitate insertion of a catheter postoperatively in the event that renal pelvic irrigation is necessary. Occasionally, a lower pole partial nephrectomy is also done to ensure a wide pyeloileal anastomosis through which calculi can pass spontaneously.

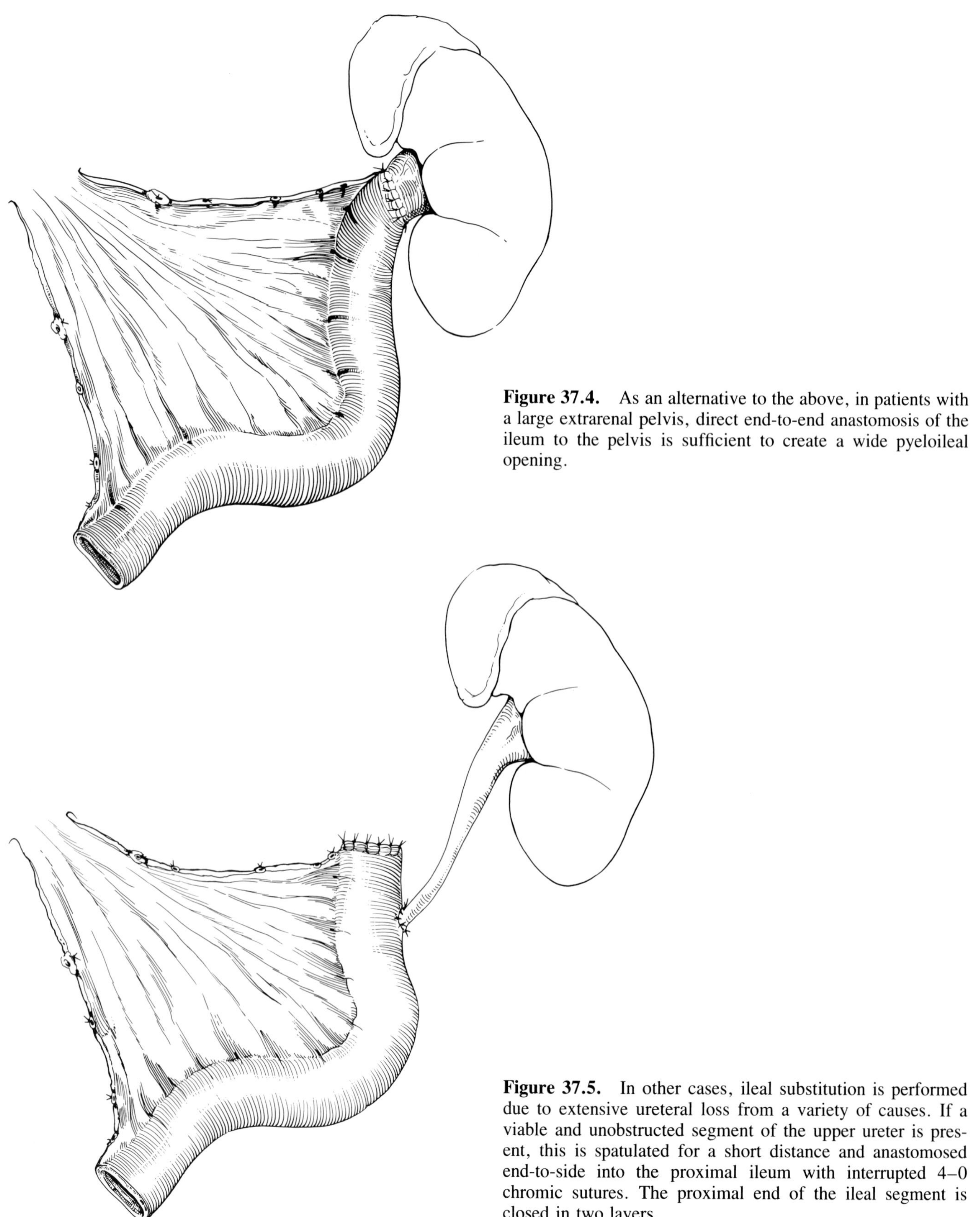

Figure 37.4. As an alternative to the above, in patients with a large extrarenal pelvis, direct end-to-end anastomosis of the ileum to the pelvis is sufficient to create a wide pyeloileal opening.

Figure 37.5. In other cases, ileal substitution is performed due to extensive ureteral loss from a variety of causes. If a viable and unobstructed segment of the upper ureter is present, this is spatulated for a short distance and anastomosed end-to-side into the proximal ileum with interrupted 4–0 chromic sutures. The proximal end of the ileal segment is closed in two layers.

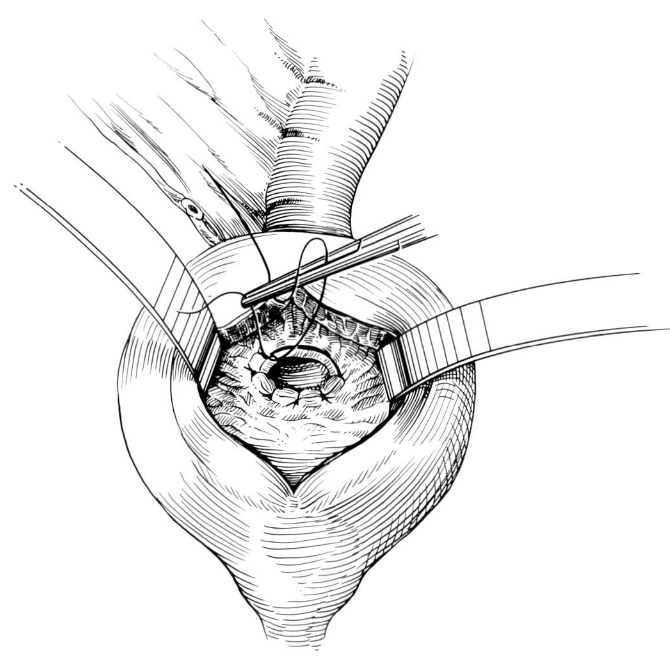

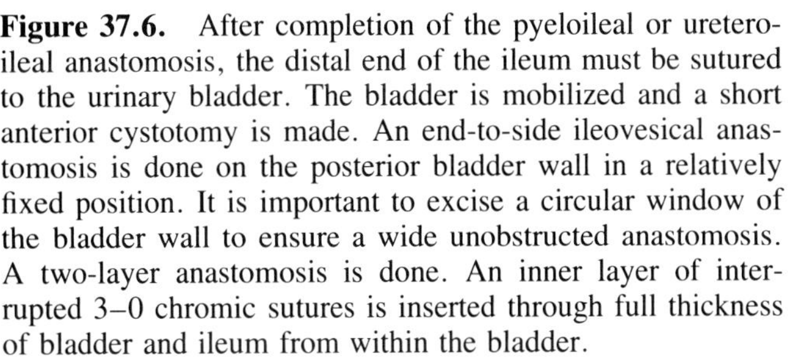

Figure 37.6. After completion of the pyeloileal or uretero-ileal anastomosis, the distal end of the ileum must be sutured to the urinary bladder. The bladder is mobilized and a short anterior cystotomy is made. An end-to-side ileovesical anastomosis is done on the posterior bladder wall in a relatively fixed position. It is important to excise a circular window of the bladder wall to ensure a wide unobstructed anastomosis. A two-layer anastomosis is done. An inner layer of interrupted 3–0 chromic sutures is inserted through full thickness of bladder and ileum from within the bladder.

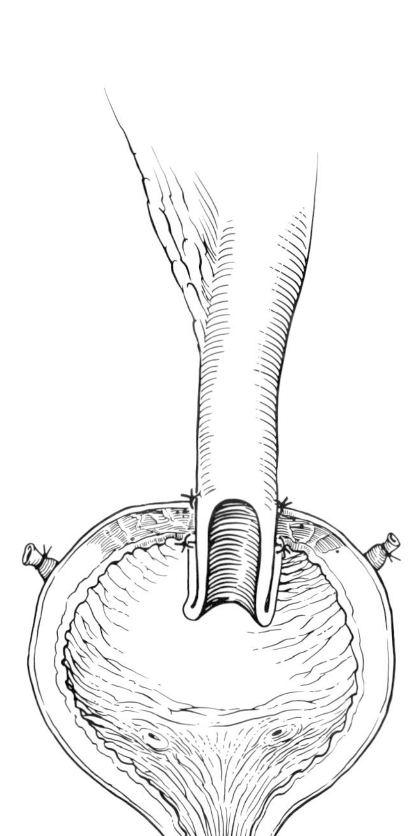

Figure 37.7. An outer reinforcing layer of interrupted seromuscular 3–0 chromic sutures is then inserted from outside the bladder. The cystotomy incision is closed in two layers. A no. 24 French urethral catheter is left indwelling and all anastomotic sites are drained.

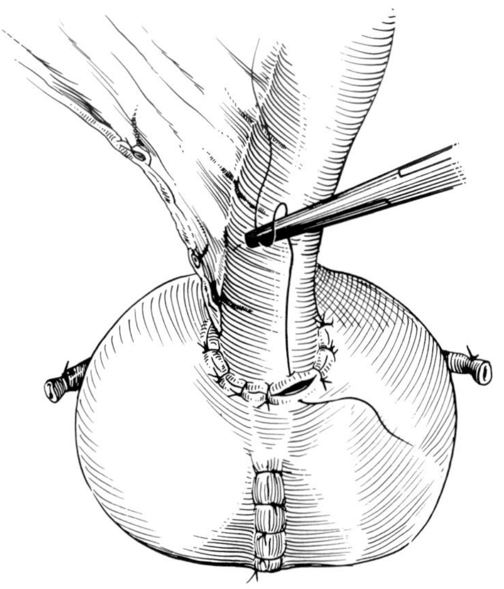

Figure 37.8. An alternative technique for performing the ileovesical anastomosis involves intussusccepting the distal 5 cm of ileum into the bladder to create a nipple that is approximately 2.5 cm in length. The intussuception is done after completing the inner layer of sutures, and the nipple is maintained in its proper position by inserting a second outer circumferential layer of interrupted seromuscular 3–0 chromic sutures. The theoretical advantage of this technique is in reducing or preventing vesicoileal reflux postoperatively. This technique is specifically contraindicated in patients with recurrent renal calculi because the narrower ileovesical anastomosis may inhibit passage of larger stones.

Figure 37.9. This illustrates a completed ileal ureteral replacement operation where the ileal segment has been positioned retroperitoneally by passage through the colonic mesentery.

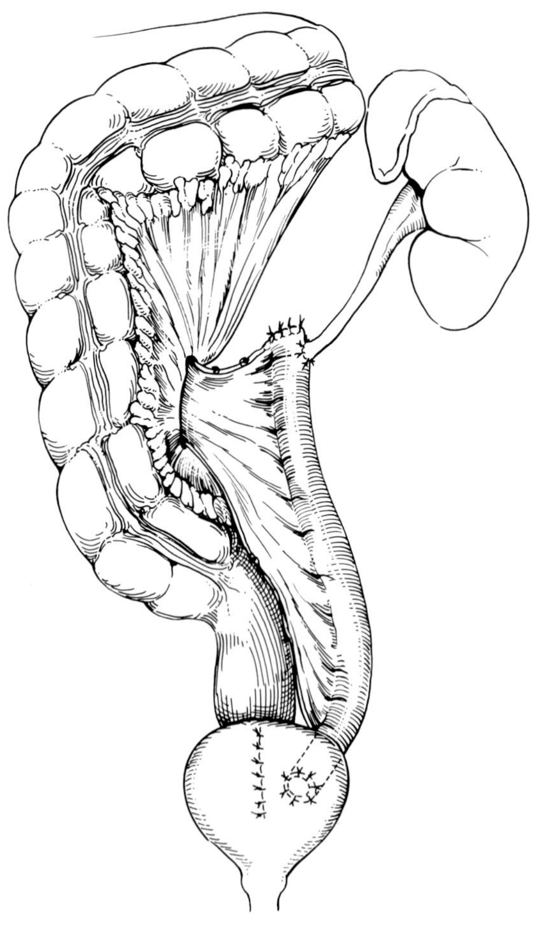

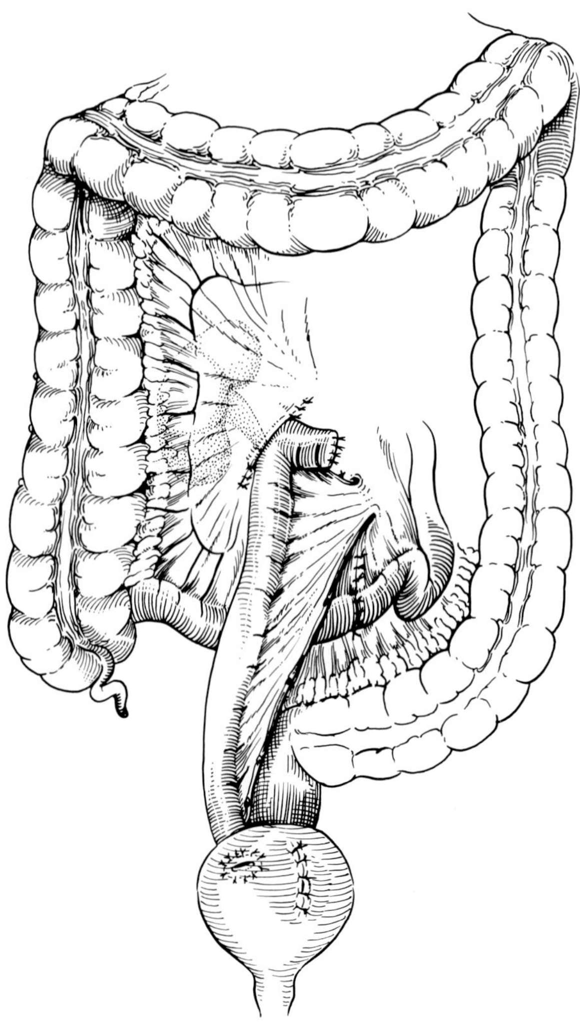

Figure 37.10. This illustrates a completed ileal ureteral replacement operation where only the proximal end of the ileum has been brought through the colonic mesentery for anastomosis to the upper urinary tract. In this situation, the ileal segment is predominantly intraperitoneal in location.

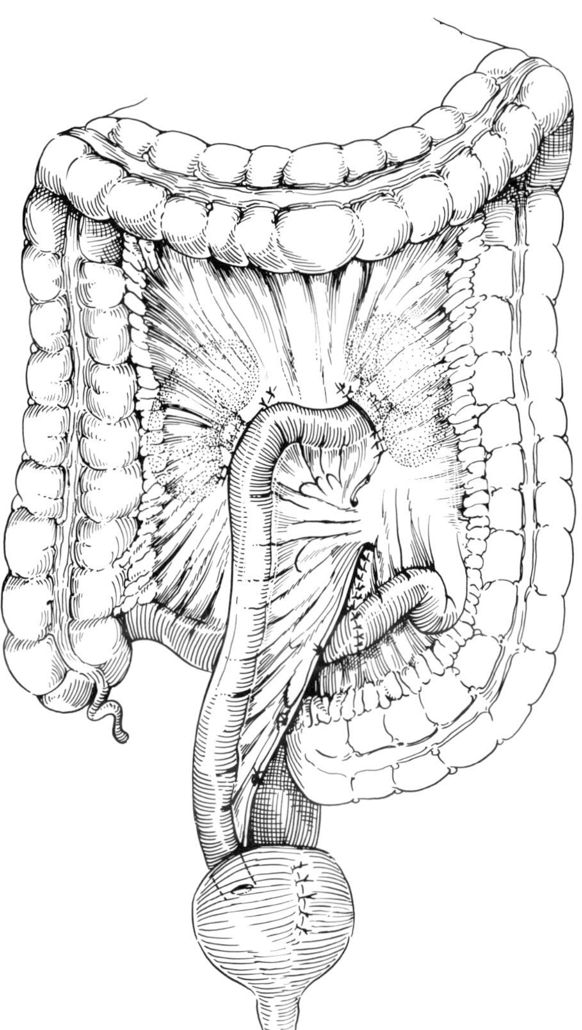

Figure 37.11. A single segment of ileum also may be used to replace both ureters as illustrated in this diagram.

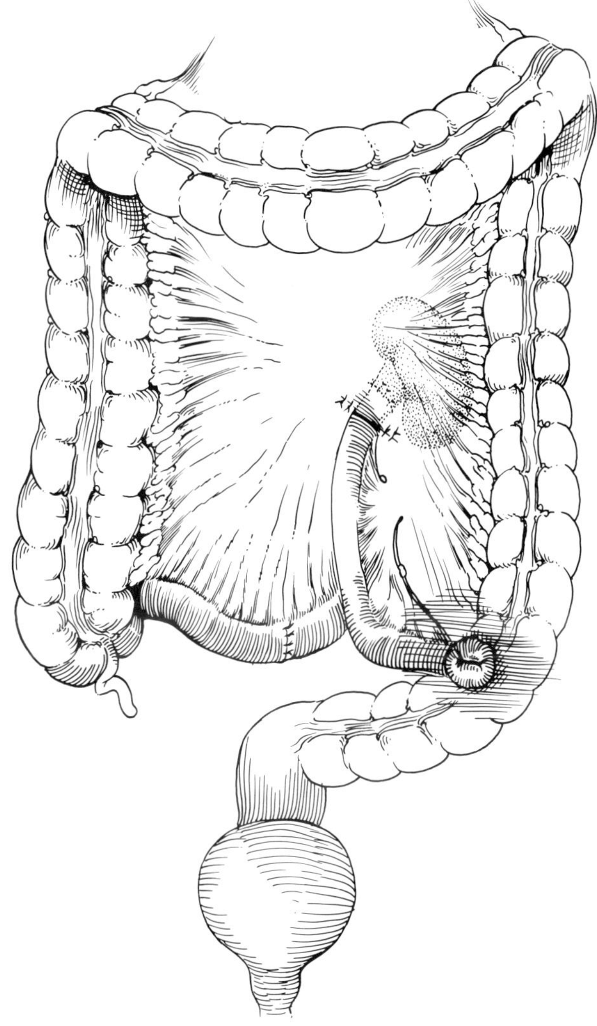

Figure 37.12. In patients with impaired renal function or a nonusable bladder, ileal ureteral replacement is done in conjunction with supravesical urinary diversion. In these cases, the ileal segment generally will lie intraperitoneally and an ileostomy stoma is created in either the right or left lower quadrant.

POSTOPERATIVE CARE

After surgery, urine cultures are obtained on a regular basis and organism-specific antibiotic therapy is administered to treat any existing infection. One week postoperatively, a nephrostogram and cystogram are obtained to ensure no extravasation and unobstructed drainage from the upper urinary tract to the bladder through the ileal segment. The urethral catheter is then removed and the nephrostomy tube is clamped. If this is well tolerated, the nephrostomy tube is removed 48 hours later. The anastomotic drains are then mobilized and removed as well. Six weeks postoperatively, an intravenous pyelogram, serum creatinine, creatinine clearance, residual urine determination, and urine culture are obtained. Patients are advised to void frequently to prevent overdistension of the bladder and dilatation of the ileal segment. Occasionally, mucus secretion from intestinal mucosa may collect in the bladder and predispose to urinary infection, stone formation, or difficulty voiding. Generally, there is progressive atrophy of the ileal mucosa during the initial postoperative months, which leads to a reduction in the amount of mucus secretion.

Suggested Readings

Boxer RJ, Fritzsche P, Skinner DG, Kaufman JJ, Belt E, Smith RB, Goodwin WE: Replacement of the ureter by small intestine: Clinical application and results of the ileal ureter in 89 patients. *J Urol* 121:728, 1979.

Creevy CD: Misadvantages following replacement of ureters with ileum. *Surgery* 58:497, 1965.

Fritzsche P, Skinner DG, Goodwin WE, Craven JD, Cahill P: Longterm radiographic changes of the kidney following the ileal ureter operation. *J Urol* 114:843, 1975.

Goodwin WE, Cockett ATK: Surgical treatment of multiple, recurrent branches, renal (staghorn) calculi by pyelo-nephro-ileovesical anastomosis. *J Urol* 85:214, 1961.

Moore EV, Weber R, Woodward ER, Moore JG, Goodwin WE: Isolated ileal loops for ureteral repair. *Surg Gynecol Obstet* 102:87, 1956.

Prout GR, Stuart WT, Witus WS: Utilization of ileal segments for extensive ureteral loss. *J Urol* 90:541, 1963.

Schoemaker J: Discussie op voordracht van J. M. van dam over intrabdominale plasticken. *Ned Tijdschr Geneeskd,* 1911, Pg. 386.

Skinner DG, Goodwin WE: Indications for the use of intestinal segments in management of nephrocalcinosis. *J Urol* 113:436, 1975.

Struthers NJ, Scott R: Reconstruction of the upper ureter with colon. *J Urol* 112:179, 1974.

Tanagho EA: A case against incorporation of bowel segments into the closed urinary system. *J Urol* 113:796, 1975.

CHAPTER 38

Endourologic Techniques for the Ureter

STEVAN B. STREEM

The recent development of endoscopic equipment designed to provide the urologist with access to the upper tract has already revolutionized the management of many common urologic disorders, such as ureteral calculus disease and stricture. Furthermore, this technology is now being applied with increasing frequency to the diagnosis and management of urothelial malignancies. Whereas upper tract endoscopy offers several advantages both diagnostically and therapeutically for many patients, there are inherent risks in the procedure. In most cases, potential complications are best avoided by careful patient selection, thorough familiarity and experience with the equipment, and patience on the part of the endoscopist.

PATIENT PREPARATION

Ureteroscopy is generally performed with a general, spinal, or epidural anesthetic. Therefore, the patient is placed "NPO" (nothing by mouth) after midnight. Urinary infection is treated vigorously before instrumentation as the continuous irrigation required for the procedure otherwise could result in bacteremia, sepsis, or pyelonephritis. In fact, patients presenting with urinary sepsis resulting from a ureteral calculus or other obstructing lesions often are managed best initially simply by establishing percutaneous nephrostomy drainage. In patients without urinary tract infection, prophylactic antibiotics have not yet proven to be required.

As ureteral perforation or even disruption are well-defined complications of this procedure, the patient should be counseled preoperatively as to the potential need for an emergent procedure, such as percutaneous nephrostomy placement or even "open" intervention. The patient should also be warned that ureteroscopy is not always successful in gaining adequate access to the lesion, be it a stone, stricture, or tumor. In that way, the endoscopist will not feel compelled to force the instruments cephaled in those cases where it does not go easily. Perhaps the single most successful way to prevent the complications of ureteroscopy is knowing when to terminate the procedure.

MANAGEMENT OF UPPER AND MIDURETERAL CALCULI

As mentioned in chapter 15, most upper and midureteral calculi are managed best by retrograde flushing of the calculus and placement of internal stents followed by extracorporeal shock wave lithotripsy (ESWL). However, in some patients, an impacted stone will be resistant to such treatment and ureteroscopic management is required. Ureteroscopy is also valuable for patients requiring intervention for obstructing ureteral fragments after ESWL.

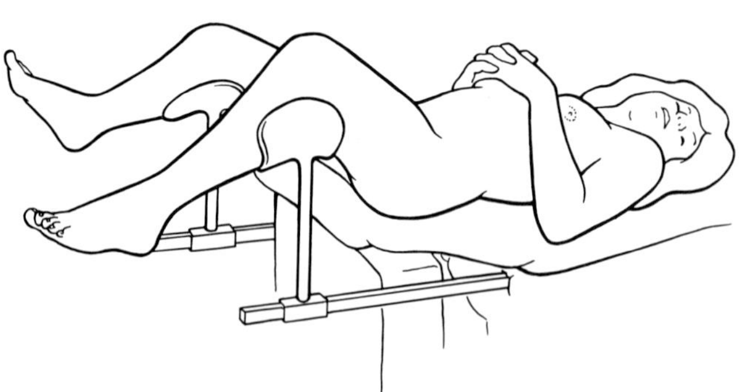

Figure 38.1. The patient is placed in the dorsal lithotomy position. Exaggerated abduction of the contralateral leg will facilitate introduction of the ureterscope. After cystoscopic examination, a ''bulb tip'' retrograde pyelogram is attained to define the pathology and course of the ureter. Fluoroscopic monitoring will be essential throughout the procedure.

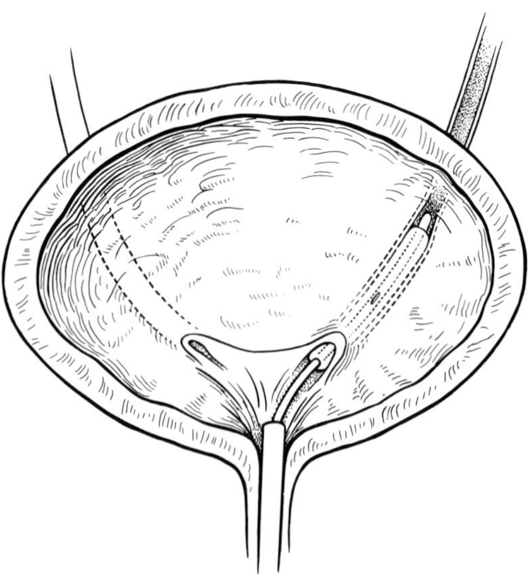

Figure 38.2. The intramural ureter is dilated with a balloon catheter. For most patients, a 5-mm diameter, 4-cm length balloon is adequate. In some cases, introduction of the balloon catheter is facilitated by passing it over a .038-inch flexible tip guidewire, although we no longer utilize that routinely.

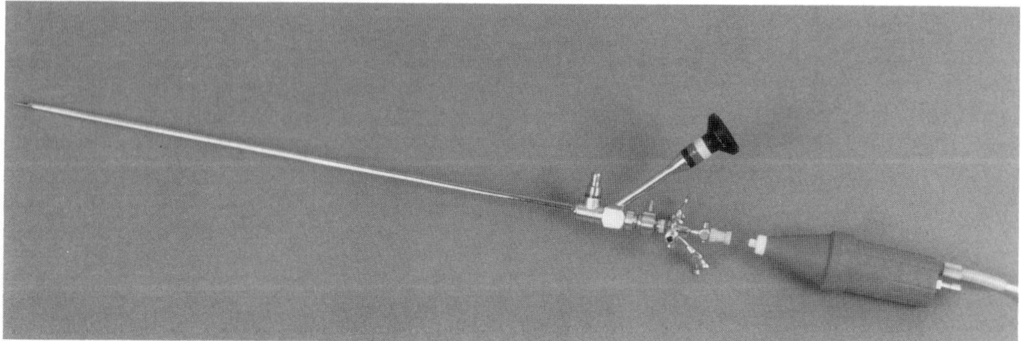

Figure 38.3. The cystoscope and balloon catheter are replaced with the ureteroscope. Stones lodged in the upper ureter will almost always require ultrasonic fragmentation for safe removal. Therefore, a ureteroscope with an offset lens that allows ultrasonic fragmentation under direct vision is utilized.

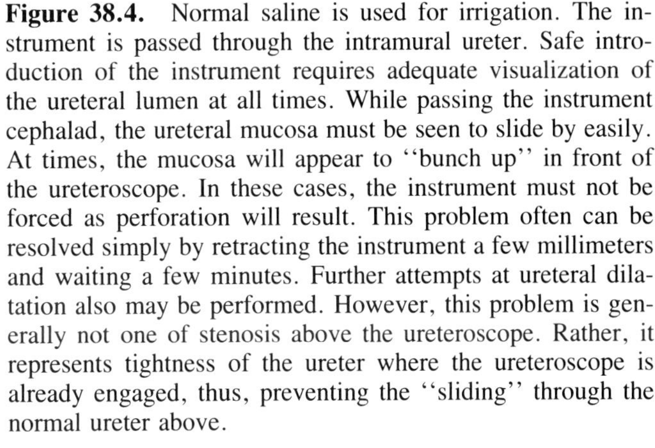

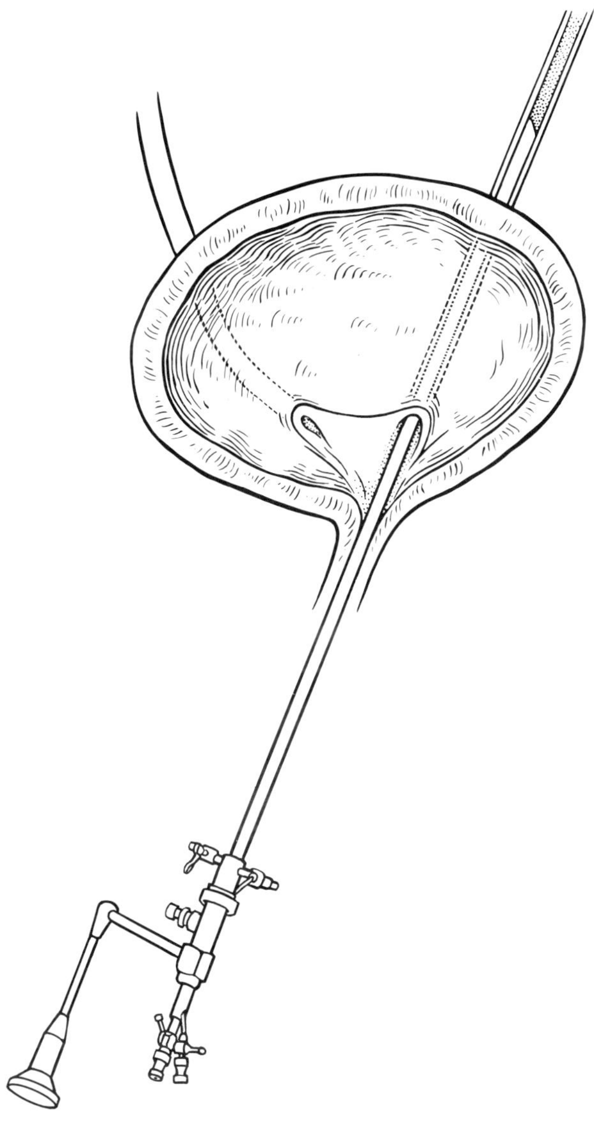

Figure 38.4. Normal saline is used for irrigation. The instrument is passed through the intramural ureter. Safe introduction of the instrument requires adequate visualization of the ureteral lumen at all times. While passing the instrument cephalad, the ureteral mucosa must be seen to slide by easily. At times, the mucosa will appear to ''bunch up'' in front of the ureteroscope. In these cases, the instrument must not be forced as perforation will result. This problem often can be resolved simply by retracting the instrument a few millimeters and waiting a few minutes. Further attempts at ureteral dilatation also may be performed. However, this problem is generally not one of stenosis above the ureteroscope. Rather, it represents tightness of the ureter where the ureteroscope is already engaged, thus, preventing the ''sliding'' through the normal ureter above.

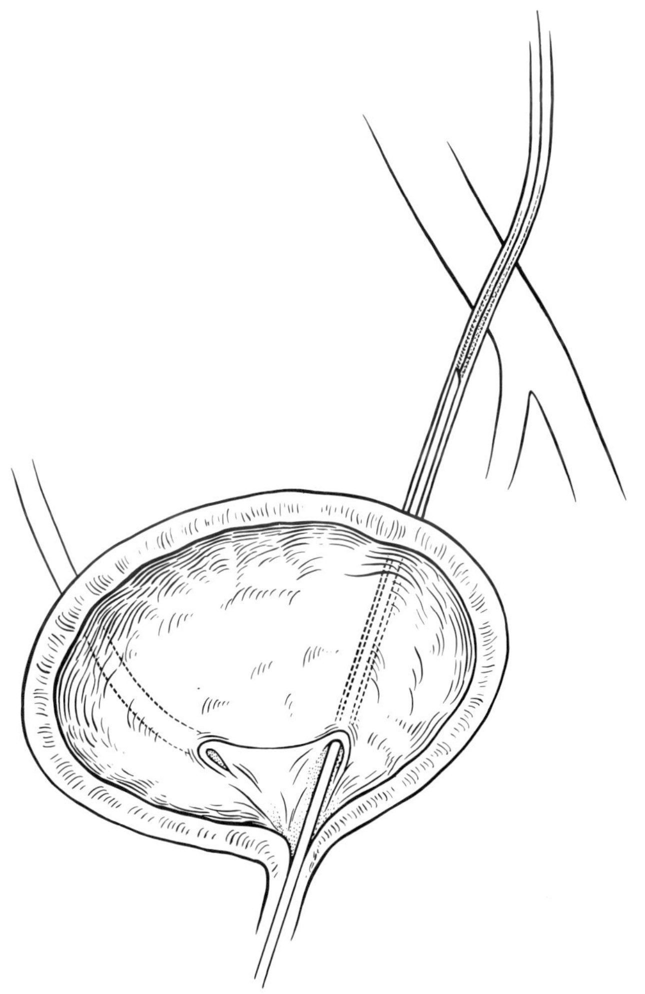

Figure 38.5. Once the intramural ureter is negotiated, difficulty may be noted at the level of the iliac vessels. Further dilation is rarely of value as the problem is not one of ureteral stenosis. Rather, the problem is one of angulation of the ureter over the vessels. This problem, if it becomes evident, is best overcome by passing a flexible tip guidewire through the ureteroscope under direct vision. This will result in straightening of the ureter and further introduction of the ureteroscope will be facilitated.

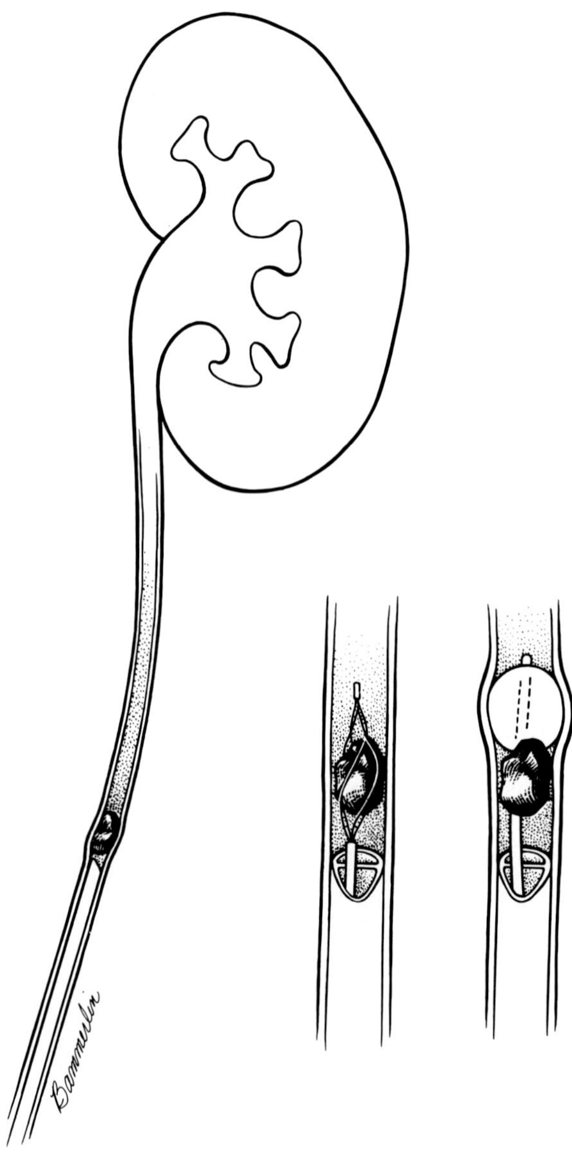

Figure 38.6. Once the ureteroscope is introduced proximal to the iliac vessels, the manipulation will be relatively easy as the midureter is more accommodating to the ureteroscope. The instrument is passed to the level of the stone. At this time, a basket is placed through the lower working port of the ureteroscope and the entrapped stone. This will prevent proximal migration of fragments during ultrasonic disintegration. Alternatively, a balloon catheter may be passed proximal to the stone. In some cases, a basket or catheter cannot be manipulated beyond the stone until at least some fragmentation has been accomplished.

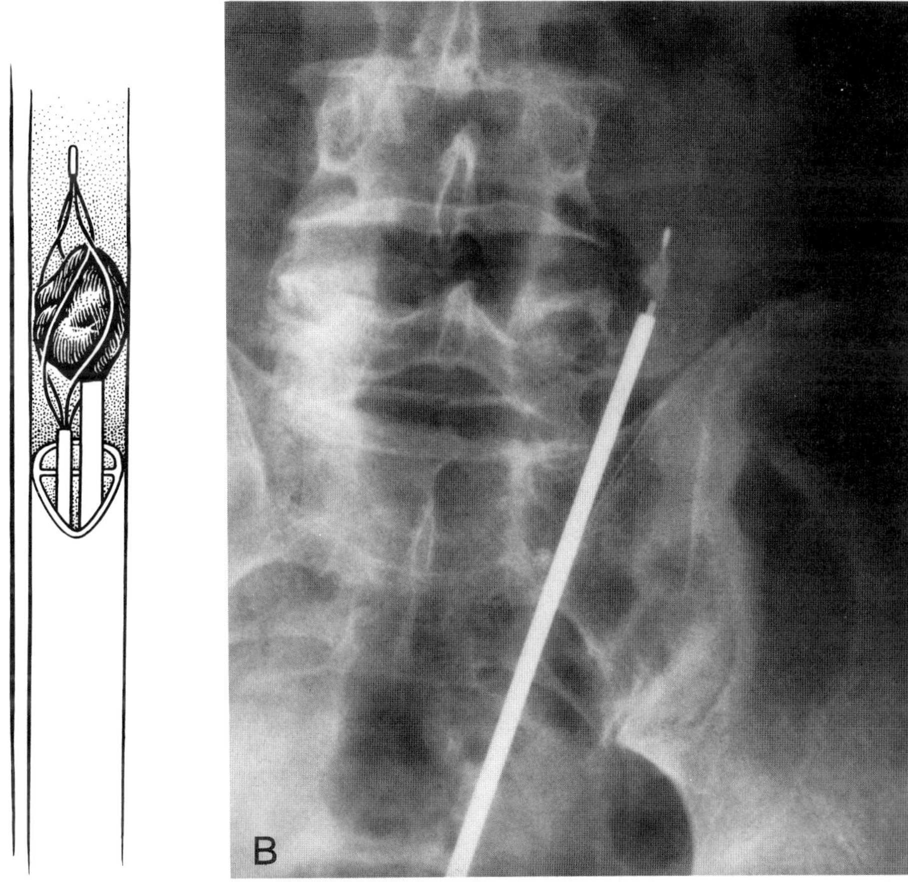

Figure 38.7. When the stone is well visualized and controlled proximally, the ultrasound wand (lithotrite) is passed through the second working port. Normal saline irrigation is continued through the ureteroscope while suction is applied to the stone through the wand. The wand is abutted against the stone, which is then fragmented with application of ultrasonic energy. The pieces will be suctioned out as they break off. Unfortunately, the small diameter wand often gets plugged with stone fragments. This will require intermittent passage of a stylet through the wand to clear it of debris. Ultrasonic fragmentation is continued until the stone is gone or until the remaining few pieces are of a size small enough to pass spontaneously. (From Streem SB, et al: Endourologic management of upper and mid ureteral calculi. *Urology* 31:34, 1988.)

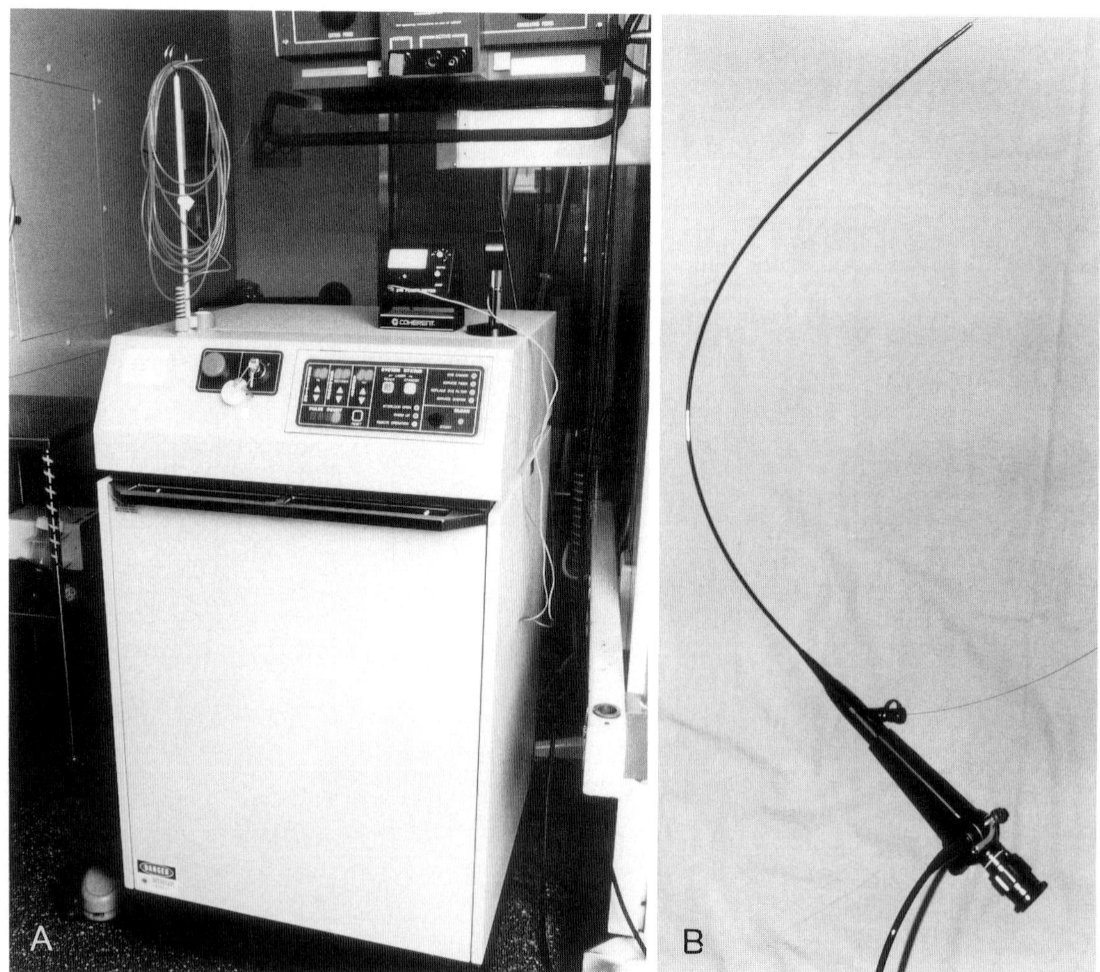

Figure 38.8. An excellent alternative to ultrasound for fragmentation is the tunable pulsed dye laser. Because the laser fiber is flexible and only 250 μ in diameter, it can be passed through a variety of small rigid or flexible ureteroscopes.

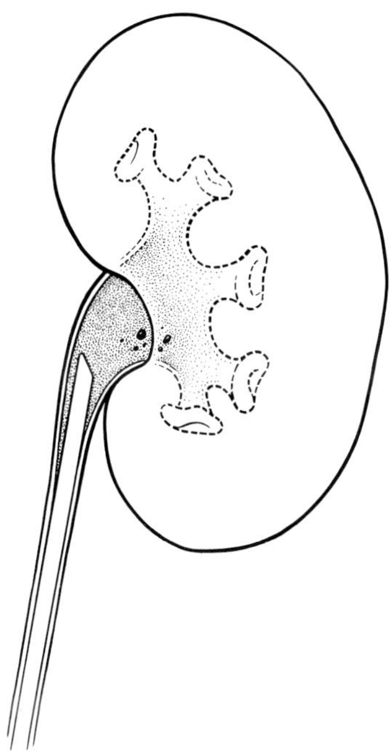

Figure 38.9. When the stone appears resolved, the ureteroscope is passed further cephalad to inspect the more proximal ureter and renal pelvis. At times, despite proximal control with a basket or balloon catheter, some small pieces will be seen to have migrated to the proximal ureter or pelvis. These are often of no consequence but larger fragments can be retrieved and further fragmented as necessary, or treated subsequently with ESWL.

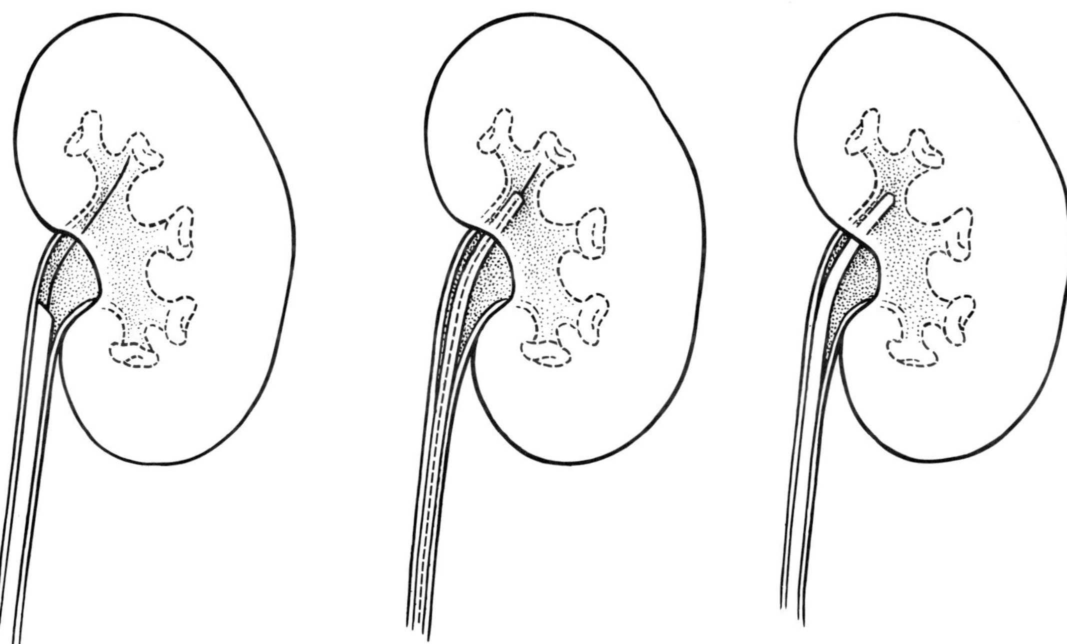

Figure 38.10. At the termination of the procedure, a guidewire is placed through the ureteroscope and the instrument is removed. In uncomplicated cases, drainage postureteroscopic manipulation is accomplished by passing a no. 6 French open-end whistle-tip catheter over the guidewire and leaving it indwelling for 24 to 48 hours. Alternatively, when more extensive stone manipulation was required, or where minor perforations or extravasation have been evident, an indwelling ureteral stent is placed and removed in an outpatient setting 2–4 weeks later.

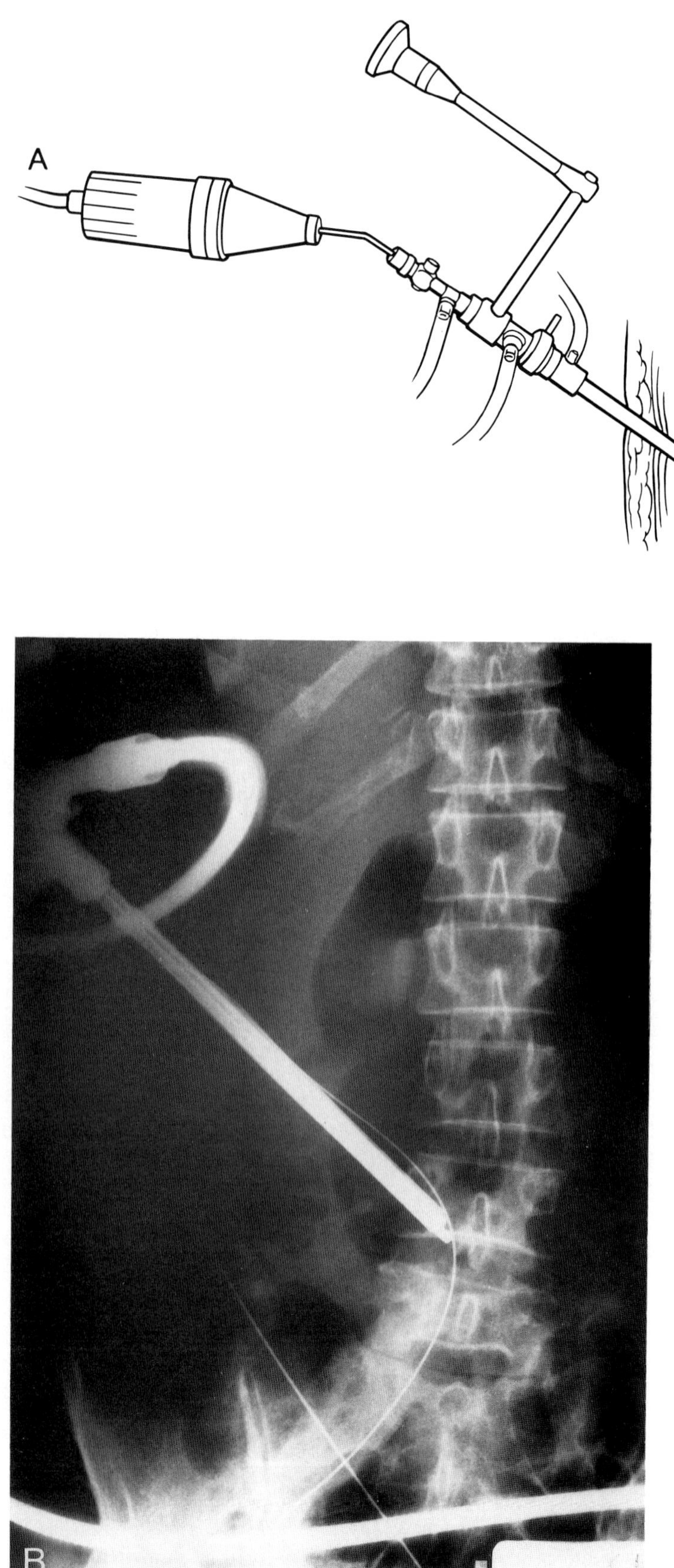

Figure 38.11. At times, upper or midureteral calculi are better managed percutaneously, in an antegrade fashion. This is especially true if there is significant ureteral dilatation above the calculus.

Percutaneous access is attained as described in chapter 13. In these cases, the approach should be through a lateral calyx or infundibulum to provide better access down the ureter. The tract is dilated as in chapter 14. For dilated systems, the rigid nephroscope may be guided under vision antegrade through the ureteropelvic junction to the calculus. Small stones are then grasped with a forceps or basket, while larger ones are fragmented with the ultrasonic lithotrite. (From Streem SB, et al: Endourologic management of upper and mid ureteral calculi. *Urology* 31:34, 1988.)

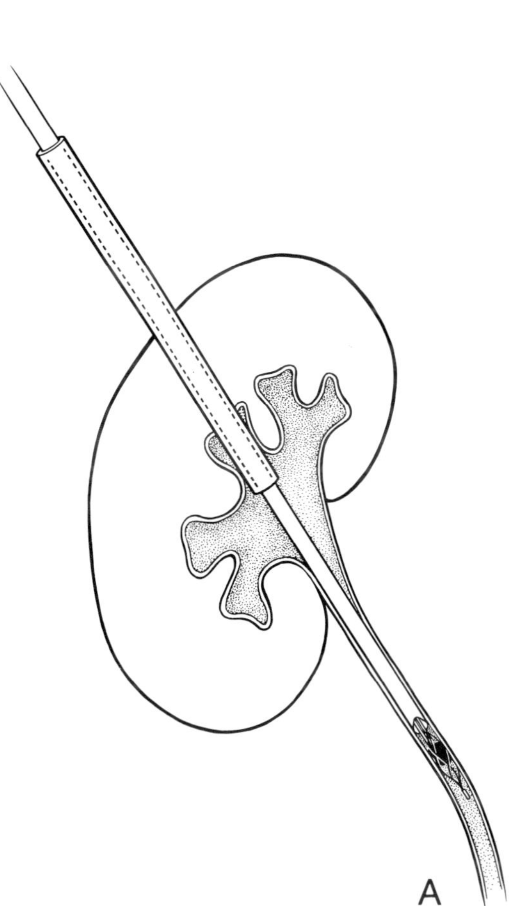

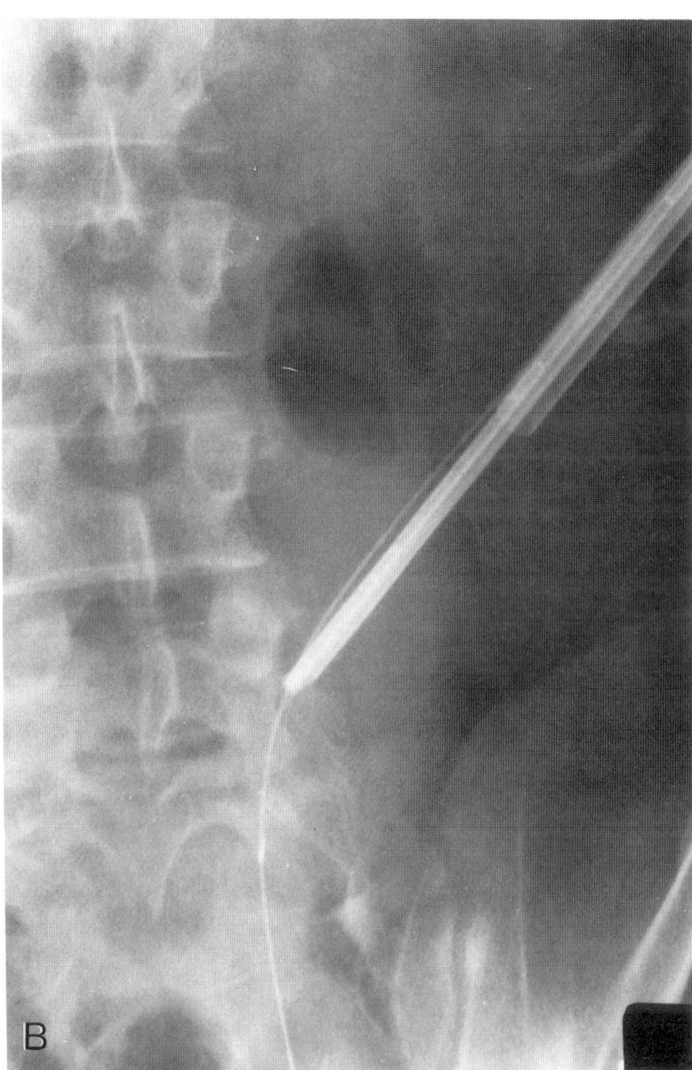

Figure 38.12. Where the ureter is not significantly dilated, passage of the nephroscope across the ureteropelvic junction and down the ureter could be traumatic. The best alternative in these cases is to pass a rigid ureteroscope. This should be done through a working sheath or the sheath of the rigid nephroscope. The offset lens ureteroscope is passed under the direct visual control to the level of the stone. Small stones then may be engaged with a basket. Larger stones should be fragmented first with the lithotrite. However, most ureteral stones can be extracted in an antegrade fashion without lithotripsy as the ureter above the stone has already proven itself capable of accommodating the calculus.

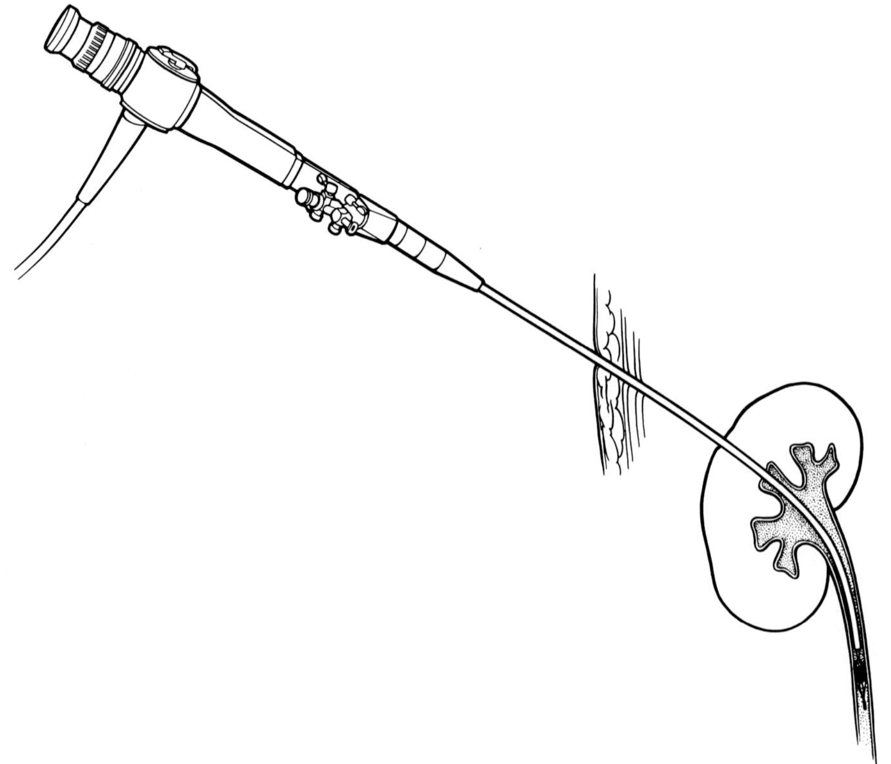

Figure 38.13. A flexible nephroscope may be used as an alternative to either the rigid ureteroscope or rigid nephroscope for simple antegrade basketing under vision.

MANAGEMENT OF URETERAL TUMORS

Ureterorenoscopy has gained an important role in the diagnosis of tumors anywhere in the upper tracts. In some instances, ureteroscopic techniques may be utilized therapeutically.

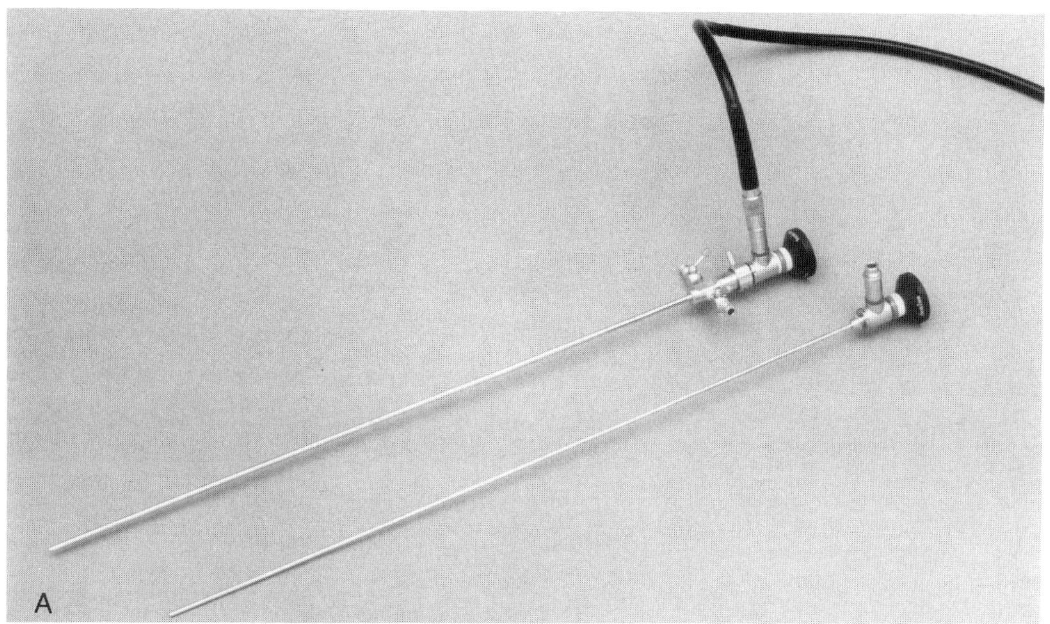

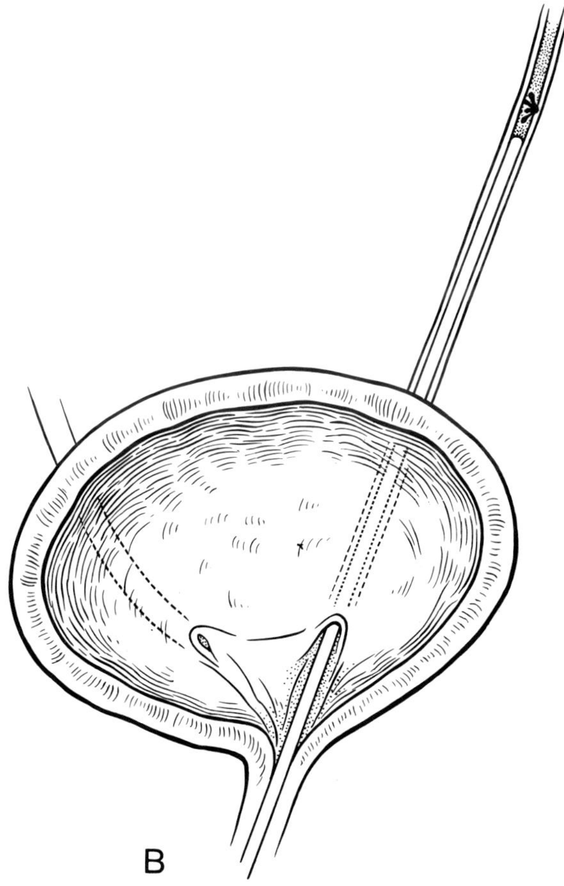

Figure 38.19. The initial steps are the same as those utilized for managing calculi. **A,** a "bulb tip" retrograde study is obtained, after which the intramural ureter is dilated. For strictly diagnostic purposes, a small ureteroscope may be utilized. **B,** with the 5° lens in place, it is guided through the intramural ureter up to the level of the lesion using the same precautions as for a stone.

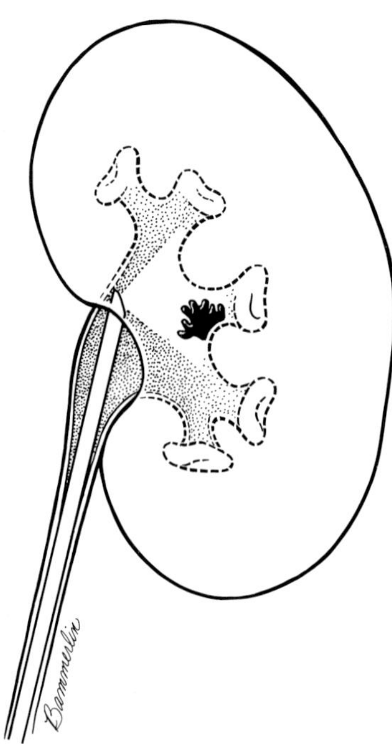

Figure 38.20. For lesions in the renal pelvis, infundibula, or calyces, the 5° lens is replaced with a 70° lens for full-field visualization once the ureteropelvic junction has been traversed.

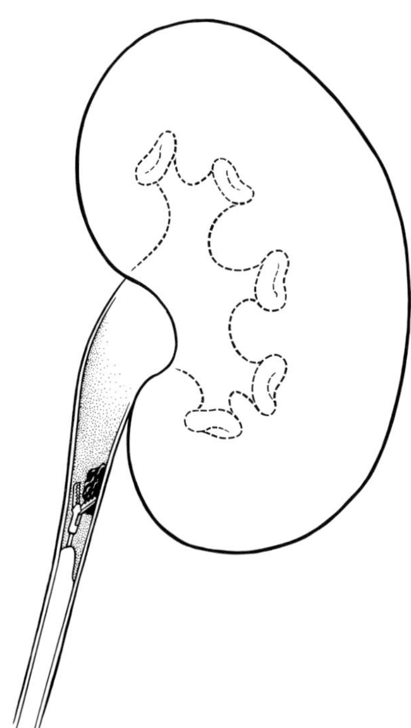

Figure 38.21. While histologic confirmation may not be necessary in all cases, we have found transureteroscopic biopsy to be helpful in confirming the clinical diagnosis. Furthermore, tumor grading may also be possible by this route so that appropriate subsequent operative intervention can be better planned.

To perform transureteroscopic biopsy, the ureteroscope with a working port is utilized. This is again guided to the level of the lesion. Under direct vision, ''alligator'' forceps are utilized for biopsy. Care is taken not to perforate the full thickness of the ureter.

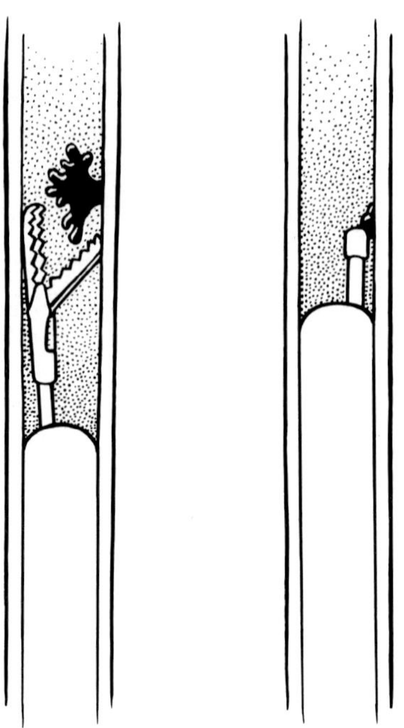

Figure 38.22. At times, a ''conservative'' approach to managing these tumors is indicated. For small, superficial lesions, a definitive procedure may be performed ureteroscopically. In such cases, the alligator forceps is used to ''debulk'' the tumor as much as possible, after which a Bugbee electrode is used to coagulate the base thoroughly. In such cases, the irrigant must be changed to 1.5% glycine or distilled water. A ureteral catheter or internal self-retaining stent is left after the procedure to circumvent local edema.

In the near future, a ureteroscopic resectoscope will be available for such lesions.

MANAGEMENT OF STRICTURE—BALLOON DILATION

Patients with ureteral strictures are often amenable to "nonoperative" endourologic management. In these cases, balloon dilatation is our initial procedure of choice.

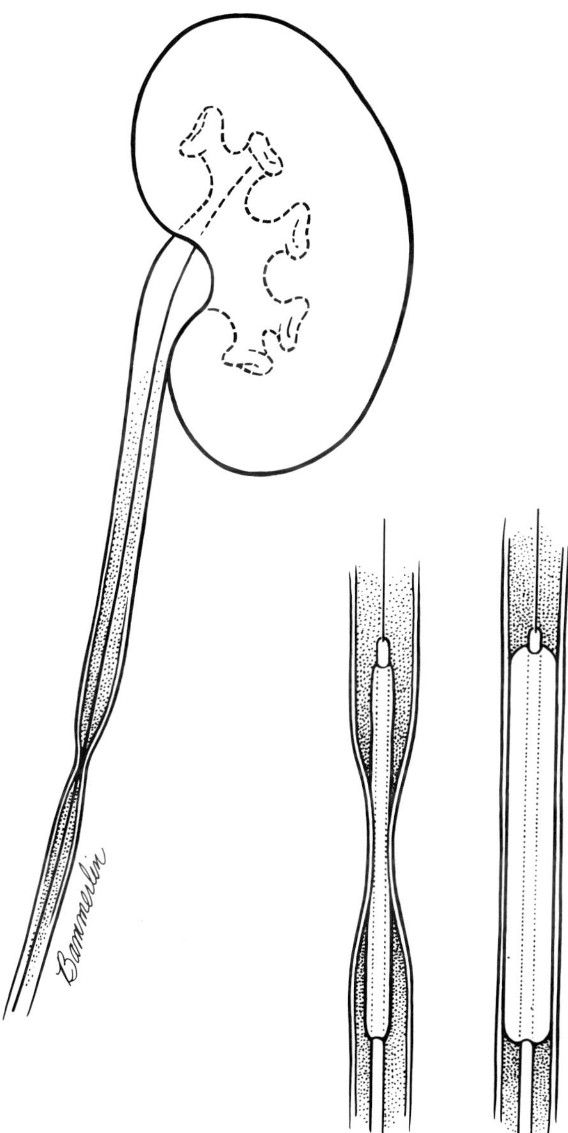

Figure 38.23. Whenever possible, the stricture is managed transurethrally. Cystoscopy and retrograde pyelography are performed to define the site and extent of the stricture accurately. Short strictures are more amenable to this therapy. After the retrograde study, a flexible-tip .038-inch guidewire is passed through the stricture, into the renal pelvis. An angiographic balloon-dilating catheter is then passed over the guidewire and positioned at the appropriate site using fluoroscopic control. The balloon is then inflated until the "waist" at the site of the stricture is gone. The balloon is inflated for 5–10 min. Generally, a 5-mm diameter, 4-cm length balloon is adequate, providing dilatation to approximately no. 15 French. Over the .038-inch guidewire, the balloon catheter is removed and replaced with a no. 8 French self-retaining internal ureteral stent, which is removed 4–6 weeks later.

Figure 38.24. At times, the guidewire cannot be negotiated retrograde through the stricture using fluoroscopy alone. In those cases, ureteroscopy can be useful and is performed as described previously. When the structured area is visualized, a guidewire is passed under direct vision and dilatation proceeds as above.

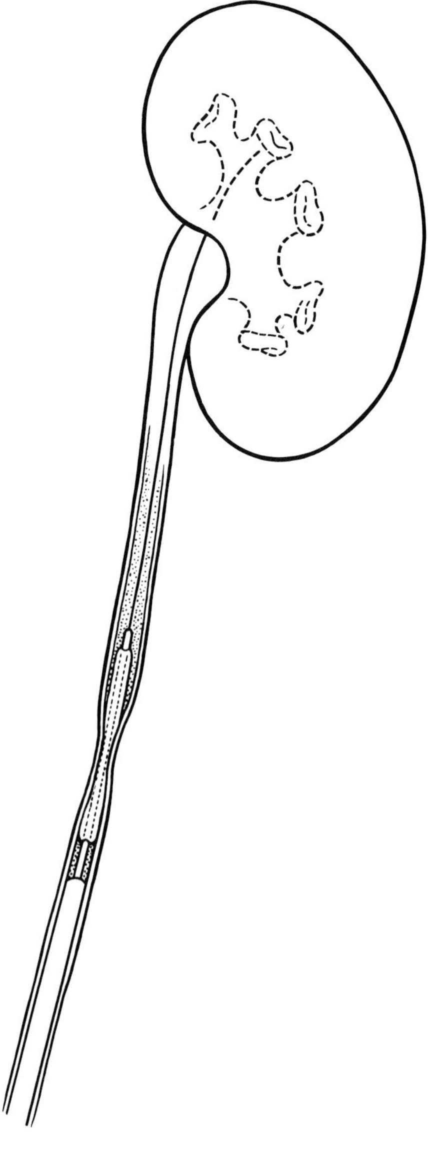

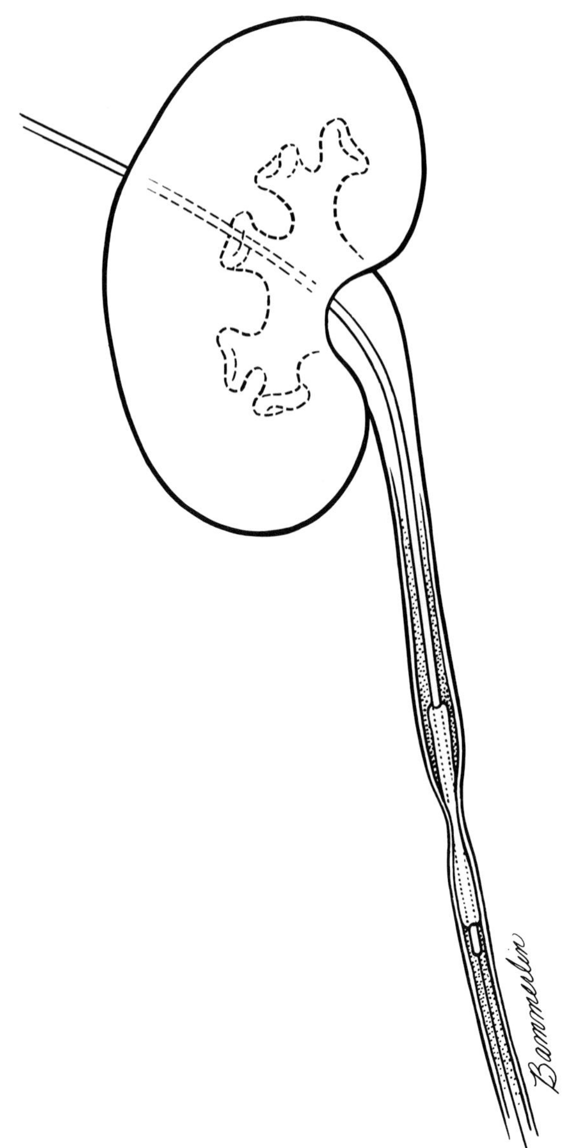

Figure 38.25. In some patients, retrograde access is impossible. This is frequently the case for patients who have undergone diversion and have ureteroileal or ureterocolic strictures, or in transplant recipients after ureteroneocystostomy. In these cases, antegrade balloon dilatation is performed.

Access is attained as described in chapter 13. Again, this should be through a middle calyx or infundibulum for better access down the ureter. A .038-inch flexible-tip guidewire is guided through the stricture and the balloon-dilating catheter is passed over that. Fluoroscopic monitoring assures proper positioning and the balloon is inflated. The balloon catheter is then substituted with an internal or internal/external stent that is left in place for 4–6 weeks.

Suggested Readings

Bagley DH, Huffman JL, Lyon ES: Flexible ureteropyeloscopy: Diagnosis and treatment in the upper urinary tract. *J Urol* 138:280, 1987.

Chang R, Marshall FF: Management of ureteroscopic injuries. *J Urol* 137:1132, 1987.

Chang R, Marshall FF, Mitchell S: Percutaneous management of benign ureteral strictures and fistulas. *J Urol* 137:1126, 1987.

Coptcoat MJ, Webb DR, Kellett MJ, Whitfield HN, Wickham JEA: The treatment of 100 consecutive patients with ureteral calculi in a British Stone Center. *J Urol* 137:1122, 1987.

Dretler SP, Keating MA, Riley J: An algorithm for the management of ureteral calculi. *J Urol* 136:1190, 1986.

Gumpinger R, Miller K, Fuchs G, Eisenberger F: Antegrade ureteroscopy for stone removal. *Eur Urol* 11:199, 1985.

Huffman JL, Bagley DH, Lyon ES: Extending cystoscopic techniques into the ureter and renal pelvis. *JAMA* 250:2002, 1983.

Huffman JL, Bagley DH, Lyon ES, Morse MJ, Herr HW, Whitmore WF Jr: Endoscopic diagnosis and treatment of upper-tract urothelial tumors. *Cancer* 55:1422, 1985.

Huffman JL, Bagley DH, Schoenberg HW, Lyon ES: Transurethral removal of large ureteral and renal pelvic calculi using ureteroscopic ultrasonic lithotripsy. *J Urol* 130:31, 1983.

Kramolowsky EV: Ureteral perforation during ureterorenoscopy: Treatment and management. *J Urol* 138:36, 1987.

King LR, Coughlin PWF, Ford KK, Brown MW, Van Moore A: Initial experience with percutaneous and transurethral oblation of postoperative ureteral strictures in children. *J Urol* 131:1167, 1984.

Lingeman JE, Sonda LP, Kahnoski RJ, Coury TA, Newman DM, Mosbaugh PG, Mertz Jack HO, Steele RE, Frank B: Ureteral stone management: Emerging concepts. *J Urol* 135:1172, 1987.

Lytton B, Weiss RM, Green DF: Complications of ureteral endoscopy. *J Urol* 137:649, 1987.

Miller K, Fuchs G, Rassweiler J, Eisenberger F: Treatment of ureteral stone disease: The role of ESWL and endourology. *World J Urol* 3:53, 1985.

Mitty HA, Train JS, Dan SJ: Antegrade ureteral stenting in the management of fistulas, strictures and calculi. *Radiology* 149:433, 1983.

Perez-Castro Ellendt E, Martinez-Pineiro JA: Ureteral and renal endoscopy: A new approach. *Eur Urol* 8:117, 1982.

Smith AD, Reinke DB, Miller RP, Lange PH: Percutaneous nephrostomy in the management of ureteral and renal calculi. *Radiology* 133:49, 1979.

Streem SB, Hall P, Zelch MA, Risius B, Geisinger MA: Endourologic management of upper and mid ureteral calculi: Percutaneous antegrade extraction versus transurethral ureteroscopy. *Urology* (in press).

Streem SB, Pontes JE, Novick AC, Montie JE: Ureteropyeloscopy in the evaluation of upper tract filling defects. *J Urol* 136:383, 1986.

Streem SB, Novick AC, Steinmuller DR, Zelch MG, Risius B, Geisinger MA: Long term efficacy of ureteral dilatation for transplant ureteral obstruction. *J Urol* (in press).

SECTION 9

Supravesical Urinary Diversion

CHAPTER 39

Ureterosigmoidostomy

RALPH A. STRAFFON

There has long been a need for a method of supravesical diversion that does not require an external appliance. The knowledge that certain animals can live normal lives with a cloacal arrangement led clinical investigators to the use of ureterosigmoidostomy.

The first ureterosigmoidostomy was reported by John Simon in 1852 for the treatment of bladder exstrophy. He used a transfixion suture between the ureter and the rectum, and noted urine coming from the rectum on the 10th postoperative day. The patient did well for about 7 months, then became ill, and died 1 year after the operation.

Since this first attempt at ureterosigmoidostomy, over 100 different techniques have been tried with varying degrees of success. The history of the development of ureterosigmoidostomy until 1936 is well documented by Hinman and Weyrauch. Until the era of antibiotics the chief concern of the surgeon was to avoid spillage of bowel content and to prevent sepsis. There are some important contributions that should be listed in the development of the current technique for bilateral ureterosigmoidostomy.

In 1909, Coffey described a method of submucosal transplantation of the common bile duct into the intestine. He mentioned in his paper that the same principle might solve the problem of ureterosigmoidostomy. The Coffey I technique was an intraperitoneal operation usually done in stages. It consisted of a submucosal tunnel, an opening in the bowel mucosa at the lower end of the tunnel through which the ureter was passed into the lumen. Fixation was by means of a chromic suture with needle on both ends that passed through the bowel wall and tied below the tunnel. The Coffey II method was simply a one-stage bilateral ureterosigmoidostomy using stenting catheters. The Coffey III technique combined the submucosal tunnel with a transfixion suture in an attempt to avoid fecal contamination.

In 1949, Nesbit described the direct elliptical anastomosis of the ureter to the full thickness of the sigmoid colon with no submucosal tunnel. The following year, Cordonnier also described the direct anastomosis of the ureter to the sigmoid, again without a submucosal tunnel. Reflux of fecal material with infection was a problem with both of these techniques.

Mathesin, in 1953, recognized that, in birds, the ureter opened into the cloaca as a small nipple that would be occluded by intraluminal intestinal pressure. He reported 18 cases in man using the protruding nipple technique. Goodwin and associates in the same year, reported a technique in which the colon was opened and a submucosal tunnel created with direct mucosal anastomosis.

Leadbetter, in reviewing his own experience with the Coffey I technique, found three problems: *(a)* stricture of the ureter at the point where it made contact with the bowel lumen; *(b)* stenosis due to periureteral scarring as the ureter passed through the bowel wall; and *(c)* obstruction of the ureter due to angulation at the site of entry of the ureter into the bowel wall. He described the combined techniques utilizing Coffey's submucosal tunnel and Nesbit's direct elliptical anastomosis to the intestinal mucosa at the lower end of the tunnel. It is basically this technique that we use at the Cleveland Clinic in doing bilateral ureterosigmoidostomy.

INDICATIONS FOR URETEROSIGMOIDOSTOMY

The patients who are to have bilateral ureterosigmoidostomy must be selected carefully. They should have a normal upper urinary tract, preferably without a chronic urinary tract infection. The anal sphincter must be competent to contain the urine, which immediately rules out the use of this operation in children with neurogenic bladders secondary to myelodysplasia or myelomeningoceles. Children in general seem to do better with the operation than do adults.

Exstrophy of the Bladder

In a child with exstrophy of the bladder and an essentially normal upper urinary tract, bilateral ureterosigmoidostomy remains our operation of choice. It is important to discuss this operation and the potential complications with the parents preoperatively, because if the child does poorly, he or she may have to be converted to an ileal conduit.

Urinary Incontinence

In selected individuals with urinary incontinence that cannot be corrected surgically, ureterosigmoidostomy may be the procedure of choice. This might be used if the patient is very obese or in the patient who is unwilling to have a stoma and wear an external appliance.

Bladder Carcinoma

In the occasional obese patient with operable bladder carcinoma, ureterosigmoidostomy may be the operation of choice. It also may be used in certain patients who are candidates for anterior exenteration for pelvic neoplasia. It should not be used as a method of diversion in a patient with inoperable bladder cancer who is to receive therapeutic or palliative irradiation therapy.

PREOPERATIVE PREPARATION

Preoperatively, a barium enema and sigmoidoscopy should be performed to rule out diverticulosis and to identify any other lesion of the colon. This is particularly important in adults. Baseline renal function studies should be done, and the serum creatinine and serum electrolytes should be measured.

Proper preparation of the bowel is extremely important in the patient who is to have ureterosigmoidostomy. The patient is placed on a low residue diet for 3–4 days with only clear liquids by mouth during the 24 hrs preceding the operation.

Polyethylene glycal electrolyte solution for gastrointestinal lavage (GoLYTELY) is given the evening before the operation. Four liters are administered at the rate of 240 ml/10 min until completed. This is a very effective cleansing agent for the bowel. Then cefotaxime sodium (Claforan) and metronidazole hydrochloride (Flagyl), 1 gm of each, are given to the patient intravenously at the time they are called to the operating room. There are other types of bowel preparations that may be used and are equally effective.

In the operating room while under anesthesia, a rectal tube may be placed into the rectum and rectosigmoid area and this area may be lavaged with 1% neomycin to complete the mechanical cleansing of the colon. A no. 30 French Pezzer catheter is left in the rectum and connected to dependent drainage. A nasogastric tube is placed in the stomach.

OPERATIVE PROCEDURE

A midline incision extending from the symphysis pubis to above the umbilicus may be used, but it is our preference to use the classic Cherney incision, which gives wide exposure to the pelvic viscera. The peritoneal cavity is entered and its contents are explored.

The rectosigmoid area of the colon is identified and the rest of the bowel is packed off from the pelvic area. The use of the Smith ring retractor, combined with the patient in a mild Trendelenberg position, is helpful in achieving good exposure.

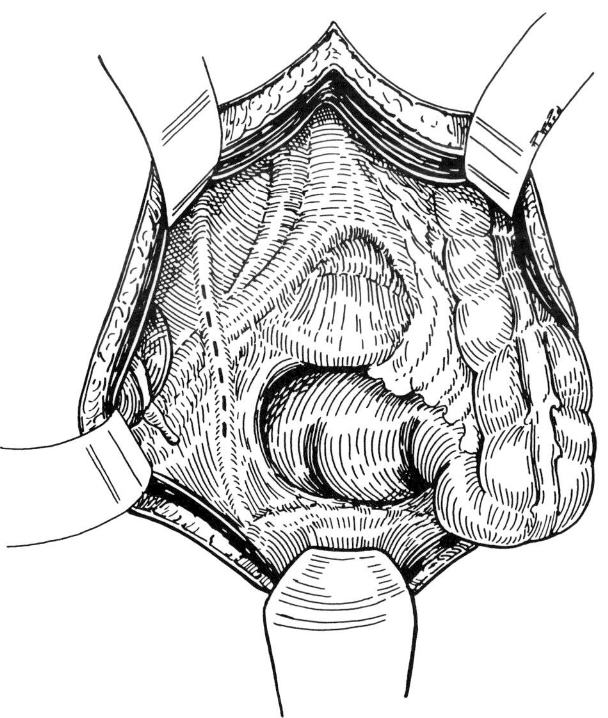

Identification of the Right Ureter

Figure 39.1. The peritoneum overlying the right ureter is incised starting at the point where the ureter crosses the iliac vessels and is extended downward following the course of the ureter. Peritoneal flaps are elevated on each side of the ureter and the ureter is dissected free from surrounding tissue.

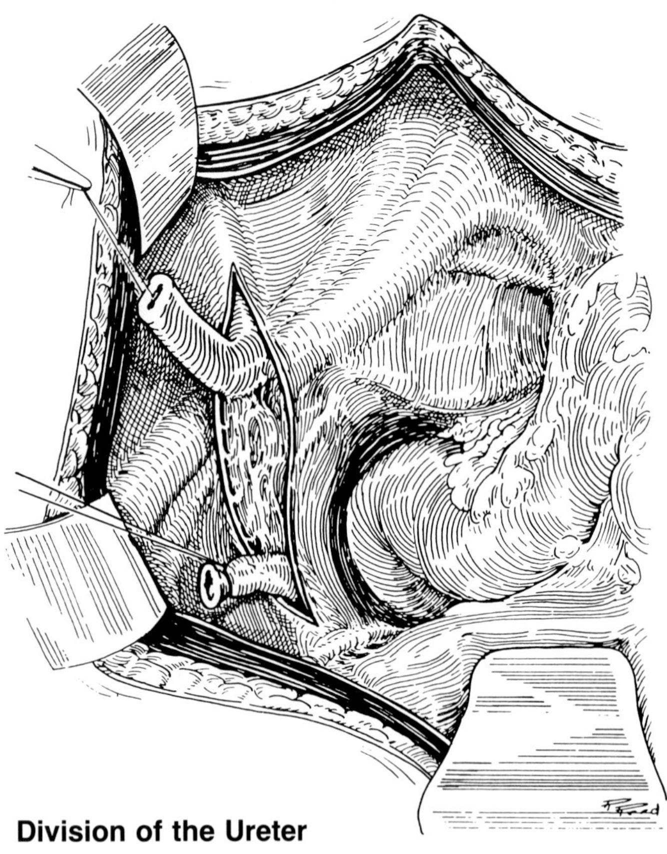

Division of the Ureter

Figure 39.2. The ureter is dissected downward to the right ureterovesical junction and a 2–0 chromic ligature is placed around it at this point. It is then divided and a 4–0 chromic suture is placed in the proximal end of the ureter to facilitate handling the ureter.

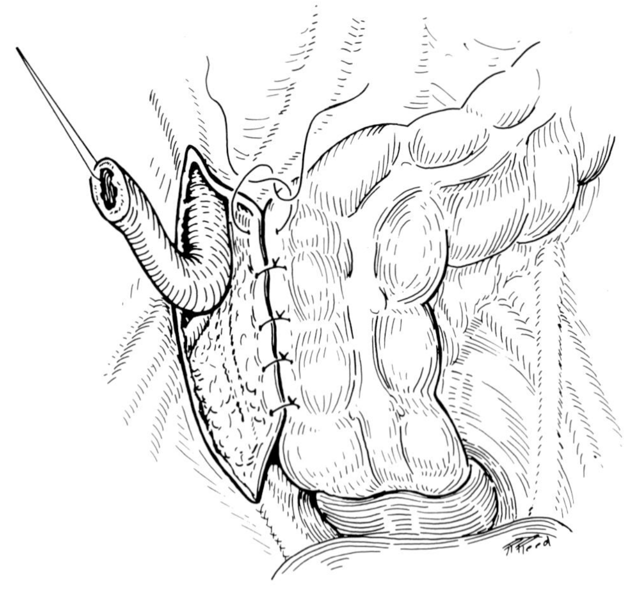

Fixation of Rectosigmoid Colon

Figure 39.3. The rectosigmoid area of the colon is pulled upward and the medial side of the peritoneal flap sutured to the seromuscular layers of the colon with interrupted 3–0 chromic sutures. The site of this line of sutures should be selected so as to exclude the epiploic appendages and to expose an area between the taeniae coli for the formation of the submucosal tunnel.

Incision in the Muscularis of Colon

Figure 39.4. Using a long-handled knife with a no. 15 Bard-Parker blade, an incision is made in the muscularis externa of the colon. This incision is made between the taeniae coli in an area where the inner circular muscle is well developed, but the outer longitudinal muscle, while present, is thinner than the area of the taeniae coli. The incision is carried down to the mucosa, which will protrude outward when all the muscular layers are incised. This incision should be 8–10 cm in length. Once the circular muscle bands are incised, taking care to avoid entering the lumen of the bowel, lateral flaps of muscularis externa can be developed on either side of the incision, using the blunt end of the knife. These flaps should be at least 0.5 cm wide on each side to allow accommodation of the ureter without compression when the muscular flaps are approximated.

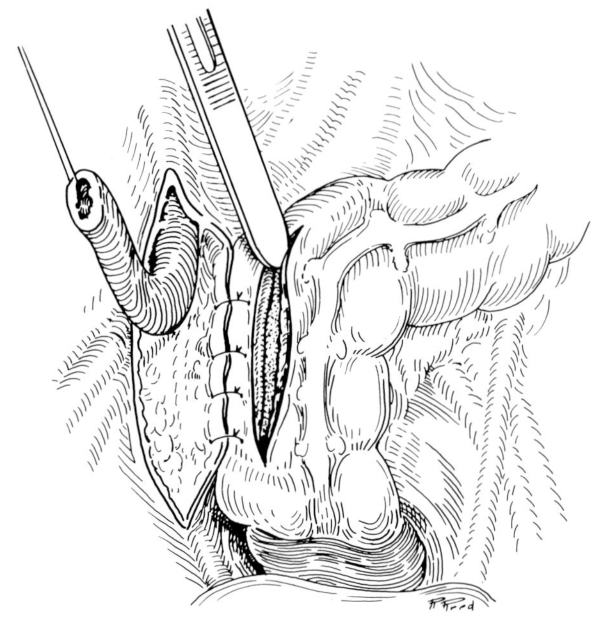

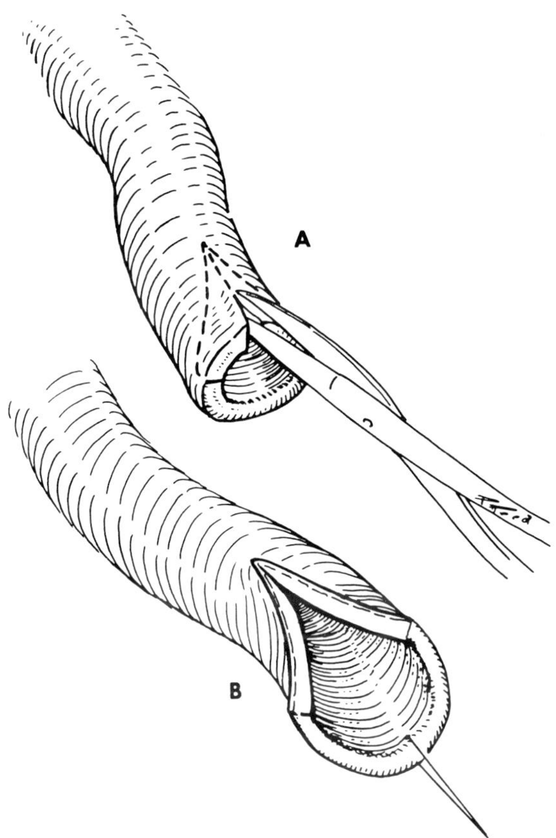

Preparation of the Ureter

Figure 39.5. The ureter is then placed along the tunnel in the colon and divided so its lower end easily reaches the lower end of the tunnel. A longitudinal incision is then made in the medial wall of the ureter, and the sharp corners on each side of the ureter are rounded off before doing an elliptic uretero-sigmoid anastomosis.

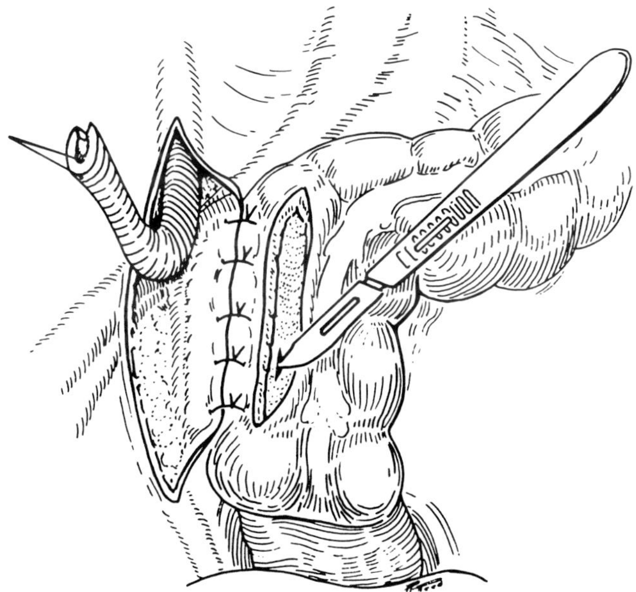

Figure 39.6. A small opening is then made in the mucosa of the colon at the lower end of the muscular tunnel. Since the mucosa stretches easily, this opening should be quite small and can be enlarged if necessary to equal the size of the spatulated ureter.

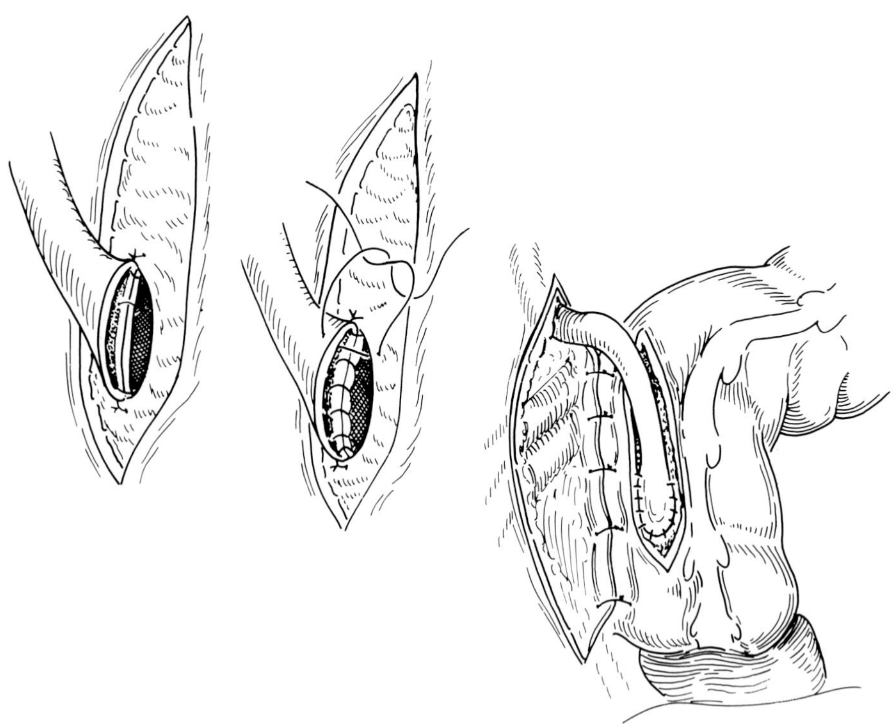

Ureterosigmoid Anastomosis

Figure 39.7. The anastomosis of the ureter to the colon is a direct elliptical anastomosis, using interrupted 5–0 chromic sutures through the full thickness of the ureter and the mucosa of the colon. A stay suture is placed initially at the apex of the longitudinal incision in the ureter and through the upper end of the incision in the colon mucosa, and this is tied in place. A second stay suture then is passed through the midpoint of the distal end of the ureter, through the lower end of the bowel mucosa, and tied in place. Interrupted sutures then may be placed on either side of the two stay sutures using 5–0 chromic and being sure not to occlude the lumen of the ureter with these sutures. Usually, four or five sutures are required on each side of the stay sutures to complete the anastomosis. If the bowel has been well prepared there should be very little if any spillage of bowel contents. We have not routinely used stenting catheters, but these may be used in selected patients and are passed out through the rectum.

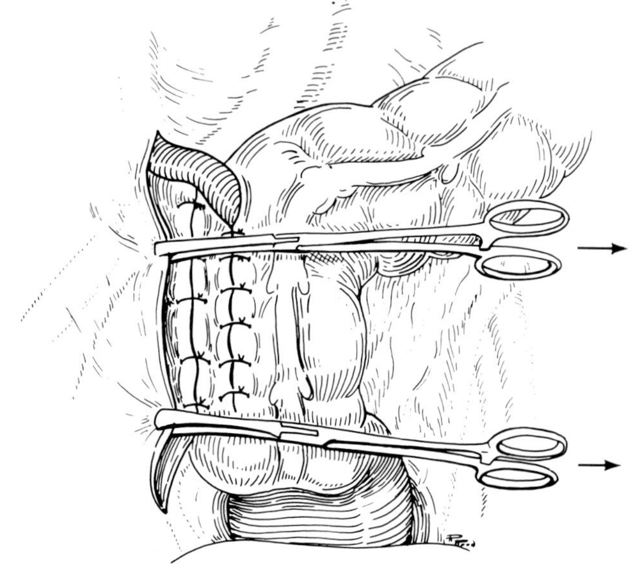

Closure of Muscularis Tunnel

Figure 39.8. Once the ureterosigmoid anastomosis is completed, the muscular flaps are approximated over the ureter using interrupted 3–0 or 4–0 chromic sutures. The ureter should lie loosely in the tunnel without compression.

Retroperitonealization of Ureterosigmoid Anastomosis

Figure 39.9. Once the muscularis externa of the colon is closed over the ureter, the entire anastomosis is retroperitonealized. This is done by suturing the lateral portion of the peritoneal flap to the seromuscular layer of the colon, medial to the ureterosigmoid anastomosis, with interrupted 3–0 chromic sutures. This maneuver fixes the area of the ureterosigmoid anastomosis and prevents any undue tension on the suture line. Before closure of the lateral flap of peritoneum, a Penrose drain may be placed extraperitoneally and brought out through a stab wound below the main abdominal incision.

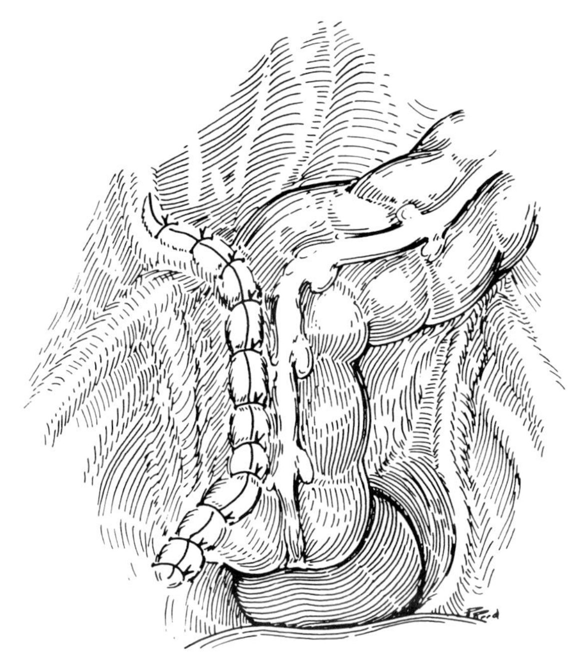

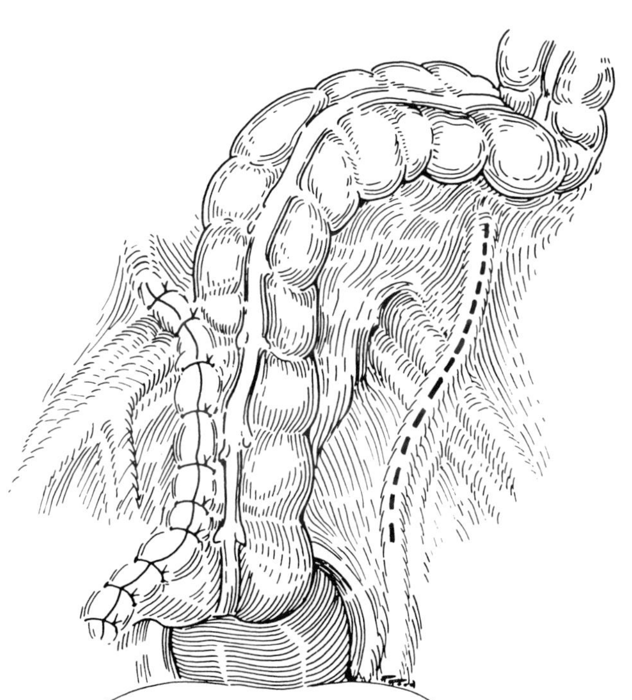

Identification of the Left Ureter

Figure 39.10. On the left side, the incision in the posterior peritoneum to expose the left ureter is made lateral to the mesosigmoid and somewhat higher than on the right side. The ureter is dissected down to the ureterovesical junction and divided.

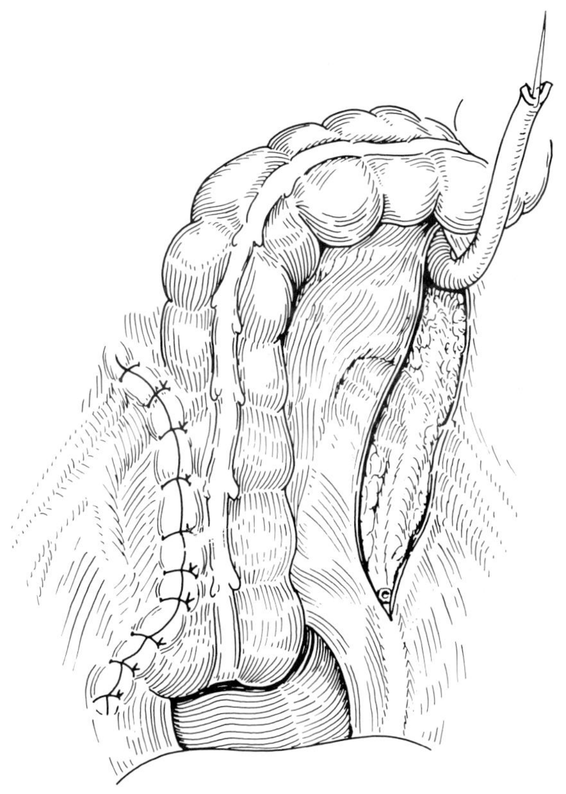

Figure 39.11. The ureterosigmoid anastomosis on the left is done exactly as described for the right side.

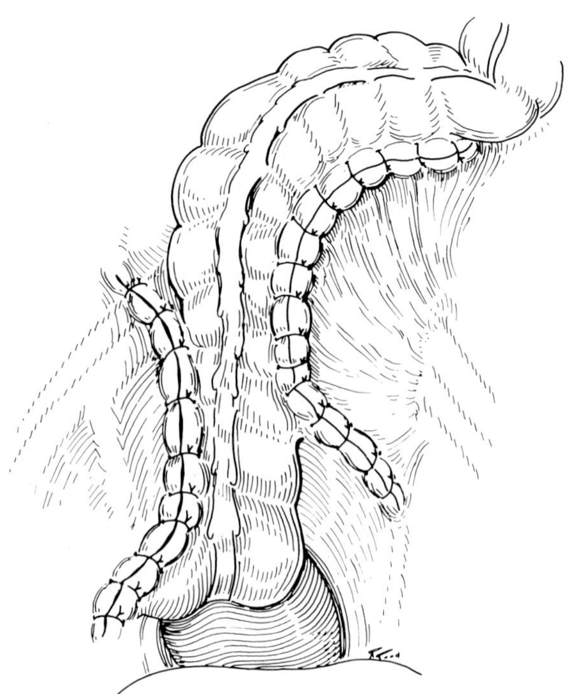

Completed Bilateral Ureterosigmoidostomy

Figure 39.12. The completed bilateral ureterosigmoidostomy is shown above. Both sides are retroperitonealized. The incision is closed in layers in the usual manner.

POSTOPERATIVE CARE

The nasogastric tube is left in place until the patient has good bowel sounds; then it may be removed. The rectal catheter is left in place as long as it drains well. This is usually for 4–5 days.

The patient is instructed to empty the colon at 2 to 3 hr intervals to minimize the absorption of urinary constituents from the colon. Long-term chemotherapy with nitrofurantoin (50 mg twice daily) is prescribed for the patient. Also, patients are routinely given additional fixed base, such as Eisenberg's solution, 15 ml three times daily.

At 1 month after the operation, the patient is evaluated to be sure the incision is well healed and the colon is being evacuated at 2- to 3-hr intervals. The serum creatinine and serum electrolytes are measured and compared with the preoperative values.

At 6 months after the operation an intravenous pyelogram is obtained, in addition to determining the serum creatinine and serum electrolytes.

COMPLICATIONS

In 1950, Ferris and Odel reported the occurrence of hyperchloremic acidosis after ureterosigmoidostomy. They studied 141 patients with bilateral ureterosigmoidostomy, and reported hyperchloremic acidosis in 80% of these patients. The use of supplemental alkali plus frequent evacuation of urine from the rectum will minimize these findings. Hyperchloremic acidosis seldom becomes a problem in the patient with good renal function.

Recurrent or persistent pyelonephritis is another complication often seen in ureterosigmoidostomy. This can be minimized using the combined antireflux techniques described above, plus the use of small-dose long-term chemotherapy.

An occasional patient will have some degree of urinary incontinence. This usually occurs at night, but those patients with normal anal musculature are usually able to adapt to this problem.

Suggested Readings

Coffey RC: Transplantation of the ureters into the large intestine in the absence of a functioning urinary bladder. *Surg Gynecol Obstet* 32:383, 1921.

Coffey RC: Cystectomy with bilateral transplantation of ureters in one operation. Preliminary report of five cases. *Northwest Med* 29:443, 1930.

Cordonnier JJ: Ureterosigmoid anastomosis. *J Urol* 63:275, 1950.

Ferris DZ, and Odel HM: electrolyte pattern of the blood after bilateral ureterosigmoidostomy. *JAMA*, 142:634, 1950.

Goodwin WE, Harris AP, Kaufman JJ, Beal JM: Open transcolonic ureterointestinal anastomosis: A new approach. *Surg Gynecol Obstet* 97:295, 1953.

Hinman F, Weyrauch HM Jr: A critical study of the different principles of surgery which have been used in ureterointestinal implantation. *Trans Am Assoc Genitourin Surg* 29:15, 1936.

Leadbetter WF: Considerations of problems incident to performance of uretero-enterostomy: Report of a technique. *J Urol* 68:818, 1951.

Mathesin W: New method for ureterointestinal anastomosis. Preliminary report. *Surg Gynecol Obstet* 96:255, 1953.

Nesbit RM: Ureterosigmoid anastomosis by the direct elliptical technique. *J Urol* 61:728, 1949.

Simon J: Ectropia vesicae; operation for directing the orifices of the ureters into the rectum; temporary success; subsequent death, autopsy. *Lancet* 2:568, 1952.

CHAPTER 40

Cutaneous Ureterostomy

RALPH A. STRAFFON

Cutaneous ureterostomy offers an effective, simple method of supravesical urinary diversion, provided the ureters can be exteriorized as a single stoma, and placed so they can be fitted with a good collection device with the avoidance of intubation. This goal is difficult to achieve with normal ureters because of the poor intrinsic blood supply to the distal ends. In the obstructed, dilated ureter, a sufficient length of ureter can be mobilized without jeopardizing blood supply, to reach the skin the maintain a patent stoma. Because gravity plays only a small role in the transport of urine from the renal pelvis down the ureters, the dilated, aperistaltic ureter should not be used for cutaneous ureterostomy and, instead, a segment of ileum should be substituted for the ureter as the conduit of urine.

TECHNIQUES

There are several techniques appropriate to cutaneous ureterostomy. The procedure used must meet the condition of the patient. For patients who require permanent supravesical diversion, there are three techniques: *(a)* for the single ureter—U-shaped skin-flap cutaneous ureterostomy; *(b)* for dilated ureter on one side and a normal sized ureter on the opposite side—U-shaped skin flap cutaneous ureterostomy and transureteroureterostomy; and *(c)* for bilateral, dilated ureters—bilateral cutaneous ureterostomy through a single stoma.

In some patients, temporary supravesical diversion may be needed, so that, hopefully, the urinary tract later can be reconstituted. The loop cutaneous ureterostomy is performed in the patient with a solitary kidney and it is combined with a transureteroureterostomy when two kidneys are present. The stoma is made in either the right or left lower quadrant of the abdomen, and the ureter from the kidney to the stoma is straightened to provide good drainage. Proper placement of the stoma when using the loop cutaneous ureterostomy allows application of an appliance to collect the urine. This may function as a permanent diversion procedure or, perhaps at a later date, the diversion may be take down and the urinary tract reconstituted by straightening and reimplanting the lower end of the ureter into the bladder.

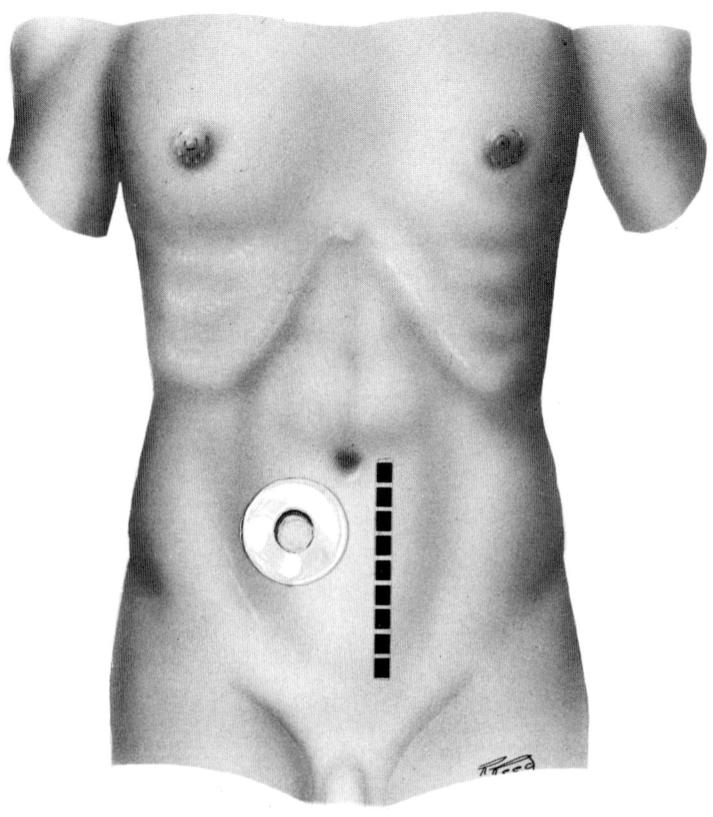

Stomal Site

Figure 40.1. The site of the urinary stoma must be selected with care, for it must allow the fitting of a single appliance that will collect the urine from both ureters without leaking. The most desirable spot for the stoma is in the right lower quadrant of the abdomen, although the left lower quadrant may be used if a better fit can be obtained. A standard appliance plate, which is available in various sizes depending on the size of the patient, is placed in the right lower quadrant so that the upper border of the plate is below the umbilicus, and the medial border overlies the midline.

The site is marked by penetrating the skin with a hypodermic needle dipped in gentian violet. When the stoma is selected in this way, it ensures that the ureters will pass through the rectus muscle, the position where the best fit of an appliance is obtained. The full urinary pouch then will be accommodated in the hollow of the groin near the pubis. It is important that the stoma is not placed at the lateral border of the rectus muscle, as a natural hollow in the skin over the linea semilunaris in this area makes adherence of the appliance difficult.

In patients with various degrees of rotoscoliosis, the stomal site must be selected with great care, and it is wise to test the site selected both in the supine and in the upright position to be sure the best position for the stoma is obtained. In general, midline stomas are more difficult to fit with an appliance and should be avoided.

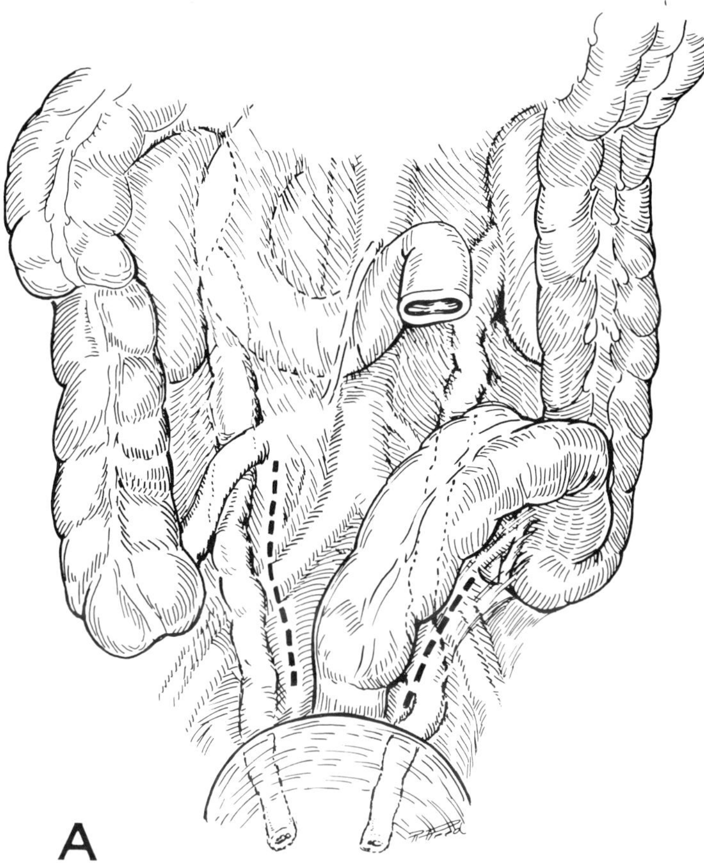

Exposure of the Ureters

Figure 40.2. **A,** a left paramedian incision is usually used for exposure of the ureters, thus keeping the incision away from the region where the appliance will be placed, yet allowing good exposure of both ureters, renal pelves, and ureterovesical junctions. The left ureter is exposed by incising the posterior peritoneum lateral to the mesosigmoid and descending colon, and retracting the colon medially. The ureter is freed from surrounding tissue and dissected down to the ureterovesical junction where it is divided and the lower end is ligated. The ureters are often dilated and tortuous, and must be straightened all the way to the renal pelvis to provide good drainage. Care must be taken to avoid interference with the intrinsic blood supply to the ureter. A minimal amount of dissection is usually done medially, except at the lower end of the ureter where great mobility is needed. On the right side, a small incision is made in the retroperitoneal region just medial to the right ureter. This ureter is mobilized to the ureterovesical junction in a similar fashion.

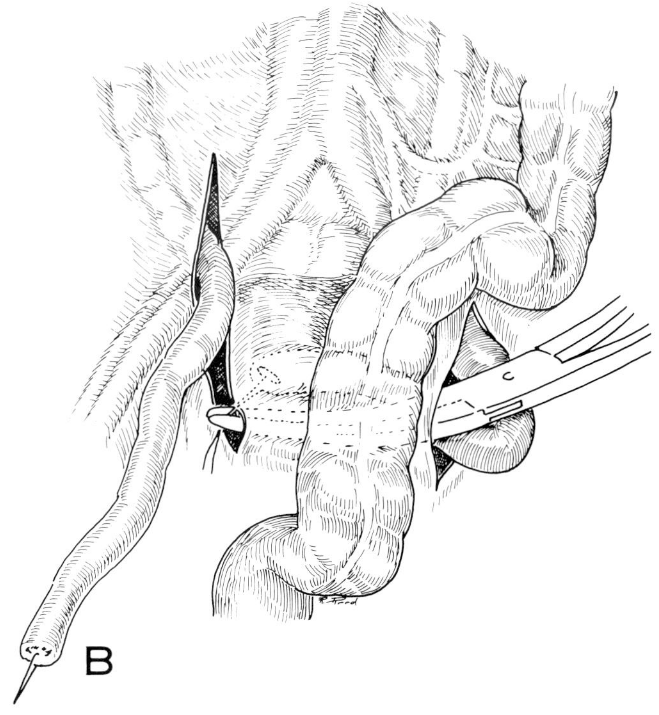

Figure 40.2. **B,** the left ureter is then brought behind the mesosigmoid, in front of the great vessels and through the opening in the retroperitoneal region on the right side. The limiting factor upward for the ureter is the inferior mesenteric artery. The surgeon should be sure that the movement of the ureter across the midline is a gentle one from renal pelvis to the distal end of the ureter to avoid acute angulation. This is easily done by blunt dissection in the avascular space in front of the great vessels.

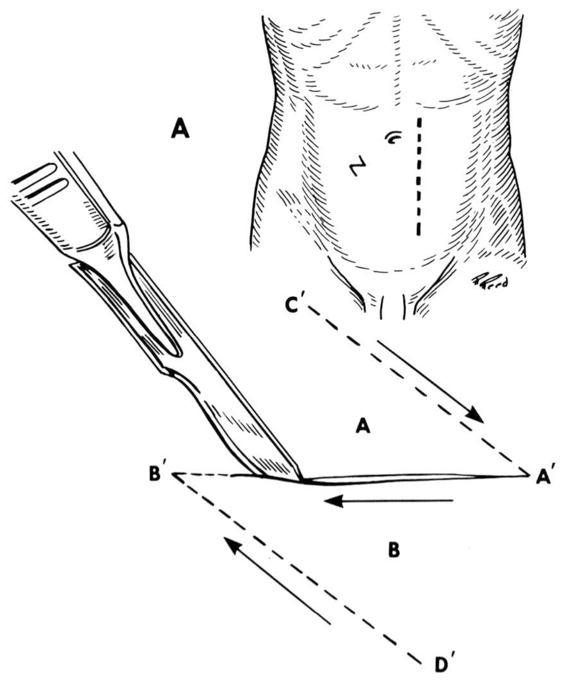

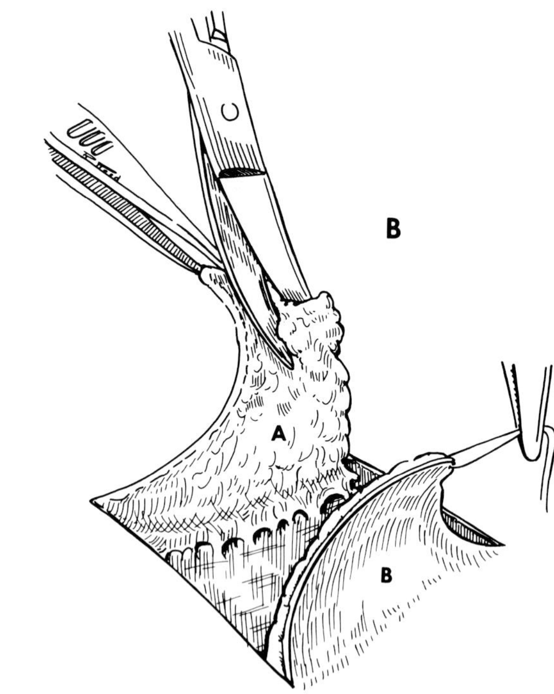

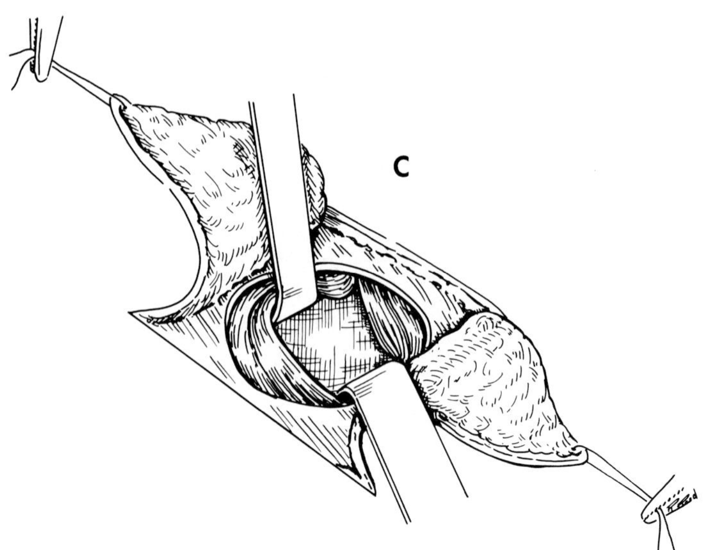

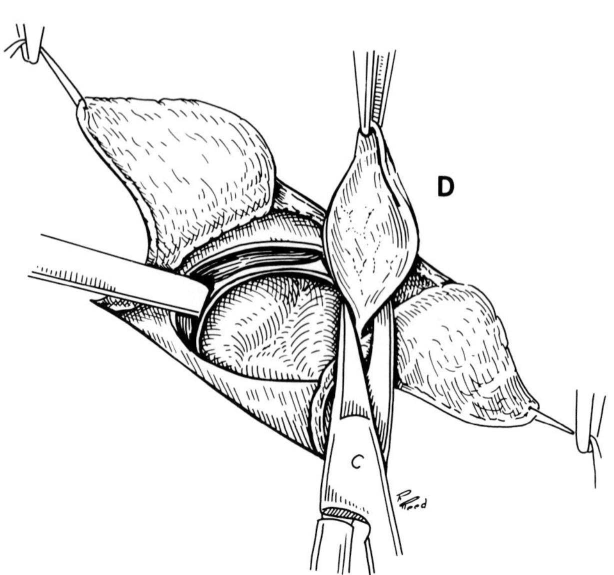

Bilateral Cutaneous Ureterostomy Through a Single Stoma

Figure 40.3. A Z-plasty is outlined on the skin with gentian violet in the area of the previously selected stomal site **(A).** After the skin is incised and trimmed **(B),** a circular button of subcutaneous fat and the anterior rectus sheath is removed, exposing the rectus muscle **(C).** The rectus muscle then is separated bluntly and another button of transversalis fascia and peritoneum is removed posteriorly **(D).** The size of the opening in the abdominal wall will depend upon the size of the two ureters, but in general, when the ureters are greatly dilated, two fingers should pass easily through the opening.

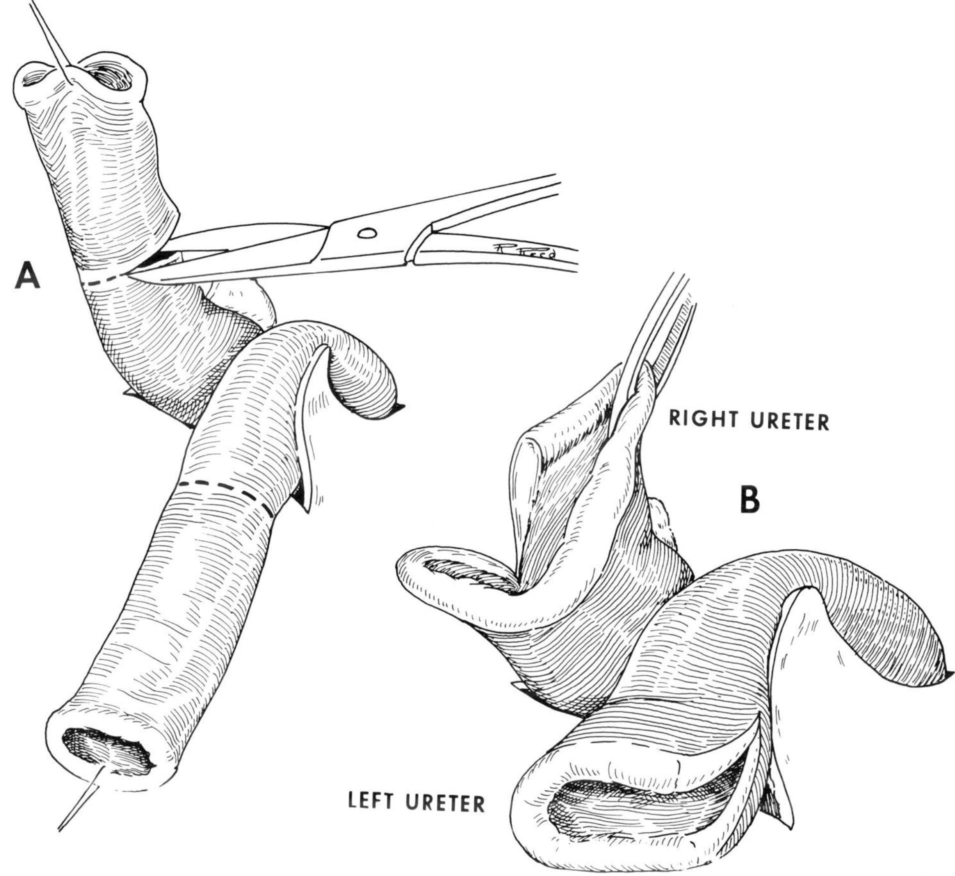

Figure 40.4. Because ureters that are suitable candidates for cutaneous ureterostomy are dilated and usually tortuous, when straightened they are much longer than is necessary to reach the skin level **(A).** In straightening the ureters, we try to avoid the major blood supply that comes into the ureters medially. There is usually an excellent intrinsic blood supply in these obstructed ureters and they can be straightened safely all the way to the renal pelvis. The excess ureter is cut off about 2 cm above the skin level and a longitudinal incision is made in the lateral border of each ureter **(B).**

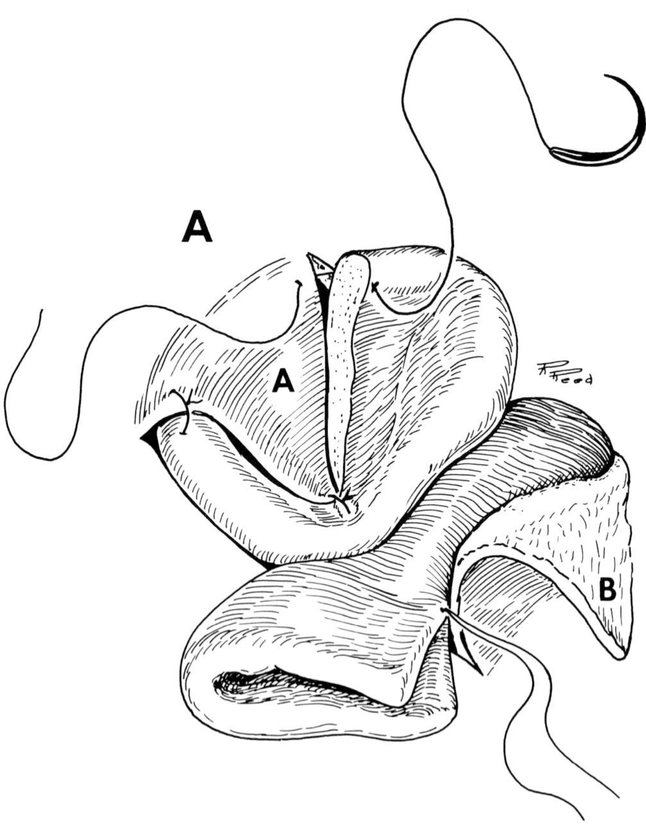

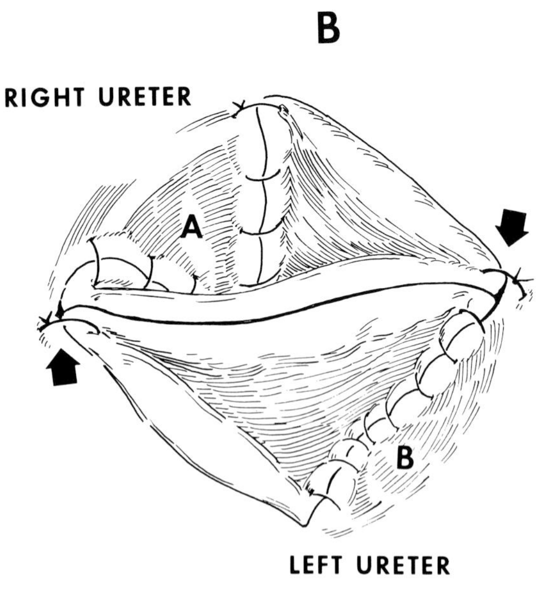

Figure 40.5. The skin flaps of the Z-plasty then are sutured into the longitudinal incision made into the ureter using either 4–0 or 5–0 interrupted chromic sutures **(A).** The midpoint of each ureter opposite the longitudinal incision is sutured to the base of the opposite skin flap as indicated by the arrows in **(B)** with interrupted 4–0 chromic sutures. The ureters then are sutured to the adjacent skin edges of the stoma with interrupted chromic sutures.

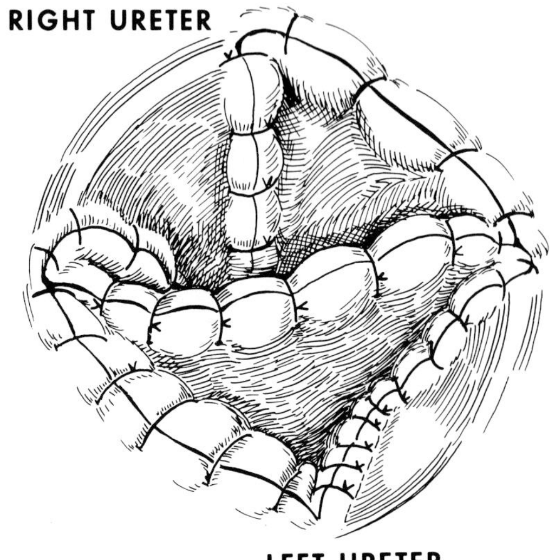

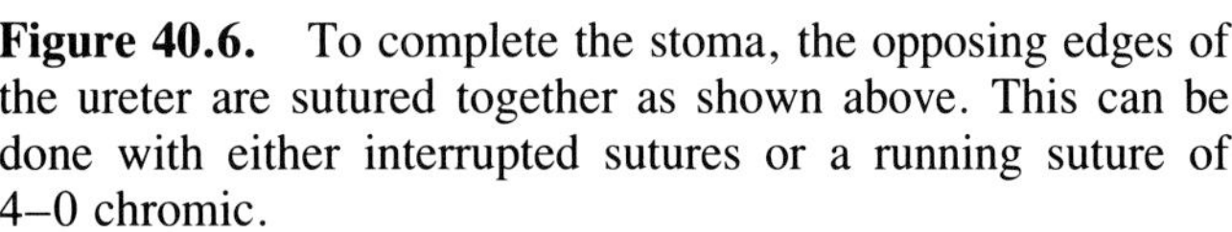

Figure 40.6. To complete the stoma, the opposing edges of the ureter are sutured together as shown above. This can be done with either interrupted sutures or a running suture of 4–0 chromic.

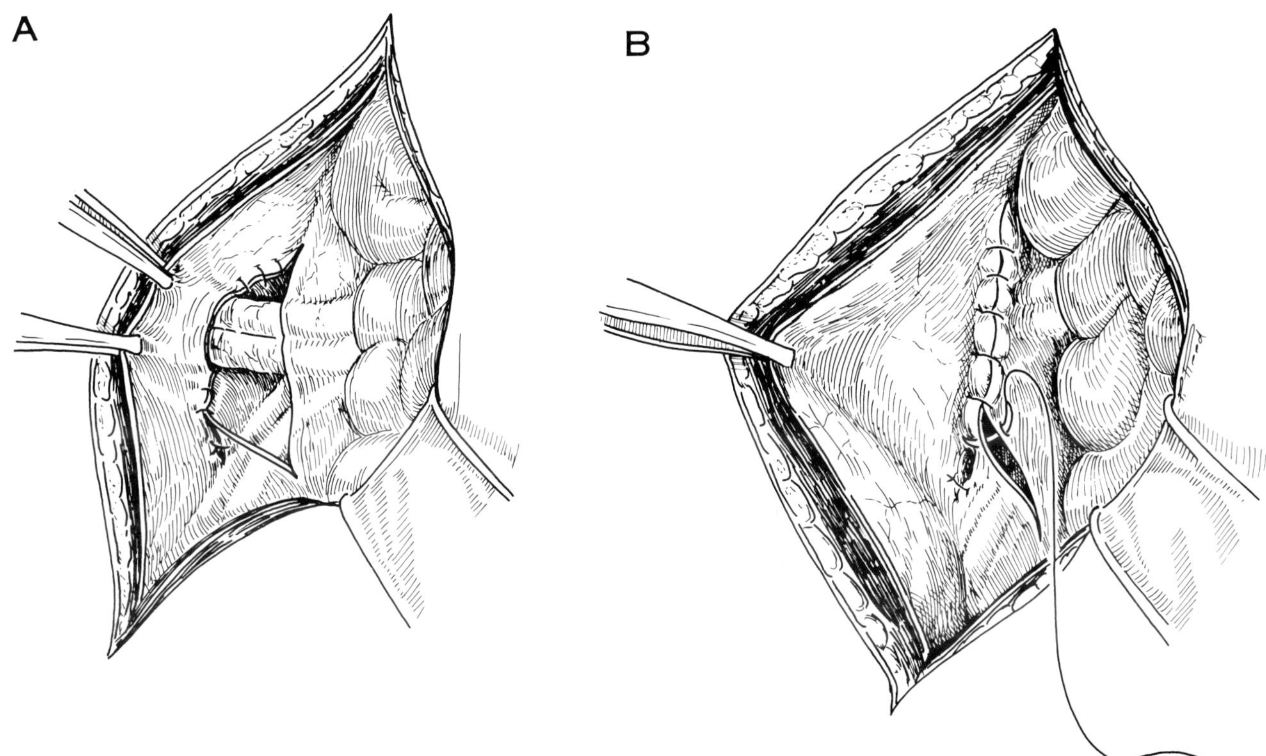

Figure 40.7. **A,** before bringing the ureters through the stoma, the lateral peritoneal margin of the incision in the posterior peritoneum is sutured to the lateral margin of the defect in the anterior peritoneum that was made for the stoma with interrupted 3–0 chromic sutures. The space lateral to this is also closed by suturing the anterior and posterior peritoneum together. The creates a cul-de-sac laterally and prevents herniation of small bowel into this space, which might occur and produce intestinal obstruction.

40.7. **B,** when the ureters have been fixed to the skin and the stoma completed, the medial margin of the incision in the posterior peritoneum is sutured to the medial side of the defect in the anterior peritoneum. The remaining defect in the posterior peritoneum simply is sutured together with a running suture of 3–0 chromic. Thus, in effect, it is creating a flap of peritoneum around the ureters. In essence, this means that the ureters in their course through the peritoneal cavity are surrounded by posterior peritoneum. This also provides a shorter and more direct course to the stoma than can be provided by bringing the ureters retroperitoneally around the abdominal wall to a midline stoma.

The incision in the posterior peritoneum lateral to the descending colon that was used in initially mobilizing the left ureter is closed with a running suture of 3–0 chromic catgut. The abdominal incision is closed in layers. No drains or stenting catheters are used and a temporary collection device is applied immediately to the stoma.

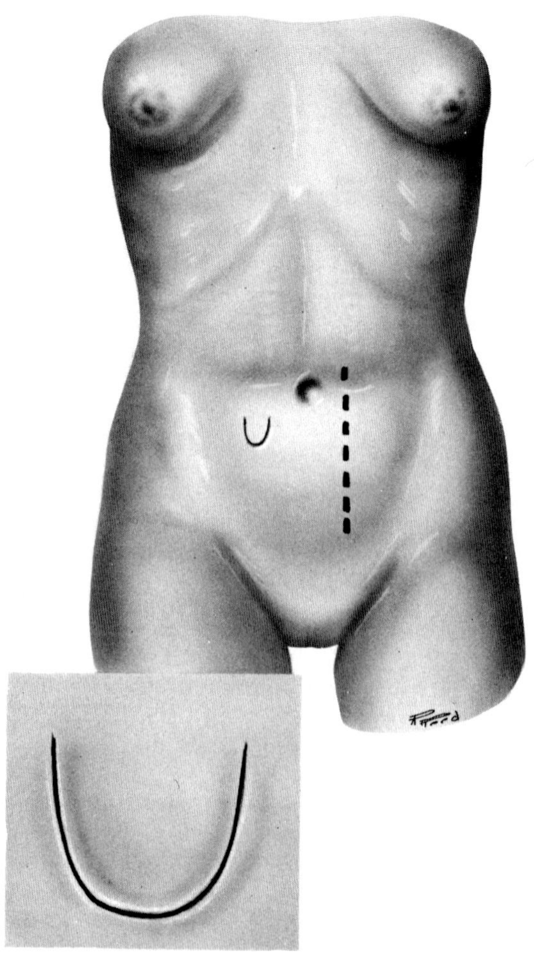

LOOP CUTANEOUS URETEROSTOMY

Figure 40.8. The loop cutaneous ureterostomy is performed according to the basic principles just presented for bilateral cutaneous ureterostomy but using a different skin incision. A U-shaped skin flap is outlined at the selected stoma site and is dissected from the underlying subcutaneous tissue. This same type of skin incision and skin flap is also used for the permanent single stoma cutaneous ureterostomy, which will be described later.

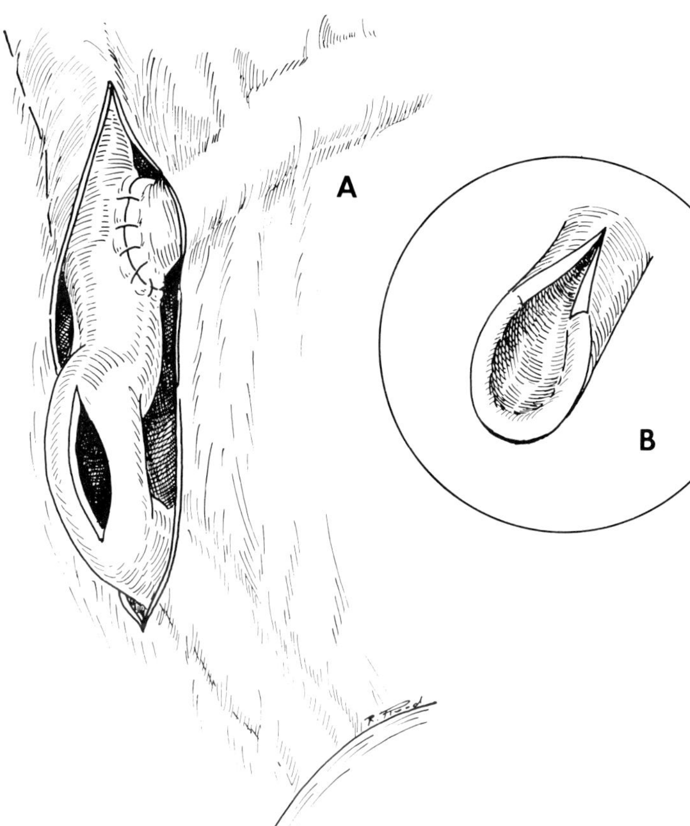

Figure 40.9. A and B, in fashioning the loop cutaneous ureterostomy, the ureter to be brought to the stoma, usually the right one, is dissected free from surrounding tissue and straightened from the renal pelvis downward until it can easily reach the skin. Again, because these ureters are thick-walled, dilated, and tortuous, they have an excellent intrinsic blood supply. Great mobility can be achieved easily. The lower end of the ureter is left in situ attached to the bladder. A longitudinal incision is made in the anterior wall of the ureter where it is to be sutured to the skin flap **(A).**

When there are two kidneys present, a transureteroureterostomy is performed using an elliptical **(B)** end-to-side anastomosis. A running suture of 4–0 or 5–0 chromic is used to form the anastomosis, much as one would do a vascular anastomosis. The left ureter is brought behind the mesosigmoid in a gentle curve from left to right and the excess ureter is trimmed away. The lower end of the left ureter is ligated near the ureterovesical junction.

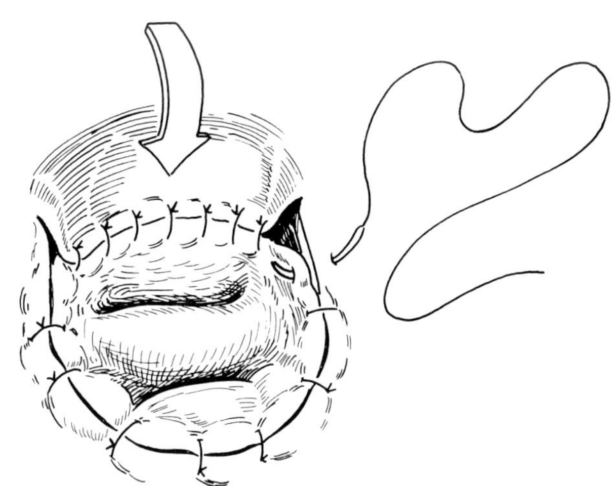

Figure 40.10. The skin flap is sutured into the upper end of the longitudinal incision in the ureter and the rest of the ureteral opening is sutured to the skin edges. This, in effect, creates a double-barreled ureterostomy in which only the upper lumen is functional. Peritoneal flaps are fashioned to surround the loop ureterostomy as it passes through the peritoneal cavity, as has been previously described.

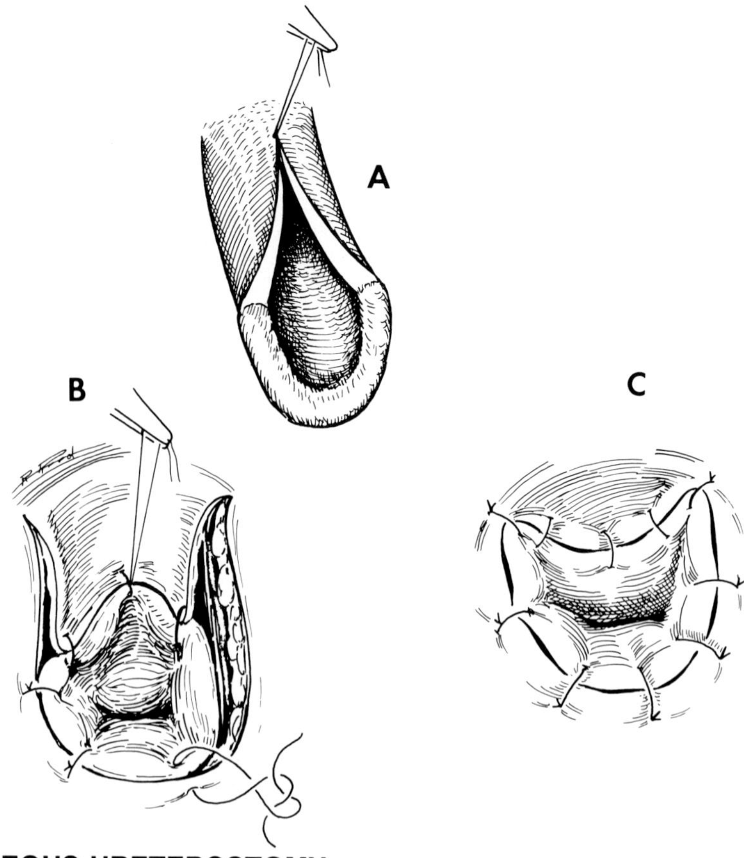

UNILATERAL CUTANEOUS URETEROSTOMY, WITH U-SHAPED SKIN FLAP

Figure 40.11. A permanent end ureterostomy for a single dilated ureter is performed by using the U-shaped skin flap (Fig. 40.8). The dilated ureter is dissected free from surrounding tissue and divided near the ureterovesical junction. The lower end of the ureter is ligated. The ureter is then straightened so the distance from the renal pelvis to the stoma is as short as possible and the excess ureter is discarded. A longitudinal incision is made in the anterior wall of the ureter **(A).** The skin flap is then sutured into the longitudinal incision **(B).** The stoma is completed by suturing the rest of the ureter to the skin margins with interrupted 4–0 chromic sutures **(C).**

When there are two kidneys and one ureter is dilated and the other is normal in size, the dilated ureter should be mobilized and brought to the skin. The normal ureter should be joined to the dilated ureter by a transureteroureterostomy.

POSTOPERATIVE CARE

The stoma is measured for a permanent appliance on the 3rd postoperative day and the appliance is in place by the time the patient is ready for discharge. Instructions are given by an Enterostomal Therapist to the patient and/or parents in fitting the appliance and care of the stoma and the peristomal skin. Each patient is seen daily by the Enterostomal Therapist during the postoperative period and at subsequent postoperative visits to be sure a proper fitting of the appliance is obtained and to help the patient with any special problems that may develop.

All patients are seen for follow-up examinations at 1 month and at 4–6 months, at which time renal function studies and an excretory urogram are obtained. In addition, after carefully cleaning the stoma, a catheter is passed up each ureter and the residual urine is obtained for measurement and for culture and sensitivity studies. Additional postoperative visits are usually at 6-month to 1-year intervals depending on how well the patient does.

Suggested Readings

Lapides J: Butterfly cutaneous ureterostomy. *J Urol* 88:735, 1962.

Mingledorff WE, Rinker JR, Owen G: Experimental study of the blood supply of the distal ureter with reference to cutaneous ureterostomy. *J Urol* 92:424, 1964.

Rinker JR, Blanchard TW: Improvement of the circulation of the ureter prior to cutaneous ureterostomy: A clinical study. *J Urol* 96:44, 1966.

Turnbull R, Weakley F: *Atlas of Intestinal Stomas.* St. Louis, CV Mosby, 1967.

CHAPTER 41

Cutaneous Urinary Diversion

JAMES E. MONTIE

Supravesical urinary diversion occasionally becomes necessary in the management of urologic disorders in adults and, less commonly, in children. The goals of the diversion must be to provide good drainage to the upper tract, to avoid upper tract infections, and to provide means of collecting the urine to preclude incontinence. The ileal conduit, as initially described by Bricker (1), has been the mainstay of urinary diversions over the last 35 years. In our opinion, it still remains the preferred method of diversion in most situations. In selected circumstances, a continent reservoir, a reservoir anastomosed to the urethra after removal of the bladder and prostate, ureterosigmoidostomy, or cutaneous ureterostomy may be appropriate choices. Patient education relative to the advantages and disadvantages of a diversion with an appliance or a continent cutaneous reservoir is the key to lasting acceptance and optimal rehabilitation.

INDICATIONS FOR A CUTANEOUS URINARY DIVERSION

Neoplasm

Carcinoma of the bladder is by far the most common indication for upper tract diversion at this time. In some situations, other pelvic malignancies such as carcinoma of the cervix, carcinoma of the rectum, or carcinoma of the prostate, might provide an indication for removal of the bladder and the need for a diversion.

Neuropathic Bladder

Bladder dysfunction secondary to congenital malformations of the sacral spinal cord used to be the primary indication for supravesical diversion. Surgery is uncommonly performed for this reason now. It would be used in a patient who had failed conservative management with intermittent catheterization and anticholinergic medications, possibly failed augmentation, and who is having deterioration of the upper tracts.

Exstrophy of the Bladder

Attempts are now made to preserve bladder function with or without a bladder augmentation in most individuals with exstrophy of the bladder. In some situations, a supravesical urinary diversion will be necessary if reconstruction of the bladder fails.

Obstructive Uropathy

Occasionally, patients with obstructive uropathy from external radiation therapy to a pelvic malignancy may need to have a urinary diversion. There can be an obstruction or a vesicovaginal or enterovesical fistula as a consequence of the disease or from previous radiation therapy or surgery.

PREOPERATIVE CARE

Well-trained enterostomal therapy support is mandatory to provide successful postoperative care for a stoma patient. The long-term success of the procedure may depend on how well the patient is instructed in caring for the stoma. The patient must be aware of the consequences of wearing an external appliance and, often, it is necessary for both the husband and wife or other family members to be involved in the preoperative education.

A 24-hr bowel prep is currently used at the Cleveland Clinic. Four liters of GoLYTLEY solution is given orally on the afternoon before surgery. No enemas are given. The patient receives a single dose of a broad spectrum antibiotic intravenously before the operation and for 24–48 hr postoperatively. This antibiotic regimen is purely aimed at wound infection prophylaxis. Some surgeons administer oral nonabsorbable antibiotics as well but the need for this over and above systemic antibiotics is debatable.

It is mandatory that an appropriate stoma site be marked before the operation. As otherwise technically successful operation can become a disaster if the stoma site has not been appropriately chosen and the patient has difficulties wearing an appliance. The patient must be comfortable in the management of the stoma before discharge.

The choice of the method of urinary diversion is based on a mutual decision by the patient and physician. Table 41.1 lists the variables that are important in the decision-making process.

Table 41.1
Issues to Consider in Choice of Urinary Diversion Method

Ileal Conduit	Continent Reservoir
Must wear appliance	Stoma still present
Low incidence upper tract infection in adults	Must perform intermittent catheterization of stoma
Few perioperative complications	Efferent valve malfunction in 20–30%
5–10% late stoma problems	Longer, more tedious operation

Postoperative care of a continent reservoir includes irrigation every 2 hr for 1 week and every 4 hr after that with gradually increasing intervals. Proper nursing education and support is mandatory. Stents and intubation of the pouch are maintained for 3 weeks.

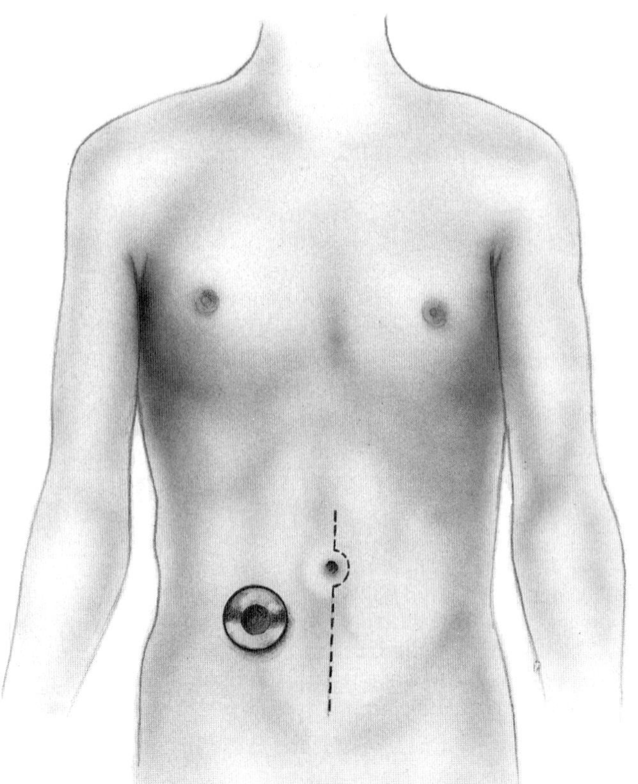

OPERATIVE TECHNIQUE FOR AN ILEAL CONDUIT

Figure 41.1. A midline incision extending from the pubis to above the umbilicus is used in preference to a low transverse incision. The transverse incision gives adequate exposure but may interfere with the site for the stoma placement by producing irregularity of the skin surface, which will interfere with adherence of the collecting device. The stoma should pass through the center of rectus muscle to minimize the risk for a parastomal hernia.

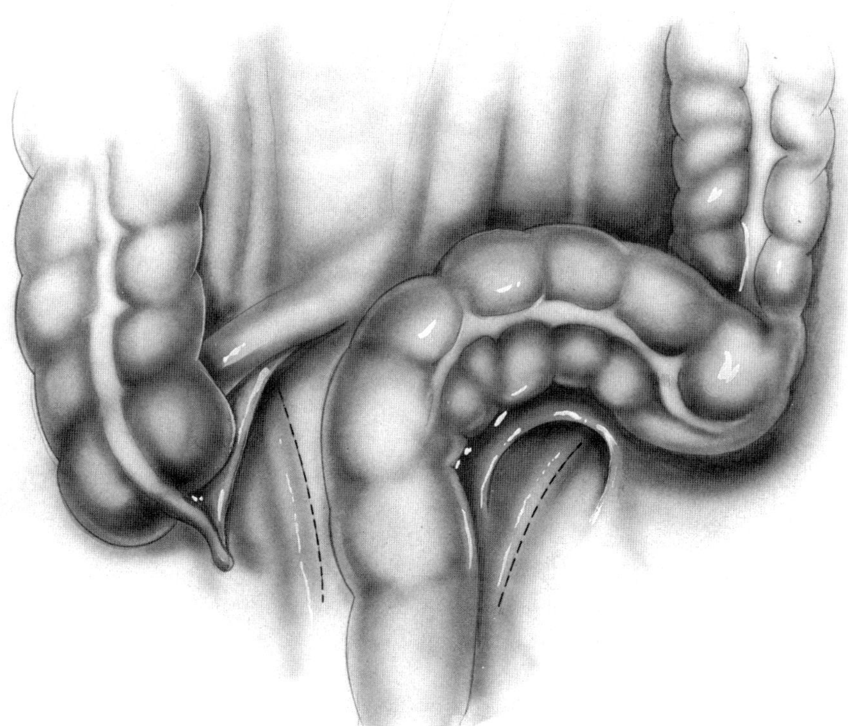

Figure 41.2. The left ureter is exposed through an incision lateral to the sigmoid colon, mobilizing the sigmoid and its mesentery in a medial direction. The right ureter is exposed through an incision in the posterior peritoneum somewhat medial to the course of the right ureter just above the brim of the pelvis. The ureters are mobilized to the ureterovesical junction, taking care to include a large amount of periureteral adventitial tissue along with the ureter to optimize collateral blood supply.

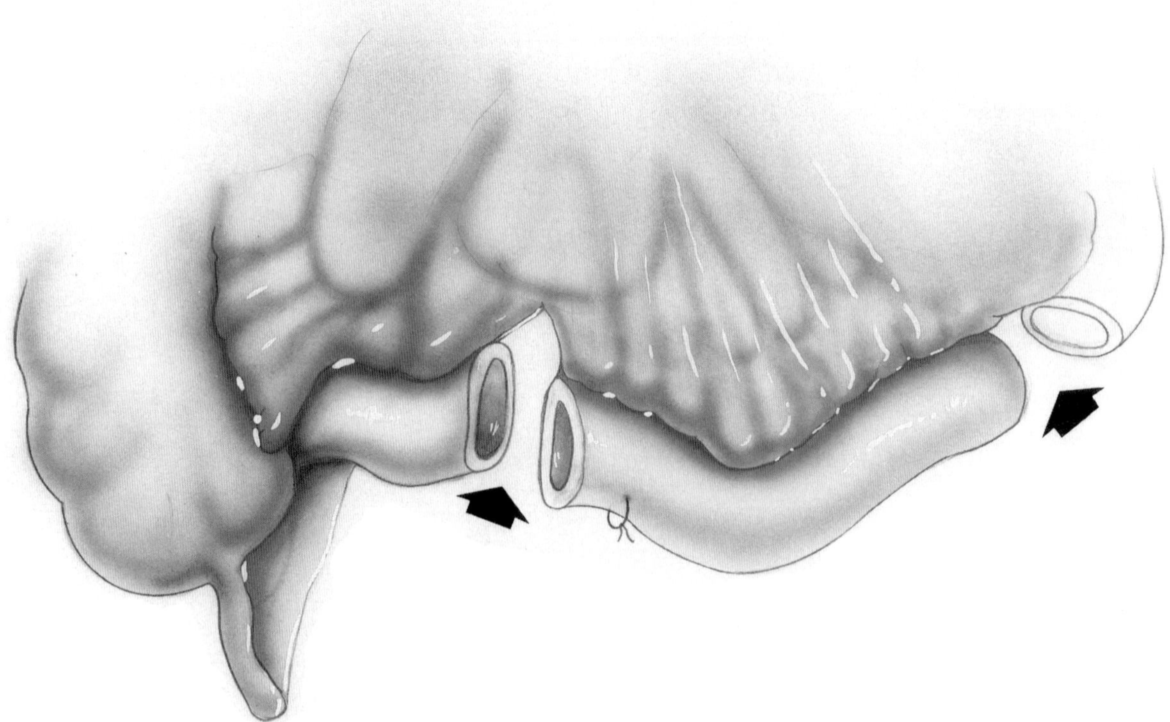

Figure 41.3. The ileocecal valve is identified and a suitable segment of the terminal ileum identified. There is an avascular segment 8–10 cm from the ileocecal valve that can be identified between the ileocolic artery and the last intestinal branch of the superior mesentery artery. The small arcade near the bowel of these vessels can be divided without impacting the blood supply to the conduit. When a loop stoma is used, it is often not necessary to divide the mesentery more than a distance of 2 or 3 cm and, thus, it is frequently possible to avoid interruption of any significant blood vessels in the mesentery. The incision in the mesentery at the more proximal site of the division of the bowel can also be quite short because less mobility is needed in this area. Care should be taken to avoid basing the vascular pedicle of the conduit on too narrow a mesenteric base, which can predispose to rotation of the conduit. The length of the conduit ranges from 15–20 cm depending on the body habitus of the patient. An appendectomy is not routinely performed.

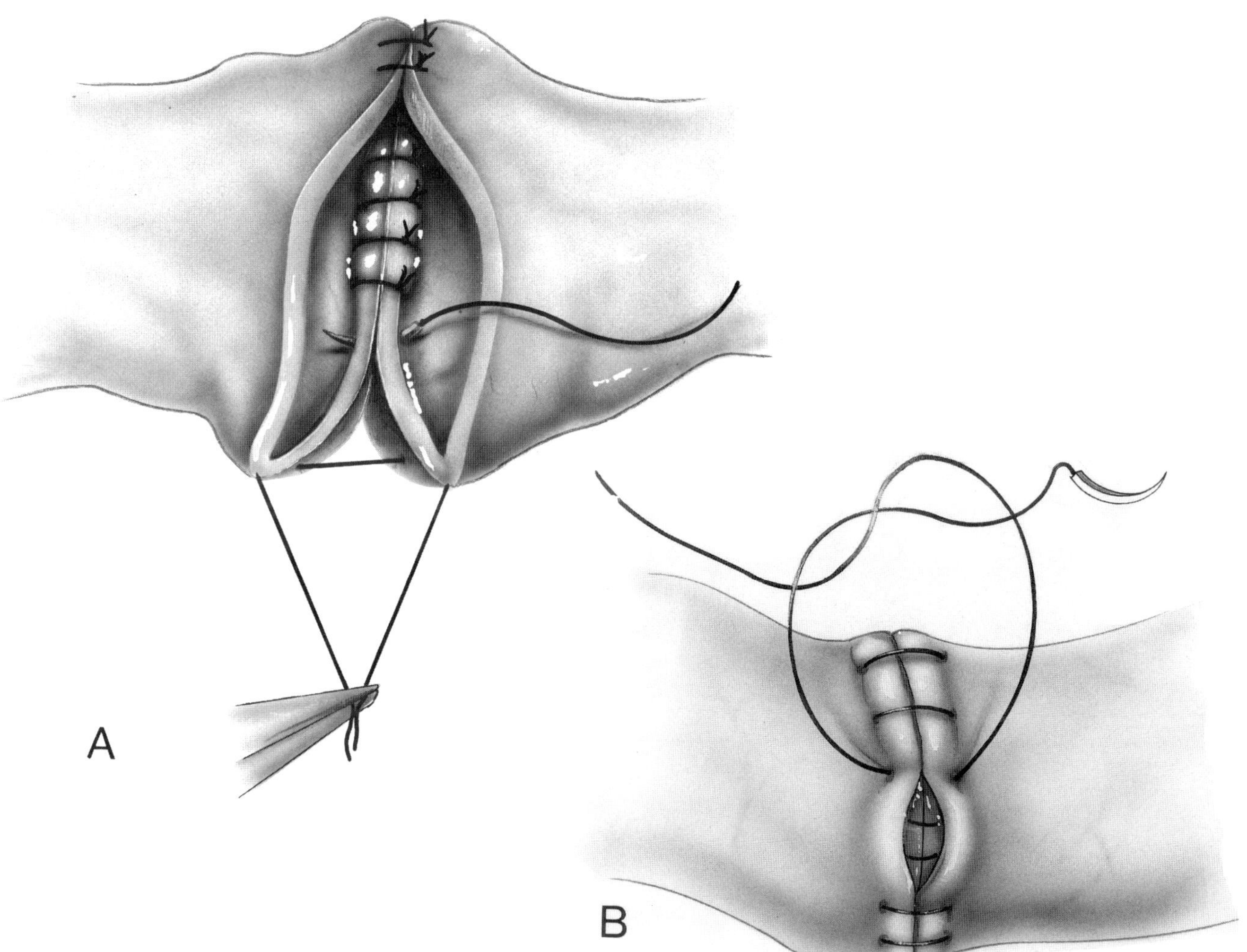

Figure 41.4. **A,** the enteroenterostomy should be performed cephalad to the conduit. Generally, a two-layered hand anastomosis has been used but many different types of bowel anastomoses can be performed successfully in normal bowel. The inner layer can be running or interrupted absorbable chromic suture through all layers of the bowel. Interrupted sutures are a personal preference in that the lumen of the bowel tends to be narrowed less with this technique. **B,** a second layer of seromuscular sutures with 3–0 nonabsorbable material is used to reinforce the anastomosis.

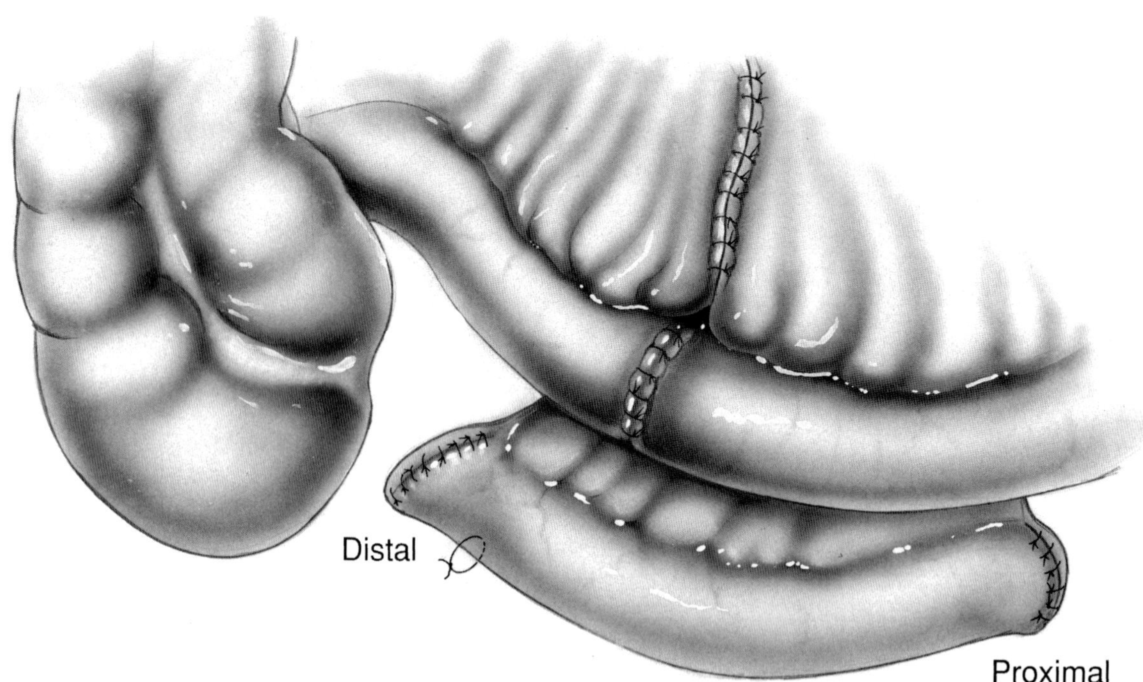

Figure 41.5. The defect in the mesentery at the site of the enteroenterostomy is closed with interrupted 4–0 nonabsorbable sutures. Care should be taken to avoid restricting the mobility of the loop itself with this closure.

The proximal (butt) and distal ends of the conduit are both oversewn in two layers of nonabsorbable suture; staples should not be used because of possible calculus formation. It is important to mark the distal end of the conduit with a seromuscular tagging stitch to eliminate the possibility of confusion or rotation of the segments later in the procedure.

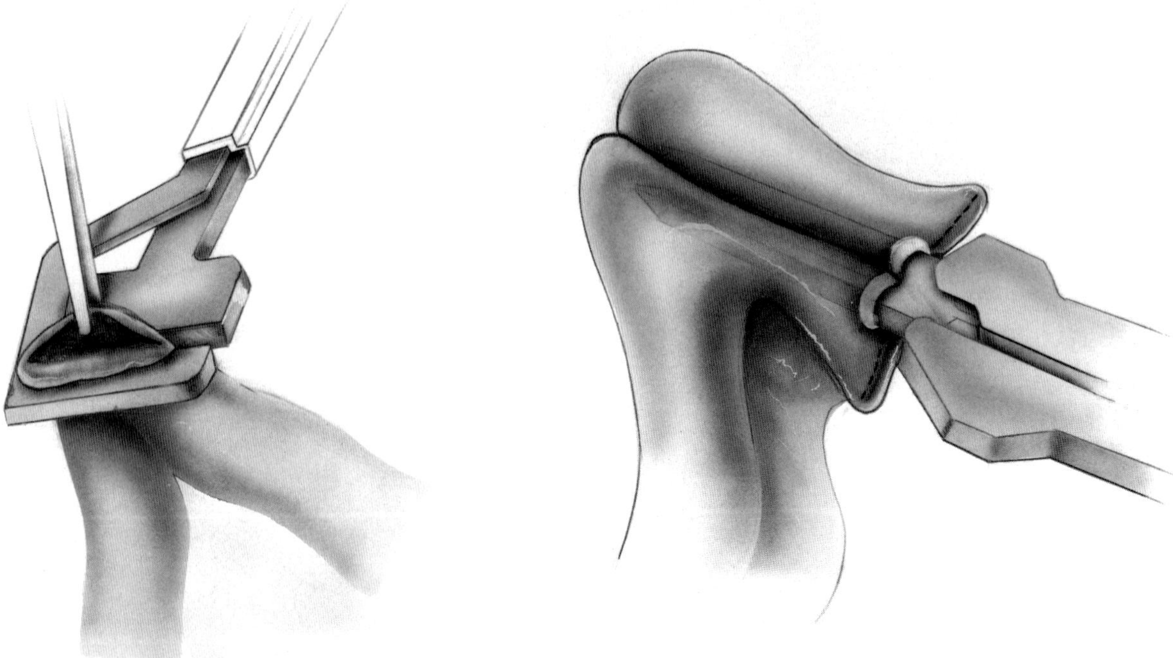

Figure 41.6. An alternative form of enteroenterostomy can be performed using staples. A GIA stapler is used to divide the bowel and to perform the enteroenterostomy. A TA55 can be used to complete the anastomosis. A stapled anastomosis does save time during the procedure but experience with the stapling equipment and knowledge of potential complications are needed.

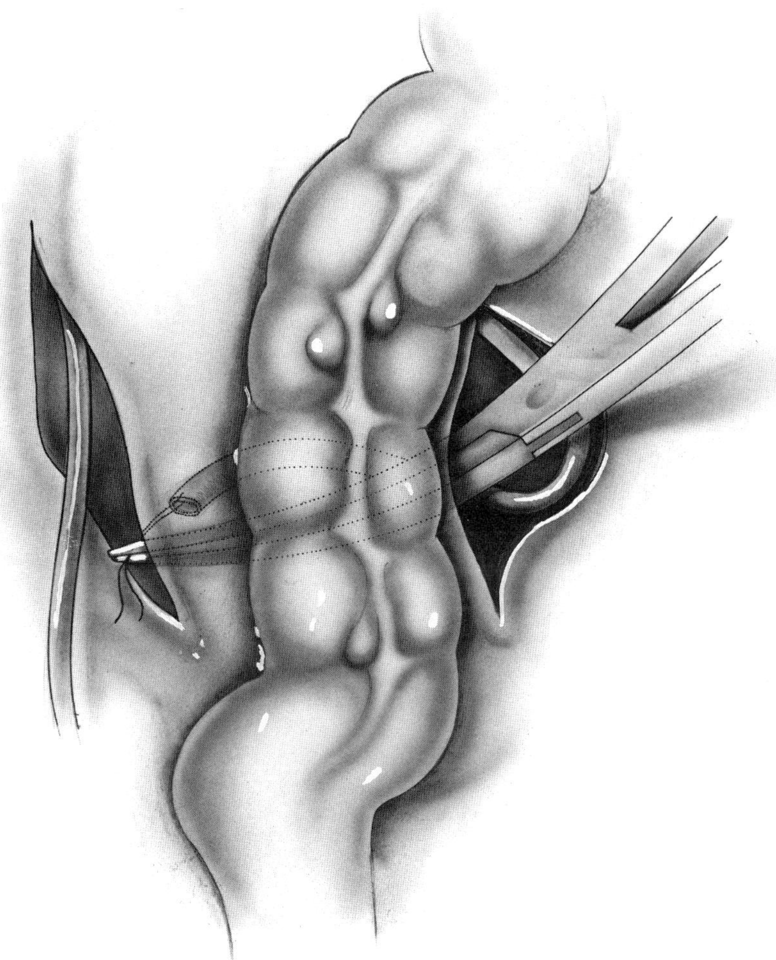

Figure 41.7. The left ureter is divided near the ureterovesical junction and the distal segment is ligated. The left ureter is passed behind the sigmoid mesentery in an avascular space in front of the great vessels, so it will emerge through the incision in the posterior peritoneum on the right side. Care must be taken to ensure that the ureter is neither rotated nor angulated but comes over in a gentle curve to the right side of the retroperitoneum. The right lower ureter is also divided near the ureterovesical junction.

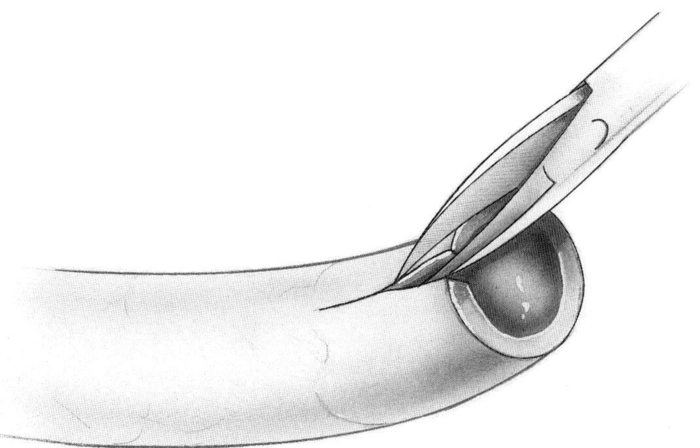

Figure 41.8. The ureter is spatulated on its medial aspect for distance of 5–6 mm.

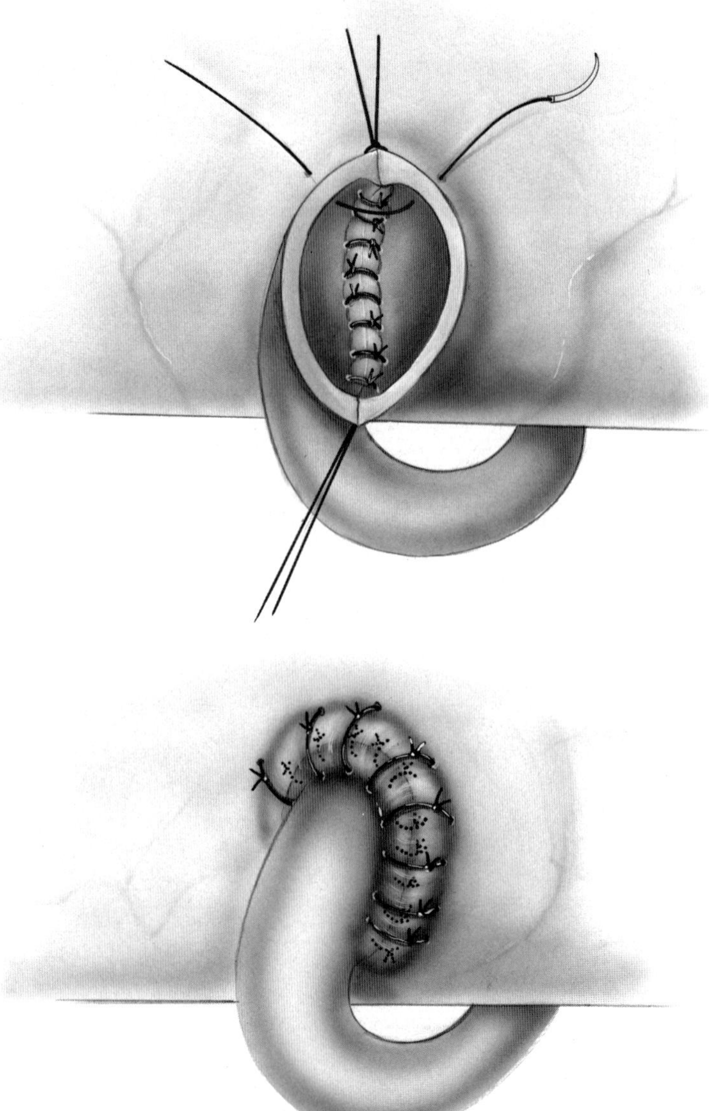

Figure 41.9. The ureteroileal anastomosis is performed in two layers. The anastomosis is very similar to an interrupted vascular anastomosis using interrupted 5–0 absorbable sutures. A watertight anastomosis is the goal. A second layer of stitches from the seromuscular portion of the bowel to the periureteral adventitial tissues is helpful in inverting the anastomosis and providing extra security for a watertight closure. Ureteral stents are not used routinely but certainly can be used if this is the surgeon's preference.

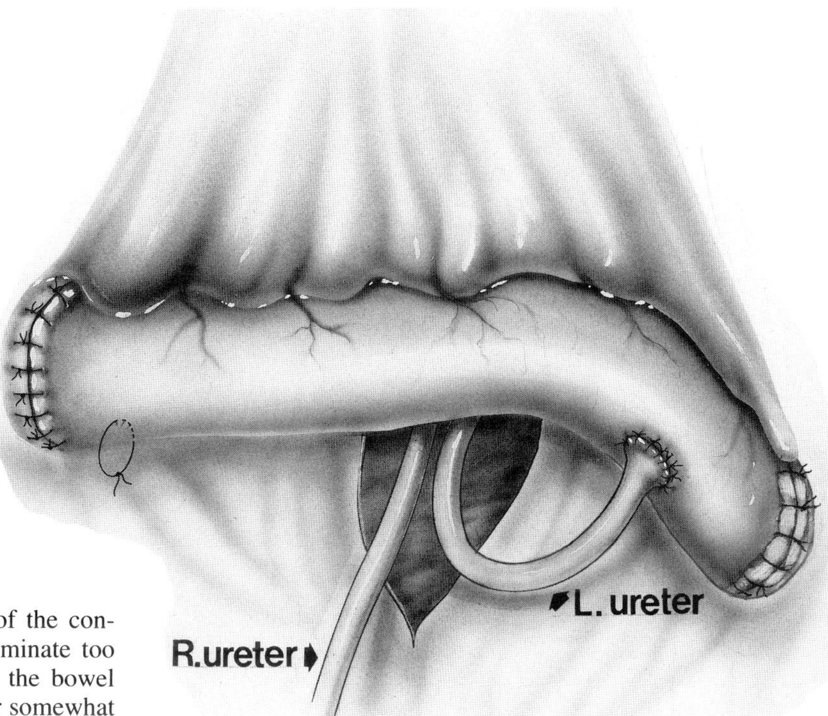

Figure 41.10. It is important that the butt end of the conduit be tacked down to the retroperitoneum to eliminate too much mobility. The left ureter is anastomosed to the bowel near the butt end of the conduit and the right ureter somewhat more distally to the conduit.

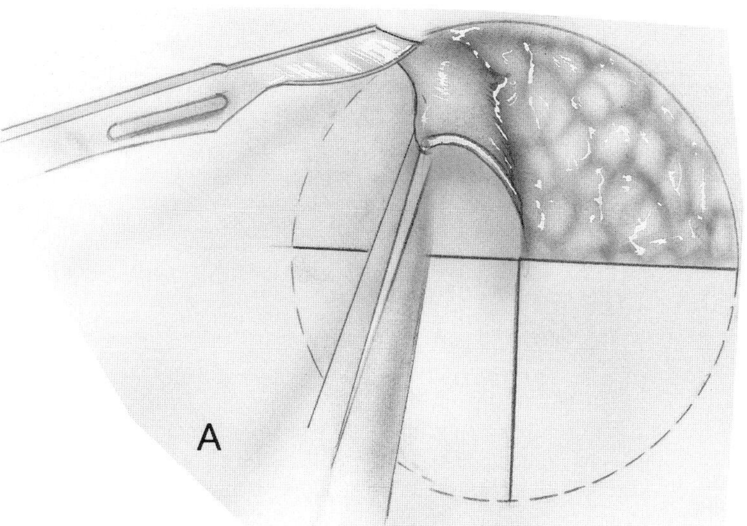

Figure 41.11. A, attention is now turned to creation of the abdominal wall aperture at the previously marked stoma site. It is imperative that the stoma site is marked before the operation by an enterostomal therapist with the patient evaluated in both the supine and sitting position. A quarter-size button of skin is removed and the subcutaneous tissue is incised, exposing the anterior rectus fascia.

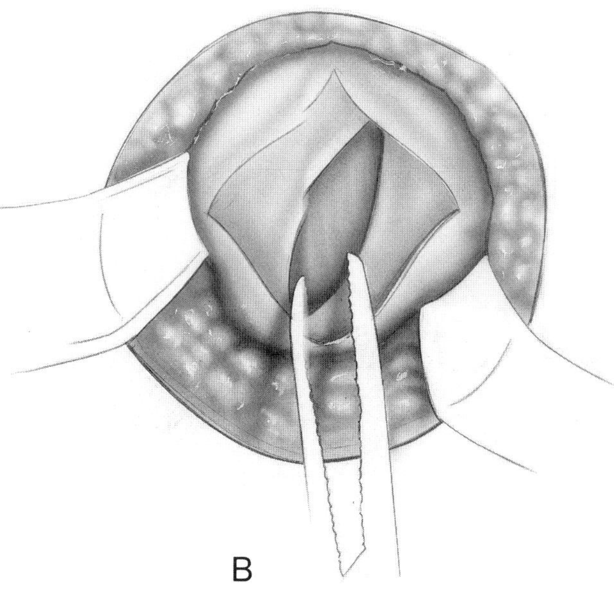

Figure 41.11. B, a similar quarter-size incision is made in the anterior rectus fascia and then the rectus muscle fibers are split in their longitudinal direction and the posterior peritoneum is perforated with a Kelly clamp. The aperture in the abdominal wall should easily admit two fingers.

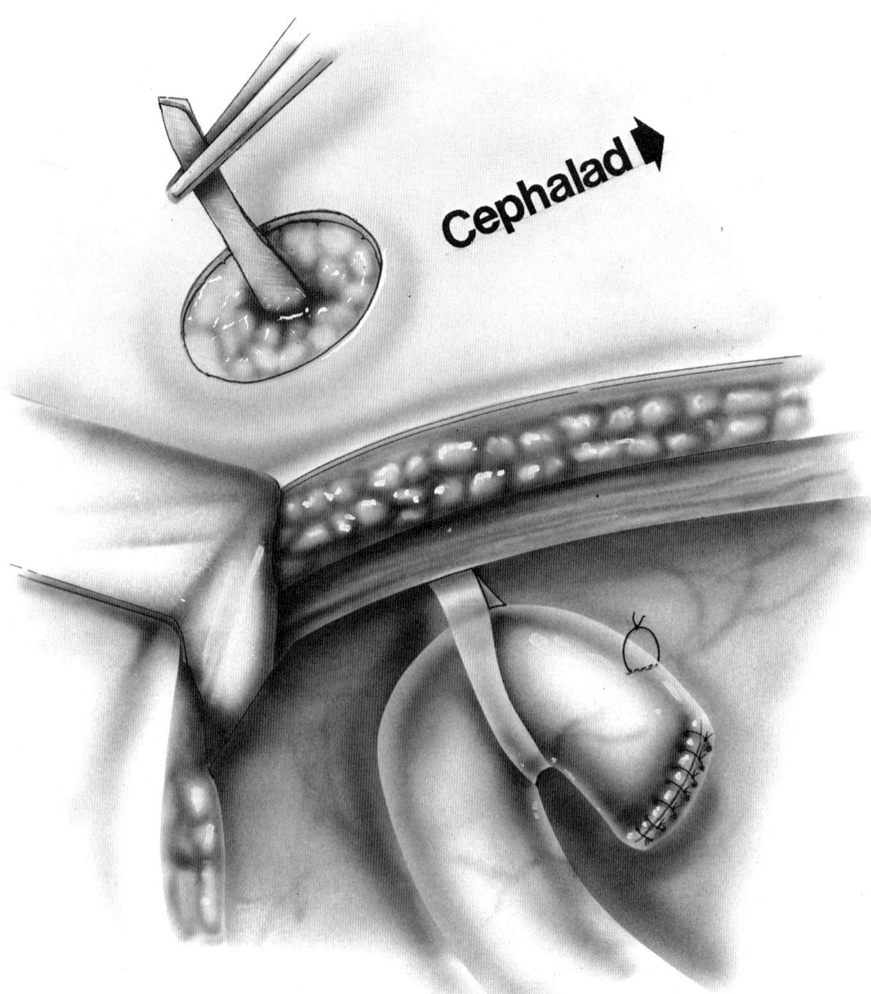

Figure 41.12. A loop stoma is used routinely. The distal portion of the conduit should be the cephalad portion of the loop stoma (i.e., the functional segment of conduit is inferior). An umbilical tape is placed through the mesentery just under the bowel approximately 3 cm proximal to the distal end of the conduit. This loop is then brought through the abdominal wall aperture, taking care to avoid tension on the bowel during this maneuver.

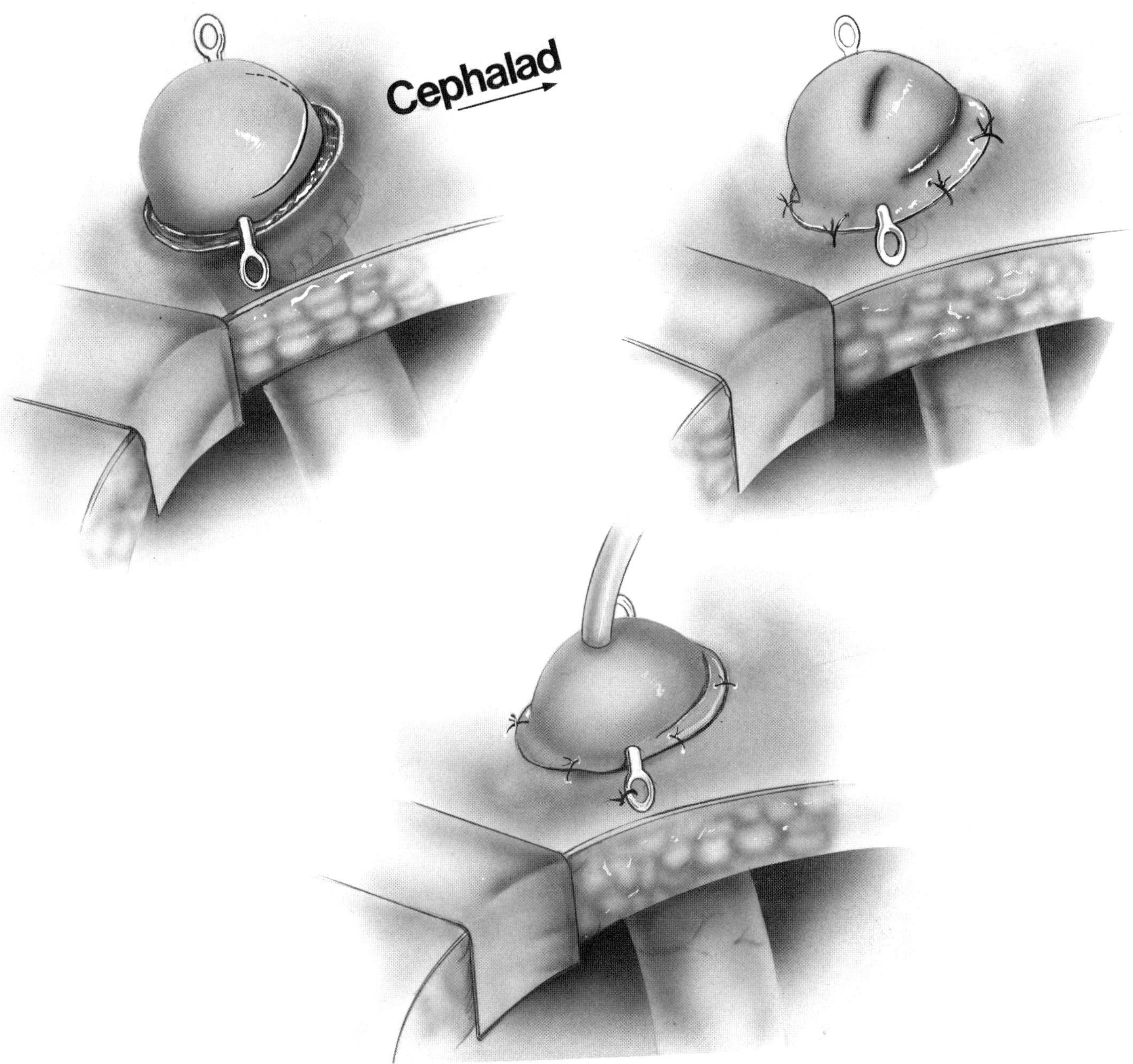

Figure 41.13. The umbilical tape is then replaced with a small plastic ileostomy rod. The ileostomy rod is sutured to the skin. The stoma is matured by incising the ileum approximately ⅘ of the way around on the cephalad aspect of the loop. This allows the stoma to be everted to create a typical "rosebud" stoma. A stoma is matured on the functional end with interrupted 3–0 chromic sutures with bites being taken of full thickness through the bowel, a seromuscular bite farther down, and then the subcutaneous tissue. On the nonfunctional end of the loop, sutures are only placed from the bowel to the subcutaneous tissue; this end ultimately will retract and be flush with the abdominal wall. A no. 24 French catheter is placed into the conduit and sutured to the ileostomy rod. The balloon is not inflated. This allows the conduit to be decompressed until adequate healing has taken place. The loop stoma is particularly advantageous in obese patients or patients who have had previous radiation therapy and in whom the blood supply to the conduit may not be ideal. Because it has such a reliable blood supply, we have used it routinely in more recent years.

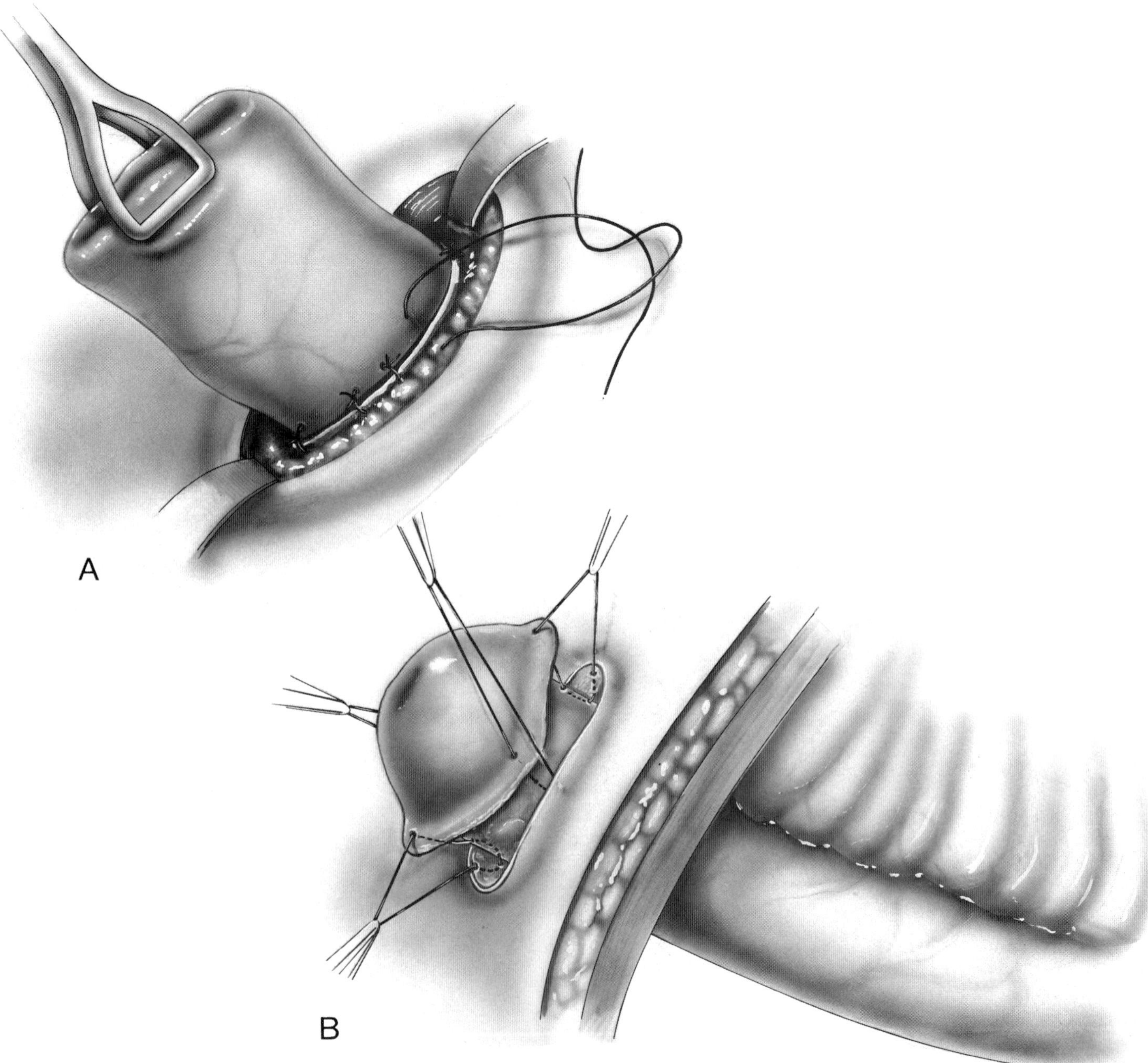

Figure 41.14. **A,** in many patients, an end stoma remains a satisfactory option. In this situation, the terminal portion of the conduit is brought directly through the anterior abdominal wall after a small amount of mesentery has been freed off the end. The nonabsorbable stitches are placed from the anterior rectus fascia to the seromuscular wall of the bowel. **B,** the stoma is matured by everting the stoma with interrupted 3–0 chromic sutures through the end of the stoma, the seromuscular bowel wall, and then to the subcutaneous tissue. The ideal stoma should project 2 cm above the skin level.

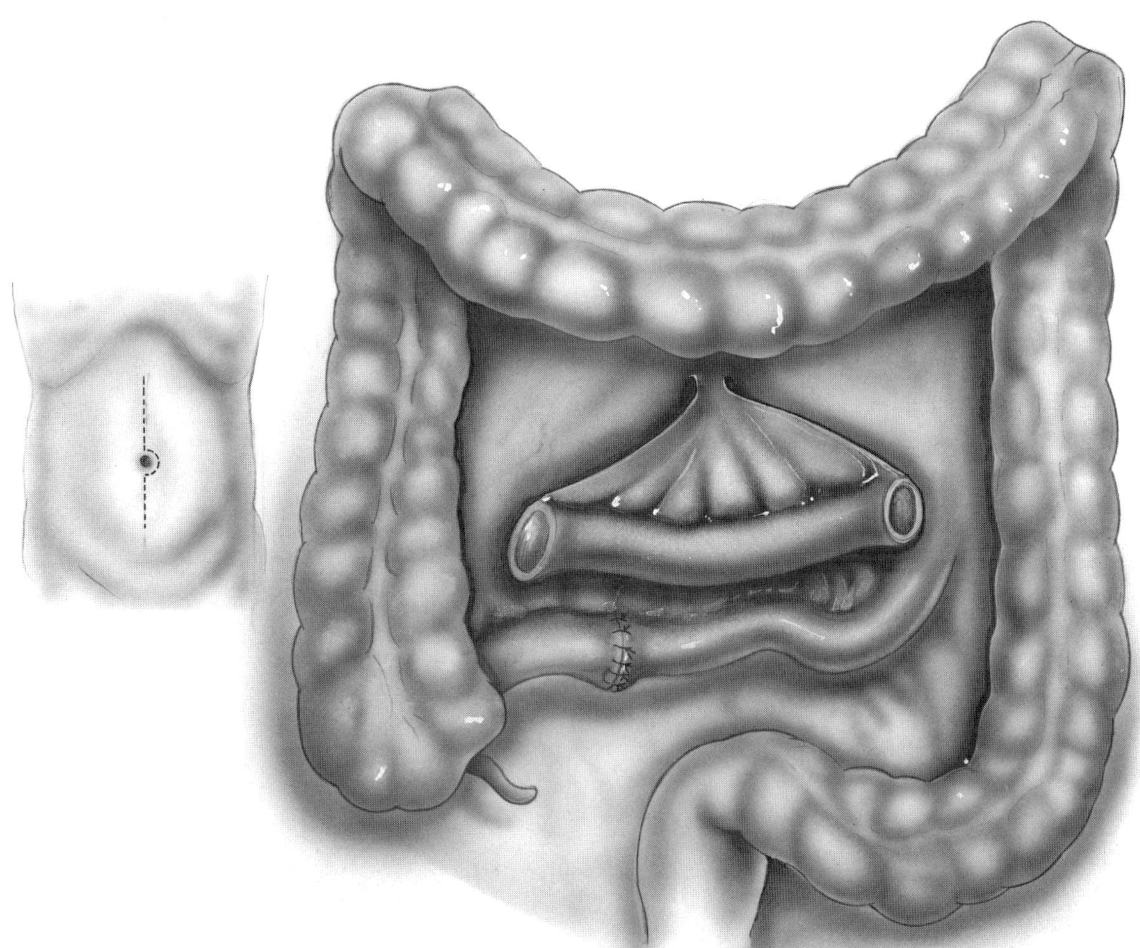

Figure 41.15. In some circumstances, it is necessary to perform a ''high'' ileal conduit. In this situation, the conduit can go from one renal pelvis or upper ureter to the opposite side and then to the skin. Most commonly, the stoma site is maintained in the right lower quadrant and the ileal segment goes from the left renal pelvis to the right renal pelvis and then to the skin. Care is taken to keep the loop as short as possible but it is frequently necessary to have a longer loop than usual to allow this diversion to be performed.

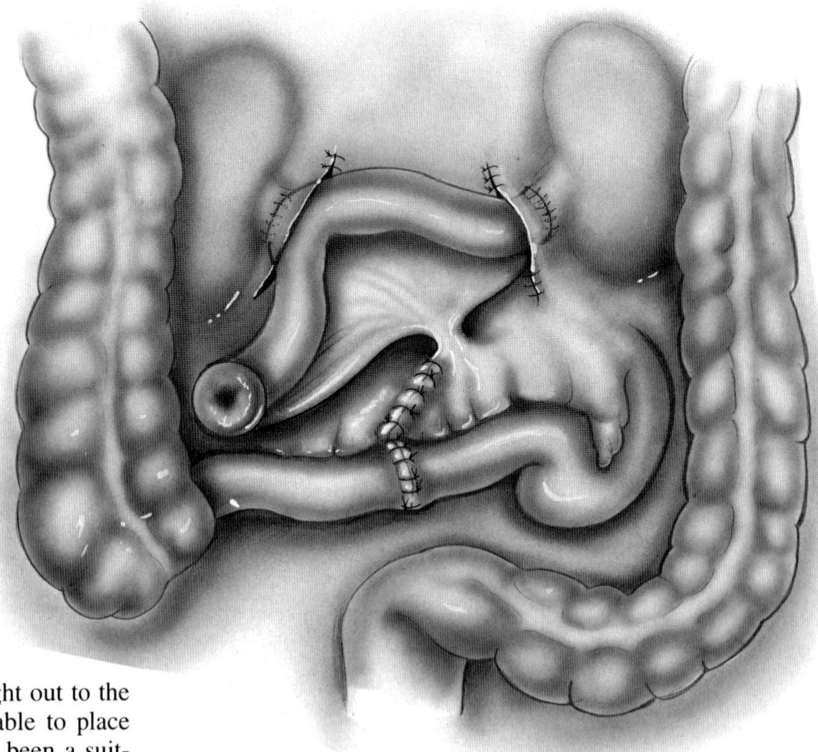

Figure 41.16. The distal portion is again brought out to the skin as an everted stoma. It is perfectly reasonable to place the stoma in the right upper quadrant if this has been a suitable site as determined by the preoperative marking.

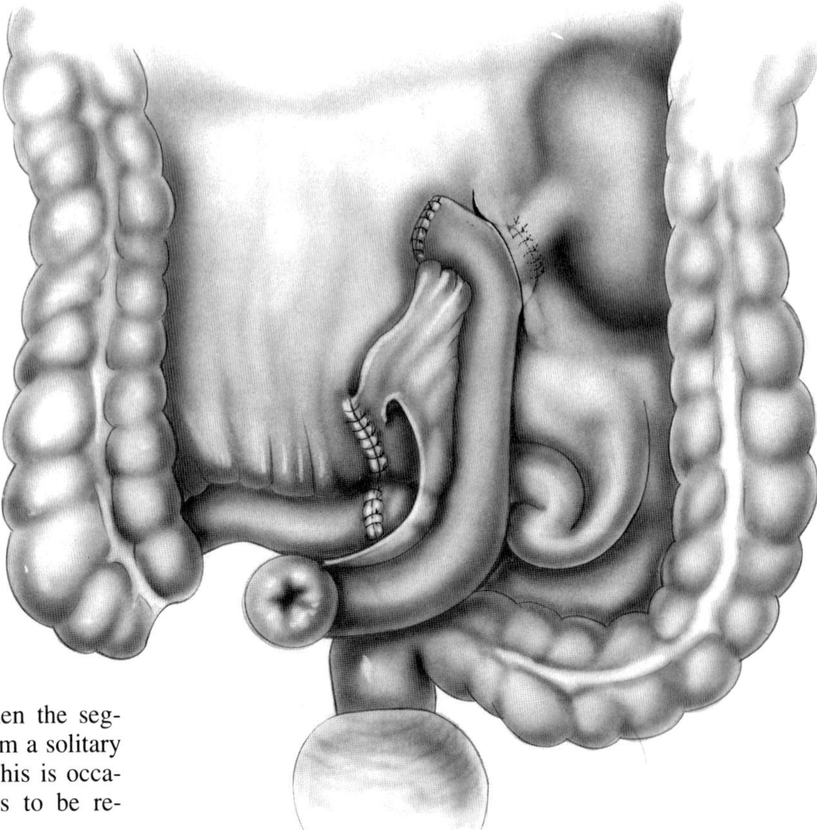

Figure 41.17. A similar procedure is used when the segment of ileum is used to function as a conduit from a solitary kidney with an external appliance on the skin. This is occasionally needed when much of the ureter needs to be removed.

OPERATIVE TECHNIQUE FOR ILEAL RESERVOIR

The following technique described is that developed by Skinner (3) based on Kock's (2) original operation. Intravenous administration of Papaverine, 300 mg in 500 ml D5 normal saline, to a dose sufficient to decrease the systolic blood pressure by 20 mm is very helpful in preventing bowel spasms during manipulation to create the reservoir.

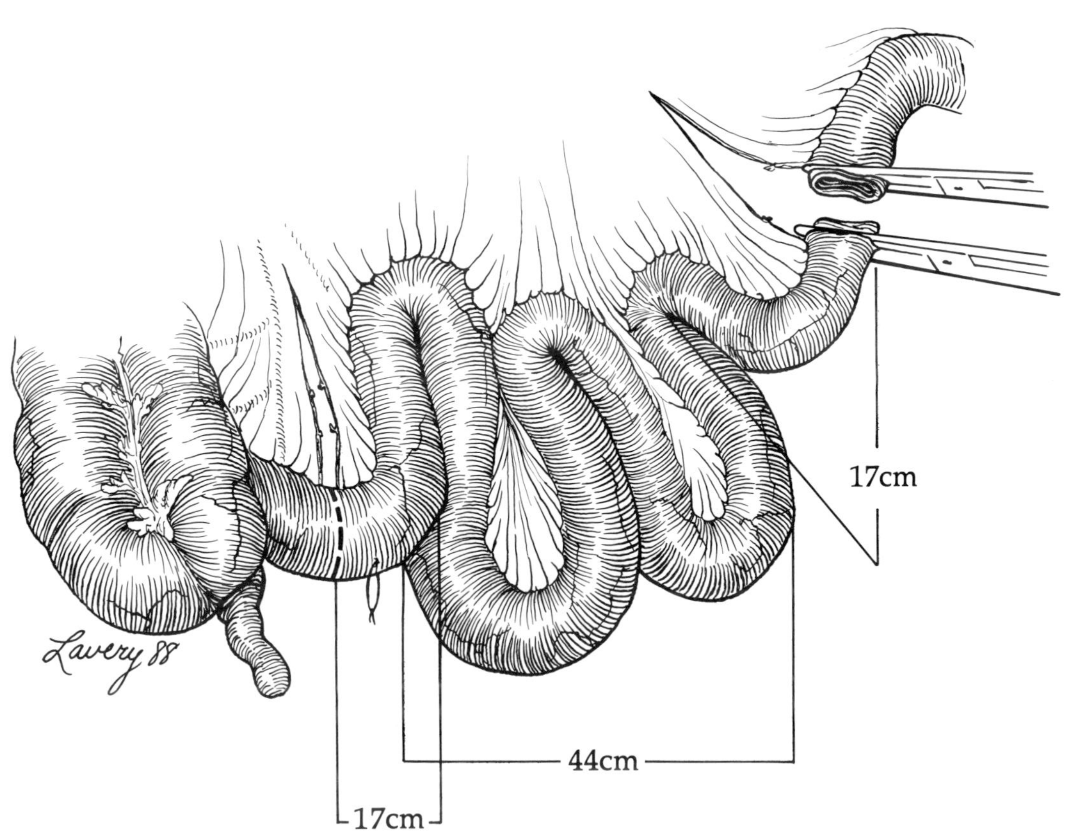

Figure 41.18. The appropriate bowel segments must be measured in the terminal ileum. The reservoir itself is composed of a 44-cm segment of ileum with both a proximal and distal limb of 17 cm each.

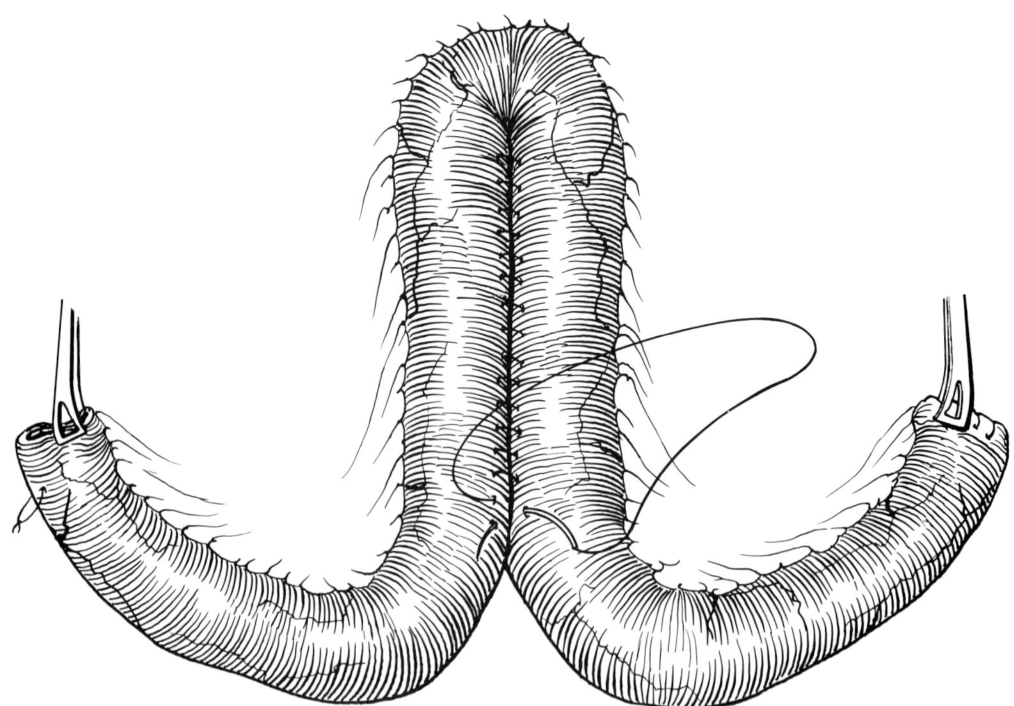

Figure 41.19. The two limbs of bowel that will be the reservoir are approximated and the back wall is sutured together with a running 4–0 nonabsorbable suture.

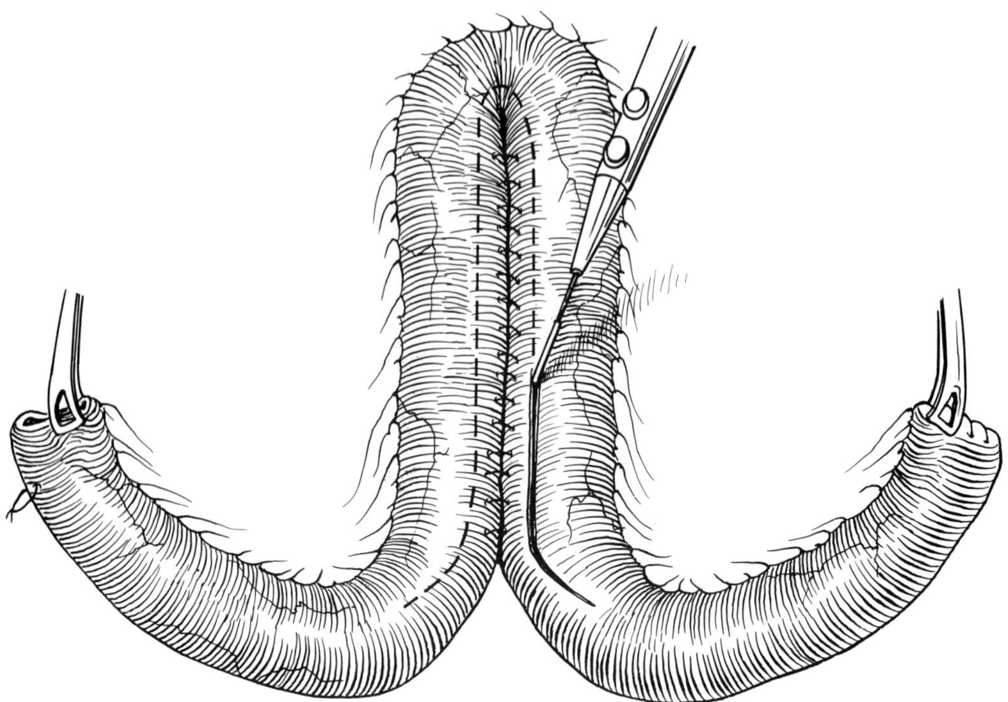

Figure 41.20. The bowel is opened on each limb above the previously placed suture line. The incision is carried on to the afferent and efferent limb for a distance of approximately 2 cm curving away from the mesentery.

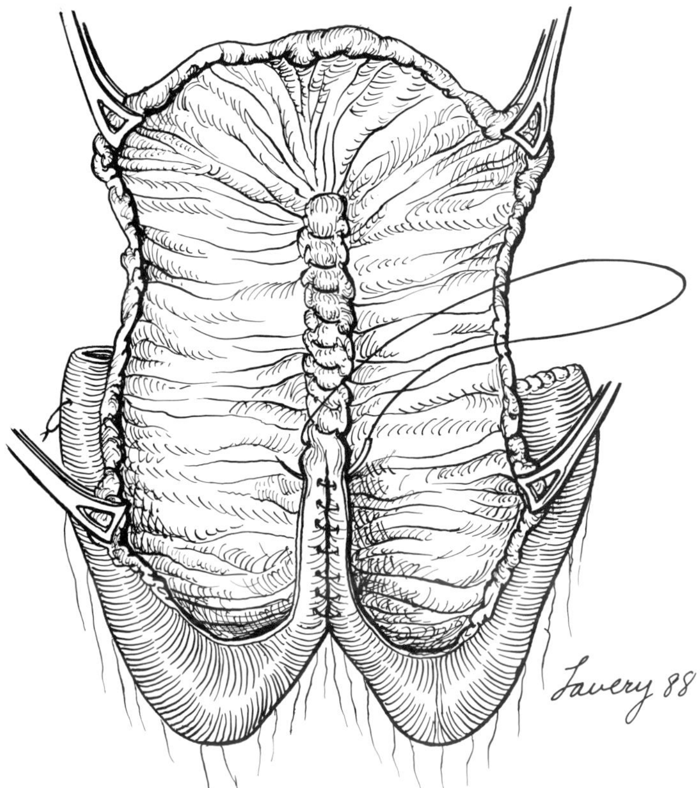

Figure 41.21. The approximated lumens of the bowel are then sutured with running 4–0 chromic sutures. This completes the closure of the back wall of the reservoir.

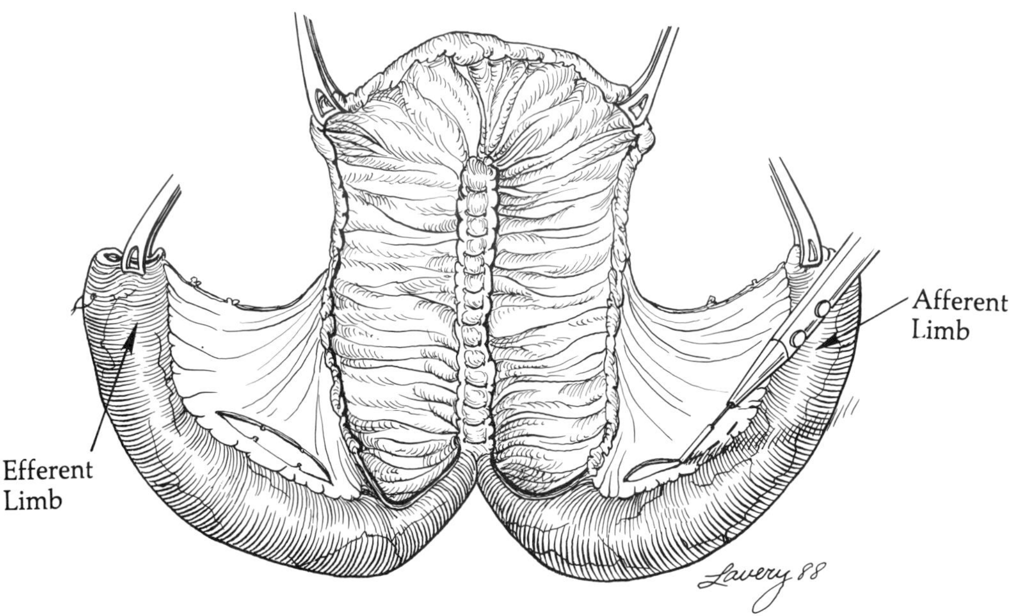

Figure 41.22. With the electrocautery, the mesentery is divided adjacent to the ileum, opening the window of Deaver on both the afferent and efferent limbs for a length of 8 cm. This allows mobility of the bowel to create the nipple.

Figure 41.23. Allis clamps are placed into the lumen of the bowel and the bowel wall is grasped approximately two-thirds of the way up of the area that has been mobilized. The bowel is intussuscepted creating an approximately 5- to 6-cm nipple.

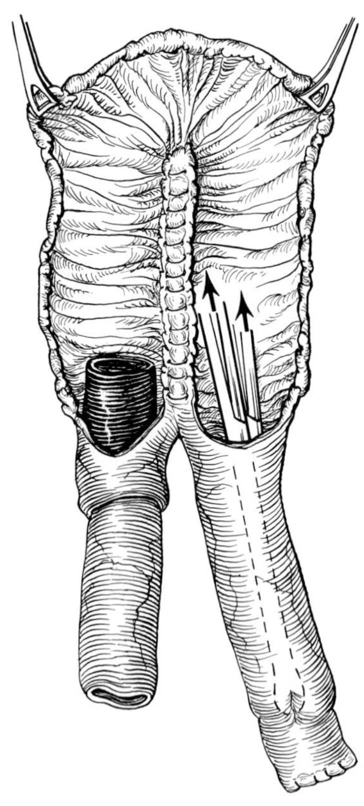

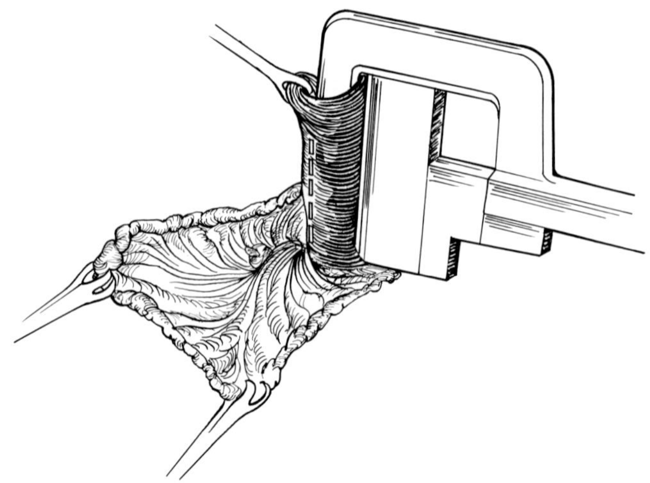

Figure 41.24. The nipple is fixed with two TA55 4.8-mm rows of staples with five staples having been removed from the distal portion of the cartridge. This removes exposed staples from the end of the nipple. The hole created by guide pin must be closed separately.

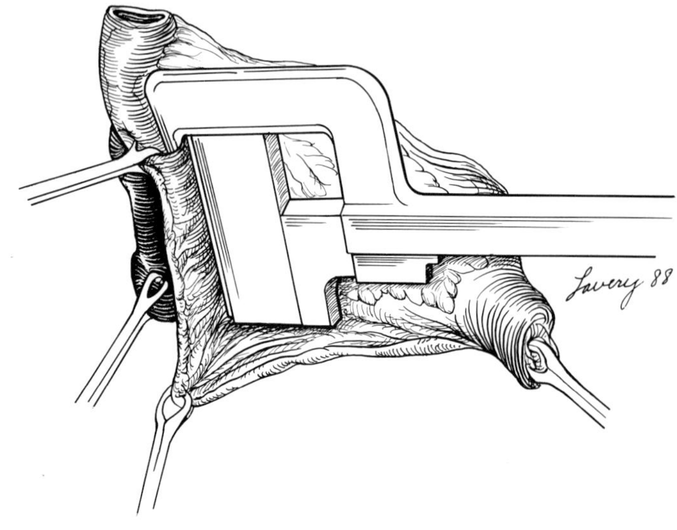

Figure 41.25. With a full cartridge in the stapling device, the anvil is slipped on the inside of the nipple along the mesentery and the nipple is then fixed to the back wall of the reservoir. Although a mersilene mesh cuff was used in our early experience with both continent ileal urinary reservoirs and continent ileostomies, the late complication of erosion of the mesh through the bowel wall has prompted us to abandon this portion of the technique.

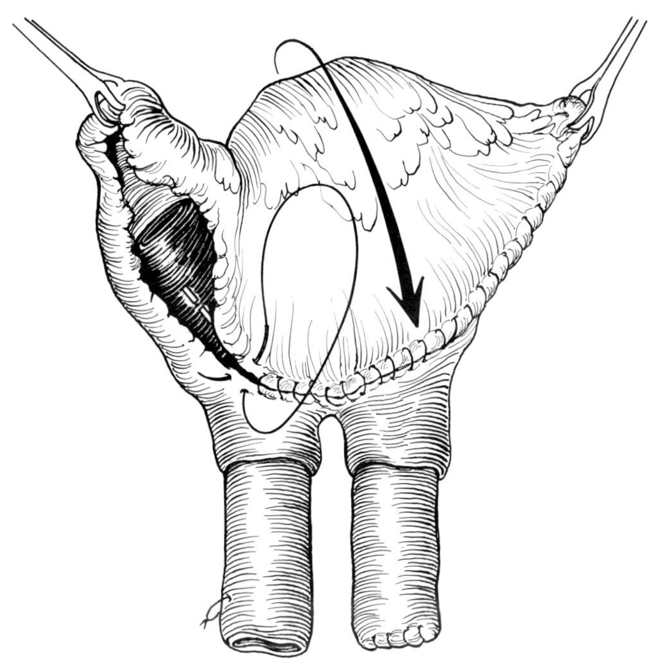

Figure 41.26. The anterior wall of the pouch is then closed in two layers with the inner layer being running 4–0 chromic and the outer layer being running or interrupted nonabsorbable sutures. A watertight closure must be ensured. The butt end of the afferent limb is closed with two layers with nonabsorbable sutures. The reservoir is rotated and the butt end of the conduit is tacked down to the retroperitoneum in the right side of the pelvis. A standard ureteroileal anastomosis is performed in the same fashion as used in the ileal conduit. It is important to use stents into the upper tract through the afferent nipple valve because edema can increase the pressure in the upper tracts or lead to a leak from the ureteroileal anastomosis. Stents are curled up in the reservoir and removed 3 weeks postoperatively in the office with ''pouchoscopy.''

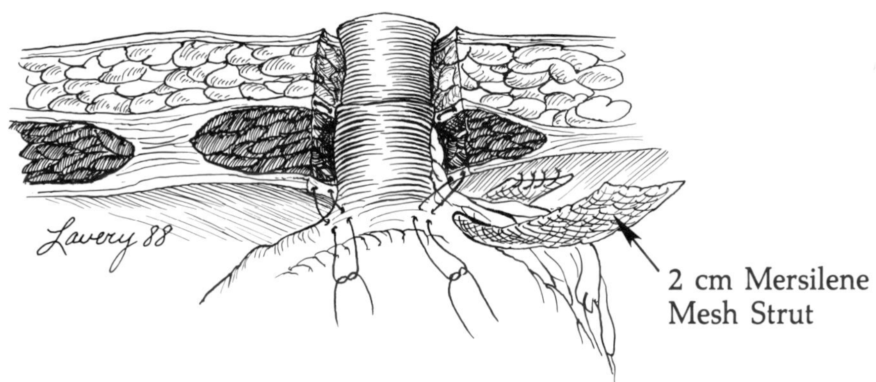

Figure 41.27. The abdominal wall aperture is similar to that made for an ileal conduit, although the skin and fascial incision may be slightly smaller than that needed for the conduit. A 2-cm wide strip of mersilene mesh is tacked to the posterior aspect of the anterior abdominal wall cephalad and lateral to the abdominal wall aperture. This will be used later to provide a strut for the mesentery to the efferent limb to provide additional stability. The efferent limb is brought through the abdominal wall aperture and the fundus of the pouch and the efferent limb is fixed to the rectus fascia with interrupted horizontal mattress sutures. The continence and ease of catheterization of the reservoir is now tested with a no. 30 Medena tube. The redundant segment of efferent limb is excised and the stoma matured with interrupted chromic sutures with a flush stoma being created. The Medena tube is left indwelling into the reservoir and sutured to the surrounding skin with tripod sutures. A closed rubber drain system is placed through a separate stab wound in the lower abdomen to drain the ureteroileal anastomosis and the pouch itself.

The mersilene strut is brought under the mesentery of the efferent limb and sutured to the posterior aspect of the anterior abdominal wall just lateral to the midline. This prevents traction on the efferent limb and fundus of the pouch, which can result in distortion of the nipple valve and loss of continence.

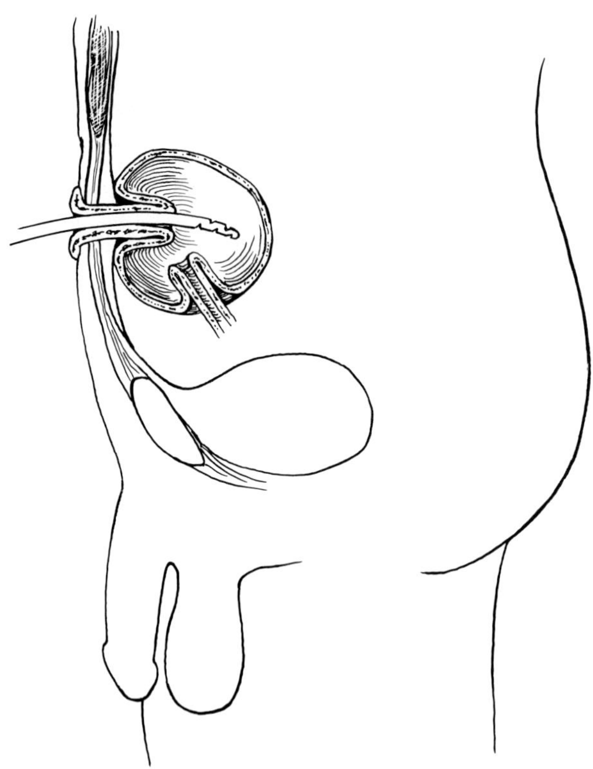

Figure 41.28. A cross-sectional schematic view shows the relations between the afferent and efferent limbs and nipples and the intubating catheter through stoma.

References

1. Bricker EM: Bladder substitution after pelvic exenteration. *Surg Clin North Am* 30:1511, 1950.
2. Kock NG, Nilsson AE, Norlen LJ, et al: Urinary diversion via a continent ileal reservoir: Clinical results in 12 patients. *J Urol* 128:469, 1982.
3. Skinner DG, Liekovsky G, Boyd SD: Technique of creation of a continent internal ileal reservoir (Kock pouch) for urinary diversion. *Urol Clin North Am* 11:741, 1984.

Suggested Readings

Bloom DA, Lieskovsky G, Rainwater G, Skinner DG: The Turnbull loop stoma. *J Urol* 129:715, 1983.

Kaiser AB: Antimicrobial prophylaxis in surgery. *N Engl J Med* 315:1129, 1986.

Klein EA, Montie JE, Montague DE, et al: Jejunal conduit urinary diversion. *J Urol* 135:244, 1986.

Montie JE: Technique of radical cystectomy. *Semin Urol* 1:42, 1983.

Wishnow KI, Johnson DE, Babaian RJ, et al: Effective outpatient use of polyethylene glycol-electrolyte bowel preparation for radical cystectomy and ileal conduit urinary diversion. *Urology* 31:7, 1988.

CHAPTER 42

Colon Conduit

ROBERT KAY

Bladder substitution has long been recognized as a necessity in some patients with neuropathic bladders or in patients with cancer requiring bladder removal. The use of intestine was clinically applied in 1894 when Chaput first described a ureterocolostomy (1). Further modification of this procedure evolved into ureterosigmoidostomy, first performed by Mayo and Coffey in 1912 (2). This procedure became widely accepted in the first half of the 20th century (2). Because of renal deterioration and electrolyte imbalance, a search for a better form of urine diversion continued. Bricker, in 1950, introduced the isolated ileum as a conduit in an effort to avoid many of the problems of the reservoir concept of the ureterosigmoidostomy (3).

Long-term results of the ileal conduit revealed a high incidence of complications (4, 5). Renal deterioration, which many have related to ureteric reflux and stomal stenosis in children, prompted continued refinements. Mogg, in 1957, began using the isolated colon conduit in an effort to decrease intraluminal pressure (6). Because reflux could be prevented in ureterosigmoidostomy as demonstrated by Leadbetter and Clark in 1954, it was recognized that reflux could be prevented in a colon conduit independent of the fecal stream, thereby avoiding electrolyte problems and, hopefully, upper tract deterioration (7). Experimentally, Richie et al. in 1974 demonstrated an increased incidence of histologic pyelonephritis in dogs occurring in 84% of freely refluxing ileal conduits as compared to 7% in the nonrefluxing colonic conduits (8).

Long-term results of colon conduits are controversial and remain to be critically analyzed in large series (9–12). There are, however, two potential complications may occur that are unique to the use of colon as opposed to ileum. The risk of obstruction of the ureteral colonic anastomosis is increased when performing a reflux preventing anastomosis. This must be guarded against intraoperatively and detected early in the postoperative period. Mogg, in a series of mixed refluxing and nonrefluxing ureteric colonic anastomoses, reported a 22% incidence of ureterocolonic anastomosis (12). Although these will vary statistically from surgeon to surgeon, the risk of obstruction will clearly be higher in a colon conduit when attempting to prevent reflux than in a standard refluxing ileal conduit.

The risk of carcinoma in the intact ureterosigmoidostomy was first described by Hammer in 1929 (13). Since the initial report, the incidence of colonic carcinoma associated with ureterosigmoidostomy has been calculated to be 500 times greater than the incidence of carcinoma of the colon in the normal population (14). Although it was previously noted that the intact fecal stream was a prerequisite for carcinoma, Chiang et al. have reported an adenocarcinoma in a colon conduit created in a child at age 3 years (15). The mean lag period for development of carcinoma of the colon has been estimated to be 8.7 years with a range of 5–14 years to patients having implantation of their ureters after the age of 40 years. This increases to a lag period of 21 years with a range of 14–50 years for those patients who had a ureterosigmoidostomy at an age younger than 40 years (14). Because the colon conduit procedure has been popular only recently, it will be one to two decades before one can determine if there is truly a significant risk of carcinoma in the colon conduit as previously seen in the ureterosigmoidostomy.

INDICATIONS

The colon conduit may be used in any clinical condition requiring supravesical diversion. Neurogenic bladder, exstrophy of the bladder, or any benign disease, such as tuberculous or interstitial cystitis requiring diversion, is a suitable indication for a sigmoid colon. Any disease with pelvic radiation requiring diversion would require a transverse colon conduit and may not be suitable for a sigmoid conduit, as the sigmoid colon may be in the field of radiation. In addition, transverse colon as opposed to sigmoid colon may be used in conjunction with a radical cystectomy. Sigmoid colon should not be used in this setting because the subsequent colonic anastomosis depends on blood supply that receives some collateral circulation from the inferior hemorrhoidal artery. The inferior hemorrhoidal artery arises from the hypogastric artery and may be ligated during cystectomy. Although Loening et al. have reported a series using transverse colon conduit with cystectomy, our current preference for noncontinent urinary diversion in conjuction with a cystectomy continues to be the ileal conduit (16).

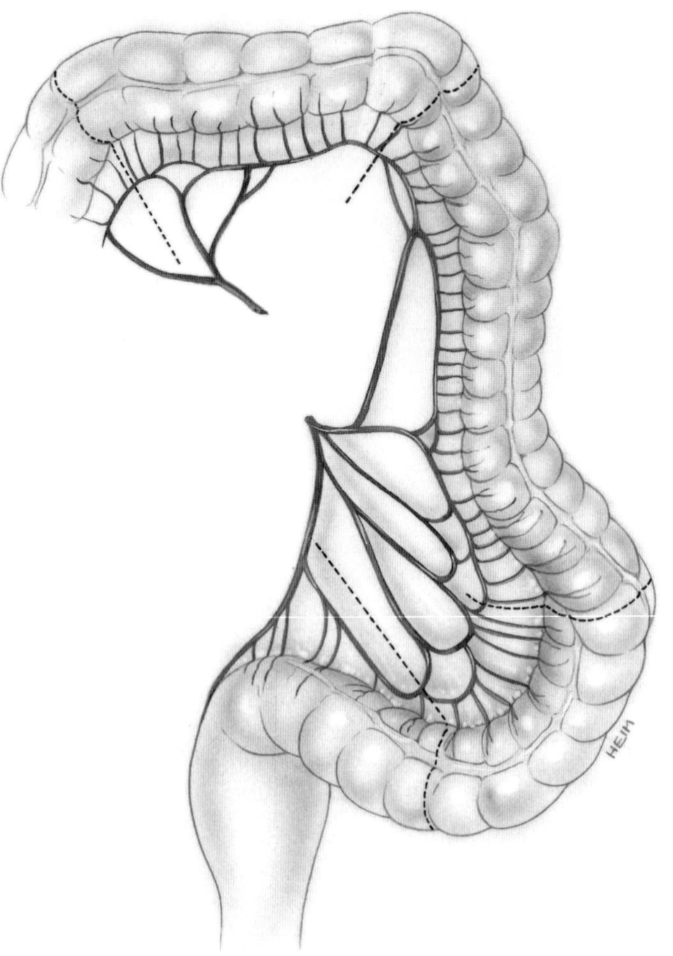

Figure 42.1. The portion of colon to be selected for the colon conduit is usually the sigmoid colon. This relatively mobile portion is easily removed from colon continuity and its vascular pedicle is preserved. In selected cases, the transverse colon may be used. It is preferable to the sigmoid colon in patients who have had preoperative pelvic radiation. In addition, in malignant disease requiring cystectomy or extensive pelvic surgery, the transverse colon is also preferable to the sigmoid colon because of its collateral circulation and potential interference with the blood supply to the distal colon in performing a cystectomy. In addition, the transverse colon may be used in direct pyelocolonic anastomoses when colon as opposed to ileum is selected. The blood supply to the colon must be studied and understood before selecting a portion of colon so that viability of the conduit is ensured.

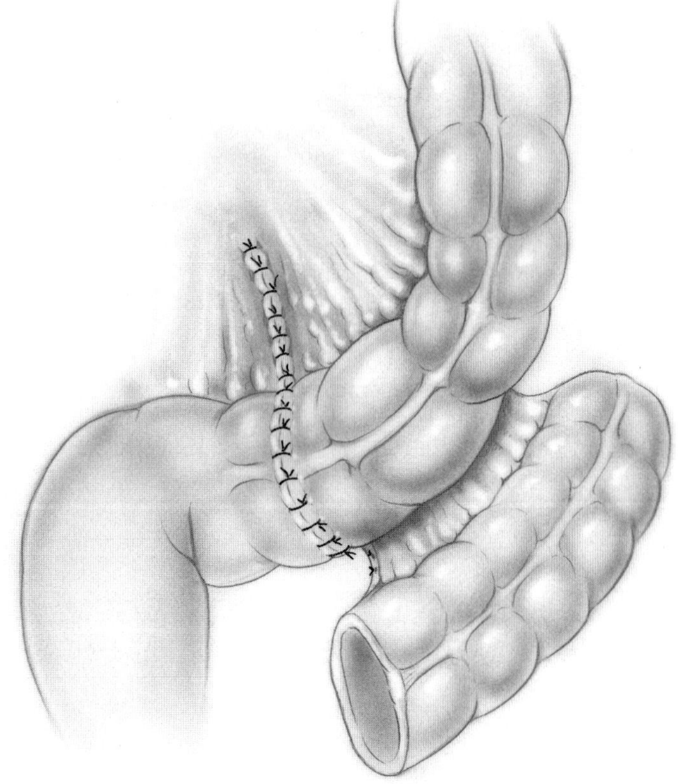

Figure 42.2. The isolated sigmoid conduit is freed with its mesenteric blood supply and excluded from the fecal stream. A standard two-layer bowel anastomosis is performed as described in chapter 41. The mesentery is also closed using interrupted 3–0 silk. The conduit may be placed lateral to the colocolostomy filling the left colic gutter or may be brought medial to the anastomosis if the anatomy of the patient and the placement of the stoma dictate such a course.

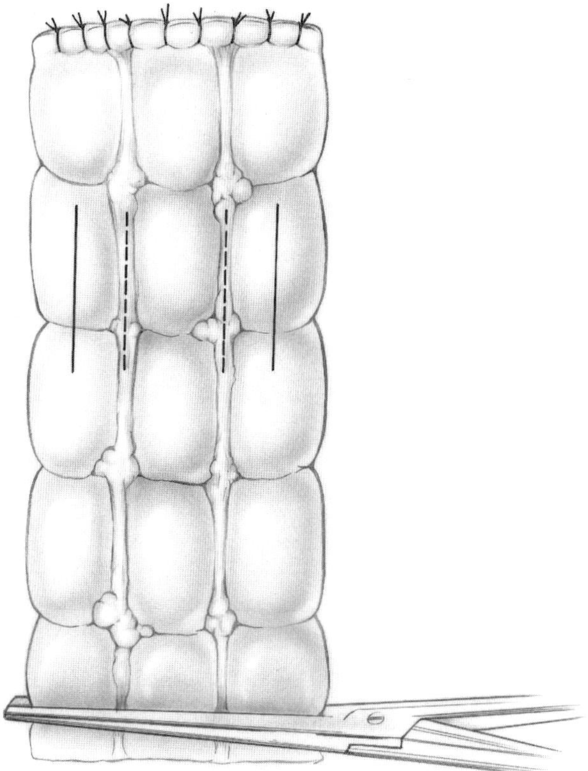

Figure 42.3. The isolated sigmoid conduit is now ready for the ureteral colonic anastomoses. The butt end of the conduit has been closed using a two-layer anastomosis of a running Connell suture of 3–0 chromic and imbricating Lembert sutures of 3–0 silk. The selection of sites for the ureteral anastomosis is normally placed in the widely separated teniae coli. There is normally a well-developed seromuscular layer. In some patients, we have placed the ureteral anastomosis in the colon between the teniae in an area where it sits freely without any angulation. We have found that we are able to develop a muscular layer for an antirefluxing anastomosis in areas separate from the teniae.

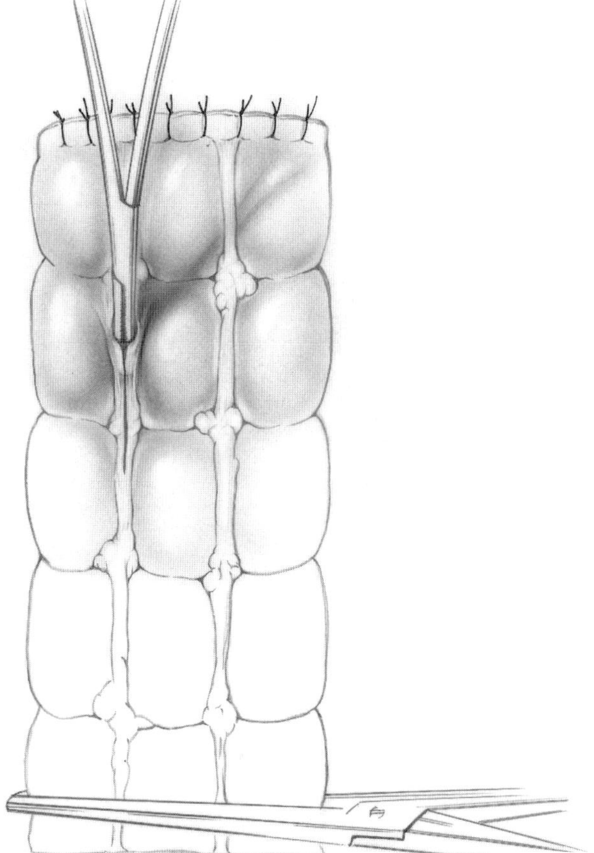

Figure 42.4. The incision is made into the teniae for the approximately 4–5 cm. Using a right-angle instrument, dissection is carried out lifting the muscular layer from the mucosa. It is important at this step to avoid entering the mucosa. In most cases, the bulging mucosa will be apparent and one can separate the muscle off the mucosa.

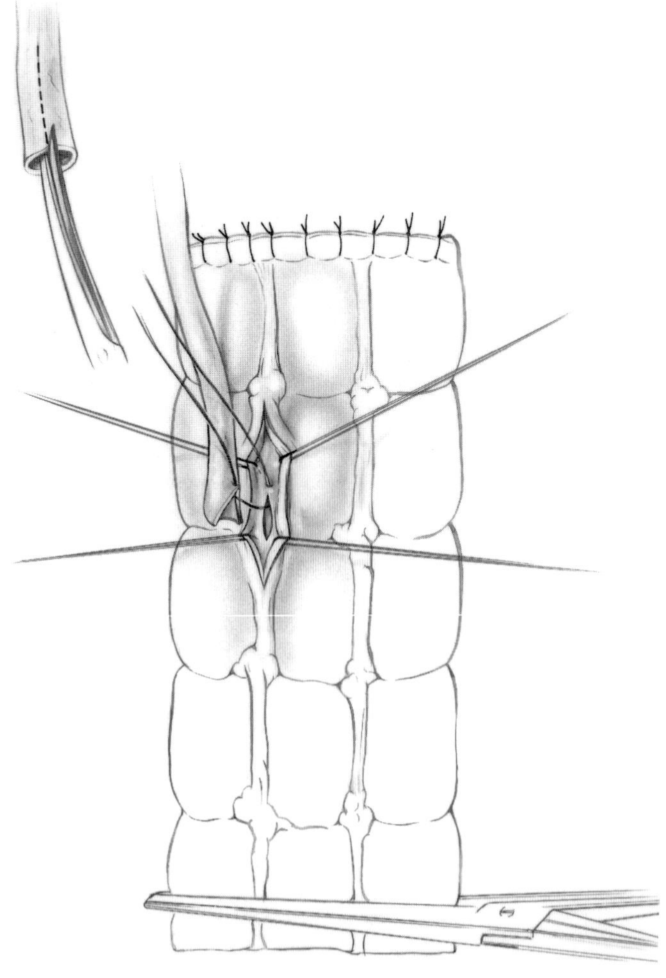

Figure 42.5. With traction sutures holding the seromuscular layer apart, the mucosal bed is carefully examined. A no. 15 blade is used to incise the mucosa at its apex for approximately 1 cm.

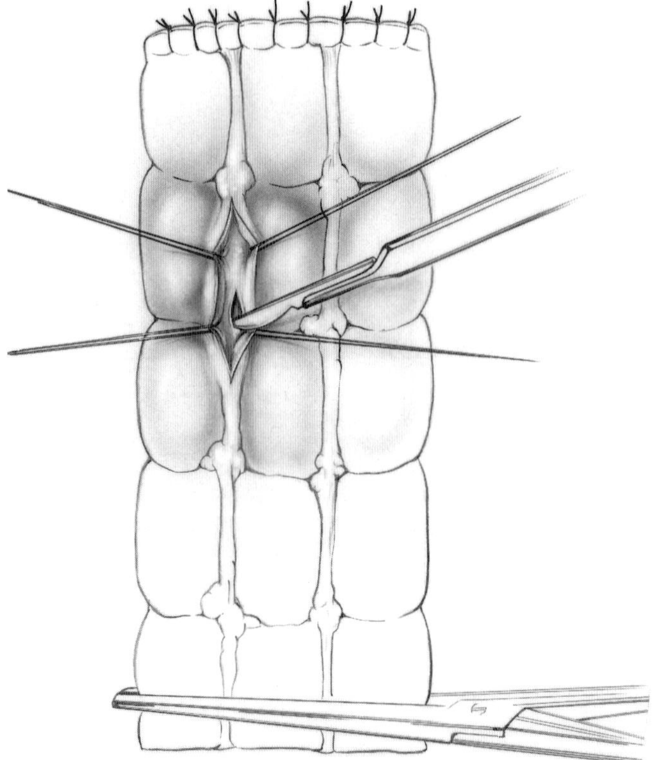

Figure 42.6. The ureter that has previously been dissected, carefully preserving its blood supply, is brought to the level of the colonic incision. The ureter is spatulated in the medial aspect for approximately 1–2 cm. A 4–0 or 5–0 chromic suture is placed through the apex of the ureter and the apex of the colonic mucosal incision. A 5–0 feeding tube is then placed through the colonic mucosa into the conduit and into the ureter to the renal pelvis.

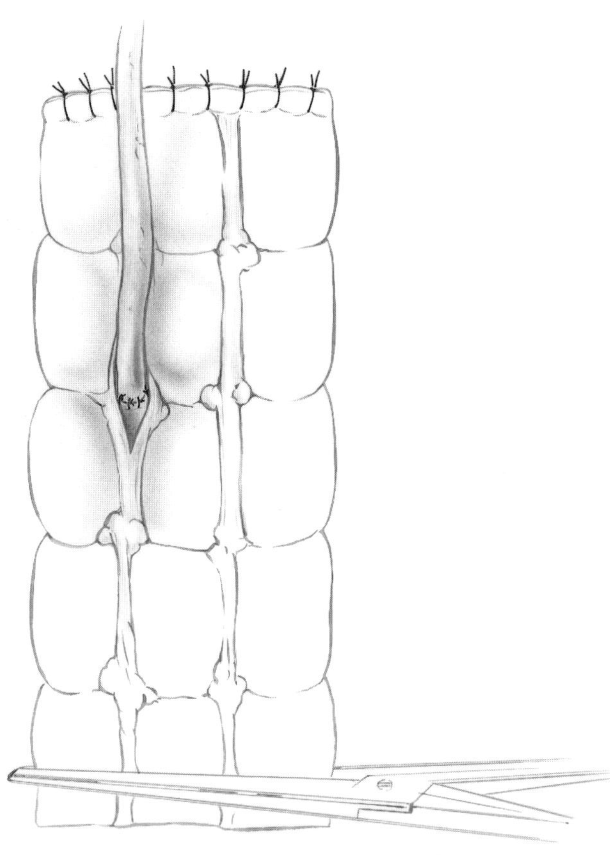

Figure 42.7. The remaining ureteral mucosal anastomosis is then performed using interrupted 5–0 chromic. Although we prefer to do this over a stenting 5–0 feeding catheter that is brought out through the conduit, this may be done with no stents according to the surgeon's desires.

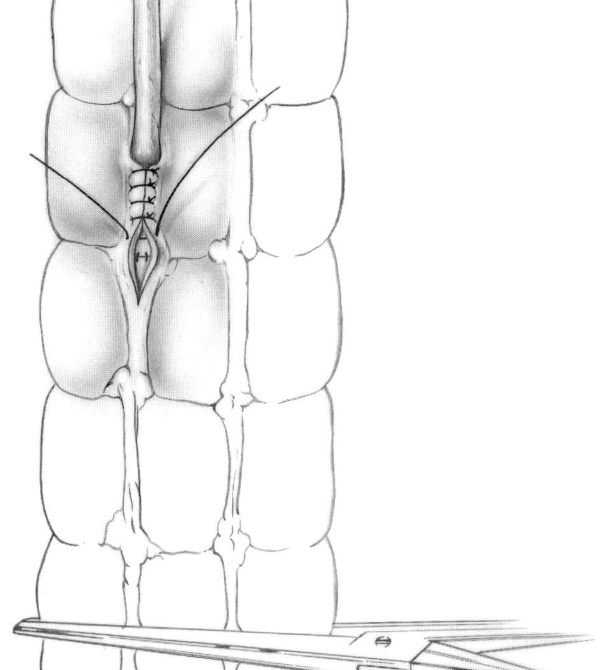

Figure 42.8. The seromuscular layer is then closed over the ureter using 4–0 chromic in interrupted fashion. Care must be taken to avoid constricting the ureter at this point.

Figure 42.9. The contralateral ureter is then placed into the opposite teniae in a similar fashion with the appropriate steps being taken.

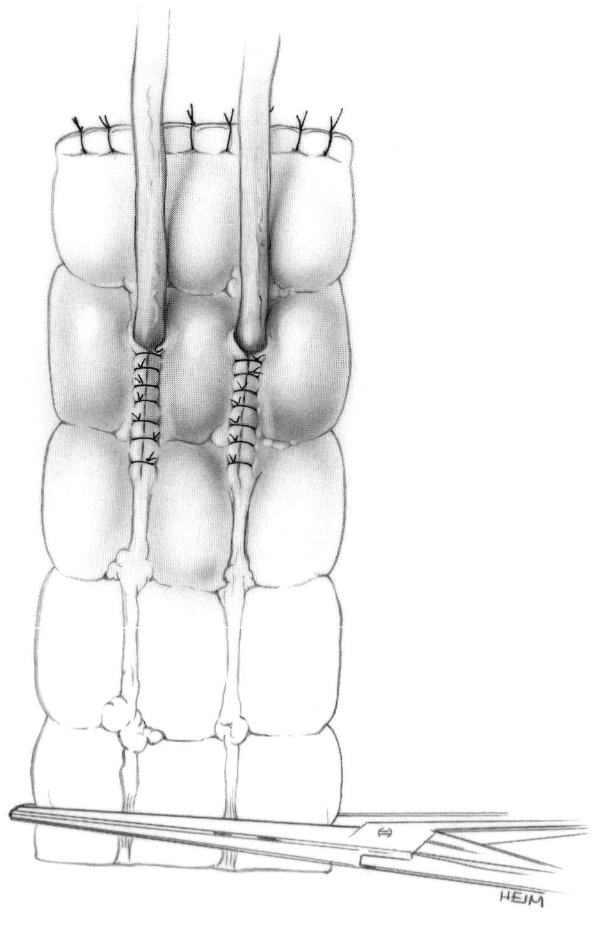

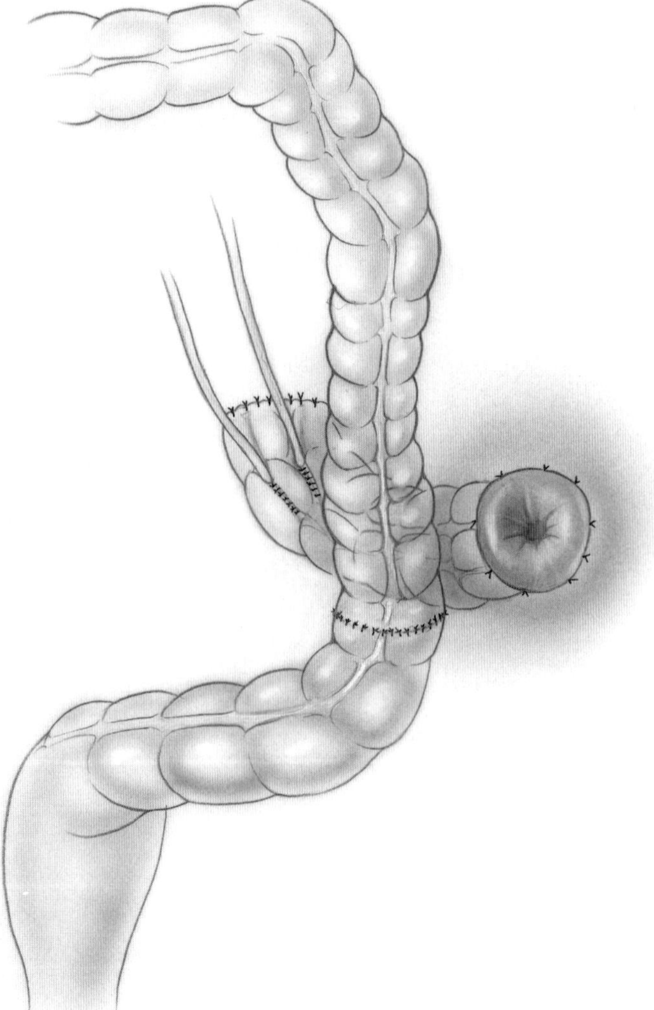

Figure 42.10. The closed end of the conduit is then secured to the posterior peritoneum using 3–0 silk over the sacral promontory. The stomal end of the conduit is then brought through the peritoneum and fascia, and a stoma is created at the previously determined site. A rosebud stoma or a loop stoma may be created as described in chapter 41.

References

1. Chaput H: D l'abouchement des ureters dans l'intestin. *Arch Gen Med* 1:5, 1894.
2. Coffey RC: Transplantation of the ureters into the large intestine. *Surg Gynecol Obstet* 47:593, 1928.
3. Bricker E: Bladder substitution after pelvic exenteration. *Surg Clin North Am* 30:1511, 1950.
4. Schwarz GR, Jeffs RD: Ileal conduit urinary diversion in children: Computer analysis of follow-up from 2 to 16 years. *J Urol* 114:285, 1975.
5. Shapiro SR, Lebowitz R, Colodny AH: Fate of 90 children with ileal conduit urinary diversion a decade later: Analysis of complications, pyelography, renal function and bacteriology. *J Urol* 114:289, 1975.
6. Mogg RA: The treatment of neurogenic urinary incontinence using a colonic conduit. *Br J Urol* 37:681, 1965.
7. Leadbetter WF, Clark BG: Five years experience with ureteroenterostomy by the "combined technique." *J Urol* 73:67, 1954.
8. Richie JP, Skinner DG, Waisman J: The effect of reflux on the development of pyelonephritis in urinary diversion: An experimental study. *J Surg Res* 16:256, 1974.
9. Althausen AF, Hagen-Cook K, Hendren WH: Non-refluxing colon conduit—experience with 70 cases. *J Urol* 120:35, 1978.
10. Arap S, Giron AM, Abrao EG, Mitre AI, Menezes de Goes G: Non refluxing colonic conduit efficiency and complications of ureteral colic anastomosis. *Eur Urol* 8:196, 1982.
11. Elver BD, Moisey CU, Rees RWM: A long term follow-up of colonic conduit operations in children. *Br J Urol* 51:462, 1979.
12. Mogg RA, Syme RR: The results of urinary diversion using the colonic conduit. *Br J Urol* 41:434, 1969.
13. Hammer E: Cancer du colon sigmoide dix ans apres implantation des ureteres d'une vessie exstrophiee. *J Urol Nephrol* (Paris) 28:260, 1948.
14. Leadbetter GW, Zickerman P, Pierce E: Ureterosigmoidostomy and carcinoma of the colon. *J Urol* 121:732, 1979.
15. Chiang NS, Minton JP, Clausen K, Clatworthy HW, Wise HA: Carcinoma in a colon conduit urinary diversion. *J Urol* 127:1185, 1982.
16. Loening SA, Navarre RJ, Narayana AS, Culp DA: Transverse colon conduit urinary diversion. *J Urol* 127:37, 1982.

INDEX

F

G

H

V

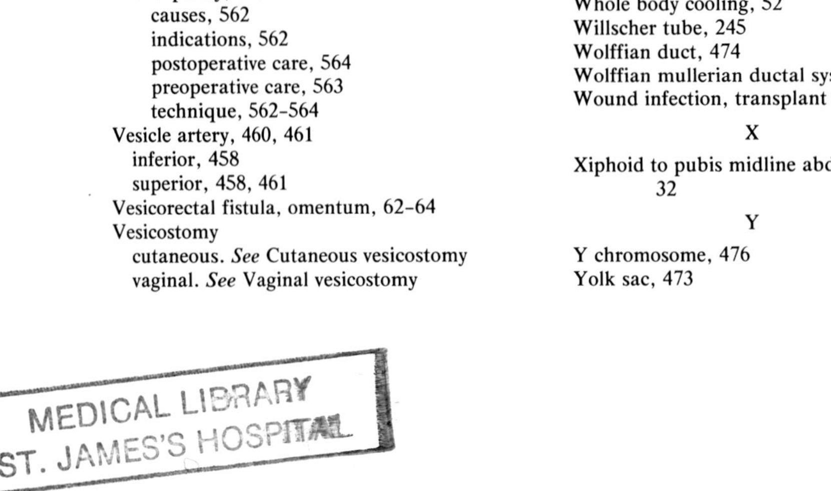